Pharmacology and
Dental Therapeutics

Library

Pharmacology and Dental Therapeutics

Third Edition

Robin A. Seymour

Professor of Restorative Dentistry,
Newcastle Dental School, University of Newcastle

John G. Meechan

Senior Lecturer and Honorary Consultant
in Oral and Maxillofacial Surgery,
Newcastle Dental School, University of Newcastle

and

Michael S. Yates

Senior Lecturer in Pharmacology,
School of Biomedical Sciences, University of Leeds

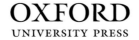

OXFORD
UNIVERSITY PRESS

OXFORD

UNIVERSITY PRESS

Great Clarendon Street, Oxford OX2 6DP

Oxford New York

Athens Auckland Bangkok Bogota Buenos Aires Calcutta
Cape Town Chennai Dar es Salaam Delhi Florence Hong Kong Istanbul
Karachi Kuala Lumpur Madrid Melbourne Mexico City Mumbai
Nairobi Paris São Paulo Taipei Tokyo Toronto Warsaw

Oxford is a trade mark of Oxford University Press

Published in the United States
by Oxford University Press, Inc., New York

A catalogue record for this book is available from the British Library

Library of Congress Cataloging in Publication Data

Seymour, R. A.
Pharmacology and dental therapeutics.—3rd ed. / Robin A.
Seymour, John Meechan, and Michael S. Yates.
Rev. ed. of: Textbook of dental pharmacology and therapeutics /
John G. Walton, John W. Thompson, and Robin A. Seymour. 2nd ed. 1994.
Includes bibliographical references and index.
1. Dental therapeutics. I. Meechan, J. G. II. Yates, M. S.
III. Walton, J. G. Textbook of dental pharmacology and therapeutics. IV. Title.
[DNLM: 1. Dentistry. 2. Pharmacology. QV 50 S521d 1999]
RK701.W35 1999 615'.1'0246176—dc21 99-24161

ISBN 978-0-19-262952-4

8 10 9 7

Typeset by Best-set Typesetter Ltd., Hong Kong
Printed in England on acid free paper by
CPI Antony Rowe, Chippenham, Wiltshire

This book is dedicated to

Gayle, Tom, and Oliver (R.A.S)
Janice, Robert, and Simon (J.G.M)
Nicola, Matthew, and Jonathan (M.S.Y)

Preface to the third edition

Pharmacology, be it either in the form of drug development or application, can make headline news. Thus, the subject seems to be growing at an amazing pace and it was not surprising that a third edition of this textbook was required. Two of the authors of the first and second editions (J.G.W and J.W.T) have now retired, although both have kept a lively interest in the development of the third edition.

Over the years, both John Thompson and John Walton have made significant contributions to the whole subject area which covers pharmacology and dentistry. They produced a series of articles in the *British Dental Journal* (Pharmacology for the dental practitioner) that formed the basis of the 2nd edition of this textbook. We would like to take this opportunity of thanking them for their support as well as the contributions they have made to this subject, and for their work as previous editors of this book.

As a result of their retirement, there was a need to find replacements for the two original authors, and at the same time retain the balance of the book between dentistry and pharmacology. It was a great pleasure that both Dr John Meechan and Dr Michael Yates accepted the invitation to co-author this new third edition.

Dr John Meechan is a Senior Lecturer in Oral and Maxillofacial Surgery at Newcastle Dental School. His research interests are in the field of local anaesthesia and he has provided a sound clinical basis to the several chapters that were under his editorship.

Dr Michael Yates is a Senior Lecturer in Pharmacology, School of Biomedical Sciences, at the University of Leeds. He has been involved extensively in teaching pharmacology, especially to dental students. His research interests are in cardiovascular pharmacology and he has provided a sound background knowledge in basic pharmacology to all the chapters.

As the remaining author, I am extremely grateful to both Dr Meechan and Dr Yates for their excellent contribution to this textbook.

All chapters have been revised, updated, and some have been rewritten. New diagrams have been added and some chapters have been totally rewritten. To help revision, we have added key fact boxes throughout the text. In spite of these changes, the format of the 3rd edition remains the same with a particular emphasis on those drugs and topics relevant to the practice of dentistry.

The first edition of this textbook appeared just over 10 years ago. The book has been well received by undergraduates, postgraduates, and teachers of pharmacology to dental students. We hope that the third edition is likewise well received.

R.A.S
J.G.M
M.S.Y

Preface to the second edition

The subject of pharmacology continues to develop at an ever increasing pace. During recent years, new techniques in molecular and cellular biology have made important contributions to the subject. As a consequence, there is now a greater understanding of how drugs work and also of new ways in which these agents may be applied to the treatment of disease, including to dental therapeutics. Nearly five years have elapsed since the first edition of this book was published and for this reason the authors considered it to be both timely and appropriate to prepare this second edition.

Some significant changes have been made from the first edition. A new chapter on 'The pharmacology of pain' has been added. The two chapters on 'Pharmacological control of caries and periodontal disease' and 'Treatments for common dental conditions' have been completely re-written. The remaining chapters have all been revised and brought up to date, so as to be in line with the latest developments. In spite of these changes, the format of the book remains the same with the emphasis placed on those topics which are particularly relevant to the practice of dentistry.

In the preface to the first edition of this book it was mentioned that this publication is based on an earlier and shorter book written by two of the authors (J.G.W. and J.W.T.). In fact, the earlier book first appeared during 1971–72 in the form of fifteen articles

which had been commissioned by the then Editor of the *British Dental Journal*, Mr. J. A. Donaldson, OBE, BA, FDS. In addition to giving the authors strong support, he was also keen that the earlier publication should be expanded into the comprehensive textbook that it has now become; and he was very pleased when the first edition was published in 1989. Sadly, he will not see this second edition because he died in February of this year. The authors wish to place on record their deep gratitude to Archie Donaldson for having started the whole exercise.

As with the first edition, the preparation of this second edition has been greatly assisted by the willing and generous help which the authors have received from colleagues and for which they are most grateful; their names are listed in Acknowledgements. The first edition of this textbook was well received and we hope that the second edition will also prove of value to undergraduates, postgraduates, and dental practitioners alike. The authors wish to thank those readers and reviewers who made comments, criticisms, and suggestions about the first edition; and we hope that this second edition will provoke a similar helpful response.

Newcastle upon Tyne J.G.W.
May 1994 J.W.T.
R.A.S.

Preface to the first edition

Over the past 30 years or so the subject of pharmacology has developed explosively with the result that there are now many groups of potent drugs used for the treatment of disease. This has had two important consequences for dentistry. First, a number of the newer drugs have found important roles in dental treatment. Second, many patients who attend for dental treatment are taking drugs for the treatment of medical conditions and it is therefore important for the dentist to be aware of this fact and to be fully conversant with the pharmacology and rationale behind the use of these drugs. Furthermore, it is previously important for the dentist to be aware of the unwanted effects that may be produced by the drugs prescribed, some directly concerned with the mouth. Of equal importance is the need to know about possible interactions that might occur (and must therefore be avoided) in the event that the dental practitioner prescribes one or more drugs for dental treatment that have the potential to interact with those already being taken by the patient for medical reasons. Thus the need for the present-day dental student and dental practitioner to have a sound working knowledge of pharmacology and therapeutics is processing one, and this book has been written to meet these needs.

The book is divided into two sections. The first deals with general pharmacological principles together with these drugs that are part of the day-to-day pharmacological armamentarium of the dental practitioner. The second part deals with the pharmacology and therapeutics related to drugs which, though unlikely to be prescribed by the dental practitioner, are nevertheless of considerable importance of reasons already given.

This book is based on an earlier and much shorter book entitled *Pharmacology for the Dental Practitioner*, which was written by two of the authors of the present book (J.G.W. and J.W.T.). That original book has now been expanded into a comprehensive textbook for dental students and dental practitioners and, in duckling this difficult and lengthy task, the original authors have had the good fortune to acquire the valuable help of Dr Robin Seymour, who has for some time assisted his colleagues in the teaching of pharmacology to dental students.

The authors are grateful to many colleagues and others who have willingly helped in various ways, had the names of these individuals are listed in the Acknowledgements. However, the authors alone are responsible for any errors of omission or commission that are to be found in this book. Furthermore, they could be most grateful to any reader who takes the trouble to point out mistakes or to make suggestions to a further edition.

Newcastle upon Tyne J.G.W.
February 1988 J.W.T.
 R.A.S.

Acknowledgements

In the preparation of this third edition, the authors would like to acknowledge the help and support of the following colleagues for their comments and criticism: Dr C. J. Bowmer, Dr I. E. Hughes, and Dr H. A. Pearson (University of Leeds). We are also extremely grateful to the following for updating chapters: Dr J. Smith, Regional Pharmaceutical Advisory, NHS Executive Northern and Yorkshire Regional Drug and Therapeutics Centre, Wolfson Unit, Newcastle upon Tyne, for updating Chapter 3; Emeritus Professor J. W. Thompson for updating Chapter 5; and Dr N. Girdler, Senior Lecturer in Dental Sedation, the Dental School, Newcastle upon Tyne, for updating Chapter 9.

We would also like to express our thanks to the *Pharmaceutical Press* for allowing us to reproduce the table on 'Drugs to be avoided in renal disease'.

Figures and tables acknowledgements

The authors of this book wish to thank the following authors, editors, and publishers for kindly granting permission to reproduce published material for this third edition.

Fig. 5.1: Definitions of pain threshold and pain tolerance from IASP Sub-Committee on Taxonomy, *Pain*, 6, 249–52. Definitions of pain, analgesia, causalgesia, dysaethesia, hyperalgesia, hyperaesthesia, neuralgia, neuritis, neuropathy, and nociceptor as published in Classification of chronic pain. IASP Sub-Committee on taxonomy of pain. *Pain* (1986), Suppl. 3, S216–221. **Fig. 5.2:** Adapted from Johnson, M. I. (1991) Factors influencing the analgesic effects and clinical efficacy of transcutaneous electrical nerve stimulation (TENS). PhD Thesis, University of Newcastle upon Tyne. **Table 5.3:** Classification of opioid peptides and opioid receptors (p.25) from Thompson, J. W. (1990). Clinical pharmacology of opioid agonist and partial agonists. In *Opioids in the treatment of cancer pain* (ed. D. Doyle), pp. 17–38, Royal Society of Medicine Services International Congress and Symposium Series No. 146. Royal Society of Medicine Services, London. **Table 5.4:** In modified form from Thompson, J. W. (1984). Chapter 1—Pain mechanisms and principles of management. In *Advanced geriatric medicine*, 4, (ed. J. Grimley Evans and F. I. Caird), pp. 3–16. Pitman, London.

Contents

27. Treatments for common dental conditions

Abbreviations

1,25-DHCC	1,25-dihydroxycholecalciferol
25(OH)D$_3$	25-hydroxy-vitamin D$_3$
5-HT	5-hydroxytryptamine; serotonin
A–V	arteriovenous
ABPI	Association of the British Pharmaceutical Industry
ACE	angiotensin-converting enzyme
ACTH	adrenocorticotrophic hormone
ADH	antidiuretic hormone
ADP	adenosine diphosphate
ANUG	acute necrotizing ulcerative gingivitis
AT	angiotensin
ATP	adenosine triphosphate
AUC	area under the curve (e.g. concentration–time curve)
AV	atrioventricular
BIPP	bismuth iodoform paraffin paste
BNF	*British national formulary*
BP	blood pressure
BSE	bovine spongiform encephalitis
C_0	concentration (of a drug) at time zero
cAMP	cyclic 3′,5′-adenosine monophosphate
CCK	cholecystokinin
Cedeta	cell demodulated electronic targeted anaesthesia
CFSH	chorionic follicle-stimulating hormone
CG	chorionic gonadotrophin
cGMP	cyclic guanosine 5′-monophosphate
Cl_p	plasma clearance
CMCP	camphorated paramonochlorphenol
CMV	cytomegalovirus
CNS	central nervous system
COMT	catechol-o-methyl transferase
COP(A)D	chronic obstructive pulmonary (airway) disease
COX-1, -2	cyclo-oxygenase enzymes 1 and 2
CRF	corticotropin-releasing factor
CGRP	calcitonin gene-related peptide
CSF	cerebrospinal fluid
CSM	Committee on the Safety of Medicines (UK)
C_{ss}	steady-state concentration

CTL	cytotoxic T lymphocytes
CTZ	chemoreceptor trigger zone
D	dopamine receptors
Δ^1THC	Δ^1 tetrahydrocannabinol
DAG	diacyglycerol
DME	drug-metabolizing enzymes
DNA	deoxyribonucleic acid
DOMA	dihydroxymandelic acid
DOPA	dihydroxyphenylalanine
DPDPE D-penicillamine	D-penicillamine enkephalin
DPF	*Dental practitioners' formulary*
EC$_{50}$	the effective concentration that produces a 50% maximal response
ECG	electrocardiogram
ECL	enterochromaffin-like
ECP	eosinophil cationic protein
ECT	electroconvulsive therapy
ED$_{50}$	the dose that has the desired effect in 50% of animals
EMLA	eutectic mixture of local anaesthetics
ENK	enkephalinergic neurone
EP	eosinophil peroxidase
Fab	antibody fragment
FSH	follicle-stimulating hormone
G-protein	guanine-nucleotide binding protein
GABA	gamma-aminobutyric acid
GDP	guanosine 5′-diphosphate
GFR	glomerular filtration rate
GIT	gastrointestinal tract
GMP	guanosine 5′-monophosphate
GSL	General sales list
GTF	glycosyl transferase
GTP	guanosine 5′-triphosphate
Hb	haemoglobin
Hb$_s$	sickle form of haemoglobin
HETE	hydroxyeicosatetraenoic acid
HIV	human immunodeficiency virus
HPETE	hydroperoxyeicosatetraenoic acid
HRT	hormone replacement therapy
hsp	heat-shock protein
HSV	herpes simplex virus

Hz	hertz	NO	nitric oxide
ICSH	interstitial-cell stimulating hormone	NREM	non-rapid eye movement type (sleep)
IFN	interferon	NSAIDs	non-steroidal anti-inflammatory drugs
IGF	insulin-like growth factor	OP	opioid peptide
IgG	immunoglobulin G	p.p.m.	parts per million
IL	interleukin	p.s.i.	pounds per square inch
INR	International Normalized Ratio	PABA	para-aminobenzoic acid
IP_3	inositol (1,4,5)-triphosphate	PAF	platelet-activating factor
IU	international units	PDGF	platelet-derived growth factor
k	any constant	PG	prostaglandin
k_{-1}	backward rate constant	PGE	prostaglandin E
k_{+1}	forward rate constant	PGF	prostaglandin F
K_B	equilibrium dissociation constant for an antagonist (see also pK_B)	PGG	prostaglandin G
		PGH	prostaglandin H
KCCT	kaolin–cephalin clotting time	PILs	Patient information leaflets
K_D	equilibrium dissociation constant	pK_B	it is normal practice to convert the value of K_B to the negative logarithm, which has the advantage of producing simple numbers
L-dopa	levodopa		
LD_{50}	the dose that is lethal in 50% of animals		
leu	leucine	PMN	polymorphonuclear leucocyte
Leu-enkephalin	leucine enkephalin	POM	prescription-only medicines
LH	luteinizing hormone	PR	proportion of receptors occupied
LMWH	low molecular weight heparin	PGI_2	prostacyclin
LSD	lysergic acid diethylamide	PTH	parathyroid hormone
LT	leukotriene	PVM/MA	polyvinylmethylether maleic acid
LTA	lipoteichoic acid	QACs	quaternary ammonium compounds
LTB	leukotriene B	RAS	reticular activating system
m.p.h.	miles per hour	REM	rapid eye movement (sleep)
MAC	minimum alveolar concentration	RNA	ribonucleic acid
MAO	monoamine oxidase	rRNA	ribosomal RNA
MAOI	monoamine oxidase inhibitor	S	Svedberg unit
MBP	major basic protein	SA	sinoatrial
MCHC	mean corpuscular haemoglobin concentration	SG	substantia gelatinosa
		SH2	Src homology 2 domain
MCV	mean corpuscular volume	SP	substance P
MDMA	3,4-methylenedioxymethamfetamine; ecstasy	SPC	Summary of Product Characteristics
		SSRIs	selective serotonin reuptake inhibitors
MEC	minimum effective concentration	t	time
met	methionine	T	transmission cell
Met-enkephalin	methionine enkephalin	t-PA	tissue plasminogen activator
MIC	minimum inhibitory concentration	$t_{0.5}$	half-life; i.e. time required to reduce the drug concentration by 50% of its former value
mRNA	messenger RNA		
MRSA	methicillin-resistant *Staphylococcus aureus*		
		TCA	tricyclic antidepressants
MW	molecular weight	TENS	transcutaneous electrical nerve stimulation
NAD	nicotinamide adenine dinucleotide		
NADP	nicotinamide adenine dinucleotide phosphate	T_H	helper T-cells (lymphocyte)
		TIA	transient ischaemic attack
NANC	non-adrenergic non-cholinergic (nervous system)	TNF	tumour necrosis factor
		TRH	thyrotrophin-releasing hormone
NGF	nerve growth factor	tRNA	transfer RNA
NK1	neurokinin-1	TSE	transcutaneous spinal electroanalgesia
NMDA	*N*-methyl-D-aspartate	TSH	thyroid-stimulating hormone

TXA_2	thromboxane A_2	VMA	vanillylmandelic acid
UDPGA	uridine diphosphate glucuronic acid	W	Waldeyer cell
V_d	apparent volume of distribution	WBC	white blood cell
VIP	vasoactive intestinal peptide		

Drug nomenclature

A change to the naming of drugs has recently occurred in order to ensure consistency of drug names in the European Union. European law requires the use of the 'Recommended International Nonproprietary Name'—the 'rINN'. The UK has its own well-established naming system for drugs—'BP monograph title/British approved Name (BAN)'. The majority of BANs are identical to the corresponding rINN but there are some differences. The best known example of substances affected is adrenaline (BAN), the corresponding rINN of which is epinephrine. rINNs have been used throughout the book although when the drug is first mentioned in a chapter or table, the BAN, if different, is given in parenthesis. Occasionally, a drug name will be followed in parenthesis by its proprietary/trade name, for example fluoxetine (Prozac). A proprietary name can be distinguished from a BAN by the upper case first letter.

1

Fate of a drug in the body

Fate of a drug in the body

Introduction

Pharmacology is the study of the effects of drugs on living systems whilst therapeutics can be defined as the use of drugs in the treatment or prevention of disease. Consequently, it is a knowledge of pharmacology that is the foundation for the application of therapeutics. Whilst the dental practitioner directly uses and prescribes a limited range of drugs, many patients who present for dental treatment will be taking drugs prescribed by their medical practitioners or even by themselves. The action of such drugs may impinge upon dental treatment, e.g. anticoagulants, or they may produce an adverse interaction with those prescribed by the dental practitioner. Therefore a broad knowledge of pharmacology and therapeutics is a prerequisite to a sound and safe dental practice.

For a drug to produce its therapeutic effect, it must be present in sufficient concentration at its site of action. Although dose is an important factor, the concentration of a drug at its site of action is a function of the extent and rate of its absorption, distribution, metabolism, and excretion (Fig. 1.1). These are termed *pharmacokinetic* processes (what the body does to the drug), whilst the term *pharmacodynamics* is used to describe the mode of action of drugs

(what the drug does to the body). This chapter will examine the various individual pharmacokinetic processes and, on a quantitative basis, examine the kinetic behaviour of drugs in biological fluids when these processes are operating simultaneously, a study of which is simply referred to as pharmacokinetics.

Absorption, distribution, metabolism, and excretion all involve the movement of a drug across cell membranes. It is therefore useful to first examine the structure of cell membranes and how the physiochemical properties of drug molecules (molecular size, lipid solubility, and degree of ionization) influence their transmembrane movement.

The cell membrane

The major part of the plasma membrane of mammalian cells consists of a double layer of phospholipid molecules oriented so that their hydrophilic head groups are situated at the inner and outer surfaces of the membrane, whilst their hydrophobic hydrocarbon chains occupy the central core (Fig. 1.2). Proteins also form an important component of the plasma membrane and are present in two forms: integral (intrinsic) and peripheral (extrinsic) proteins.

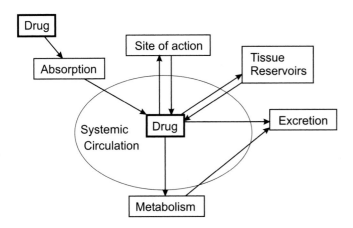

Fig. 1.1 A representation of the interrelationship between the processes of drug absorption, distribution, metabolism, and excretion, and how this determines the concentration of a drug at its site of action.

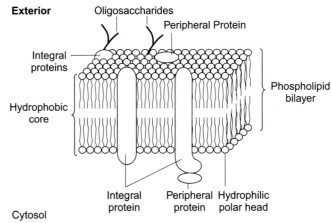

Fig. 1.2 Schematic diagram of a cell membrane showing: the two layers of phospholipid whose fatty-acid tails form the hydrophobic core with their hydrophilic head groups lining the exterior and interior surfaces; integral and peripheral proteins; and oligosaccharides bound to membrane proteins or phospholipid.

Integral proteins span the lipid bilayer and include transporter molecules and receptors for hormones and neurotransmitters. Peripheral proteins, for example some types of enzymes, unlike integral proteins, do not interact with the hydrophobic core of the phospholipid bilayer but are attached to either an integral protein on the inner aspect of the membrane or to the hydrophilic phospholipid head groups at the external or internal surfaces. In addition, oligosaccharides may be attached to membrane proteins or lipid on the external surface of the plasma membrane, thus forming glycoproteins or glycolipids. These various components of the cell plasma membrane do not result in a rigid structure, but a fluid one in which the various components are mobile.

The movement of drugs across cell membranes

There are four main routes by which drugs cross cell membranes (Fig. 1.3):

(1) passive diffusion through the phospholipid bilayer;
(2) diffusion through aqueous pores in the membrane;
(3) diffusion through intercellular pores;
(4) carrier-mediated transport.

Passive diffusion through lipid

The majority of drugs pass through cell membranes by simple passive diffusion, i.e. the tendency for molecules to move down a concentration gradient as a result of random thermal motion. Most drugs have a molecular mass of less than 500 daltons (Da) and, as such, molecular size has little effect on diffusion through lipid membranes. The rate of passive diffusion of a drug across a cell membrane is proportional to its lipid solubility (the ability to dissolve in fat-like substances), the area of the membrane, and the magnitude of the concentration gradient across the membrane.

Lipid solubility can be determined by measuring the distribution of a drug between an immiscible organic solvent and an aqueous solution, an oil:water partition coefficient. The higher the partition coefficient, the greater the lipid solubility and this means that the drug will diffuse more rapidly across the lipid cell membrane. Many non-polar drug molecules, i.e. those with no separation of positive and negative charges, freely dissolve in lipids and therefore easily pass across cell membranes. However, the majority of drugs are either weak acids or weak bases and can exist in either an unionized lipid-soluble form or an ionized relatively lipid-insoluble form, the relative proportions of which are dependent upon the drug's intrinsic tendency to ionize and the pH of the solution in which it is dissolved.

pH and drug ionization

The fractions of the ionized and unionized form of a drug in a particular pH environment depend upon its dissociation constant, pK_a, which is given by the Henderson–Hasselbach equation (shown below). The pK_a of a drug represents the pH at which 50% of the drug is in the ionized form and therefore 50% is in the unionized form. Thus for acidic drugs:

$$HA \rightleftharpoons H^+ + A^-,$$

and:

$$pK_a = pH + \log(HA/A^-).$$

Whilst for basic drugs:

$$BH^+ \rightleftharpoons B + H^+,$$

and

$$pK_a = pH + \log(BH^+/B).$$

The lipid solubility of the uncharged species will depend upon its oil:water partition coefficient although, for the majority of drugs, the uncharged species is sufficiently lipid-soluble to rapidly diffuse across cell membranes. The pK_a values of drugs

Outside

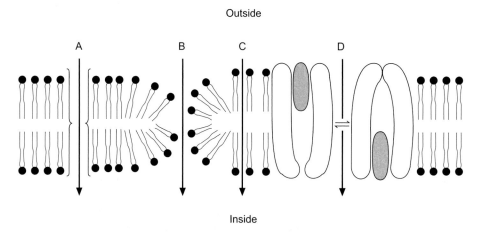

Inside

Fig. 1.3 The principal mechanisms by which drugs cross cell membranes: (A) diffusion between cells; (B) diffusion through aqueous pores; (C) diffusion through phospholipid; and (D) transport by carriers.

show considerable variation; for example acidic drugs such as aspirin and phenytoin have values of 3.5 and 8.5, respectively, whilst basic drugs such as diazepam and propranolol have values of 3.3 and 9.5, respectively. Such differences in pK_a values will be reflected in varying proportions of ionized and unionized species of drugs present in the pH environment of biological fluids. The fraction of a drug in the ionized form will be greater when present in its opposite pH environment, i.e. an acidic drug will be predominately ionized in basic conditions and basic drugs will be largely ionized in acidic conditions. The effect of pH on the fractions of a drug in its ionized and unionized forms has consequences for its absorption and excretion (see below).

Diffusion through pores

Cells are permeable to water that passes across the membrane via small pores (aquaporins, 0.4 nm in diameter), and such a bulk flow of water can carry small molecules of less than 100 Da in diameter such as urea and ethanol. However, most drug molecules are too large to cross cell membranes by this route. Furthermore, inorganic ions do not transfer across cell membranes through the aqueous pores since their hydrated radius is too large. Inorganic ions move across membranes via selective ion channels—such as the sodium channel in nerve membranes or carrier-mediated mechanisms e.g. Na^+/ K^+-ATPase.

Some drugs are large proteins (e.g. insulin) and have difficulty penetrating cells by diffusion across the cell membrane. However, such large molecules can move across membranes by diffusing through the intercellular pores (50–100 nm in diameter) that exist between cells, this is termed the paracellular route.

Carrier-mediated transport

Cells possess many specialized transport mechanisms for the transmembrane movement of substances such as sugars, amino acids, and neurotransmitters which are not very soluble in lipids. These transport systems involve a transmembrane carrier protein that undergoes a conformational change on binding the substrate (transported molecule). This change allows the substrate to dissociate from the carrier on the opposite side of the membrane (Fig. 1.3). Moreover, these systems can operate solely on the concentration gradient across the membrane, with the substrate moving from the side of low to high concentration until equilibrium is reached. Such a transport system is termed facilitated diffusion. Some carrier-mediated transport systems are directly coupled to a supply of energy provided by the hydrolysis of ATP and can transport substrates against a concentration gradient and/or an electrical gradient (an electrochemical gradient)—these are called active transport systems. In addition, there are a number of carrier-mediated transport systems, most notably in the kidney, that, whilst not directly linked to ATP hydrolysis, are dependent upon the establishment of an electrochemical gradient for another substance. For example, in the kidney, glucose and Na^+ are co-transported by a carrier in the luminal membrane. The whole process is driven by a low intracellular Na^+ concentration produced by the activity of Na^+/ K^+-ATPase present in the opposite cell membrane that moves three Na^+ ions out of the cell whilst transporting two K^+ ions into the cell.

In contrast to diffusion through lipid membrane, which increases in relation to the concentration gradient across the membrane, carrier-mediated diffusion is saturable such that a maximum rate of transport is reached at high substrate concentrations. Drugs that have a similar structure to the natural substrate can cross cell membranes via a carrier: such carrier-mediated transport is present in the gastrointestinal tract, blood–brain barrier (see later), renal tubules, and the biliary tract. For example, L-dopa/levodopa, used in the treatment of Parkinson's disease, is actively absorbed from the gastrointestinal tract and transported into the brain by an aromatic amino acid, carrier-mediated transport pathway. In addition to transporting some drugs across cell membranes, protein carriers are also sites of drug action since inhibition of these transport mechanisms is responsible for the pharmacological effects of some drugs (see Chapter 2).

Key facts
Passage of drugs across cell membranes

- Most drugs cross cell membranes by passive diffusion through lipid.

- The rate of diffusion through lipid membranes is determined by a drug's lipid solubility, the area of membrane available for diffusion, and the concentration gradient of the drug across the membrane.

- Most drugs are weak acids or bases, and the proportions of drug in the unionized lipid-soluble form and the ionized lipid-insoluble form are dependent on the drug's pK_a as well as the pH of the surrounding environment.

- Carrier-mediated transport across membranes occurs for some drugs that are chemically similar to the endogenous substrate.

Drug absorption and routes of administration

The absorption of a drug is the movement of that drug from its site of administration into the plasma from where it is distributed throughout the body. Absorption is required for a drug to reach its site of action following administration via the majority of routes, with the exception of intravenous injections and some instances of topical application. Drugs that are administered with the intention of acting within the body are described as being given systemically, as opposed to local administration when drugs are applied to a particular site with the intention of acting solely at that site. Routes of administration can be divided into two classes:

(1) *enteral* (a gastrointestinal route):
- oral,
- sublingual/buccal,
- rectal;

(2) *parenteral* (a non-gastrointestinal route):
- injection,
- inhalation,
- topical.

Enteral routes of administration

Oral

DISSOLUTION

Most drugs are given orally in solid form, usually as tablets or capsules for reasons of convenience and economy. Since absorption will take place only after the drug is in solution, the drug must first dissolve in gut fluids. Dissolution of a solid drug is limited by the small surface area from which the drug can dissolve. Factors which limit the dissolution of a drug are particle size, the dosage form, the pH conditions in the gastrointestinal tract, and the influence of additives (excipients). The rate of dissolution of a drug in solid form is inversely proportional to particle size, and therefore a decrease in particle size, which will increase surface area, will increase its dissolution rate. The dosage form of a drug that is given orally may affect the extent and rate of absorption into the general circulation. Clearly, a drug given in an aqueous solution will remove the dissolution stage, but this is not always convenient or practical. The relative rates of release of other oral dosage forms are suspension > capsules > tablets > coated tablets. Tablets are often coated to mask taste or smell, to prevent atmospheric degradation of drug, and to control sites of release (see below).

Since many drugs are weak acids or bases, their solubility will be affected by the pH environment present in a particular part of the gastrointestinal tract. A weak acid will be poorly soluble in the acidic conditions of the stomach, whereas a weak base will be readily soluble. Thus, for example, aspirin, which is a weak acid, is poorly soluble in the stomach and one technique to aid dissolution is to add buffering ingredients to the formulation. Dissolution is enhanced by the addition of sodium bicarbonate, magnesium carbonate, etc. to the formulation to raise the pH of the immediate environment surrounding the dissolving solid particle.

Excipients are substances added to the formulation of a drug that act as disintegration agents, fillers, binders, and flavourings. Such additives have no therapeutic action and are considered to be inert, although they may affect the absorption of a drug. One dramatic example of the influence of excipients is a study in which epileptic patients previously stabilized on a dosage regimen of phenytoin capsules suddenly developed features of phenytoin toxicity. It was found that the majority of these patients had blood levels of phenytoin in the toxic range although the quantity of active drug was unaltered. It was subsequently discovered that the manufacturer had changed the primary excipient in its capsules and this had resulted in increased absorption of phenytoin with resultant toxicity.

ABSORPTION IN THE GASTROINTESTINAL TRACT

Since the pH of the contents of the stomach varies between 1 and 3, most weak acids are in the unionized form and are able to be absorbed *once they have dissolved*. By contrast, most weak bases are largely ionized and are poorly absorbed from the stomach. The area of the stomach available for absorption (1 m^2) and its blood flow (0.15 L min^{-1}) are modest, particularly when compared to the small intestine. As a result, the absorption of neutral drugs and even weak acids is often slow. In addition, gastric emptying occurs and its frequency, which varies between 1 and 3 hours, determines the time available for gastric absorption.

The small intestine has a large surface area available for absorption (estimated to be 200 m^2) and a blood flow of 1 L min^{-1}, with the pH of its contents varying from 5 (duodenum) to 7 (ileum). The pH of small intestine therefore favours the absorption of weak bases with less favourable conditions for the absorption of weak acids. Nevertheless, the absorption of weak acids is faster in the small intestine than the stomach because of the much larger surface area and blood flow, and thus the small intestine is the major site of absorption of all drugs given orally. The large intestine is of much lesser importance in the absorption of orally administered drugs since few drugs are absorbed here unless they have escaped absorption in the small intestine.

The overall conditions in the gastrointestinal tract are more favourable for the absorption of weak bases since the site for dissolution of a weak base (the stomach) precedes the site where the pH conditions are conducive for its absorption (the small intestine). Conversely, for a weak acid, the anatomical site favouring dissolution (the small intestine) follows the site where pH conditions favour its absorption (the stomach) and are therefore opposite to the desired order. As a result, the rate of dissolution of weak acids more often limits the rate of absorption than for weak bases.

Modification of the dissolution rates of drugs in the gut can be used to produce sustained-release (timed-release) preparations designed to give slow uniform absorption over periods of 8 hours or longer. The advantage of such preparations is a reduction in the frequency of drug administration with a possible improvement in patient compliance (see below) or maintained therapeutic effect overnight. However, caution is necessary when using such preparations since there may be either failure of adequate release with a loss of therapeutic effect or an excessive release with possible toxicity—this is because these preparations necessarily contain multiples of the normal dose.

The presence of food in the gastrointestinal tract may also affect the absorption of drugs. In general, a drug taken following a meal is more slowly absorbed because its progress to the small intestine is delayed. In some instances, the nature of the food may reduce absorption. For example, tetracycline antibacterial drugs chelate calcium ions to produce an insoluble complex, and therefore the presence of calcium-rich foods such as milk and cheese will reduce or prevent absorption of these drugs.

LIMITATIONS TO THE ORAL ADMINISTRATION OF DRUGS

There a number of factors that limit or preclude the use of oral administration, including:

- delay in absorption;
- destruction of the drug by gastric acid;
- irritation of the gastrointestinal tract;
- hepatic first-pass metabolism;
- patient compliance.

1 **DELAY IN ABSORPTION:** As discussed above, various factors affect the rate of absorption of a drug and there is a delay, ranging from 30 minutes to 2 hours, between oral administration and achieving effective concentrations of a drug at its site of action. Whilst, in many cases, this delay is of little consequence, in emergency situations where the patient is unconscious and/or effective blood concentrations need to be achieved quickly then parenteral administration of drugs is necessary.

2 **DESTRUCTION OF THE DRUG BY GASTRIC ACID:** Some drugs are broken down by the acidic contents of the stomach—for example benzylpenicillin—and consequently these are not given by the oral route.

3 **IRRITATION OF THE GASTROINTESTINAL TRACT:** Some drugs produce irritation of the gastrointestinal tract resulting in vomiting (for example >1.5 g of erythromycin) and diarrhoea (for instance broad-spectrum antibiotics). Whilst these side-effects are obviously distressing to the patient, such reactions do not allow adequate time for effective quantities of the drug to be absorbed. In addition, some drugs can directly damage the gastrointestinal tract: for example aspirin can produce focal erosions and bleeding, and therefore is contraindicated in patients with peptic ulcers. A strategy to protect the gastric mucosa from a drug or to protect a drug from gastric acid is to use enteric-coated tablets, these are coated in a film designed to resist the effects of gastric acid and to permit disintegration of the tablet in the small intestine.

4 **HEPATIC FIRST-PASS METABOLISM:** Before entering the general circulation, drugs absorbed from the stomach and small intestine are delivered to the liver via the portal vein. Some drugs are rapidly metabolized by enzymes in the liver with the result that only a fraction of the absorbed dose reaches the general circulation. These drugs are described as undergoing hepatic first-pass metabolism ('the first-pass effect') or presystemic elimination. Metabolism of some drugs may occur within the gastrointestinal epithelium and this will also contribute to presystemic elimination. There is considerable interindividual variation in hepatic first-pass metabolism and, because of this, wide differences in plasma concentrations can be seen in any group of patients following the administration of a standard dose. An example of a drug which undergoes hepatic first-pass metabolism is the β-adrenoceptor antagonist propranolol, only a third to a quarter of which reaches the circulation following oral administration. Furthermore, interindividual variation in the hepatic first-pass effect accounts for the variability in plasma concentrations of propranolol (up to 20-fold) in patients given a comparable oral dose. Morphine also undergoes considerable first-pass metabolism and therefore, when compared to an intramuscular injection, a much higher oral dose is required to produce an equivalent analgesic effect. Hepatic first-pass metabolism can be so extensive that a drug is ineffective when given orally and therefore must be given by a non-oral route, e.g. sublingual administration of glyceryl trinitrate.

5 **PATIENT COMPLIANCE:** The oral administration of drugs, along with some other modes of administration, requires co-operation on the part of the patient. The simplest cause of an apparent failure to respond to drug treatment is because the patient has failed to take an adequate quantity of the drug. In one extreme case, it was found that 75% of epileptic patients who were considered refractory to treatment with phenytoin were not taking the drug as prescribed. There are a number of reasons for patient non-compliance, including failure on the practitioner's part: to explain how the drug should be taken; to advise the patient of the possibility of minor adverse effects; or to explain the length of time drug treatment is required before a beneficial effect is evident. Alternatively, non-compliance may result from failure on the patient's part as a result of: wilful determination not to take the drug; failure to comply with clear dosing instructions (more likely in elderly patients or with multiple drug therapy); or the deterrent effect of minor adverse effects.

Sublingual/buccal

This mode of drug administration involves tablets being placed beneath the tongue (sublingual) or inside the cheek (buccal). These areas have a good blood supply and allow the rapid absorption of lipid-soluble drugs such as glyceryl trinitrate, which is used in the symptomatic relief of an anginal attack. The venous drainage from these tissues is to the heart via the jugular vein and hence the liver is bypassed. Therefore these routes of administration are potentially useful for drugs subject to extensive hepatic first-pass metabolism or those destroyed in the gut.

Rectal

Drugs administered rectally are usually in the form of suppositories and this route is useful when oral administration is difficult, such as in young children or if the patient is unconscious, vomiting, or unable to swallow. A significant proportion of the venous drainage from the rectum avoids the liver and therefore, in comparison to oral administration, there is reduced hepatic first-pass metabolism. Disadvantages to this route of administration are that absorption of drugs is often irregular and incomplete. In addition, this route of drug administration is unacceptable to certain patients.

Parenteral routes of administration

Injection of drugs by either intravenous, intramuscular, or subcutaneous routes is required when effective plasma concentrations need to be achieved quickly or when the oral route is not possible. Figure 1.4 shows how ineffective oral administration can be for a drug, e.g. benzylpenicillin, compared to intravenous and intramuscular routes such that effective therapeutic concentrations are not achieved following oral administration. This figure also demonstrates the slower rate of absorption following oral administration compared to intramuscular injections since peak drug concentrations are achieved later when the drug is given via the oral route.

The disadvantages to injections are:

• strict asepsis must be maintained to avoid infection;

• injections can cause pain;

• the inconvenience and greater cost compared to the oral route.

INTRAVENOUS (IV)

Administration by intravenous injection produces rapid plasma concentrations since there is no absorption phase. Injections are

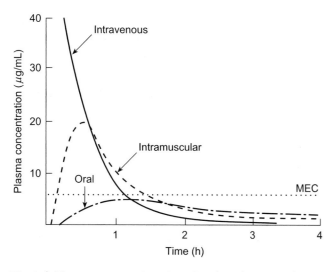

Fig. 1.4 Plasma concentration–time plots for a drug given by the intravenous, intramuscular, and oral routes. These plots show: (1) absence of an absorption phase following intravenous administration; (2) the slower rate of absorption following oral compared to intramuscular administration—as shown by the shorter time to achieve peak concentration with the latter; and (3) the low bioavailability following oral administration of the drug such that the minimum effective concentration (MEC) is not attained.

made into a peripheral vein, most commonly a vein in the antecubital region of the arm, and are frequently given over a period of minutes to prevent excessively high concentrations in the blood that could produce toxic effects. Whilst suspensions of relatively insoluble drugs can not be given because of the risk of embolism, intravenous administration can be used for drugs that are irritants by intramuscular and subcutaneous injection.

INTRAMUSCULAR (IM) AND SUBCUTANEOUS (SC)

Although poorly soluble drugs can be injected in suspensions, the drugs must eventually dissolve in the interstitial fluid before absorption can occur. Highly ionized and therefore poorly lipid-soluble drugs such as gentamicin and large molecular weight drugs (e.g. insulin), which cannot be given orally, are absorbed after intramuscular/subcutaneous injection as a result of diffusion through large intercellular pores in the capillary membrane. The action of a drug can be prolonged using depot preparations given either subcutaneously or intramuscularly. Dissolution and absorption of a drug implanted subcutaneously as a solid pellet occurs slowly over a period of weeks or months, for example the estradiol (oestradiol) implants used in hormone replacement therapy. The deep intramuscular injection of a drug dissolved in an oil, from which the drug is slowly absorbed, can produce an action which lasts for four weeks. This technique is employed for the administration of neuroleptic drugs such as flupentixol (flupenthixol), which is used in the treatment of schizophrenia.

Drugs that are injected intramuscularly are usually given into the upper arm (deltoid), thigh, (vastus lateralis), or buttocks (gluteus maximus). In a resting patient the deltoid muscle has the greatest blood supply and absorption is more rapid from this site than from the other two. Absorption from intramuscular sites is usually faster than from subcutaneous sites because of the poorer blood flow to the latter.

With the exception of the administration of local anaesthetics in dentistry, drugs that are administered subcutaneously are usually injected into the upper arm or thigh. Absorption may be increased by co-injecting the enzyme hyaluronidase, which breaks down connective tissue, allowing the drug solution to spread over a greater area. Alternatively, absorption can be slowed by co-injecting a vasoconstrictor such as epinephrine (adrenaline), which is frequently used in dentistry to prolong the action of local anaesthetics.

OTHER INJECTION ROUTES

Other less common routes of injection include intra-arterial, spinal, epidural, and intrathecal. Antibacterial drugs, such as gentamicin, are sometimes given by intrathecal injection in meningeal infection to bypass the blood–brain barrier (see later).

Inhalation

There are two important classes of drug given by inhalation: anaesthetic gases and drugs used in the treatment of asthma. Anaesthetic gases are small lipophilic molecules that are readily absorbed by passive diffusion through the lungs: an organ designed to promote the efficient exchange of gases with a large surface area ($70\,m^2$) and a high blood flow—100% of cardiac output. Venous drainage from the lungs is directly to the heart so first-pass metabolism by the liver is avoided. Most anti-asthma drugs, such as salbutamol and beclometasone (beclomethasone), are delivered as aerosols (suspension of a solid or liquid in a gaseous vehicle) designed to deposit drug on the airways (bronchioles). Anti-asthma drugs are thus given to produce a local effect on the bronchiolar smooth muscle and mucosa with little absorption into blood, whilst anaesthetic gases produce systemic effects. Particle or droplet size is important for the efficient delivery of drugs to their site of action within the pulmonary tree. Large particles or droplets ($20\,\mu m$ in diameter) deposit too high up in the respiratory tract, whereas small particles ($>1\,\mu m$) penetrate into the alveoli, with particles of intermediate size (2–$6\,\mu m$) impacting mainly on the bronchioles.

Topical

This mode of drug administration is an efficient way of delivering drugs to sites such as the oral and nasal mucosa, skin, eye, and vagina although topical application can be used to achieve either a local action or a systemic effect. Topical application is used to produce a local action in, for example, the treatment of dermatological conditions such as eczema or aphthous ulceration (triamcinolone paste or hydrocortisone lozenges) with the aim of avoiding systemic effects. However, the oral mucosa is an excellent surface for the absorption of a wide variety of substances. In this case, systemic side-effects are avoided by applying a small quantity of drug to the site of the lesion, this produces relatively high local concentrations but low blood concentrations following absorption. Application of drugs to the nasal mucosa can result in a local action (such as that produced by nasal decongestants) or a systemic effect (for example midazolam can be administered intranasally to produce sedation in children). Systemic effects can also be achieved following topical application to the skin with a transdermal delivery system, an adhesive patch containing the drug. This is applied to the skin and can supply drug for up to 24 hours. Examples of such a delivery system are patches containing glyceryl trinitrate for the prophylaxis of angina and nicotine used as an aid to stopping smoking. The skin is not uniformly permeable over the entire body surface, as illustrated by the use of hyoscine to treat motion sickness which is more quickly absorbed from behind the ear than when applied to the chest.

Bioavailability

This is a term used to describe the proportion of administered drug reaching the systemic circulation. Bioavailability can be determined from the blood/plasma concentration–time data, since the total area under the blood/plasma concentration–time curve (AUC) after a single dose reflects the amount of drug reaching the systemic circulation. After intravenous administration there is no elimination of a drug before it reaches the systemic circulation. Thus the fraction of drug absorbed is 1.0 and the AUC

is the maximum that can be obtained because all the drug enters the bloodstream. A comparison of the AUC after oral administration with that obtained after intravenous administration allows the fraction of drug absorbed (F) to be calculated, i.e.

$$F = AUC_{oral}/AUC_{IV},$$

which is normally expressed as a percentage value (see Table 1.1).

If only half the drug reaches the general circulation, then oral bioavailability = 50%; whilst for the drug shown in Fig. 1.4, the oral bioavailability is 20%. Such a low value could be a result of destruction by gastric acid (benzylpenicillin), poor absorption (gentamicin), or extensive first-pass metabolism (lidocaine (lignocaine)) as discussed above. Bioavailability only gives an estimate of the fraction of a drug that enters the systemic circulation and not the extent to which a drug achieves effective therapeutic concentrations, since following oral administration these are not achieved for the drug shown in Fig. 1.4.

Key facts
Drug absorption and routes of administration

- Oral administration is the most convenient route of drug administration but is limited for some drugs by:
  - poor absorption due to low lipid solubility;
  - destruction of drug by gastric acid;
  - gastric irritation;
  - "the first-pass effect" where a significant proportion of the drug is metabolized in the liver before reaching the systemic circulation.

- Oral bioavailability of a drug is the fraction of the dose that reaches the systemic circulation. Low bioavailability results from incomplete absorption from the gut and/or a large first-pass effect.

- Sublingual administration of drugs avoids the first-pass effect.

- Intravenous administration has no absorption phase but cannot be used for poorly soluble drugs.

- The action of a local anaesthetic agent injected subcutaneously can be prolonged by the co-injection of a drug that produces vasoconstriction.

- A prolongation of drug action can be produced by oral sustained-release preparations or intramuscular or subcutaneous depot preparations.

- Topical administration can be used to produce local or systemic effects.

Distribution

After a drug is absorbed or injected into the bloodstream, it is available for distribution to interstitial and cellular fluids. The capillaries, with the exception of those in the brain and placenta, have endothelial membranes with intercellular pores so most drugs quickly diffuse out of the vascular system and reach the interstitial fluid that bathes the cells, although this process may be modified by binding to plasma proteins. The penetration of drugs into cells depends upon the same factors that determine absorption from the gut—molecular size, lipid solubility, and the degree of ionization. Hydrophilic (water-soluble but poorly lipid-soluble) drugs cannot penetrate cells easily, unless by carrier-mediated transport, and their distribution is often limited to the extracellular fluid, e.g. gentamicin. By contrast, lipid-soluble drugs can diffuse through cell membranes and enter the intracellular fluid.

Blood–brain barrier

The central nervous system (CNS) is surrounded by a specialized barrier which is an obstacle to the penetration of hydrophilic substances into the CNS. Unlike capillaries in most tissues, endothelial cells in the brain do not possess intercellular pores and are described as having tight junctions. In addition, glial cells are often associated with the capillaries in the brain and these present an additional lipid barrier to the diffusion of poorly lipid-soluble drugs. Thus, drugs must be lipid-soluble in order to diffuse quickly into the brain. Rapid penetration into the brain is important for drugs used to treat disorders of the CNS (such as anticonvulsant drugs) and therefore these drugs must be lipid-soluble. However, some hydrophilic drugs such as L-dopa do gain access to the brain via carrier-mediated transport.

Placenta

This structure separates fetal and maternal blood flow and regulates the exchange of many substances between the two circulations. The placental membranes behave like a lipid membrane, such that hydrophilic drugs traverse the membrane much more slowly than unionized lipid-soluble drugs.

The effect of blood flow

Cell membranes present no barrier to the entry of highly lipid-soluble drugs into tissues and the rate of entry of these drugs is determined by their rate of delivery to tissues. Thus, blood flow is the rate-limiting step in the distribution of lipid-soluble drugs; however, blood flow does not influence the rate of entry into cells of poorly lipid-soluble drugs or drugs with a large molecular mass. Lipid-soluble drugs rapidly equilibrate in well-perfused tissues such as the brain, kidneys, liver, and heart. Equilibration is slower for moderately well, perfused tissues (muscle) and much slower for poorly perfused tissues such as adipose tissue and skin. However, loss of the drug from tissues will occur in the order: well perfused > moderately well perfused > poorly perfused.

The redistribution of a highly lipid-soluble drug into less-well perfused tissues can have a marked effect on the duration of drug action. Thiopental (thiopentone) induces anaesthesia within 30–50 seconds of intravenous injection; but its duration of action is only several minutes. Thiopental is highly lipid-soluble and

rapidly crosses the blood–brain barrier and distributes into the CNS. However, the concentration of drug in the brain rapidly falls, despite the fact that the drug is only slowly metabolized. This decline in concentration is due to its redistribution into other tissues (skeletal muscle and fat) which are less-well perfused than the brain.

Drug binding in blood (protein binding)

Many drugs bind reversibly to plasma proteins, the major binding protein being albumin that constitutes about 50% of total plasma proteins. This protein can bind a wide variety of neutral, acidic, and basic drugs. Some basic drugs, however, can also bind to another type of plasma protein, α_1-acid glycoprotein. Binding to plasma proteins affects the distribution and elimination of drugs and, as a result, their pharmacological effects. Drug bound to plasma proteins is restricted to plasma because the high molecular weight of proteins impairs their passage across the capillary endothelium. Consequently, only unbound drug is available for diffusion into tissues to exert its action (Fig. 1.5). The extent of protein binding can be as high as 95–99% (for example, diazepam and warfarin), whilst 49% of aspirin and 70% of lidocaine are bound to plasma proteins (see Table 1.1). Extensively bound drugs, such as warfarin, may be displaced by drugs that show moderate degrees of protein binding; this has the effect of producing a rise in the free concentration of the extensively bound drug. Since it is free and not bound drug that is pharmacologically active, the displacement of an extensively protein-bound drug can, under some circumstances, result in an increased drug response (see Chapter 24).

Drug binding in tissues

In addition to plasma proteins, drugs may also bind to tissue components such as proteins, phospholipids, and nucleic acids. A drug may bind to plasma proteins but may still be located mainly in tissue, if the tissue components have an affinity for the drug greater than that of plasma proteins. Some drugs accumulate in muscle and other cells in higher concentrations than in the

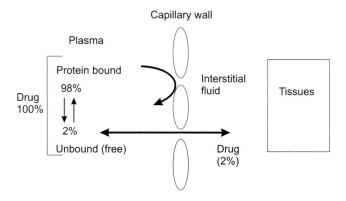

Fig. 1.5 The effect of protein binding of a drug on its distribution between plasma and interstitial fluid. Only the unbound fraction gains access to the interstitial fluid.

extracellular fluid. If the binding is reversible and high intracellular concentrations are achieved, the tissue may act as a drug reservoir (particularly if the tissue represents a significant proportion of body mass) from which the drug can diffuse back into plasma when plasma concentrations decline.

Apparent volume of distribution

The concentration of a drug in plasma after distribution to tissues is complete is dependent on the dose given and the extent of tissue distribution. The apparent volume of distribution, V_d, relates the amount of drug in the body to plasma concentration according to the following formula:

$$V_d = A/C;$$

where A is the amount of drug in the body and C is the plasma drug concentration.

V_d can be estimated from plasma concentration–time plots when a bolus dose of drug is given intravenously and blood samples are taken at various times after administration. The concentration of drug in plasma is measured and plotted as a log value against time (t) (see Fig 1.10(a)) The linear portion of this graph is extrapolated to the intercept on the y axis, when $t = 0$. The antilog of this intercept value gives C_0, the concentration of drug immediately after injection. Since the amount of drug in the body at $t = 0$ is nearly equal to the dose, V_d can be calculated by modifying the above equation to:

$$V_d = IV\ dose/C_0.$$

The magnitude of V_d does not necessarily correspond to a real anatomical value such as plasma volume (3.5 L), extracellular fluid volume (15 L), or total body water (42 L) but can vary between several litres to many hundreds of litres. Some drugs such as warfarin have low apparent volumes of distribution because they are preferentially bound to plasma proteins rather than to extravascular sites. Although these drugs distribute throughout the body water, the bulk of the drug remains in the plasma and V_d is small, ranging from 10 to 15 L. By contrast, some drugs such as propranolol have large volumes of distribution ranging from a few hundred to several thousand litres (see Table 1.1). These drugs are extensively bound to extravascular sites with little drug remaining in plasma.

Key facts
Distribution of drugs

- The blood–brain barrier only allows lipid-soluble drugs to diffuse into the brain.

- Many drugs bind reversibly to plasma proteins, the major binding protein being albumin. Only unbound drug can diffuse into tissues.

- Some drugs accumulate in tissues such as muscle, and these tissues can act as drug reservoirs.

- The apparent volume of distribution (V_d) of a drug is a calculated volume in to which a drug appears to distribute, but it does not necessarily correspond to an anatomical volume. It can vary from several litres to hundreds of litres. Extensive binding to plasma protein reduces V_d, whilst binding to extravascular sites increases V_d.

Drug metabolism (biotransformation)

The process of drug metabolism is an attempt by the body to transform a drug into forms (metabolites) that are less pharmacologically active and more hydrophilic, the latter effect enabling excretion in urine and bile (see later). Drug metabolism can occur in the skin, lungs, gut wall, plasma, and kidney; but by far the most important organ is the liver. Drug metabolism involves two principal types of reaction: phase I reactions in which a chemically reactive group is added or uncovered and phase II reactions, also termed conjugation reactions, which involve the addition of a pharmacologically inactive group. Figure 1.6 shows the various pathways of drug metabolism in which a drug undergoes either phase I or phase II metabolism only or a combination of these. Some drugs are not metabolized and are excreted unchanged as the parent compound, examples of which include benzylpenicillin and gentamicin. These pathways of drug metabolism are not mutually exclusive such that a number of different metabolites can arise from one drug. For example, a fraction of a particular drug may undergo phase I metabolism only, another fraction of the same drug may be metabolized by both phase I and phase 2 reactions, whilst a further fraction of this same drug may be excreted

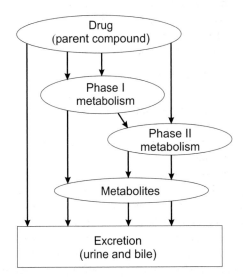

Fig. 1.6 The various pathways of drug metabolism. A drug can undergo either phase I or phase II metabolism only, or phase I metabolism followed by phase II metabolism. Some drugs such as benzylpenicillin do not undergo metabolism and are excreted unchanged.

unchanged. Within the liver, phase I and phase II reactions are carried out by intracellular enzymes, many of which are attached to the smooth endoplasmic reticulum. These enzymes are referred to as microsomal enzymes—so-called because the endoplasmic reticulum sediments obtained on homogenization and centrifugation are very small fragments called microsomes.

Phase I reactions

These reactions include oxidative and reductive reactions, although the latter reactions are less common. Oxidative reactions include N- and O-dealkylation, S-oxidation, hydroxylation, and oxidative deamination (S-oxidation is illustrated in Fig. 1.7(a)). Drug oxidation reactions are generally catalysed by the mixed-function enzyme system, of which the most important enzymes are the cytochrome oxidases. These are haemoproteins which bind the drug substrate and transfer electrons to molecular oxygen. Cytochrome P450—so-called because it absorbs light maximally at 450 nm—is present as numerous isoenzymes, and plays a critical role in the different types of oxidative reactions by producing an intermediate product from which the final oxidative metabolite is derived.

The mixed-function oxidase system does not account for all drug oxidation reactions. One example is ethanol which is metabolized in the cytosol by the soluble enzyme alcohol dehydrogenase. In addition, hydrolytic reactions are not catalysed by microsomal enzymes but take place in plasma and in a variety of tissues in addition to the liver. Drugs that contain ester and amide bonds are susceptible to hydrolysis, although amide bonds are the more resistant. One example of ester hydrolysis is suxamethonium, a neuromuscular blocking drug metabolized by the enzyme pseudocholinesterase, which is present in plasma.

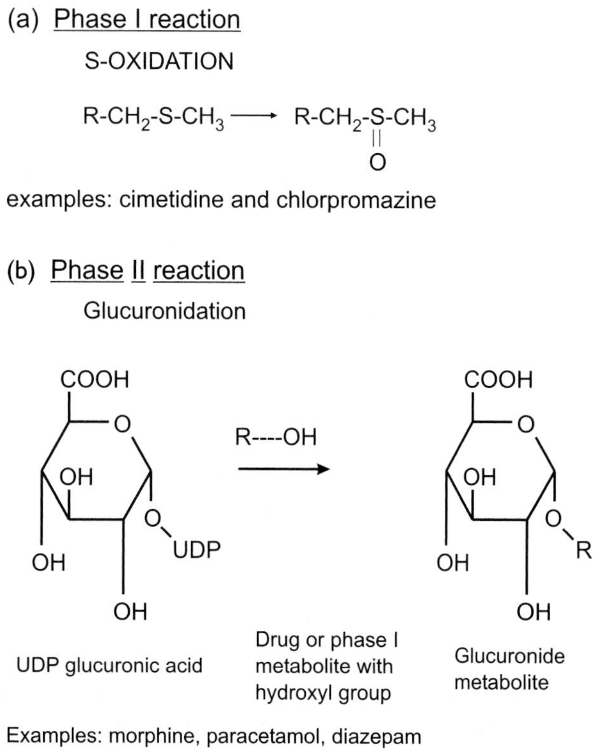

Phase II reactions

Drugs containing reactive groups (such as a thiol, hydroxyl, or amino group) are candidates for the attachment of an additional chemical group. Reactive groups, such as hydroxyl, may be present in the parent compound or have resulted from phase I reactions. The conjugates resulting from phase II reactions are usually pharmacologically inactive and less lipid-soluble than the initial substrate. The chemical groups added in conjugation reactions are sulfate, glutathione, methyl, acetyl, glycyl, glucuronyl, and glutamyl—with glucuronide formation illustrated in Fig. 1.7(b).

Glucuronide formation involves the compound uridine diphosphate glucuronic acid (UDPGA) from which the glucuronic acid component is transferred to the parent drug, or its phase I metabolite, by the action of the enzyme UDP glucuronyl transferase. This enzyme has a broad substrate specificity and therefore glucuronide conjugates are formed from a wide variety of drugs.

Pharmacologically or toxicologically active drug metabolites

In some instances, the process of drug metabolism generates metabolites that are pharmacologically active. Metabolism of benzodiazepine drugs (used as sedatives, anxiolytics, and anticonvulsants) results in metabolites that have pharmacological actions similar to the parent compound, but with a longer duration of action. As a result, the pharmacological action of these drugs can persist after the parent compound has disappeared. Some drugs are inactive as the parent compound but only produce a pharmacological action following metabolism. Such drugs are referred to as pro-drugs, with one example being the angiotensin-converting enzyme inhibitor enalapril which is hydrolysed to the pharmacological active metabolite enalaprilat. Phase I metabolism can also generate toxic metabolites. An example is the metabolism of paracetamol to N-acetyl-p-benzoquinone which is normally inactivated by conjugation with glutathione. However, in cases of paracetamol overdose the supply of glutathione is depleted and the toxic metabolite accumulates which results in hepatic necrosis (see Chapter 6).

Factors that influence drug metabolism

Drug interactions during metabolism

A number of drugs, such as phenytoin, carbamazepine, ethanol, and rifampicin, when repeatedly administered increase the activity of the mixed-function oxidase system and conjugating systems. The mechanism involves the stimulation of gene transcription leading to increased synthesis of drug metabolizing enzymes, an effect which is termed enzyme induction. The result is not only increased metabolism of the inducing agent with the possible loss of its therapeutic effect, but increased metabolism of other drugs a patient may be taking if the drugs share a similar metabolic pathway.

(a) Phase I reaction

S-OXIDATION

$$R\text{-}CH_2\text{-}S\text{-}CH_3 \longrightarrow R\text{-}CH_2\text{-}\underset{\underset{O}{\|}}{S}\text{-}CH_3$$

examples: cimetidine and chlorpromazine

(b) Phase II reaction

Glucuronidation

UDP glucuronic acid   Drug or phase I metabolite with hydroxyl group   Glucuronide metabolite

Examples: morphine, paracetamol, diazepam

Fig. 1.7 Examples of (a) phase I and (b) phase II drug metabolism.

In contrast to the induction of microsomal enzymes, the simultaneous administration of two or more drugs can result in the impaired metabolism of the more slowly metabolized drug. The histamine H_2 receptor antagonist cimetidine has an inhibitory effect on the mixed-function oxidase system, and as a result inhibits the metabolism of warfarin and benzodiazepine drugs with potentiation of their pharmacological actions. Inhibition of drug metabolism can also result from competition between drugs for a particular metabolic pathway. For example, erythromycin inhibits the metabolism of theophylline, resulting in increased theophylline plasma concentrations.

The effect of one drug on the metabolism of another is the major cause of adverse drug interactions, and those which are relevant to dentistry are detailed in Chapter 24.

Age

At either end of the age spectrum, the absorption, distribution, metabolism, and excretion of drugs (pharmacokinetic processes) differ from young and middle-aged adults on whom drugs are normally tested. In addition, the very young and elderly may also respond differently to drugs (pharmacodynamics).

In the newborn, drug metabolic pathways are limited, although these develop in a variable fashion during the first year of life. One unwanted effect of this restricted drug metabolism was the 'grey baby' syndrome in which chloramphenicol produced circulatory collapse when given to young babies. This arose from inadequate glucuronidation of chloramphenicol with resulting drug accumulation.

The removal (clearance) of many drugs is reduced in the elderly (> 70 years of age), a group of people who are of more direct concern to the dental surgeon. This reduction in the removal of drugs results from a decline in renal function, hepatic blood flow, and the activity of drug metabolizing enzymes. The activities of the cytochrome-P450 enzyme system are reduced in the elderly, whilst phase II metabolism is normally well maintained. As a general rule, the elderly should initially be prescribed 50% of the normal adult dose of a drug, with subsequent small increases in dose, if required, until the desired therapeutic effect is achieved.

Disease

The capacity of the liver to metabolize drugs is very great and, as a consequence, liver disease needs to be severe before a significant impairment of drug metabolism is evident. However, severe hepatic dysfunction can occur with alcoholic and fatty liver disease, which results in the reduced metabolism of drugs such as diazepam and morphine, with enhanced pharmacological responses. Moreover, decreases in liver blood flow can result from cardiac failure or from the administration of β-adrenoceptor antagonists which reduce cardiac output. A decline in liver blood flow can reduce the metabolism of drugs such as lidocaine and verapamil—these types of drugs are rapidly removed from the circulation by the liver and their metabolism is therefore limited by hepatic blood flow.

Genetic factors

Genetic differences in the ability to metabolize a drug through a particular pathway is an important factor underlying individual differences in drug metabolism. Phenotypic differences in the amount of drug metabolized via a particular route of metabolism has led to individuals being classified as slow or fast metabolizers, with an increased incidence of adverse effects noted in slow metabolizers. Major deficiencies in drug metabolism are inherited as autosomal recessive characteristics.

Genetic polymorphism accounts for the variable rates of N-acetylation of isoniazid (a drug used in the treatment of tuberculosis) with decreased levels of functional enzymes found in the livers of slow acetylators. Genetic polymorphism in N-acetylation shows racial differences, with a 60–70% incidence of slow acetylators in Northern Europeans compared to a 5–10% incidence in Asians. Isoniazid is likely to accumulate to toxic levels when given in normal doses to slow acetylators such that adverse effects, particularly peripheral neuropathy, are more common in these people. Similar problems will arise when other drugs, which are primarily inactivated by acetylation, are administered to slow acetylators: these drugs include procainamide (an antidysrhythmic drug) and hydralazine (a vasodilator drug).

The administration of the short-acting neuromuscular blocking drug suxamethonium is occasionally followed by prolonged apnoea. This is a result of genetic variants that result in an atypical form of pseudocholinesterase which hydrolyses suxamethonium. In such individuals suxamethonium produces muscle paralysis which can last for 2 hours or more; whilst in normal individuals, the duration of action is less than 5 minutes.

Key facts
Drug metabolism

- The process of drug metabolism, in general, produces metabolites which are less pharmacologically active and more water soluble than the parent compound. However, there are exceptions, with metabolites produced with equivalent or greater pharmacological activity than the parent compound.

- Phase I reactions uncover or add a chemical reactive group, sometimes producing toxic metabolites. Phase I reactions include oxidation, reduction, and hydrolysis. Oxidation reactions often involve the mixed-function oxygenase system in which cytochromes P450 play an important role.

- Phase II reactions (conjugation) involve the attachment of an additional chemical group, e.g. glucuronidation and sulfation.

- One drug may increase or decrease the metabolism of another drug, effects which are common causes of adverse drug interactions.

Excretion of drugs

Drugs are eliminated from the body by a combination of metabolism and excretion. As discussed above, the liver is the main site of drug metabolism; this organ may also contribute to excretion because some drugs and their metabolites are excreted in bile and removed from the body in faeces. The kidneys, however, play a central role in the excretion of most drugs and their metabolites.

Renal excretion

Whilst some drugs, like benzylpenicillin and gentamicin, are eliminated almost entirely by renal excretion, most are eliminated by a mixture of renal excretion and hepatic metabolism. Even when the drug is inactivated entirely by metabolism, the resulting metabolites are usually cleared from the body by the kidneys. Renal excretion involves three basic processes (Fig. 1.8):

- glomerular filtration;
- active tubular secretion;
- passive tubular reabsorption.

The relationship between these processes is given by:

rate of renal excretion = (rate of filtration + rate of secretion)
− rate of reabsorption.

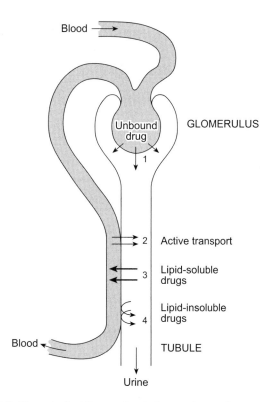

Fig. 1.8 The principal factors that influence the renal excretion of drugs. (1) Unbound drugs are filtered at the glomerulus; (2) active secretion of drugs into the proximal tubule; (3) lipid-soluble drugs are reabsorbed into plasma; and (4) lipid-insoluble drugs are retained in the tubule and excreted in urine.

Glomerular filtration

The kidneys receive about 25% of cardiac output and about 10% of this is filtered at the glomeruli. This means that about 130 mL of plasma is filtered each minute—this is known as the glomerular filtration rate (GFR). The glomerular filter is semipermeable and allows an almost protein-free ultrafiltrate to pass from the glomerular capillaries into Bowman's capsule. The main driving force for filtration is the hydrostatic pressure in the glomerular capillaries.

Molecular mass is the main determinant of a whether a substance will be filtered, with the molecular mass cut-off being about 70 kDa. Albumin has a molecular mass of 69 kDa and passes through the filter in only minute amounts, whilst molecules with a molecular mass of < 2 kDa, which includes most drugs, are freely permeable. Since plasma proteins such as albumin are not filtered, only the unbound fraction of a drug is filtered at the glomerulus. Therefore drugs that are highly bound to plasma proteins, such as warfarin, undergo little glomerular filtration compared to drugs with low protein binding.

Active secretion

Mechanisms exist in the proximal tubule for the active secretion of organic acids (anions such as benzylpenicillin) and bases (cations such as pethidine) from plasma. Both mechanisms are able to transport a wide variety of drugs, and the acid pathway is not only responsible for the secretion of anionic drugs but also for the products of phase II metabolism such as glucuronide, sulfate, and amino-acid conjugates. The secretory mechanisms are active and as such can transport drugs against a concentration gradient. Furthermore, tubular secretion for most drugs, unlike glomerular filtration, is not limited by binding to plasma proteins. This is because tubular transport is so efficient that dissociation of drug from the drug–protein complex is sufficiently rapid not to restrict the secretory process. Competition for the carriers involved in tubular secretion can occur which will reduce renal excretion. Probenecid (anion) will competitively inhibit the secretion of benzylpenicillin and other penicillins, and reduce their urinary excretion rate. In the past, probenecid was co-administered with benzylpenicillin to increase its duration of action.

Reabsorption

Most drugs are subject to some degree of reabsorption: a passive process that occurs along the length of the nephron. GFR is about 130 mL min^{-1}, whilst normal urine flow is about 1–2 mL min^{-1}, demonstrating that most of the water in the filtrate is reabsorbed. This leads to concentration of drugs in the filtrate and to a large concentration gradient between drug in the tubular fluid and drug in plasma. Consequently, if a drug is lipid-soluble it will diffuse from the tubular fluid back into plasma.

Tubular reabsorption of weak acids and bases is dependent on their pK_a and urinary pH, which may vary between 4.5 and 8.0. Acidification of urine will promote the reabsorption of weak acids (greater fraction unionized) and decrease their excretion rate. By contrast, acidification will reduce the reabsorption of weak bases (greater fraction ionized) and facilitate their renal excretion. The opposite effect will result if the urine is made alkaline: enhanced excretion of weak acids (greater fraction ionized) and enhanced reabsorption of weak bases (greater fraction unionized).

The pH of urine can be manipulated to facilitate the excretion of weak acids/bases in patients who have taken drug overdoses. Infusion of sodium bicarbonate will produce an alkaline diuresis to promote the excretion of weak acids (barbiturates and aspirin). In contrast, acidification of urine by administering ascorbic acid will enhance the excretion of a weak base such as amfetamine (amphetamine). However, this is seldom used clinically since it may exacerbate the renal complications associated with amfetamine overdose.

Drug excretion in the presence of renal impairment

When glomerular filtration is impaired as a result of renal disease or age (i.e. in the elderly), this will have potentially serious implications for the excretion of any drug that is eliminated predominantly by the renal route. GFR is commonly measured by the clearance of creatinine (see below for an explanation of clearance). Creatinine is a breakdown product derived from the amino acids of muscle, and, in a healthy adult, the clearance of creatinine is approximately $140 \, \text{mL min}^{-1}$. In a patient suffering from renal impairment this figure will be reduced, and an allowance for this is necessary when calculating the dosage of any drug that depends mainly upon renal excretion for its removal from the body. The simplest way to calculate the appropriate amended dosage is by means of available nomograms.

Biliary excretion

Liver cells may excrete drug and their metabolites (particularly conjugates) into the bile, which is stored in the gall bladder before its release into the small intestine. Biliary excretion is an active process and occurs via transport systems for organic anions (e.g. cromoglycate), cations (e.g. erythromycin), and neutral substances (e.g. digitoxin). The most important factor influencing biliary excretion by these systems is molecular mass—when this exceeds 300 Da, biliary excretion becomes significant (>10% of the dose is excreted by this route); and above 400 Da, biliary excretion can be pronounced. Drug conjugation (phase II metabolism), particularly with glucuronic acid and glutathione, is important in biliary excretion for two reasons. First, it increases molecular mass (glucuronide by 176 Da and glutathione by 306 Da) and second, it makes non-polar compounds much more polar (lipid insoluble) which restricts diffusion from bile canaliculi back into blood.

Following biliary excretion into the small intestine, drug conjugates are not reabsorbed because they are usually too polar and faecal excretion occurs. However, a proportion of some conjugates, particularly glucuronides, may be deconjugated by the enzyme β-glucuronidase (present in the gut) to release the parent drug which is then reabsorbed. This process is called enterohepatic recycling (Fig. 1.9) and it can be repeated many times until other metabolic routes, urinary excretion, and faecal loss eliminate the drug from the body. Such recycling may also occur for any parent drug that undergoes biliary excretion, the overall effect being that the drug persists in the body. One example of a drug that undergoes enterohepatic cycling is indometacin (indomethacin), a non-steroidal, anti-inflammatory agent.

Key facts
Renal excretion of drugs

- The kidneys play a central role in the excretion of most drugs and their metabolites.

- Drug that is not bound to plasma proteins is freely filtered at the glomerulus.

- Drugs can be actively secreted into the proximal tubule by transport mechanisms for acids and bases.

- Lipid-soluble drugs are reabsorbed across the tubule membrane, which reduces their renal excretion.

- Weak acids are more readily excreted in alkaline urine where a greater proportion of drug is in the unionized lipid-insoluble form and *vice versa* for weak bases.

- Toxicity, due to the accumulation of a drug, may occur in patients with renal disease for those drugs primarily eliminated by the kidneys.

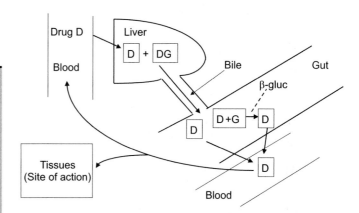

Fig. 1.9 An example of the enterohepatic cycling of a drug. Drug (D) is taken up into the liver where some is conjugated with glucuronide. Drug and its glucuronide metabolite (DG) are excreted into bile and enter the gut. Here the glucuronide metabolite is hydrolysed by the enzyme β-glucuronidase (β-gluc) which generates the parent drug. The drug can be reabsorbed back into plasma to be distributed to its site of action and to the liver where the cycle starts again.

Indometacin and its conjugates are excreted in bile; the conjugates are deconjugated in the gut and the liberated drug, together with drug already present, are reabsorbed.

Other routes of drug excretion

Excretion of drugs may also occur in sweat, tears, and saliva, although these routes are quantitatively unimportant. Drugs may also be excreted in breast milk and, whilst the amounts are small, they may produce unwanted effects in the nursing infant. Pulmonary excretion is important for the elimination of anaesthetic gases and vapours and is dealt with in Chapter 9. Occasionally small quantities of drugs and/or their metabolites are excreted via this route e.g. ethanol.

Pharmacokinetics

This is the study of the absorption, distribution, metabolism, and excretion of a drug on a quantitative basis. In practice, this consists of measuring the concentration of a drug in body fluids, such as plasma and urine, and using this data to analyse the kinetic behaviour of the drug, which affects the intensity and duration of drug action. The information gained from pharmacokinetic studies is used to design dosage regimens and the way in which the drug is formulated. Pharmacokinetics can also be used to aid the safe and effective management of individual patients, for example, the treatment of transplant patients with the immunosuppressant drug cyclosporin.

The pharmacokinetic parameters for various drugs are shown in Table 1.1.

Intravenous administration

Most drugs, when given as a bolus IV injection, distribute so rapidly that within a few minutes of administration only the rate of elimination determines the amount of drug in the body. Usually elimination follows simple first-order kinetics, that is the rate of elimination (dA/dt, rate of change of amount of drug in the body) is proportional to the amount of drug in the body at a given time (A). When this occurs, the amount of drug in the body falls exponentially. It follows that:

$$-dA/dt \propto A,$$

and:

$$-dA/dt = kA; \tag{1.1}$$

where k is the first-order rate constant for elimination which has units of reciprocal time, i.e. h^{-1} or min^{-1}. The negative sign in eqn 1.1 indicates that drug is lost from the body. The elimination rate constant, denoted as k_{el}, is the sum of all the individual processes that contribute to elimination, i.e. metabolism, renal excretion, and biliary excretion.

The amount of drug in the body (A) is related to plasma concentration (C) by the apparent volume of distribution (V_d) such that $A = V_d \times C$. Substituting $V_d \times C$ (V_dC) for A in eqn 1.1 gives:

Table 1.1 Pharmacokinetic parameters for selected drugs

Drug	Oral bioavailability (%)	Bound to plasma proteins (%)	*Apparent volume of distribution, V_d (L)	Clearance ($mL\,min^{-1}\,kg^{-1}$)	Half-life, $t_{0.5}$ (h)
Amitriptyline	48	95	1050	12.00	21.00
Ampicillin	62	18	20	1.9	1.3
Aspirin	68	49	11	9.0	0.25
Captopril	65	30	57	12.00	2.2
Carbamazepine	70	74	98	1.3	15.00
Cimetidine	62	19	70	8.3	2.0
Diazepam	100	99	77	0.38	43.00
Digoxin	70	25	440	1.2	39.00
Erythromycin	35	84	55	9.1	1.6
Indometacin	98	90	20	1.4	2.4
Lidocaine	35	70	77	9.2	1.8
Pethidine	52	58	308	17.00	3.2
Metronidazole	99	11	52	1.3	8.5
Midazolam	44	95	77	6.6	1.9
Morphine	24	35	231	24.00	1.9
Phenytoin	90	89	45	CD**	CD**
Propranolol	26	87	301	16.00	3.9
Tetracycline	77	65	105	1.7	11.00
Warfarin	93	99	10	0.05	37.00

* Estimated for a 70 kg male.

** CD = concentration-dependent since phenytoin exhibits saturation kinetics.

$$-\mathrm{d}(V_{\mathrm{d}}C)\big/\mathrm{d}t = k(V_{\mathrm{d}}C),$$

or:

$$-\mathrm{d}C\big/\mathrm{d}t = kC. \tag{1.2}$$

Equation 1.2 describes the rate of change of drug concentration in blood or plasma with time. Integration of this equation yields:

$$\log C = \log C_0 - kt\big/2.303;$$

where C_0 is the concentration of drug immediately after injection and t is the time after injection. This equation indicates that a plot of $\log C$ versus t should be linear since it has the form of an equation for a straight line ($y = mx + c$) and this is shown in Fig. 1.10(a). By contrast, a curve results when C is plotted on a linear scale against t (Fig. 1.10(b)). The slope of the log plot is equal to $k_{\mathrm{el}}/2.303$, and the intercept at $t = 0$ gives C_0 which, as discussed earlier, can be used to calculate the apparent volume of distribution ($V_{\mathrm{d}} = dose/C_0$).

Half-life

From the value of k_{el} alone, it is not easy to comprehend how fast or slow elimination is for a particular drug. To solve this problem the rate of elimination is often described by the half-life ($t_{0.5}$) of the drug. This is the time required to reduce the drug concentration by 50% of its former value. This can be estimated directly from the plot of C vs t (see Fig. 1.10), but it can also be calculated from k_{el} since:

$$t_{0.5} = 0.693\big/k_{\mathrm{el}}.$$

Examples of the half-lives for a number of drug are shown in Table 1.1 which illustrates the variability in the rate of elimination of drugs.

Clearance

The concept of clearance can be applied to describe the elimination of a drug from plasma. Plasma clearance (Cl_{p}) can be visualized as the volume of plasma cleared per unit time and is related to the rate of elimination ($\mathrm{d}A/\mathrm{d}t$) and plasma concentration (C) by:

$$Cl_{\mathrm{p}} = (\mathrm{d}A\big/\mathrm{d}t)\big/C;$$

from eqn 1.1, $\mathrm{d}A/\mathrm{d}t = kA$ and $C = A/V_{\mathrm{d}}$, hence:

$$Cl_{\mathrm{p}} = kA\big/(A\big/V_{\mathrm{d}}),$$

and:

$$Cl_{\mathrm{p}} = k \times V_{\mathrm{d}}.$$

Therefore, Cl_{p} which has units of flow (mL min^{-1}, etc.), can be calculated from the product of k (k_{el}, i.e. the elimination rate constant) and V_{d} the apparent volume of distribution. Cl_{p}, like k, is the sum of the processes that contribute to the clearance of drug from plasma. It follows that $Cl_{\mathrm{p}} = Cl_{\mathrm{metab}} + Cl_{\mathrm{renal}} + Cl_{\mathrm{biliary}} + Cl_{\mathrm{other}}$. The clearance values for a number of drugs are shown in Table 1.1.

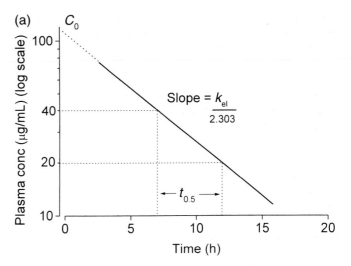

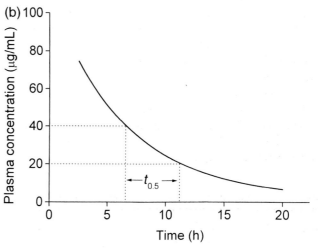

Fig. 1.10 (a) Log plasma concentration–time plot for a drug given intravenously whose elimination is a first-order process. The elimination rate constant (k_{el}) can be calculated from the slope as indicated, and the half-life of the drug ($t_{0.5}$) can be estimated from the plot or from k_{el} ($t_{0.5} = 0.693/k_{\mathrm{el}}$). Extrapolation of the line to time zero gives an estimate of the initial drug concentration (C_0) assuming distribution was instantaneous. (b) A plot of the data in (a) but with plasma concentration on a linear scale. The curve indicates that disappearance from plasma is an exponential process, with a constant fraction of drug eliminated in unit time.

Curvilinear log plasma concentration–time plots

For many drugs, a log plasma concentration–time plot produces not a straight line but a curvilinear relationship (Fig. 1.11), which indicates that the decline in plasma concentration is described by two exponential processes. The early phase is known as the distribution phase, when distribution of drug into tissues primarily determines the initial rapid decline in plasma concentration. The later phase (terminal phase) is referred to as the elimination phase,

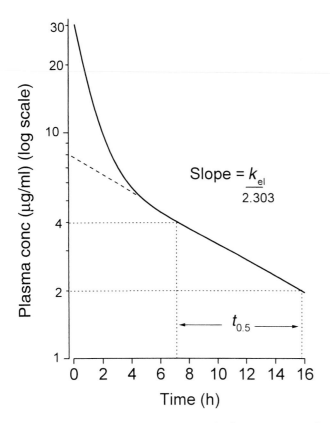

Fig. 1.11 Log plasma concentration–time plot for an intravenously administered drug with a significant distribution phase as indicated by a curve with two exponential phases. The slope of the slow terminal phase provides a way of estimating the elimination rate constant. The plasma half-life can be estimated directly from the plot or from k_{el} ($t_{0.5} = 0.693/k_{el}$).

since at these times the decline in plasma concentration reflects the elimination of drug from the body. The slope of the terminal phase allows an estimate of the elimination rate constant, k_{el}, from which can be calculated a terminal half-life as described above, or it can be estimated directly from the graph. Cl_p can be calculated from this form of log plasma concentration–time curve plot by measuring the area under the curve (AUC). Such that:

$$Cl_p = dose/AUC.$$

The apparent volume of distribution cannot be simply estimated from C_0. However V_d can be estimated from Cl_p from the equation:

$$V_d = Cl_p/k_{el}.$$

Oral administration

The plasma concentration–time profiles seen after oral administration, or parenteral routes other than intravenous, are biphasic: an initial absorptive phase is followed by a postabsorptive phase (Fig. 1.12). If the distribution phase is rapid, the postabsorptive

phase is linear and can be used to estimate k_{el} and $t_{0.5}$. It is not possible to estimate V_d by extrapolation to C_0 because of an interaction between the rates of absorption and elimination. The rate of absorption is indicated by the peak plasma concentration and the time to reach this peak. The peak concentration increases and the time to achieve this decreases as the rate of absorption increases.

Repeated dosing

Most drugs are given as repeated doses rather than a single dose. For drugs with first-order kinetics the total amount of drug in the body increases until the amount eliminated is equal to the dose administered. At this point, the amount of drug in body, and therefore the plasma concentration, has reached a steady state or plateau which remains constant as long as the dosing regimen is maintained. The time taken to reach steady-state concentration (C_{ss}) depends only on the terminal half-life which, from a practical point of view, occurs within 3–5 half-lives (Fig. 1.13). The more frequently the dose is given, the higher will be the steady-state concentration and the less will be the variation between peak and trough concentrations.

In some situations, it may be desirable to rapidly achieve a therapeutic steady-state concentration; for example the administration of digoxin to a patient with atrial fibrillation. In order to reduce the time to steady-state concentration, it is possible to give a loading dose, i.e. an initial dose greater than the maintenance dose. Such a loading dose can be calculated from the following formula:

$$loading\ dose = V_d \times C_{ss}.$$

Whilst subsequent maintenance doses can be determined from:

$$maintenance\ dose = Cl_p \times C_{ss} \times t;$$

where t is the interval between doses.

Saturation kinetics (zero-order kinetics)

For a limited number of drugs that are eliminated by metabolism, the decline in plasma concentration occurs at a constant rate and is independent of the amount of drug in the body. Such drugs are described as exhibiting saturation or zero-order kinetics, which differs from the majority of drugs which show first-order kinetics where the rate of elimination is proportional to the amount of drug in the body at a given time, as discussed above. One example of a drug that exhibits saturation kinetics is ethanol, which is metabolized to ethanal (acetaldehyde) by the enzyme alcohol dehydrogenase. Fig. 1.14 shows that the rate of decline in plasma concentration of ethanol is constant (about $10\,g\,h^{-1}$ for a $70\,kg$ male) irrespective of its plasma concentration as shown by the parallel elimination phases. This occurs because the rate of oxidation of ethanol reaches a maximum at low ethanol concentrations.

One consequence of saturation kinetics is that on repeated dosing the concentration of a drug does not attain a predictable steady-state concentration. A steady-state concentration will be achieved eventually since, at high plasma concentrations, non-

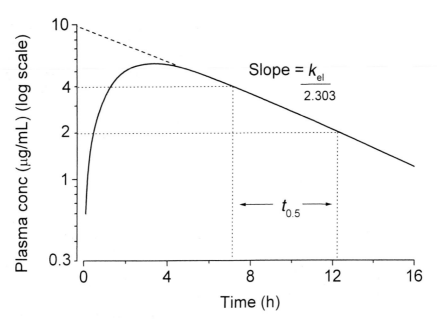

Fig. 1.12 Log plasma concentration–time plot for an orally administered drug which shows an absorptive phase. If distribution is rapid, k_{el} can be estimated from the slope of the postabsorptive linear phase.

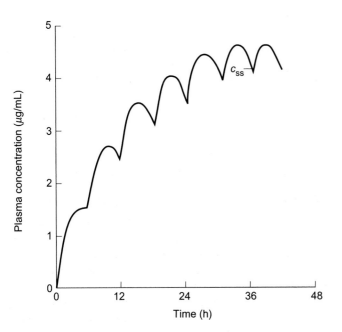

Fig. 1.13 Linear plasma concentration–time plot for a drug given orally at a dose of 50 mg every 6 hours. The half-life of the drug is 12 hours. Note the steady-state concentration (C_{ss}) is achieved after 3 half-lives, i.e. 36 hours.

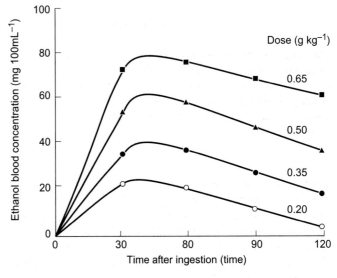

Fig. 1.14 Saturation kinetics of alcohol elimination in man (from Drew *et al.* 1958). Note the linear rather than exponential fall in blood ethanol concentrations and that the rate of elimination does not alter with dose. Compare the linear decline in concentration with the curve shown in Fig. 1.10(b) which shows the disappearance from plasma of a drug with first-order elimination kinetics.

saturating metabolic pathways or renal excretion will contribute to the drug's elimination. However, the steady-state plasma concentration of drugs with saturation kinetics is much less predictable and varies widely with dose compared to drugs which show first-order kinetics. One drug with saturation kinetics is the antiepileptic drug phenytoin which shows large increases in plasma concentrations for small increases in dose. For example, a fourfold increase in steady-state plasma concentration has been noted in one patient following a 50% increase in dose. As a result of its saturation kinetics, it is necessary to monitor the plasma concentrations of phenytoin. A radioimmunoassay for phenytoin in plasma is available and is used to adjust the dose in an individual patient to ensure that plasma concentrations lie within the therapeutic range, i.e. above the minimum effective concentration but below the toxic concentration.

Key facts
Pharmacokinetics

- Most drug are eliminated from the body as a constant fraction of their plasma concentration, a first-order process. Their disappearance from plasma follows an exponential time course which is characterized by a plasma half-life.

- For drugs that show first-order kinetics, clearance (volume of plasma cleared of drug per unit time) is constant irrespective of dose, and this can be calculated from the dose divided by the area under the plasma concentration–time plot.

- On repeated dosing, the time to achieve steady-state concentration depends only on the rate of elimination.

- Time to steady-state concentration is 3–5 plasma half-lives.

- Some drugs exhibit saturation kinetics (zero-order kinetics), such that their disappearance from plasma occurs at a constant rate. These drugs show disproportionate increases in steady-state concentrations and prolonged effects following increases in dose.

Reference

Drew, G. C., Colquhoun, W. P. and Long, H. A. (1958). Effect of small doses of alchohol on a skill resembling driving. *British Medical Journal*, **ii**, 993–9.

Further reading

Benet, L. Z., Kroetz, D. L., and Sheiner, L. B. (1996). Pharmacokinetics. In *Goodman and Gilman's the pharmacological basis of therapeutics* (9th edn) (ed. J. G. Hardman, L. E. Limbird, P. B. Molinoff, R. W. Ruddon, and A. G. Gilman), pp. 3–27. McGraw Hill, New York.

Lindup, W. E. and Orme, M. C. L'E (1981). Plasma protein binding of drugs. *British Medical Journal*, **282**, 212–14.

Rang, H. P., Dale, M. M., and Ritter, J. M. (1995). Absorption, distribution and fate of drugs. In *Pharmacology* (3rd edn), pp. 66–97. Churchill Livingstone, Edinburgh.

Sitar, D. S. (1989). Human drug metabolism in vivo. *Pharmacology and Therapeutics*, **43**, 363–75.

Voet, D. and Voet, J. G. (1995). Lipids and membranes. In *Biochemistry* (2nd edn), pp. 277–329. Wiley, London.

2

Mechanisms of drug action: pharmacodynamics

Mechanisms of drug action: pharmacodynamics

Introduction

For a drug to be useful therapeutically it must act selectively on particular cells or tissues. The majority of drugs possess this selective action by binding to target proteins, which can be divided into:

- receptors (Fig. 2.1(a));
- ion channels (Fig. 2.1(b));
- enzymes (Fig. 2.1(c));
- carrier molecules (Fig. 2.1(d)).

The converse also applies in that target proteins show ligand specificity (a ligand is a molecule which binds to a target protein) in that they will only recognize and bind to ligands of a precise structure. It should be stressed, however, that no drug acts with absolute specificity and that binding to proteins other than its principal target can account for some of a drug's additional properties and adverse effects. For example, the tricyclic antidepressant drug amitriptyline binds to the carrier molecule that transports amines into nerve terminals, an action which underlies its antidepressant action. However, amitriptyline also binds to receptors for acetylcholine, which results in the adverse effects of dry mouth, blurred vision, and constipation.

Receptors

The term receptor is sometimes used to identify any molecular target with which a drug binds to produce an effect. On this basis, an enzyme could be a receptor, such that the enzyme cyclo-oxygenase would be described as the receptor for aspirin. A more restrictive term for a drug receptor is a protein which has no other function than to recognize and bind a hormone, neurotransmitter, or drug. For example, acetylcholine released from the nerve terminals of the vagus nerve in the heart stimulates muscarinic receptors to produce a fall in heart rate. Drugs may bind to this receptor to mimic the effects of acetylcholine or block the action of released acetylcholine. The more restrictive definition for a receptor will be used throughout this book. Other important definitions in relation to drugs and receptors are described below.

Agonists

An *agonist* is a drug (hormone, or neurotransmitter) that combines with its specific receptor, activates it, and initiates a sequence of events which leads to a cellular response. In the majority of cells the maximum response is produced by the stimulation of only a small proportion of the cell's receptors, i.e. there are numbers of receptors in excess of that required to produce a maximum response. The excess receptors are termed spare receptors. The coupling between binding to the receptor and the ensuing response are the result of various signal transduction mechanisms (receptor–effector pathways) used to distinguish four receptor families or superfamilies (Fig. 2.2):

(1) ligand-gated ion channels (receptor-operated channels);

(2) G-protein-coupled receptors;

(3) enzyme-linked receptors;

(4) DNA-linked receptors.

Partial agonists

A *partial agonist* can be simply described as an inefficient agonist since it produces a maximal response which is less than the maximum response produced by a full agonist. Whilst a full agonist can produce a maximum response when a small proportion of receptors are occupied, a partial agonist only produces a submaximal response (relative to a full agonist) when 100% of receptors are occupied, as discussed more fully later.

Antagonists

An *antagonist* is a drug which binds to a receptor but does not initiate a response. The effects produced by an antagonist are a result of preventing the binding of an agonist to its receptor. An example of such a drug is the muscarinic receptor antagonist atropine.

Receptor classification

Receptors have been classified according to: (a) the principal endogenous agonist that activates them (for example, adrenocep-

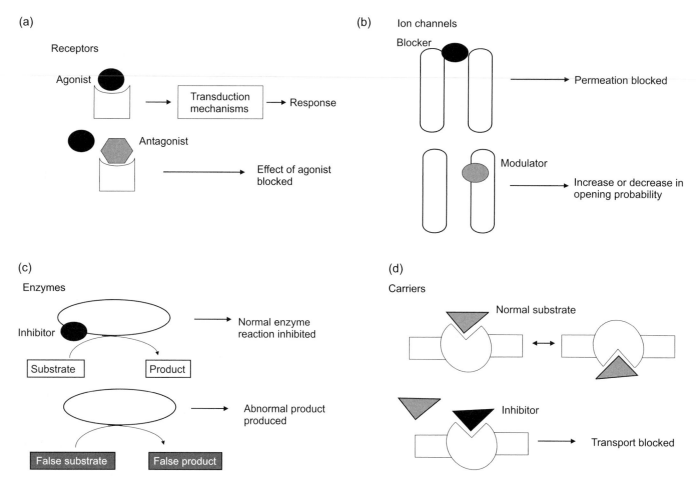

Fig. 2.1 Protein targets for drug action. (a) Receptors: drugs may act as agonists that initiate cellular responses or antagonists that block the effect of agonists. (b) Ion channels: drugs may block the passage of ions through channels or modulate the opening of channels. (c) Enzymes: drugs may inhibit enzymes or act as false substrates to produce false products. (d) Carriers: drug may bind to carriers to inhibit the transport of the normal substrate.

tors stimulated by epinephrine (adrenaline) and cholino-ceptors stimulated by acetylcholine); or (b) the first exo-genous agonist found to activate them (for example, opioid receptors and benzodiazepine receptors) whether or not an endogenous agonist is subsequently discovered. Further classification of a particular type of receptor has been based on the rank order of potency of a series of agonists and the ability of antagonists to bind more avidly to one subtype of a receptor than another. One example of such a subclassifi-cation of a receptor is that for the histamine receptor: the histamine H_1 receptor mediates the inflammatory effects of histamine, whilst stimulation of histamine H_2 receptors produces increased gastric acid secretion. The subclassification of histamine receptors led to the development of selective H_2 receptor antagonists for the treatment of peptic ulcers. In addition to classifying receptors based on the pharmacological

Fig. 2.2 Schematic representation of the structure of the four receptor superfamilies. The rectangular sections represent the hydrophobic α-helical membrane-spanning domains of the recep-tor. N and C indicate the free amino group (N-terminus) and free carboxyl group (the C-terminus) of the protein. The binding domain indicates the site at which agonists bind. (a) Ligand-gated ion channels: these receptors consist of 4–5 subunits of the type shown which surround a central ion channel. (b) G-protein-coupled receptor. (c) Enzyme-linked receptor; either tyrosine kinase or guanylyl cyclase. (d) Intracellular DNA-linked receptor. Agonists, such as steroid or thyroid hormones, pass through the cell mem-brane and bind to the receptor. The agonist–receptor complex translocates to the nucleus and binds to DNA to promote or inhibit gene transcription. (Adapted from Pharmacology, 3rd edn, Rang, Dale and Ritter, p 29, 1995, with permission of the publisher Churchill Livingstone, Edinburgh.)

(a) Ligand-goted ion channel

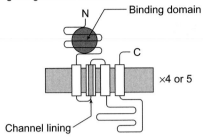

(b) G-protein-coupled receptor

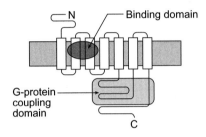

(c) Enzyme-linked receptor

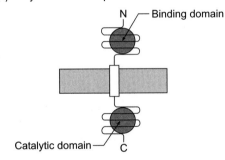

(c) Intracellular DNA-linked receptor

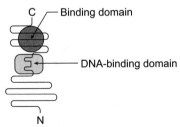

Key facts
Drug action

- Drugs produce their effects by selectively binding to target proteins which are:
  - receptors;
  - ion channels;
  - enzymes;
  - carriers (transporters).

- Drugs which bind to receptors can act as agonist or antagonists.

- Agonist binding produces a cellular response via transduction mechanisms.

- Antagonists bind to receptors but not do initiate a cellular response. The effects produced by antagonists are a result of blocking the effects of agonists, either endogenous (neurotransmitters and hormones) or exogenous (drugs), by preventing their access to the receptors.

Ligand-gated ion channels

These are receptors directly linked to ion channels, in that the receptor is an intrinsic part of the ion-channel structure (Fig. 2.2). The nicotinic acetylcholine receptor is a typical example. The structure of the receptor and the requirement for the binding of two molecules of acetylcholine in order to open the channel is illustrated in Fig. 2.3. Each of the five separate subunits—2α, β, γ, and δ, consist of four transmembrane domains (i.e. 20 transmembrane segments in all) which surround a central aqueous core. Other receptors of this type include the gamma-aminobutyric acid ($GABA_A$) and the 5-hydroxytryptamine ($5\text{-}HT_3$) receptors. Receptors of this type mediate fast synaptic transmission in the nervous system, with ligand binding and channel opening occurring within milliseconds.

G-protein-coupled receptors

This type of receptor is coupled to its effector mechanism by G-proteins, so termed because of their interaction with the guanine nucleotides GTP and GDP. All these types of receptors possess seven transmembrane α-helices with a long, third cytoplasmic loop which couples to the G-protein (Fig. 2.2). The ligand-binding domain is buried within the membrane on one or more of the α-helices, in contrast to ligand-gated ion channels where ligands bind to the extracellular N-terminal region. The response produced by the activation of G-protein-coupled receptors occurs within seconds compared to milliseconds with ligand-gated ion channels. Examples of G-protein-coupled receptors include muscarinic acetylcholine receptors and α- and β-adrenoceptors (see Chapter 14).

In the resting state, the G-protein—which consists of three

criteria described above, the molecular cloning of receptors—with the subsequent identification of their amino-acid sequence—has added a new dimension and complexity to receptor classification.

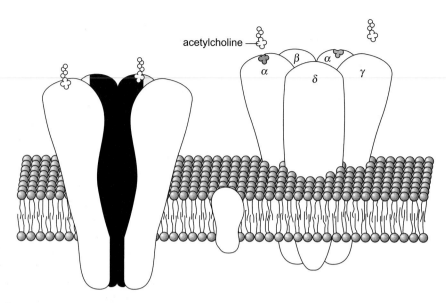

Fig. 2.3 Model of nicotinic receptor, which consists of 2α subunits and one each of β, γ, and δ subunits surrounding a central pore. Acetycholine binds to the α-subunits, and two molecules of acetylcholine must bind in order to open the channel as illustrated in the left channel.

subunits, α, β, and γ—is associated with the receptor where GDP is bound to the α-subunit. The sequence of events following binding of agonist and activation of the effector system is shown in Figs 2.4(a–c). Since a single, agonist receptor complex can activate a number of G-proteins consecutively there is in-built amplification to this system of receptor–effector coupling. Furthermore, association of the GTP-α subunit with an effector enzyme can result in a number of molecules of the product, which results in a further level of amplification of the initial signal arising from the binding of drug to receptor.

The effector systems to which G-proteins directly couple include adenylyl cyclase, phospholipase C, phospholipase A_2, and ion channels (Fig. 2.5). There a number of subtypes of G-protein, and these determine, at least in part, the effector system with which a particular G-protein interacts.

Adenylyl cyclase is stimulated or inhibited by G_s and G_i proteins, respectively. Stimulation of adenylyl cyclase results in the production of cAMP (cyclic 3',5'-adenosine monophosphate) which acts as a second messenger in that it activates protein kinases, in particular protein kinase A, and they in turn use ATP to phosphorylate various enzymes, transport proteins, and ion channels to regulate their function. G-protein activation of phospholipase C results in the breakdown of a class of phospholipids, the phosphatidyl-inositols to produce inositol (1,4,5)-triphosphate (IP_3) and diacylglycerol (DAG) which are further examples of second messengers. IP_3 produces the release of Ca^{2+} from intracellular stores by binding to a receptor on the membrane of the sarcoplasmic reticulum, whilst DAG activates protein kinase C of which there a number of subtypes. Protein kinase C phosphorylates a range of intracellular proteins whose functions

include contraction and relaxation of smooth muscle, alteration of neurotransmitter release, and ion transport. Activation of phospholipase A_2 results in the release of arachidonic acid. This is used in the synthesis of eicosanoids that are released from the cell to act as paracrine agents (local hormones) and which influence vascular smooth muscle and capillary permeability. In addition to the modulation of ion channels by second messengers such as cAMP, G-proteins may directly interact with an ion channel, independent of any second messenger. For example, acetylcholine via stimulation of muscarinic receptors produces hyperpolarization of cardiac cells, which results in inhibition of their electrical activity. The mechanism for this effect is the activation of potassium channels, with the subsequent movement of potassium ions out of the cells, produced by direct coupling of G-protein to the potassium channel. However, in this example of a G-protein-coupled receptor, it is the β- and γ-subunits, and not the α-subunit, that are the active form of the G-protein which interacts with the channel.

Enzyme-linked receptors

These receptors incorporate an enzyme in their intracellular domain that is either tyrosine kinase or guanylyl cyclase. The response to binding of an agonist to this type of receptor can produce a response within minutes. Guanylyl cyclase-linked receptors mediate the action of natriuretic peptides such as atrial natriuretic peptide. Tyrosine-kinase linked receptors mediate the actions of various growth factors, cytokines, and insulin, the general structure and transduction mechanism of which are outlined in Fig. 2.6. A single, transmembrane α-helix connects the outer receptor binding domain to the inner tyrosine-kinase domain.

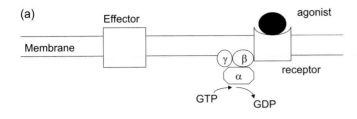

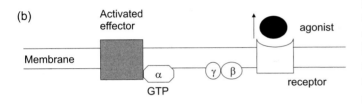

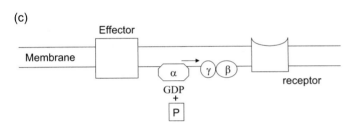

Fig. 2.4 The role of G-proteins in receptor–effector coupling. G-proteins consist of α-, β-, and γ-subunits. (a) Binding of agonist to the receptor produces a conformational change in the receptor which causes the bound GDP (guanine diphosphate) to exchange with intracellular GTP (guanine triphosphate). (b) The G-protein subunits dissociate from the receptor followed by dissociation of the α-subunit from the β-, γ-subunits. The α-subunit migrates in the membrane to bind and activate an effector protein, e.g. adenylyl cyclase. Dissociation of G-protein subunits from the receptor causes dissociation of agonist from the receptor. (c) The GTPase activity of the α-subunit increases on binding to the effector protein, which results in hydrolysis of GTP to GDP, promoting dissociation of the α-subunit which recombines with the β–γ complex. The α–β–γ complex then reassociates with the receptor. Note that when G-proteins couple directly with ion channels, it is the β–γ subunits which migrate to activate the effector.

Binding of ligand to the receptor produces receptor dimer formation, which produces autophosphorylation of the tyrosine residues in both tyrosine-kinase domains. The phosphorylated tyrosine residues then act as binding sites for intracellular proteins, which have a common conserved sequence termed the SH2 domain. Once bound, the SH2 domain proteins undergo phosphorylation and subsequent activation. The target SH2 proteins may be enzymes (including kinases), structural proteins, or regulatory proteins which affect transcription of specific genes or transport mechanisms. For example, one result of the binding of insulin to its receptor is the translocation of intracellular vesicles, contain-

ing the glucose transporter, to the plasma membrane, which facilitates the diffusion of glucose into cells.

DNA-linked receptors

These receptors regulate DNA transcription and are characteristic of steroid and thyroid hormones. The receptors for thyroid and the majority of steroid hormones reside in the nucleus, although receptors for glucocorticoids are predominantly found in the cytoplasm. The inactive glucocorticoid receptor is associated with a complex of other proteins, including heat-shock protein, which dissociate from the receptor on ligand binding (Fig. 2.7). Ligand binding also induces a conformational change in the receptor that results in the exposure of a DNA binding domain. The steroid–receptor complex migrates to the nucleus and binds to a glucocorticoid response element on DNA. One result of this interaction is the promotion of gene transcription, mRNA translation, and the subsequent synthesis of a protein such as lipocortin which has anti-inflammatory actions. In addition, glucocorticoids may have a negative effect on gene transcription, such as inhibition of the synthesis of cytokines which play key roles in immune and inflammatory responses. In contrast to other types of receptor, the response to the activation of DNA-linked receptors takes hours to develop.

Regulation of receptors and their transduction mechanisms

There is abundant evidence to show that neither the efficiency of the coupling of receptors to their effector mechanisms nor the density or the binding affinity of receptors for agonists and antagonists are fixed quantities. For example, continued stimulation of the β-adrenoceptor with a β-adrenoceptor agonist over a period of hours results in a failure to activate adenylyl cyclase, a process termed uncoupling, although the receptor retains the ability to bind the agonist molecule. This effect is a result of phosphorylation of a particular single serine residue in the β-adrenoceptor structure. Alternatively, prolonged exposure to agonists may result in a reduction of the number of receptors (down-regulation)—which can be measured directly using radioactively labelled drug molecules (ligand-binding experiments). This can also occur with β-adrenoceptors, the number of which may fall by as much as 90% over a period of 8 hours. These changes in receptor coupling or density may explain some instances when the effect of a drug diminishes when given either continuously or repeatedly. Such effects are termed tachyphylaxis (desensitization) or tolerance, and these are distinguished on the basis of the time scale—tachyphylaxis occurs within minutes or hours and tolerance occurs over a period of days or weeks—although there is considerable overlap in the use of these terms.

Receptor density as well as decreasing may also increase (up-regulation). The proliferation of receptors was first noticed following the degeneration of nerve terminals caused by cutting a nerve, with the result that the innervated tissue became

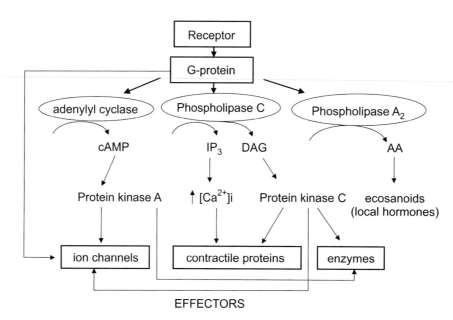

Fig. 2.5 Some of the pathways involved in the coupling of G-proteins to effector systems. cAMP (cyclic 3′,5′-adenosine monophosphate); PIP_2 (phosphatidylinositol (4,5)-biphosphate); IP_3 (inositol (1,4,5)-triphosphate); DAG (diacylglycerol); $[Ca^{2+}]i$ (intracellular calcium levels); PLs (phospholipids); AA (arachidonic acid).

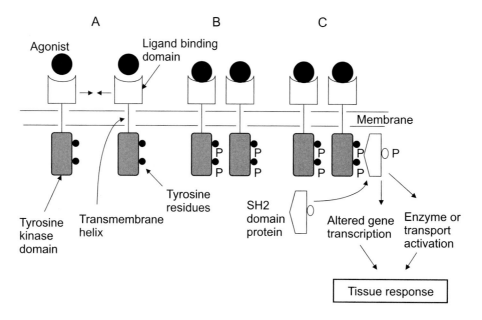

Fig. 2.6 Transduction mechanism of enzyme-linked receptors. These receptors have an extracellular ligand binding domain linked to the enzyme domain by a single transmembrane helix. (A) Binding of agonist (e.g. insulin or cytokines) produces dimerization of receptors. (B) Dimerization is followed by autophosphorylation of tyrosine residues. (C) The phosphorylated tyrosine regions of the tyrosine kinase domain then bind and phosphorylate the SH2-domain protein. Activation of the SH2-domain protein results in either enzyme activation, stimulation of transport mechanisms, or altered gene transcription.

supersensitive to the neurotransmitter previously released from the nerve terminals. Such an effect occurs with acetylcholine receptors in skeletal muscle, numbers of which can increase by up to 20-fold following denervation. Similar changes, although less pronounced than those following denervation, can occur follow-

ing treatment with a receptor antagonist. This can be of clinical importance, particularly with respect to the use of drugs which affect the central nervous system, since when the drug is removed the endogenous agonist can interact with enhanced numbers of receptors resulting in 'rebound' effects.

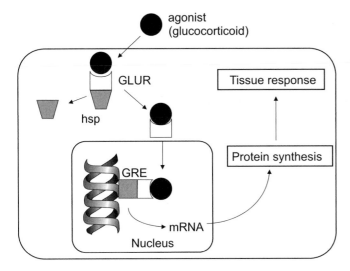

Fig. 2.7 Transduction mechanism for DNA-linked receptors. The glucocorticoid agonist crosses the cell membrane and binds to the glucocorticoid receptor (GLUR) which is associated with heat-shock protein (hsp). On binding of glucocorticoid to the receptor, the heat-shock protein dissociates and the glucocorticoid–receptor complex, with the receptor DNA-binding domain exposed, migrates to the nucleus and binds to the glucocorticoid response elements (GRE) on the target genes. This leads to gene transcription and protein synthesis, e.g. the anti-inflammatory lipocortins.

Key facts
Receptors

- There are four main groups of receptor distinguished by their transduction mechanisms.

- Ligand-gated ion channels consist of a receptor that is an intrinsic part of the ion-channel structure, e.g. nicotinic receptors. Binding of agonists produces channel opening, which occurs within milliseconds.

- G-protein-coupled receptors, e.g. β-adrenoceptors, are linked to effector systems such as enzymes and ion channels by a guanine nucleotide binding protein (G-protein), which consists of α-, β-, and γ-subunits. The response to the stimulation of this type of receptor occurs within seconds.

- Enzyme-linked receptors have an intracellular enzyme domain linked to an extracellular ligand recognition site by a single transmembrane helix. Binding of an agonist, e.g. insulin to a tyrosine-kinase linked receptor produces autophosphorylation of tyrosine residues. These residues catalyse the phosphorylation of signalling proteins, producing a tissue response which can occur within minutes.

- DNA-linked receptors are present in the nucleus or cytosol and bind agonists (thyroid and steroid hormones) following their passage across the cell membrane. The agonist–receptor complex binds to DNA and influences protein synthesis, the tissue response to which can take hours to develop.

Drug targets other than receptors
Ion channels

In addition to drugs directly affecting ion-channel function by binding to a specific receptor associated with an ion channel (ligand-gated ion channels) or indirectly via a G-protein (G-protein-coupled receptors), some drugs affect ion-channel function by binding directly to part of the ion-channel protein. Drugs that affect ion-channel function in this manner do so by either affecting ion movement through the channel, i.e. an affect on permeation, or by modulating the opening of the channel, i.e. an affect on gating of the channel (Fig 2.1). The classical example of drugs that influence ion-channel permeation are the local anaesthetics (see Chapter 8), which physically block the sodium channel in nerves and cardiac muscle. Drugs that modulate the opening of channels include drugs of the dihydropyridine type, which produce vasodilation by inhibiting the opening of calcium channels in response to depolarization in vascular smooth muscle.

Enzymes

A number of drugs exert their pharmacological effect by interacting with an enzyme (Fig. 2.1). In the majority of cases, the drug is similar in structure to the normal substrate for the enzyme and acts as a competitive inhibitor. This inhibition may be reversible, as in the case of angiotensin-converting enzyme inhibitors (such as captopril) which are used in the treatment of hypertension and heart failure, or irreversibly as exemplified by the inhibition of cyclo-oxygenase by aspirin. A less common form of drug interaction with an enzyme occurs when the drug acts as a false substrate, in which the drug undergoes chemical transformation to produce an abnormal product. Such an example is the antihypertensive drug methyldopa which is converted to methylnorepinephrine (methylnoradenaline) as a result of entering the pathway for the synthesis of norepinephrine. Methylnorepinephrine produces a lowering of blood pressure by an action in the central nervous system.

Carriers

The movement of ions and small molecules across cell membranes generally involves a protein carrier (transporter), since simple diffusion is often inadequate due to the poor lipid solubility of such molecules. These carrier molecules possess specific binding sites for the transported ions or molecules, which include Na^+, K^+, Cl^-, glucose, and neurotransmitters such as norepinephrine and 5-HT.

A number of drugs produce their pharmacological effects by binding to the recognition sites on the carrier molecule, with the result that the transport process is blocked (Fig. 2.1). Some classes of diuretic drug produce an increase in urine production by binding to carriers in the renal tubules that facilitate the reabsorption of ions from the renal tubule. For example, thiazide diuretics bind to the Na^+/Cl^- co-transporter in the distal tubule. Another example is the tricyclic antidepressant drugs which, as discussed above, bind to the carrier involved in the reuptake of amine neurotransmitters into nerve terminals.

Drug targets other than proteins

Whilst the vast majority of drugs exert their effects by interacting with specific proteins, some drugs target molecules other than proteins. One such drug target is DNA which is disrupted by some antimicrobial and anticancer agents. For example, the antibacterial drug metronidazole produces degradation of bacterial DNA (see Chapter 11). General anaesthetic agents were previously regarded as producing depression of the central nervous system by interacting with constituent lipids of nerve cell membranes to produce a fluidizing or disordering effect on the membrane. However, in recent years it has become apparent that general anaesthetics also interact with protein targets, in particular ligand-gated ion channels. There are limited number of agents that do not interact with a discrete target but produce useful actions as result of their physicochemical properties. Examples include mannitol, which produces a diuretic action by increasing the osmotic pressure of fluid in the renal tubules, and agents active in the gastrointestinal tract such as antacids and bulk laxatives.

Key facts
Drug targets other than receptors

- Drugs can bind to ion channels to either directly block movement of ions through the channels (e.g. local anaesthetics), or to modulate their opening (e.g. dihydropyridine calcium channel-blocking drugs).

- Drugs can produce their effects by inhibiting enzymes, with the result that the normal product is not produced (e.g. aspirin), or by acting as false substrates which are then converted to an abnormal product (e.g. methyldopa).

- Carriers (membrane transporters) are also targets for drug action. Binding of drugs to carriers inhibits the transport of the normal substrate. For example, diuretic drugs inhibit the reabsorption of Na^+ across the renal tubule membrane.

- A limited number of drugs have targets other than proteins. For example, the antibacterial drug metronidazole and some drugs used in cancer chemotherapy disrupt DNA.

Agonist concentration–response curves

The responses to increasing concentrations of a drug, when plotted, produce curves such as those shown in Figs 2.8(a) and (b). Note that if quantities of the drug, i.e. doses, were given, the curve would be termed a dose–response curve. With the smallest concentration or dose no effect is seen, but, above a certain threshold, a response becomes detectable. Thereafter, the response increases as the concentration is increased until a maximum is reached. Beyond this point, any further increase in concentration is not accompanied by any increase in the size of the response. The curve shown in Fig 2.8(a) is termed a rectangular hyperbola. It is more convenient to plot the logarithm of dose or concentration against response since this transforms a rectangular hyperbola to a

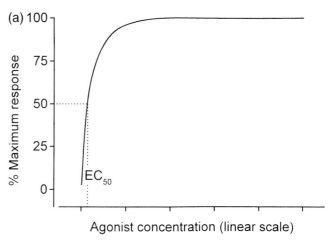

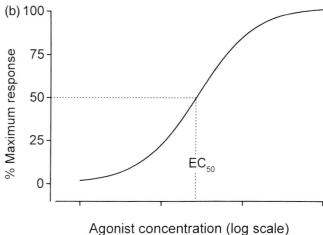

Fig. 2.8 Agonist concentration–response curves. (a) The relationship between concentration and response – when concentration is plotted on a linear scale – is described by a rectangular hyperbola, whilst (b) a sigmoid curve is produced when concentration is plotted on a log scale. EC_{50} is the concentration that produces a response which is 50% of the maximum response.

sigmoid curve, as shown in Fig 2.8(b). The sigmoid curve has the advantage that over the maximum response range of 25 to 75%, the graph is a straight line and is easier to interpret, particularly when determining the effect of a competitive antagonist on the response to an agonist (see below).

It is not necessary for the dental student or practitioner to be conversant with the detailed mathematical analysis of concentration–response curves. However, the principles of the mathematical relationships will be described since this helps to appreciate the mechanisms of action of agonist and antagonists. The interaction between a drug and receptor is as follows:

Drug + receptor k_{+1} Drug–receptor complex

$[A] + [R]$ $\overset{\longrightarrow}{k_{-1}}$ $[AR]$;

where k_{+1} and k_{-1} are the rate constants for the forward and backward reactions, respectively.

The equilibrium dissociation constant K_D for the binding of a drug to a receptor is equal to the ratio of k_{-1} to k_{+1}, i.e.:

$$K_D = k_{-1}/k_{+1}.$$

From these relationships, an equation can be derived relating the proportion of receptors occupied, PR, to the concentration of drug and the equilibrium dissociation constant:

$$PR = \frac{[A]/K_D}{[A]/K_D + 1}. \qquad (2.1)$$

The equilibrium dissociation constant, K_D, has units of concentration and is a measure of the affinity of a particular drug for its receptors since the higher the affinity, the lower will be K_D. The value of K_D is equal to the concentration of drug required to occupy 50% of its receptors at equilibrium since from eqn 2.1, when $[A] = K_D$, then $PR = 0.5$. This is indicated on curve A in Fig. 2.9, which makes the assumption that the response is directly proportional to the fraction of receptors occupied (occupancy). However, since many drugs produce a maximum response when only a small proportion of receptors are occupied and there is amplification between receptor binding and response, the actual concentration–response curve (curve B in Fig. 2.9) lies to the left of the theoretical one (curve A). The concentration that produces a 50% maximal response (EC$_{50}$), whilst not a measure of the equilibrium dissociation constant, is a measure of the agonist potency, the dependency of effect on its concentration. For example in Fig. 2.10, agonist A has a lower EC$_{50}$ than agonist B and is therefore more potent than the agonist B.

Agonists not only bind to receptors, and therefore have affinity for the receptor, but they also produce a response. The effectiveness of an agonist in producing a response is termed efficacy—or more recently, intrinsic efficacy. A full explanation and the methods used to estimate intrinsic efficacy is beyond the scope of this book, but full agonists have high values of intrinsic efficacy (e.g. 100), whilst a partial agonist has a value little more than 1. Thus, as described earlier, partial agonists have such a low efficacy that even with 100% receptor occupancy, they produce a maximum response which is less than that of a full agonist (agonist C

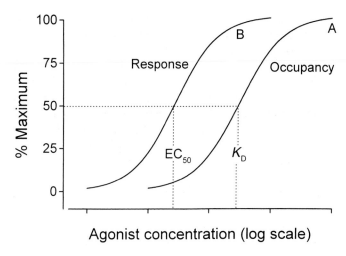

Fig. 2.9 Curve A shows the theoretical relationship between agonist concentration and response, assuming the response is directly proportional to receptor occupancy. In such a case the EC$_{50}$ would be equivalent of the value of K_D, the equilibrium dissociation constant. Curve B shows an actual relationship between agonist concentration and response, with the curve lying to the left of the theoretical one because of: (1) signal amplification between receptor occupancy and response; and (2) the lack of a direct relationship between receptor occupancy and response.

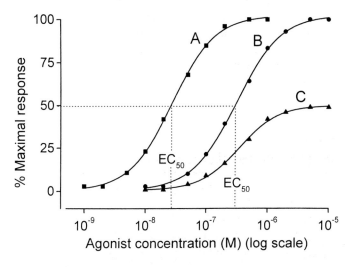

Fig. 2.10 Agonist concentration–response curves which show that agonist A is more potent than agonist B, whilst agonist C is a partial agonist since its maximum response is less than the maximum response produced by the full agonists A and B.

in Fig. 2.10). One consequence of the high receptor occupancy of partial agonists is that they can act as competitive antagonists of a full agonist. Therefore a partial agonist can block the effect of a full agonist whilst producing a low level of receptor activation. Drugs that bind to receptors and act as antagonists have affinity for the receptor but, since they do not produce a cellular response, they have zero efficacy.

Drug antagonism

Drug antagonism occurs when the effect of one drug or endogenous agonist is reduced or abolished by the presence of another drug. The mechanisms by which drug antagonism occurs are as follows:

- antagonism by receptor block;
- non-competitive antagonism;
- physiological antagonism;
- chemical antagonism;
- pharmacokinetic antagonism.

Antagonism by receptor block

This form of drug antagonism has two mechanisms:

- reversible competitive antagonism; and
- irreversible (non-equilibrium) competitive antagonism.

Reversible competitive antagonism

Many clinically useful drugs are reversible competitive antagonists, for example:

- atenolol (β_1-adrenoceptors);
- hyoscine (muscarinic receptors);
- ranitidine (H_2 histamine receptors).

The effect of reversible competitive antagonism can be overcome by increasing the concentration of agonist, i.e. the antagonism is surmountable. In this situation, the increased numbers of agonist molecules are able to occupy receptors from which the antagonist has dissociated. This hinders the reassociation of antagonist with the receptors and the overall antagonist occupancy falls. As a result, the maximal effect produced by the agonist can still be achieved if sufficient agonist is present. The log concentration–response curve for the agonist in the presence of the competitive antagonist is shifted to the right in a parallel fashion (Fig. 2.11). The extent to which the concentration–response curve is shifted to the right is termed the dose ratio (the ratio of the concentrations of agonist which produce a 50% maximal response in

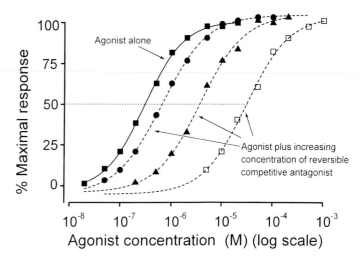

Fig. 2.11 Agonist concentration–response curves in the presence of an increasing concentration of a reversible competitive antagonist. With an increasing concentration of antagonist, the agonist concentration–response curves are shifted to the right in a parallel fashion. The extent to which the concentration–response curve is shifted to the right by each concentration of antagonist is the dose ratio (the ratio of the concentrations of agonist which produce a 50% maximal response in the absence and presence of antagonist).

the absence and presence of antagonist). The degree to which various concentrations of competitive antagonist shift the agonist concentration–response curve to the right can be used to calculate the equilibrium dissociation constant for the antagonist which is usually termed K_B. This is accomplished by plotting the log (dose ratio—1) versus the log antagonist concentration, known as a Schild plot (Fig. 2.12), which has a slope of 1 or a slope which is not statistically significant from 1. The value of K_B is given by the intercept on the x axis It is normal practice to convert the value of K_B to the negative logarithm (this has the advantage of producing simple numbers), values which are termed pK_B, e.g. a K_B of 3.2×10^{-9} M is converted a pK_B value of 8.5. An alternative term for pK_B is pA_2, however, the term pA_2 should strictly only be applied when the slope of the Schild plot is exactly unity. The value of pK_B is an estimate of the affinity of an antagonist for its receptor; the higher the value of pK_B, the greater is the affinity of the antagonist for the receptor. Furthermore, pK_B should be independent of the agonist used, provided that agonist and antagonist act at the same receptor. Estimates of pK_B are therefore widely used in receptor classification.

Irreversible (non-equilibrium) competitive antagonism

Irreversible antagonism occurs when the antagonist dissociates very slowly or not at all from the receptor as a result of the formation of covalent bonds between the drug and receptor. This form of antagonism is insurmountable since an increase in agonist concentration does not affect antagonist occupancy, which increases with incubation time. The log concentration–response curves for

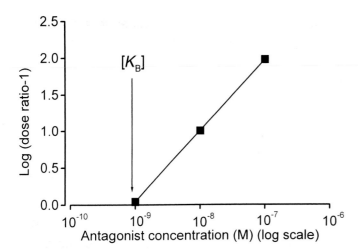

Fig. 2.12 A Schild plot of log (dose ratio–1) against antagonist concentration on a log scale. The slope of the line is unity with the equilibrium dissociation constant K_B given by the intercept on the abscissa.

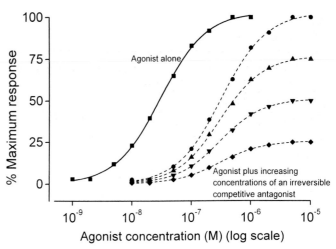

Fig. 2.13 Agonist concentration–response curves in the presence of increasing concentrations of an irreversible competitive antagonist. The antagonist produces an initial parallel shift of the curve to the right followed by curves with progressive depression of the maximum response.

an agonist in the presence of an irreversible antagonist show depression of the maximum response (Fig. 2.13). Parallel shifts of the agonist concentration–response curves with no depression of the maximum response may initially occur, as seen with a reversible competitive antagonist. This initial parallel shift occurs because of the presence of spare receptors—since, for example, if an agonist requires only 10% occupation of receptors to produce a maximum response, then more than 90% of receptors need to be irreversibly blocked before a depression of maximum response is seen. The clinical use of irreversible receptor antagonists is rare, although there are a number of drugs that act as irreversible enzyme inhibitors, for example aspirin and omeprazole irreversibly inhibit cyclo-oxygenase and H^+/K^+-ATPase, respectively. One example of an irreversible receptor antagonist is phenoxybenzamine, an α-adrenoceptor antagonist, used in the treatment of phaeochromocytoma, a tumour of chromaffin tissue, which secretes epinephrine (adrenaline) and norepinephrine (noradrenaline) causing episodes of severe hypertension.

Non-competitive antagonism

Non-competitive antagonists do not compete with an agonist for its receptor but block at some point in the transduction pathway, which produces the response to an agonist. Examples of such non-competitive antagonists are the calcium channel-blocking drugs such as nifedipine and verapamil. These drugs non-selectively block the response to agonists; they produce their effects (such as contraction of vascular smooth muscle) by activating calcium channels, thereby increasing the influx of calcium ions into cells. This type of antagonist reduces the slope and maximum of the agonist concentration–response curves in a manner similar to that produced by an irreversible competitive antagonist (see Fig. 2.13).

Physiological antagonism (functional antagonism)

Drugs can have opposing actions on a tissue by interacting with different molecular targets. In such a situation, the drugs can be described as being physiological or functional antagonists of one another. Examples of such physiological antagonism are insulin and glucagon—which respectively raise and lower blood glucose levels—and norepinephrine and acetylcholine—which respectively increase and decrease heart rate. In both pairs of examples, the physiological antagonism results from each agonist binding to a different receptor type which produce opposing effects. Physiological antagonism is of clinical importance, and can be life-saving in the treatment of bronchial asthma where bronchoconstriction produced by a range of endogenous mediators is relieved by bronchodilator drugs such as salbutamol.

Chemical antagonism

This occurs when drugs combine in solution to produce an inactive product. For example, dimercaprol forms relatively non-toxic complexes with heavy metals such as lead and mercury and so can be used to treat poisoning with these substances. Compounds such as dimercaprol, which avidly bind metal ions to produce inactive complexes, are termed chelating agents.

Pharmacokinetic antagonism

This form of antagonism occurs when one drug reduces the concentration of another drug at its site of action by interfering with its absorption, distribution, metabolism, and excretion. One example is the reduction in the anticoagulant effect of warfarin due to an increase in its rate of hepatic metabolism produced by enzyme-inducing agents such as carbamazepine and phenytoin. The principles that underlie this form of antagonism have been described in the previous chapter and are the basis of various adverse drug interactions which are important clinically and are described in more detail in Chapter 24.

Key facts
Drug antagonism

- Drug antagonism occurs when the effect of one drug or endogenous agonist is reduced or abolished by the presence of another drug.

- Antagonism can result from a competitive block at receptors, i.e. both drugs bind to the same receptor. This antagonism can be either reversible or irreversible. Many clinically useful drugs are reversible competitive antagonists, e.g. the β-adrenoceptor antagonist propranolol.

- Non-competitive antagonism occurs when one drug inhibits the effect of another by blocking its receptor–effector coupling mechanism.

- Physiological antagonism results from drugs producing opposing effects when acting by different mechanisms.

- Chemical antagonism occurs when drugs combine in solution to produce an inactive product.

- Pharmacokinetic antagonism is when one drug reduces the concentration of another drug at its site of action by interfering with its absorption, distribution, metabolism, and excretion.

Quantal responses

Responses to drugs can either be graded—for instance, the increase in heart rate to epinephrine—or all-or-nothing, as in death or sleep (hypnosis)—as determined in animals as a loss of the righting reflex when they are placed on their backs. These latter responses are termed quantal in that the response occurs or it does not. Dose-response curves can still be constructed for such responses by determining the percentage of animals, patients, or cells that respond to the drug. One example of the measurement and use of quantal responses is the determination of the therapeutic index of a drug.

Therapeutic index (ratio)

This index is an attempt to provide an estimate of the safety margin of a drug by determining (in animals) the doses that, on the one hand, produce the desired effect and on the other hand a toxic effect, i.e. death. The definition is:

$$\text{Therapeutic index} = LD_{50}/ED_{50};$$

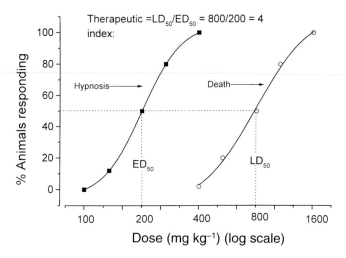

Fig. 2.14 Quantal dose-response curves which show the cumulative percentage of animals exhibiting the therapeutic effect (hypnosis) and the cumulative percentage of animals dead at various doses of a hypothetical hypnotic drug. The ED_{50} (effective dose in 50% of animals) and LD_{50} (lethal dose in 50% of animals) can be derived from the these curves in order to obtain the therapeutic index.

where LD_{50} is the dose that is lethal in 50% of animals and ED_{50} is the dose that has the desired effect in 50% of animals.

The data obtained to determine the therapeutic index of a hypothetical hypnotic drug are shown in Fig. 2.14. This index of the safety margin of a drug has obvious limitations, not least of which is that a lethal dose in animals is hardly a good indication of toxicity in man. Moreover, some drugs produce more that one therapeutic effect, e.g. codeine has antitussive and analgesic actions, and therefore the determination of a therapeutic ratio would depend upon selecting the particular therapeutic effect. A therapeutic index is not able to take into account the contraindications for a drug. One example is the non-selective β-adrenoceptor blocking drugs such as propranolol, which may produce bronchospasm in asthmatic patients although have no detrimental effects on respiratory function in normal patients. A therapeutic index can not account for adverse reactions that occur in only a small proportion of patients, such as the prolonged effect of suxamethonium in patients with an abnormal form of pseudo-cholinesterase (see Chapter 1). These limitations mean that the therapeutic index for a drug has little relevance to its clinical use, although it has some relevance to its potential dangers when taken in overdose. Whilst the general concept of a safety margin between the doses of a drug which produce toxic and therapeutic effects is useful, it can be seen from the above discussion that attempting to put a number to such a safety margin is fraught with difficulties.

Reference

Rang, Dale, and Ritter (1995). In *Pharmacology* (3rd edn), p 29. Churchill Livingstone. Edinburgh.

Further reading

Evans, R. M. (1988). The steroid and thyroid hormone receptor superfamily. *Science*, 240, 889–95.

Kenakin, T. (1984). The classification of drugs and drug–receptor antagonism. *Pharmacological Reviews*, 36, 165–222.

Kenakin, T. (1987). *Pharmacological analysis of drug–receptor interactions*. Raven Press, New York.

Milligan, G. (1993). Mechanisms of multifunctional signalling by G-protein-coupled receptors. *Trends in Pharmacological Sciences*, 14, 239–44.

Page, C. P., Curtis, M. J., Sutter, M. C., Walker, M. J. A., and Hoffman, B. B. (1997). General principles of drug action. In *Integrated pharmacology* (ed. C. P. Page, M. J. Curtis, M. C. Sutter, M. J. A. Walker, and B. B. Hoffman), pp 17–51. Mosby, London.

3

Prescribing and the law

- The Medicines Act, 1968
- Some factors influencing prescribing
- Standard reference books and data sheets
- The Misuse of Drugs Act, 1971
- Selected list regulations (NHS Act, 1977)
- Further reading

Prescribing and the law

Dental surgeons do not prescribe a wide variety of drugs, but they must have knowledge about the regulations that govern prescribing. At one time pharmacists made up elaborate prescriptions to the order of the doctor; today most drugs are conveniently prepared as tablets, capsules, and so on. Drugs have chemical names, official (approved) names, and proprietary names—the brand names provided by a manufacturer. Wherever possible it is sensible to use the official name rather than the proprietary name. If the proprietary name is used, then the pharmacist must supply that particular brand (with the exception of those drugs, for example, benzodiazepines, where generic prescribing is mandatory under the selected list regulations). If the official name is used, then the pharmacist is able to dispense whichever brand is available, for there may be many proprietary names and it would be impossible for any pharmacist to stock them all. The official name is spelt with a lower-case initial letter, and the proprietary name with an initial capital: for example Erythrocin, Erycen, and Erythroped are proprietary names for erythromycin preparations.

Prescribing is governed by a number of regulations made under the Medicines Act of 1968, the Misuse of Drugs Act of 1971, and the NHS Act, 1977 (selected list regulations). UK medicines regulation is also now governed by European Union Directives, which must be implemented through domestic acts and regulations.

The Medicines Act, 1968

This Act deals with the manufacture, distribution, and importation of medicines for human use or for administration to animals. It also deals with the advertising and promotion of drugs, the registration of pharmacies, homeopathic medicines, containers and packages for drugs, labelling regulations, pharmacopoeias, formularies, and much else.

The Medicines Act is an enabling Act that allows the appropriate Ministers (Health Ministers) to make orders or regulations interpreting the spirit of the Act in practical terms. The Health Ministers are advised by the Medicines Commission, which is a body appointed to advise them on matters related to medicines. The orders that are promulgated from time to time to interpret the meaning of the Act are known as Statutory Instruments (SI).

The Medicines Act is intended to ensure the safety, quality, and efficacy of prescription medicines. The products subject to the Act are those that fall within the definition of a medicinal product, together with certain other articles and substances incorporated in an animal feeding stuff for a medicinal purpose, or brought within the licensing provision by statutory orders under the Act.

A basic principle of the Act is that it only applies when substances are used as medicinal products or as ingredients of medicinal products. A medicinal product is defined as a substance or article sold or supplied for administration to human beings or animals for a medicinal purpose, or as an ingredient for use in a preparation in a pharmacy or in a hospital, or by a practitioner, or in the course of a retail herbal remedy business.

There are three classes of medicinal products:

1. *General sales list (GSL) medicines*: This is a list of substances that can be sold or supplied other than under the direction of a pharmacist, including such things as aspirin, paracetamol (in packs containing not more than 16 tablets or capsules), liquid paraffin, honeysuckle flowers, rock water, rose water, etc. Such substances do not have to be sold in a pharmacy, although there may be a limit on the quantity supplied if sold elsewhere.

2. *Prescription-only medicines (POM)*: These are medicinal products that can only be sold or supplied from pharmacies in accordance with a prescription given by an appropriate practitioner. For the purposes of the Act, a dental surgeon is regarded as an appropriate practitioner, as is a doctor and veterinary surgeon. The order that specifies such medicines includes drugs like lidocaine (lignocaine), antimicrobials, and psychotropic drugs.

3. *Pharmacy medicines (P)*: There is a host of substances which are called pharmacy medicines. These are medicinal products not listed as general sales list or prescription only medicines. They can be sold over the counter to the general public without prescription, but they have to be sold from a pharmacy and with the pharmacist present at the time of the sale.

The prescription for a prescription-only medicine

This has to follow certain rules, for example:

1. It must be written in indelible ink, or be typewritten.

2. It must contain the following particulars:
   - the address and usual signature of the practitioner giving it;
   - the date on which it was signed by the practitioner;
   - an indication of whether the practitioner is a dentist, doctor, or veterinary surgeon;
   - where the practitioner is a dentist or a doctor, the name, address, and the age (if under 12) of the person for whose treatment it is given.

3. The prescription shall not be dispensed later than 6 months after the date of signature.

The form of the prescription

Prescriptions should be written clearly in English. There are a number of abbreviations that have commonly been used and may still be used. These include: IM (i.m.), intramuscular injection; IV (i.v.), intravenous injection; SC (s.c.), subcutaneous injection. Many other abbreviations are best discarded, including: o.m., every morning; o.n., every night; t.d.s., three times a day; q.d.s., four times a day. Multiplicity of abbreviations leads to confusion and error.

Doses of drugs are to found in official books of reference, such as the *Dental practitioners' formulary* (DPF). The recommendations in these guides are not binding on the prescriber, but are obviously sensible indications based on experience and deliberation. A prescription is the authority for a pharmacist to supply specified drugs to a particular patient. A sample of a completed prescription is shown in Fig. 3.1.

The main body of the prescription refers to the drug(s) to be prescribed, in this instance erythromycin. The name and strength of the drug is indicated first (erythromycin tablets 250 mg), and this is followed by the amount of the drug supplied (e.g. 20 tablets). This information is immediately followed by instructions to the pharmacist as to what information is to be written on the labelled medicine. Such directions should be written in English without abbreviation, and it is of the utmost importance that these instructions are clear. There must be no possibility of confusion on the part of the dispenser, for it is these instructions that are transcribed by the dispenser to the label on the package to be received by the patient. A phrase like 'as directed' should never appear because this is far too vague and open to misinterpretation. Indeed, the Courts have found against practitioners where prescriptions have lacked clarity or been illegible.

It is not always necessary to give the strength of the drug to be supplied; prescribing can be by 'title'. Drugs that are of fixed composition and are included in the *British national formulary* (BNF) or the DPF may be prescribed by title. For example,

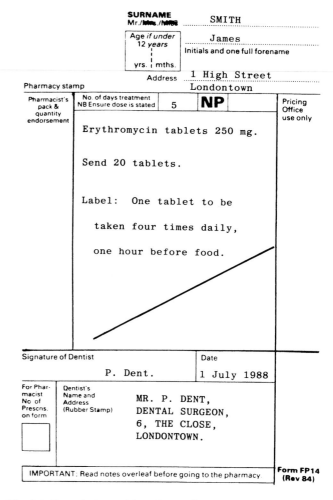

Fig. 3.1 Prescription writing. Layout for a prescription-only medicine.

instead of writing penicillin V tablets, 250 mg, it is in order to write penicillin V tablets *DPF*. Here the amount in each tablet is not specified because the inclusion of the abbreviation *DPF* indicates a standard preparation. Prescriptions for other and non-standard preparations must be written out in full.

The letters NP appear on National Health Service prescription forms. NP (*nomen proprium*) means that the drug(s) listed in the prescription will be named on the label automatically. This makes for ready identification of the drug(s). If for any reason the prescriber does not want the drugs so labelled, then the NP must be crossed out.

Although dental surgeons may issue a prescription for prescription-only drugs, they may also keep a supply to give to patients as needed. Dental surgeons can purchase such medicines. The seller, i.e. the chemist, has to keep a record of supply in the prescription-only register. The following details are required:

(1) the date on which the medicine was sold or supplied;

(2) its name, quantity, and pharmaceutical form and strength;

(3) the name and address, trade, business, or profession of the person to whom the medicine is sold or supplied.

No entry is required in the prescription-only register where the drug is a 'controlled drug' (see Misuse of Drugs Act below), as a separate entry has then to be made in another register.

The prescription-only register must be preserved by the pharmacist for 2 years from the date of the last entry. Prescriptions must also be kept for 2 years from the date when the medicine was supplied. If a dentist does purchase drugs to give to patients as needed, e.g. local anaesthetic agents, then they need to be aware of the Consumer Protection Act, 1987; this Act creates liability without fault on the part of the producer for damage caused by a defect in their product. A dental surgeon who supplied or administered a defective product and who was unable to identify the primary producer would carry liability for harm to the patient. Records should be kept for at least 10 years to be able to identify the source of drugs supplied or administered.

The dental practitioner is able to prescribe drugs listed in the *DPF* as a charge to the Health Service. For this purpose Form FP14 is used in England and Wales, and Form EC14 in Scotland. Prescribing is not limited to those drugs listed in the *Formulary* but if a drug is prescribed which is not listed it will have to be prescribed privately.

A prescription must be signed by the prescribing practitioner and an assistant must also add the name of the practitioner by whom he or she is employed.

Key facts
Medicines Act

- The Medicines Act of 1968 (which is an enabling Act) deals with the manufacture, distribution, and importation of medicines for human and animal use; it also ensures safety, quality, and efficacy of medicines to be prescribed.

- There are three classes of medicinal products: General Sales List Medicines (GSL), Prescription-only Medicine (POM), and Pharmacy Medicines (PM).

- Prescriptions must be written in ink or typewritten, contain details of the practitioner, and be signed and dated.

- Details of recommended dosing schedules are given in either the *Dental practitioner's formulary* (DPF), or in the *British national formulary* (BNF).

Some factors influencing prescribing

Age

The dose of a drug should bear some relationship to body weight. The reaction to drugs is markedly different in children, especially

Table 3.1 Age-related dosages for drugs with a high therapeutic index

Age	Percentage of adult dose
Birth	12–13
1 year	25
3 years	33
7 years	50
10 years	60
14 years	Adult dose

in the newborn, from that of adults. In the very early days of life there is limited renal filtration and detoxification of drugs is inadequate. Although doses for children based on body weight or body surface area are preferred, an age-related dosage can be used when prescribing drugs with a high therapeutic index (Table 3.1) (see Chapter 1).

Dosage for the in-between years can be adjusted accordingly. An important point to remember is that drugs should not be prescribed in liquid preparations containing sucrose, particularly for a long period, because this encourages dental caries.

The elderly also present a problem for the prescriber. In old age many factors, including the speed of absorption of drugs may be altered, as may the metabolism and excretion. These changes were explained in Chapter 1 but bear repetition. Of special importance is the decrease in renal clearance that occurs from mid-life onwards. This invariably increases, the concentration of drug in the body because of the reduction in the rate of elimination. At the same time the liver may not be so efficient in metabolizing drugs as it is in earlier life. The *British National Formulary* suggests that 'when prescribing drugs in the elderly, it is a sensible policy to limit the range of drugs used to a minimum' and that 'it is good practice to initiate treatment in aged patients with doses of little more than half that recommended for younger subjects'.

Prescribing in pregnancy and during breast-feeding

Care must be exercised in prescribing drugs to pregnant patients because of the possibility of fetal damage. It is better not to prescribe drugs to the pregnant patient at all unless it is absolutely imperative, and new drugs should be viewed with extreme caution. This subject is extensively reviewed in the combined *British national and dental practitioner formulary*, which should be possessed by all dental practitioners. Prescribing during breast-feeding is also reviewed in the combined *Formulary*.

Prescribing in renal disease

Some drugs should be avoided when the patient has reduced renal function, whilst others should be prescribed at reduced dosage

Table 3.2 Drugs in the *DPF* to be avoided or used with caution in renal impairment

Drugs	Dosage recommendations	Comments
Acyclovir	Reduce dose	Possible transient increase in plasma urea
Amoxicillin (amoxycillin)	Reduce dose	Rashes more common
Amphotericin	Use only if no alternative	Nephrotoxic
Ampicillin	Reduce dose	Rashes more common
Aspirin	Avoid	Fluid retention; deterioration in renal function; increased risk of gastrointestinal bleeding
Benzylpenicillin	Max. 6 g daily in severe impairment	Neurotoxicity—high doses may cause convulsions
Cefalexin (cephalexin)	Max. 500 mg daily in severe impairment	
Cefradine (cephradine)	Reduce dose	
Co-trimoxazole	Reduce dose	Rashes and blood disorders; may cause further deterioration in renal function
Diazepam	Start with small doses	Increased cerebral sensitivity
Diflunisal	Avoid if possible	Excreted by kidney; sodium and water retention and deterioration in renal function (**important**: see *BNF*)
Dihydrocodeine	Avoid	Increased and prolonged effect
Erythromycin	Max. 1.5 g daily in severe impairment	Ototoxicity
Ibuprofen	Avoid if possible	Sodium and water retention and deterioration in renal function (**important**: see *BNF*)
Nitrazepam	Start with small doses	Increased cerebral sensitivity
Pethidine	Avoid	Increased CNS toxicity
Temazepam	Start with small doses	Increased cerebral sensitivity
Tetracyclines (except doxycycline)	Avoid	Antianabolic effect, increased plasma urea, further deterioration in renal function

From *Dental practitioners' formulary 1998–2000*. (Published by kind permission of The Pharmaceutical Society of Great Britain.)

(Table 3.2). In the presence of renal impairment a drug, or its metabolites, may not be excreted and the accumulation of the drug may produce a toxic effect.

Prescribing in liver disease

Many factors may alter the response to drugs in a patient with liver disease. Although metabolism by the liver is probably the principal route whereby drugs are metabolized (see Chapter 1), liver disease has to be very severe before significant effects are produced on drug metabolism. The clotting factors prothrombin and fibrinogen are formed in the liver and their synthesis may be reduced in liver disease, which may lead to overactivity of oral anticoagulants such as warfarin. Furthermore, some drugs are hepatotoxic, and their effects may be dose-related or idiosyncratic. Drugs listed in the *DPF* that should be used with caution or avoided in liver disease include anti-inflammatory analgesics (e.g. aspirin, paracetamol), opioid analgesics, psychotropic drugs, and antimicrobials such as clindamycin, metronidazole, and IV tetracyclines.

Cardiovascular disease

The problems associated with the use of vasoconstrictors in cardiovascular disease will be dealt with elsewhere (see Chapter 8).

Key facts
Prescribing

- A variety of factors and systemic diseases influence prescribing, in particular the doses of drug and dosing schedules: the main factors include age, renal, and liver disease.

- Caution should be exercised when prescribing during pregnancy and to breast-feeding mothers.

- Age-related doses are required for children, and similarly for the elderly.

- Liver and renal diseases impact upon drug metabolism and excretion, respectively: alteration in drug dosage may be required for such patients depending upon the disease severity.

Standard reference books and data sheets

The *Dental practitioners' formulary*

This is perhaps the most useful reference book for the dental surgeon. It is revised every 2 years as a supplement to the *British national formulary*, which is issued every 6 months. The *DPF* is issued free to all practising dentists, and lists all preparations that the dental surgeon can prescribe as a charge to the Health Service. Information is provided on each drug listed, on adverse effects of drugs used in dentistry, and on medical problems.

Dental surgeons are not limited to prescribing drugs listed in the *Formulary*—they can prescribe other drugs provided that they observe the appropriate regulations, but the patient will have to bear the full cost of the prescription. Hospital dental surgeons are not limited to the *DPF* in NHS prescribing.

The *British national formulary*

The *BNF* is an index of preparations in common use in medicine. It contains useful information on the actions and adverse effects of important drugs. It is a useful publication for the dental practitioner, because it provides information about a drug that the patient is taking on medical prescription and information about the nature of the patient's disease. Both the *BNF* and *DPF* are now available in electronic form on CD-ROM.

MIMS (Monthly index of medical specialties)

MIMS is a useful reference booklet because it is revised monthly. It is designed as a reference and prescribing guide for doctors in general practice and lists proprietary preparations that may be prescribed or recommended. The inclusion of products in the index does not necessarily mean that they are available at NHS expense.

It is sent free of charge to all general medical practitioners, heads of hospital pharmacy departments, and on rotation to selected doctors and consultants in the UK. It is not supplied free of charge to dental practitioners, and all payments and enquiries about subscriptions should be addressed to: MIMS Subscriptions, 12–14 Ansdell Street, London W8 5TR.

Summary of Product Characteristics (SPC)

Before a medicinal product is marketed or advertised to medical or dental practitioners or any representation made, an SPC (formerly known as a data sheet) relating to the product must have been provided. An SPC is simply an information sheet, which must contain the following information about the product:

(1) its name;

(2) its presentation, i.e. a description of its appearance and pharmaceutical form;

(3) its uses, i.e. its main action and the purpose for which it is to be recommended in treatments;

(4) dosage and administration, including methods and routes of administration;

(5) contraindications and warnings.

Other information must also be contained on the sheet, but these are the main categories. The SPC is produced for each product of a manufacturer and the information contained must be fac-

tual and not promotional. It must be agreed by the National or European Regulatory Authority, and it must conform to rules on size and presentation style. As existing products come up for licence renewal (every 5 years), current data sheets will be replaced by new SPCs

Compendium of SPCs

A 'Compendium of SPCs' is compiled each year and is published by Datapharm Publications Limited in association with the Association of the British Pharmaceutical Industry (ABPI). This joint compendium is not prepared by persons or organizations concerned with manufacturing medicinal products. The individual data sheets are prepared by the companies concerned and participation in this joint compendium is open to all producing medicinal products for use under medical or dental supervision.

Patient information leaflets (PILs)

Many companies have voluntarily been providing patient leaflets in packs for some time. However, since January 1994, UK regulations implementing EU Directives have required companies to include a PIL in all packs of newly introduced products or those whose licence is being renewed. By the end of 1998, leaflets will be in all packs of licensed medicines. The Medicines Control Agency is consulting on ways to provide patients with leaflets on those medicines dispensed from bulk supplies, rather than from individual patient packs. The ABPI/Datapharm Publications publishes a 'Compendium of patient information leaflets' in parallel with the 'Compendium of SPCs'. Information leaflets are an important aid to patient safety and concordance with prescribed treatments. They are also important medicolegal safeguards for practitioners. Pharmacists will ensure that leaflets are supplied with all dispensed medicines, and dental surgeons should provide a leaflet with any medicines they supply direct to patients.

Key facts
Reference books and data sheets

- A variety of reference books and data sheets are available to the dental practitioner and patients: these include the *Dental practitioner* and *British national formularies*, *MIMS*, 'Compendium of SPCs', and patient information leaflets.

- The *DPF* is published every 2 years and is issued with the *BNF*: it provides a list of drugs the dental practitioners can prescribe and charge to the NHS.

- *MIMS* provides up-to-date information on new and existing products.

- The 'Compendium of SPCs' provides details of all medicinal products and is produced in association with the British Pharmaceutical Industry.

(cont.)

- Patient information leaflets (PILs) are produced for every licensed product and contain details of the drug, usage, and unwanted effects.

The Misuse of Drugs Act, 1971

Before 1971, drugs that were regarded as subject to abuse were regulated by the Dangerous Drugs Act. The present legislation had tidied up what had become a somewhat confused legislation.

The Misuse of Drugs Act of 1971, and its associated orders, control drugs that are liable to abuse, for example morphine and amfetamines (amphetamines). These are now described as 'controlled' drugs, whereas at one time they would have been referred to as 'dangerous' drugs.

Under this Act an Advisory Council has been set up to advise the appropriate minister (in this instance, the Secretary of State for the Home Office) on those drugs that are, or appear likely to be, misused and may thereby cause a social problem. The Council consists of at least 20 members representing various interested parties, including dentistry and medicine.

Controlled drugs are classified in the Act as Class A drugs, Class B drugs, and Class C drugs, and this division refers to the penalties for misuse awarded under the Act. Penalties for illegal use or possession of Class A drugs tend to be more severe than for the other two classes. Class A drugs (over 100 preparations) include substances such as cocaine, diamorphine, lysergide, methadone, opium, pethidine. Class B drugs include oral amfetamines (amphetamines), barbiturates, cannabis, codeine, and pentazocine. Class C drugs include most benzodiazepines.

The Misuse of Drugs Regulations, which interpret the spirit of the Act, allow certain persons or classes of persons (for example dentists) to possess, supply, prescribe, or administer controlled drugs in the *practice of their profession*. They also apply selective controls in relation to record-keeping, custody of drugs, and prescription writing. The regulations to the Act were originally stated in 1973 and were revised in 1985, *Statutory Instrument No. 2066*. These regulations include five schedules listing different categories of drugs to which varying requirements as to supply, prescribing, and record-keeping apply. A further schedule, *Schedule 6*, is simply a form of register indicating details to be kept when drugs listed under *Schedules 1* and *2* are received or supplied (see later).

Schedule 1 includes such drugs as cannabis, lysergide, and mescaline. A licence from the Home Secretary is required to possess, supply, administer, or cause to be administered, any drugs specified in this schedule. These drugs are effectively banned from mainstream medical and dental practice.

Schedule 2 lists those drugs that are used medicinally and are subject to the strictest controls. The list includes amfetamine (amphetamine), cocaine, codeine, dihydrocodeine, dextropropoxyphene, methadone, morphine, pethidine, and many others. Unless exempted in *Schedule 5*, these drugs are subject to the full control exercised by the regulations regarding prescriptions, safe custody, and record-keeping.

Schedule 3 includes the barbiturates and pentazocine. These drugs must fulfil the special prescription requirements for controlled drugs, but not the special requirements for safe custody. The *Schedule 6* type of register need not be kept for drugs so listed. Temazepam has recently been moved from *Schedule 4* into *Schedule 3* because of problems with widespread abuse. At the same time, the Secretary of State for Health used the Selected List Regulations to blacklist the liquid-filled temazepam capsules which were the main source of abuse.

Schedule 4 includes over 30 benzodiazepines, which are not subject to the strict controls regarding prescriptions, safe custody, or record-keeping indicated for drugs in the previous schedules. The benzodiazepines are prescription-only medicines and the form of prescription is as indicated on p. 40. Drugs abused in sport (anabolic steroids, growth hormone, and gonadotrophins) have recently been added to *Schedule 4*.

Schedule 5 include preparations that, because of their strength, are exempt from nearly all the controlled drug requirements. These exempt substances are not preparations for injection. Included in this list are certain preparations of dihydrocodeine or codeine. For instance, dihydrocodeine tartrate 30 mg tablet, because of the strength used, is classed simply as a prescription-only medicine, whereas dihydrocodeine for injection is a *Schedule 2* drug and therefore strictly controlled. Similarly, codeine, as contained in Codis tablets, is even less controlled than dihydrocodeine tartrate tablets, being classified as a Pharmacy Medicine. On the other hand, codeine phosphate injection would come under the regulations governing *Schedule 2* drugs.

Doctors, or dentists, may administer to a patient any drug specified in *Schedule 2*, *3*, or *4*. Furthermore, dentists may direct another person, other than a doctor or a dentist, to administer such a drug to a patient under their care. Any person may administer to another any drug specified in *Schedule 5*.

The form of the prescription for a *Schedule 2* or *3* drug

A prescription for a controlled drug listed in *Schedules 2* or *3*, and issued by a dentist or doctor, must be written in ink or otherwise indelible material. Its layout is shown in Fig. 3.2.

The whole prescription must be handwritten by the prescriber, dated, and signed with his or her usual signature. Except in the case of an NHS prescription, the address of the person issuing the prescription must be given, but this need not be handwritten. To minimize the possibility of forgery or alteration of the prescription, the following details should be in the dentist's or doctor's own handwriting:

(1) the name and address of the person for whose treatment the prescription is issued;

(2) the dose to be taken and, in the case of a prescription that is a preparation, the form, for example tablet or capsule;

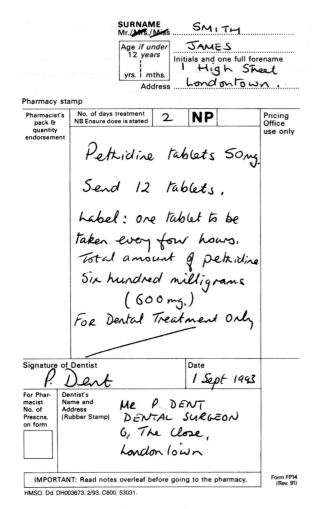

SURNAME Mr./Mrs./Miss _SMITH_

Age *if under* 12 years _JAMES_
Initials and one full forename
yrs. | mths. _1 High Street_
Address _Londontown_

Pharmacy stamp

| Pharmacist's pack & quantity endorsement | No. of days treatment NB Ensure dose is stated _2_ | **NP** | | Pricing Office use only |

Pethidine tablets 50mg.
Send 12 tablets.
Label: one tablet to be
taken every four hours.
Total amount of pethidine
Six hundred milligrams
_(600mg.)_
For Dental Treatment Only

Signature of Dentist _P. Dent_   Date _1 Sept 1993_

For Pharmacist No. of Prescns. on form

Dentist's Name and Address (Rubber Stamp) _Mr P. DENT DENTAL SURGEON 6, The Close, London Town_

IMPORTANT: Read notes overleaf before going to the pharmacy.   Form FP14 (Rev. 91)

HMSO. Dd. DH003673. 2/93. C800. 53031.

Fig. 3.2 Prescription writing. Layout for a controlled drug.

(3) the total quantity of the drug to be supplied, stated in both words and figures;

(4) a dental prescription for *Schedule 2* or *3* drugs must be endorsed with the words 'for dental treatment only'.

The requirements that a prescription is in the handwriting of the prescriber, and the total quantity of the drug is given in both words and figures, is to prevent alterations of the prescription. This elaboration is only required for drugs listed in *Schedules 1, 2,* and *3.* Even here there is some modification, in that phenobarbital (phenobarbitone) is exempt from the handwriting requirement, other than for the prescriber's usual signature.

Dental surgeons working in general hospitals may instruct staff to administer a fully controlled drug to a patient under their care. When this is done for an in-patient in a NHS hospital, it must conform to the standard prescribing procedures of the ward.

Requisition of controlled drugs

To obtain supplies of controlled drugs for use in practice, the practitioner must provide the supplier (pharmacist) with a signed requisition form giving the practitioner's name, address, and pro-

PART 1 ENTRIES TO BE MADE IN CASE OF OBTAINING			
Date on which supply received	Name and address of person or firm from whom obtained	Amount obtained	Form in which obtained

PART 2 ENTRIES TO BE MADE IN CASE OF SUPPLY				
Date on which the transaction was effected	Name and address of person or firm supplied	Particulars as to licence or authority of person or firm supplied to be in possession	Amount supplied	Form in which supplied

Fig. 3.3 Schedule 6 The misuse of drugs regulations 1985. 'Form of register'.

fession or occupation, the purpose for which the drug is required, and the total quantity of the drug to be supplied.

The supplier must be satisfied that the signature on the requisition form is genuine and that the signatory is engaged in the profession or occupation stated.

Registers for controlled drugs (*Schedule 6*)

Registers must be kept for all drugs specified in *Schedules 1* and *2* of the Regulations. A register must be kept for the receipt of drugs and another for the issue of these drugs. The 'Form of Register' is shown in Fig. 3.3. The register must be a bound book; loose-leaf books will not do. All entries must be in chronological order giving particulars of every quantity of a drug received and every quantity of a drug supplied, whether by administration or otherwise.

Entries should be made on the day the drugs are obtained or supplied. If this is not possible, the entries must be made not later than the next day. They must be made with some indelible material and must not be erased or changed in any way. If a correction is necessary, then this must be made by means of a marginal note or footnote, and the date of correction indicated. A separate part of the register must be used for each substance specified in the Act.

The registers must be kept on the premises to which they relate, so separate registers must be maintained for each set of premises. The record must be preserved for 2 years from the date of the final entry, and the registers must be available for scrutiny by the appropriate authority when required.

Storage of controlled drugs

A controlled drug must be kept in a locked receptacle, and the key held by the dentist.

Because the acquiring, possession, and storage of *Schedule 1* and *2* drugs does pose problems, it is unlikely that many dentists will feel the effort is worthwhile. The use of opioids and similar drugs in hospital practice is, of course, another matter.

Key facts
Misuse of Drugs Act, 1971

- This Act categorizes drugs into various schedules that limit their availability and prescription.
- *Schedule 1* drugs (e.g. cannabis) require a Home Office licence to possess, supply, and administer.
- *Schedule 2* and *3* drugs (e.g. cocaine, morphine, pentazocine) are subjected to the strictest control, and require the prescription to be entered into a Register.
- *Schedule 4* drugs include the benzodiazepines and drugs abused in sport.
- *Schedule 5* drugs include preparations that because of their strength or preparation are exempt from nearly all the controlled drug requirements (e.g. dihydrocodeine).

Selected list regulations (NHS Act, 1977)

From 1 April 1985 the range of drugs available for prescription on the NHS was limited by the 'Selected List Scheme'. The Government concluded that there were two areas in which action should be taken. The first was simple remedies for the relief of minor ailments and self-limiting complaints that are often bought over the counter by patients without recourse to GPs. These were laxatives, antacids, mild analgesics, cough and cold remedies, and vitamins. The second area was the use of benzodiazepines, which had escalated in recent years. Often expensive proprietary preparations were prescribed rather than generic compounds. There came into being what have come to be known as a 'white list' and a 'black list' of drugs in these areas. The list of drugs available for the medical practitioner to prescribe under the NHS is the 'white list' and the 'black list' covers the drugs no longer prescribable under the NHS. Doctors and pharmacists have a complete list of drugs no longer prescribable, which is amended from time to time. A practitioner who prescribes, or a pharmacist who dispenses, a blacklisted product is in breach of their NHS terms of service.

A further development in the operation of the selected list scheme was announced in the Autumn of 1992. Faced with an annual growth rate in primary care prescribing costs of 12–13%, Ministers announced a range of measures to attempt to contain this growth. Among these measures was a radical extension to the selected list. Proposed new categories of drugs that would be restricted under the regulations included appetite suppressants, antidiarrhoeal drugs, drugs acting on the skin, drugs acting on the ear and nose, drugs for vaginal and vulval conditions, contraceptives, drugs for allergic disorders, topical antirheumatics, hypnotics and anxiolytics, and drugs used in anaemia. Many of these proposals were subsequently withdrawn as part of Government negotiations with the ABPI on the Pharmaceutical Price Regulation Scheme which led to substantial price cuts being agreed by the industry. The selected list regulations remain a valuable tool for controlling the availabilty and costings of medicines to the NHS.

Further reading

Anon. (1978). The Medicines Act 1968 and other legislation. *British Dental Journal*, 145, 174–7.

Bateman, D. N. (1993). The Selected List. *British Medical Journal*, 306, 1141–2.

Dental Practioners' Formulary 1998–2000. British Dental Association, the British Medical Association and the Pharmaceutical Society of Great Britain, London.

Medicines Act, 1968. HMSO, London.

Misuse of Drugs Act, 1971. HMSO, London.

4

Pharmacology of inflammation and immunopharmacology

Pharmacology of inflammation and immunopharmacology

Inflammation is a complex process that can be defined as 'the reaction of the vascular and supporting elements of a tissue to injury, and results in the formation of a protein-rich exudate, provided the injury has not been so severe as to destroy the area'.

The clinical features that accompany inflammation have been known since antiquity. They include swelling (tumour), redness (rubor), hotness (calor), and pain (dolour). Inflammation is under the control of a variety of endogenous biochemical mediators produced at or near the site of injury. The biochemical and pharmacological properties of these mediators will be considered in this chapter, together with drugs that can affect the inflammatory response.

Chemical mediators of inflammation

Histamine

This vasoactive amine is found in most tissues of the body, but the major source is the granules of mast cells. Histamine is formed by the decarboxylation of the amino acid histidine. Trauma, either mechanical or chemical, causes the release of histamine from the mast cells into the extracellular fluid. Once released, histamine is rapidly metabolized by one of two enzyme systems (histamine-N-methyltransferase or diamine oxidase) to metabolites with little or no pharmacological activity (Fig. 4.1).

Pharmacological properties

Many of the properties of histamine are related to its action on smooth muscles, including relaxation of the vascular smooth muscle and contraction of the bronchi and gut wall. It is also a very potent stimulus to secretion of the exocrine glands, particularly those in the gastric mucosa. Histamine also has a direct effect on free nerve endings and is important in the production of pain and itch.

There is also evidence that histamine may function as a neurotransmitter in the CNS, being involved in the control of thirst, the secretion of antidiuretic hormone, the control of blood pressure, and pain perception.

Histamine receptors

Three types of histamine receptor, termed H_1, H_2, and H_3, have been identified. H_1 receptors are primarily involved in smooth muscle activity, i.e. vasodilatation and bronchial constriction. H_2 receptors are mainly involved with the stimulation of gastric secretions. The CNS effects of histamine may be mediated by H_3 receptors, which appear to be present on histaminergic nerve terminals. All histamine receptors have been shown to belong to the superfamily of G-protein-coupled receptors. A synopsis of the properties of the various histamine receptors is shown in Table 4.1.

Cardiovascular effects

VASODILATATION

In the peripheral circulation, histamine causes dilatation of the small blood vessels, an effect mediated by both H_1 and H_2 receptors. This leads to flushing, a lowered peripheral resistance, and a drop in blood pressure. Activation of H_1 receptors results in a rapid vascular response, which is short-lived, whereas activation of H_2 receptors results in a slower, but more sustained, vascular response. A fall in blood pressure can also occur by activation of the H_3 receptor which causes an inhibition of sympathetic outflow and subsequent vasodilatation.

CAPILLARY PERMEABILITY

Histamine-induced vasodilatation is accompanied by an increase in capillary permeability that results in oedema. The effect of histamine on the vasculature is best demonstrated by the 'triple response' described by Lewis and Grant in 1924. The features of this response to firm stroking of the skin are the red line, the flare, and the weal. Increased capillary permeability arises from the action of histamine on postcapillary venules, where it causes the contraction of endothelial cells and the exposure of the permeable basement membrane. Activation of H_1 receptors also increases polymorphonuclear leucocyte (PMN) adhesion and hence the migration of these cells.

CARDIAC EFFECTS

The effect of histamine on the heart is variable: it depends, in part, upon the concentration, the simultaneous release of catecholamines, or the reduction in blood pressure causing stimulation of the baroreceptor reflex. Cardiac effects include an increase in rate and force of contraction, which result in an increase in cardiac output. Higher concentrations of histamine may cause arrhythmias due to slowing of arteriovenous (A–V) conduction.

Smooth muscles

The bronchial muscles are the most important group of smooth muscles affected by histamine. Bronchoconstriction results from activation of the H_1 receptor and patients who suffer from asthma

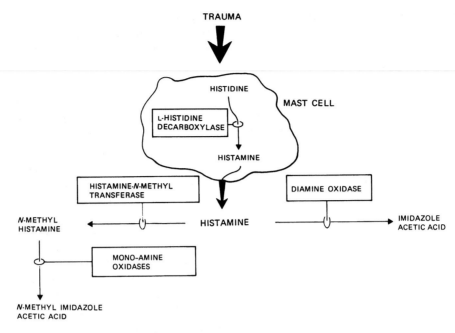

Fig. 4.1 The synthesis and metabolism of histamine.

Table 4.1 Summary of responses obtained on activation of the histamine receptors

Structures	H_1	H_2	H_3
Capillaries	Increase in capillary permeability	—	—
Vascular smooth muscle	Rapid, but short vasodilation	Slow and sustained vasodilation	Vasodilation
Bronchial muscles	Contraction	Slight relaxation	Bronchodilation
Free nerve endings (C fibres)	Pain and itch (peripheral)	—	—
Gastric mucosa	—	Secretion of gastric acid	—
CNS	—	—	Thirst control; regulation of body temperature; secretion of ADH; control of blood pressure; central pain perception, sedation

are particularly sensitive to the action of histamine on the bronchial musculature. However, antihistamines are of no value in the treatment of asthma because histamine is not the principal causative agent in this condition. Histamine-induced bronchoconstriction may also involve an additional reflex component that arises from the irritation of afferent vagal nerve endings.

Gastric secretion

The gastric secretory cells are very sensitive to histamine, with even low concentrations causing a copious secretion of gastric juices. This effect is mediated by the H_2 receptor (see Chapter 18).

Pain and itch

Histamine directly stimulates free nerve endings, which accounts for its ability to produce pain and itch when injected into the skin. A subcutaneous injection of histamine causes a sharp pain of short duration, similar to a wasp's sting. When injected into the more superficial layers of the skin, histamine causes itching.

Anaphylaxis and allergy

The release of histamine from mast cells plays a crucial role in both anaphylactic and allergic reactions. The active release is due to an antigen combining with a specific antibody (IgE) attached to the surface of the mast cell. The combination of antigen with antibody causes the extrusion of histamine from the secretory granules in the mast cells (degranulation). Histamine release is accompanied by the liberation of many other endogenous substances (see below) that contribute to the varied responses seen in such reactions.

Many substances, including drugs can act as antigens and cause anaphylactic or allergic reactions. Common examples include penicillin, animal fur, and pollen. Anaphylactic reactions can be fatal: their management is discussed in Chapter 26.

Autocoids

The term autocoid is derived from the Greek *'autos'* (self) and *'akas'* (remedy). It refers to substances that have local hormone-like activity at or near the site of production. Two distinct families of autocoids have been identified that are derived from membrane phospholipids: the eicosanoids, which are formed from certain polyunsaturated fatty acids (principally arachidonic acid) and platelet activation factor (PAF), derived from modified phospholipids.

The eicosanoids

The term eicosanoids has been used to denote the metabolites of certain 20-carbon polyunsaturated fatty acids, mainly arachidonic acid. These precursors can be converted into compounds that act as regulators and mediators of the functions of various cells.

Many different products of arachidonic acid metabolism have been identified, but they can be conveniently divided into two main groups on the basis that they are ultimately derived from the action of one of two enzymes systems (cyclo-oxygenase and lipoxygenase) on arachidonic acid (see Fig. 4.2).

Cyclo-oxygenase products can be further subdivided into three groups—the prostaglandins, the thromboxanes, and prostacyclin. Lipoxygenase products consist mainly of the leukotrienes and various compounds based on eicosatetraenoic acid.

ARACHIDONIC ACID

This is a 20-carbon polyunsaturated fatty acid. It has been suggested that there are two sources—the metabolic pool and the cell-membrane pool. The endogenous synthesis of arachidonic acid appears to be from the metabolic pool by metabolism of dietary linoleic acid, whereas stimulated synthesis (for example after trauma) comes from the cell-membrane pool. The membrane pool seems to be the major source of the eicosanoid precursor in inflammation.

In most cells and tissues it is thought that phospholipids are the major source of arachidonic acid. The first step in eicosanoid synthesis is the liberation of arachidonic acid from cell-membrane phospholipids (phosphate fraction) by the action of a group of enzymes known as the phospholipases. In particular, phospholipase A_2 is responsible for the bulk of arachidonic acid synthesis.

CYCLO-OXYGENASE PRODUCTS

The next step in the formation of cyclo-oxygenase products is the action of the enzyme cyclo-oxygenase on free arachidonic acid.

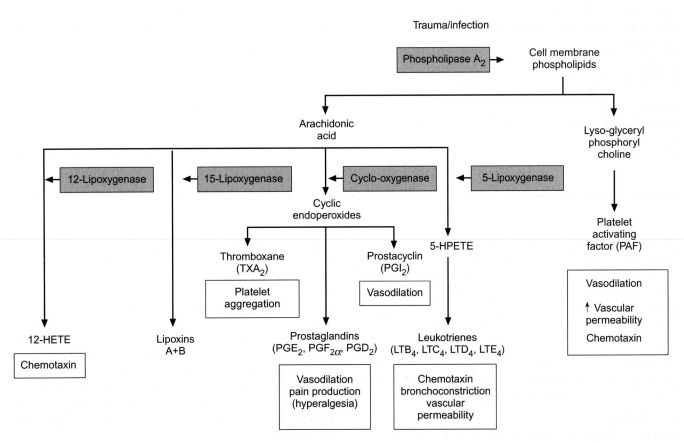

Fig. 4.2 The metabolic pathways of arachidonic acid and the synthesis of the eicosanoids. WBC, white blood cells; for other abbreviations, see text.

This action results in the insertion of two oxygen molecules into the fatty-acid carbon chain to form prostaglandin G_2 (PGG_2), which is rapidly transformed by the peroxidase-like activity of cyclo-oxygenase into the hydroxyperoxide prostaglandin H_2 (PGH_2). Following this, and depending on the particular cell and circumstances involved, one or more of the three groups—the prostaglandins, thromboxane, or prostacyclin—may be formed.

So far, two forms of the cyclo-oxygenase enzyme have been identified, now referred to as COX-1 and COX-2. COX-1 is a constitutive enzyme expressed in most cells, whereas COX-2 is induced by various cytokines and growth factors. Cytokine-induced COX-2 activity is suppressed by glucocorticoids and thus may account for some of the anti-inflammatory properties of these drugs. COX-2 also differs in its sensitivity to inhibition by other anti-inflammatory agents. Selective inhibition of COX-2 may be of clinical significance, especially in the propagation of dental pain. This enzyme is probably involved in prostaglandin production at the site of inflammation (e.g. a third molar tooth socket during and after extraction), but not at other sites such as the gastrointestinal tract. Thus inhibition of COX-2 may be anti-inflammatory without the unwanted effects of gastric irritation.

PROSTAGLANDINS

These were first identified in 1930, but it was not until the 1960s that their structure and function were elucidated. Prostaglandins occur in every tissue and body fluid. Their pharmacological properties are listed later.

THROMBOXANE AND PROSTACYCLIN

Further enzyme activity (thromboxane synthetase and prostacyclin synthetase) on PGH_2 results in the formation of thromboxane (TXA_2) and prostacyclin (prostaglandin I_2; PGI_2). The main synthesis of thromboxane occurs in platelets, whereas prostacyclin is synthesized in vessel walls. Thromboxane A_2 plays an important role in platelet aggregation. Prostacyclin is a potent vasodilator and acts as an antagonist of platelet aggregation. Thromboxane A_2 and prostacyclin are therefore biologically opposite poles of the mechanism for regulating the platelet–vessel-wall interaction and the formation of a haemostatic plug. Both thromboxane A_2 and prostacyclin are unstable, with very short half-lives. Thromboxane A_2 is broken down to thromboxane B_2, whereas prostacyclin is further metabolized to 6-keto-PGF-1α. Further details of the mechanisms of haemostasis are given in Chapter 13.

LIPOXYGENASE PRODUCTS (LEUKOTRIENES)

The action of the lipoxygenase enzyme system on arachidonic acid forms a range of hydroperoxyeicosatetraenoic acids (HPETEs), which may then be reduced to form the corresponding hydroxyeicosatetraenoic acids (HETEs). The leukotrienes are derived from 5-lipoxygenase acting on arachidonic acid to form 5-HPETE, which may then be reduced to 5-HETE or rearranged to form lipoteichoic acid LTA_4. LTA_4 can be hydrolysed enzymatically to produce LTB_4, or non-enzymatically to produce various di-HETEs. Alternatively, LTA_4 may undergo nucleophilic attack by

glutathione to produce LTC_4 from which LTD_4 and LTE_4 are generated.

Pharmacological properties of the eicosanoids

These are summarized in Table 4.2.

CARDIOVASCULAR SYSTEM

The prostaglandins are potent vasodilators and hence cause a fall in blood pressure. Cardiac output is increased by prostaglandins E and F.

Thromboxane A_2 is a potent vasoconstrictor that acts by contracting vascular smooth muscle. Conversely, prostacyclin relaxes vascular smooth muscle. The balance of actions between these two eicosanoids contributes to the control of vascular tone.

Leukotrienes C_4 and D_4 cause hypotension, which may be due to a decrease in either intravascular volume or cardiac contractility secondary to a reduction in coronary blood flow.

SMOOTH MUSCLES

Prostaglandins of the F series contract bronchial muscles, whereas prostaglandins of the E series relax them. An intravenous infusion of PGE_2 or $PGF_{2\alpha}$ causes severe contractions of the uterus.

Leukotrienes C_4 and D_4 are powerful bronchoconstrictors and are thus important mediators of asthma. The slow-reacting substance of anaphylaxis has been found to be a mixture of C_4 and D_4.

INFLAMMATION AND THE IMMUNE RESPONSE

Prostaglandins play an important role in the inflammatory process and the immune response. Prostaglandins of the E series cause a long-lasting vasodilatation accompanied by an increase in vascular permeability. PGE_1 appears to regulate the function of B lymphocytes and to inhibit the production and release of lymphokines from sensitized T lymphocytes.

Leukotriene B_4 is a powerful chemotactic attractant for polymorphonuclear leucocytes (PMN) and other white blood cells. Leukotrienes C_4 and D_4 have a potent action on the endothelial lining of the postcapillary venules and cause leakage of plasma proteins and oedema formation.

GASTRIC SECRETION

Prostaglandins of the E series and prostacyclin inhibit gastric secretion, but increase the production of mucus in the stomach and small intestines.

PAIN

The role of eicosanoids in the production of pain is discussed in Chapter 5.

Eicosanoid receptors

The many and diverse properties of the eicosanoids is explained by the discovery of a number of distinct receptors to these compounds that mediate their actions. Eicosanoid receptors are all G-proteins, and the ones identified to date have been located on smooth muscle and platelets. The receptors are named for the eicosanoid for which they have the greatest affinity. The isolation of eicosanoid receptors has afforded the opportunity to develop receptor antagonists; one such compound, montelukast—a potent

Table 4.2 Summary of pharmacological properties of the lipid-derived autocoids

Structures	Prostaglandins	Thromboxane	Prostacyclin	Leukotrienes	PAF
Cardiovascular system	Vasodilatation	Vasoconstriction	Hypotension	Hypotension	Vasodilatation
Platelets	—	Induces platelet aggregation	Inhibits platelet aggregation	—	Stimulates platelet aggregation
White blood cells	Inhibits lymphocyte function		—	—	Chemotactic for blood cells; causes release of lysosomal enzymes
				Chemotactic for leucocytes and macrophages	
Bronchial muscles	PGF and PGD_2 causes bronchoconstriction PGE_2 causes bronchodilatation	Bronchoconstriction	Bronchodilation	Bronchoconstriction	Bronchoconstriction
Uterus	Causes contraction	—	Relaxation	—	—
Gastric secretion	Inhibition	—	Inhibition	—	—
Smooth muscles of gastrointestinal tract Contraction		Contraction	Contraction	—	—
Free nerve endings	Sensitizes to histamine and bradykinin	—	Sensitizes to histamine and bradykinin	Causes hyperalgesia	—

orally active leukotriene antagonist—has recently been introduced for the treatment of asthma (see Chapter 17).

Platelet-activating factor

This lipid autocoid is synthesized mainly by platelets, leucocytes, and endothelial cells. Platelet-activating factor (PAF) is involved in many aspects of inflammation and its actions include vasodilatation, increase in vascular permeability, white blood chemotaxis, and the release of lysosomal enzymes. As its name suggests, PAF is a potent stimulator of platelet aggregation.

PAF may also be important in the pathogenesis of asthma and other allergic conditions. When inhaled, the compound produces bronchoconstriction and facilitates the accumulation of eosinophils in the lungs. However, current PAF antagonists appear to be of limited use in the treatment of asthma; this perhaps reflects the complexity of the condition. PAF is also implicated in anaphylactic reactions, since an intravenous infusion produces many of the signs and symptoms of this condition. It would appear that further development of PAF antagonists may provide a useful addition to the management of allergic conditions.

Bradykinin and kallidin

These two kinins are polypeptides formed from the plasma α_2-globulins by a complex series of proteolytic reactions (Fig. 4.3). The precursors of bradykinin and kallidin (lysyl-bradykinin) are high and low molecular weight kininogens, respectively. Low

molecular weight kininogen can be activated by tissue kallikrein which can be activated by a variety of factors, including the Hageman factor (factor XII) in the blood clotting cascade, and plasmin.

Bradykinin and kallidin have very short half-lives ($t_{0.5}$ 15 s) and are inactivated by carboxypeptidases (kinases I and II) and angiotensin-converting enzyme.

Pharmacological properties

Both bradykinin and kallidin are potent vasodilators and increase capillary permeability, leading to oedema formation. In this respect, bradykinin, is approximately 10 times more active than histamine on a molar basis. Kinin-induced systemic vasodilatation causes a sharp fall in blood pressure, which is mediated by endothelial-cell nitric oxide. As with most endogenous mediators of inflammation, both bradykinin and kallidin cause bronchoconstriction. The role of bradykinin in pain production is discussed in Chapter 5.

The effects of the kinins, including bradykinin, are mediated by receptors designated B_1 and B_2. The B_2 receptors mediate most of the pharmacological activities of bradykinin and kallidin. Trauma appears to increase the rate of formation of B_1 receptors.

5-Hydroxytryptamine

5-Hydroxytryptamine (5-HT, serotonin) is an amine formed by the hydroxylation of tryptophan, which is then decarboxylated to

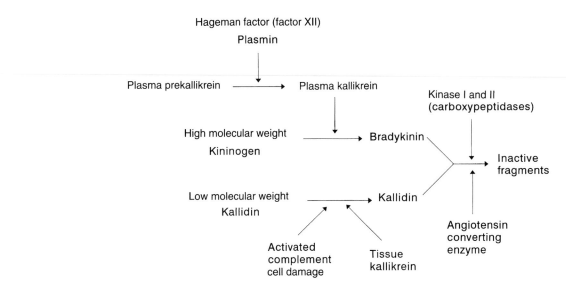

Fig. 4.3 The synthesis and metabolism of bradykinin and kallidin.

form 5-HT. After release, 5-HT is oxidized by monoamine oxidases (Fig. 4.4). The enterochromaffin cells of the gastric mucosa are the main storage site of 5-HT, and high concentrations are found in platelets.

Pharmacological properties

The role of 5-HT in inflammation is uncertain and may be insignificant. However, it has a wide and variable range of pharmacological properties that not only vary between species but also in the same individual. An important property of 5-HT is its effect on blood vessels—dilatation of arteries and constriction of veins. These effects are mediated via receptors, of which seven main types and several subtypes have been isolated

Complement

The complement system consists of a series of proteins that react in a cascade fashion (Fig. 4.5). One stimulus for the cascade reaction is the combination of antigen with antibody on a cell surface (this is known as the classical pathway). An alternate pathway can be triggered by bacterial toxins or large polysaccharides.

Fragments produced during the complement cascade are important in the inflammatory process. Fragments C3a and C5a induce the release of histamine from mast cells which, as described earlier, causes increased capillary permeability. Other components of the complement cascade are chemotactic to white blood cells (C5a, C5b, C567 complex) and enhance phagocytosis (C3b, C5b). Damage to cell membranes followed by cell lysis occurs when factors C8 and C9 are activated.

Interleukins

Interleukins (IL) are cytokines released from macrophages and lymphocytes during inflammation and the immune response. At least sixteen interleukins have been identified: referred to as inter-

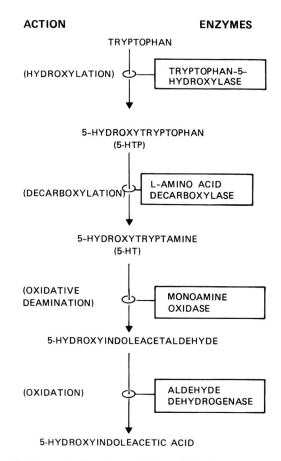

Fig. 4.4 The synthesis and metabolism of 5-hydroxytryptamine.

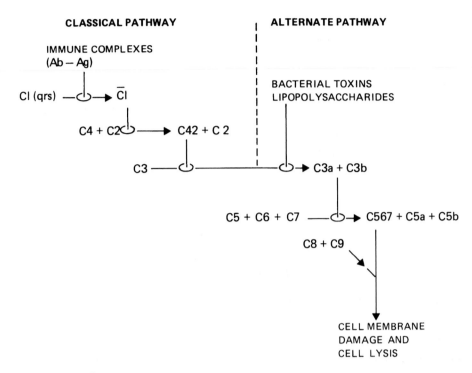

CLASSICAL PATHWAY

ALTERNATE PATHWAY

IMMUNE COMPLEXES
(Ab – Ag)

BACTERIAL TOXINS
LIPOPOLYSACCHARIDES

CI (qrs) → $\overline{CI}$

C4 + C2 → C42 + C 2

C3 → C3a + C3b

C5 + C6 + C7 → C567 + C5a + C5b

C8 + C9

CELL MEMBRANE
DAMAGE AND
CELL LYSIS

Fig. 4.5 The complement cascade.

leukins 1–16. They are involved in communication between lymphocytes, and their role in the immune system is discussed in more detail later. Interleukin-1 is produced by macrophages whilst processing antigen. It exerts a number of inflammatory actions, which include the stimulation of prostaglandin and collagenase production, chemoattraction for white blood cells, and enhancement of the hepatic synthesis of acute-phase proteins.

Key facts
Inflammatory mediators

- Mediators of inflammation include histamine, the eicosanoids (prostaglandins, thromboxane, prostacyclin, and the leukotrienes), platelet activation factor (PAF), the kinins, and to a lesser extent 5-hydroxytryptamine.

- All these mediators induce various vascular responses, leading to vasodilatation and increased vascular permeability.

- Complement proteins, lymphokines, and interleukins play specific roles in both the immune and inflammatory responses, in particular activating further cells, especially white blood cells (WBCs) to prolong the reaction.

Antihistamines

These competitively antagonize histamine at the receptor sites: they do not alter the formation or release of histamine from tissues or mast cells. Antihistamines are classified as H_1 or H_2 receptor blockers (antagonists). H_3 receptor blockers have been synthesized, but their therapeutic value has yet to be determined.

H_1 receptor antagonists

These are sometimes referred to as the classical antihistamines. Examples are chlorphenamine (chlorpheniramine), promethazine, diphenhydramine, and terfenadine.

Pharmacological properties

H_1 blockers are competitive antagonists, that is they interact with H_1 receptors on cell membranes, which results in a decrease in the availability of these receptors for the actions of histamine. Hence, H_1 blockers antagonize the action of histamine on smooth muscles and thus reduce vasodilatation, capillary permeability, and the flare and itch components of the triple response. Some H_1 blockers also have central effects, including sedation and the reduction of nausea and vomiting, that are not related to the antagonism of histamine.

H_1 blockers are well-absorbed from the gastrointestinal tract. Therapeutic effects can be observed within 15–30 minutes after dosage. The drugs are widely distributed throughout the body and are broken down in the liver.

Therapeutic uses

H_1 blockers are widely used in the treatment and prevention of a variety of allergic conditions, for example rhinitis, hay fever, and certain allergic dermatoses such as acute urticaria. Topical application of H_1 blockers is useful in relieving the itching associated with insect bites, but is not without problems (see below). H_1 blockers are widely used in common cold remedies—usually combined with a decongestant (e.g. Actifed). However, there is no evidence to suggest that H_1 blockers prevent or shorten the duration of the common cold.

The central effects of H_1 blockers make them useful in the prophylaxis of motion sickness (see Chapter 18) and as a sedative, especially in children.

H_1 blockers have no effect on bronchospasm or the severe hypotension associated with anaphylactic shock. Similarly, this group of drugs is of no value in the treatment of asthma.

Unwanted effects

Sedation is the major unwanted effect associated with the H_1 blockers, but the degree of sedation does vary between different preparations. Some, including phenindamine (Thephorin) may cause stimulation. Alcohol should be avoided whilst taking H_1 blockers as it enhances the sedative effect. The second generation of H_1 antagonists (e.g. terfenadine, astemizole, loratadine, and cetirizine) do not cause sedation since they do not cross the blood–brain barrier. However, these drugs, especially terfenadine and astemizole are rarely associated with prolongation of the QTc interval and subsequent polymorphic ventricular tachycardia. Cardiac problems from terfenadine and astemizole can occur when the drugs are taken in higher than normal doses, or when there is either a drug or disease-induced impairment in hepatic metabolism. These H_1 blockers are therefore contraindicated in patients with a pre-existing prolongation of their QTc interval or hepatic disease affecting drug metabolism. Other unwanted effects include dryness of the mouth and a variety of gastrointestinal disturbances. These unwanted effects are thought to arise as a consequence of the anticholinergic properties of the early H_1 antagonists, although the incidence of these disturbances can be reduced by taking them with meals.

Topical application of antihistamines

Antihistamine creams and lotions are widely used to relieve itching in skin conditions and after insect bites. However, these preparations are liable to produce a contact dermatitis (type IV reaction) (see Chapter 23) and their use is best avoided. Topical antihistamines act as haptens and probably conjugate with some protein of epidermal origin. If these drugs were to be applied topically in certain oral conditions, a similar sensitization might occur. Such sensitization is not only highly undesirable, but could be fatal if the patient needed urgent systemic treatment with antihistamines. If it were known that the patient was hypersensitive to antihistamines, they could not be treated with systemic antihistamine; if this vital fact were not known, and they were treated, it would be dangerous.

H_2 receptor antagonists

These competitively antagonize the action of histamine at the H_2 receptor. The two most widely used H_2 blockers are cimetidine and ranitidine. These compounds are discussed in Chapter 18.

Dental applications of antihistamines

Only H_1 blocking agents have any dental applications, and these principally make use of their central actions. Promethazine has both sedative and weak atropine-like properties, and is used as a preoperative sedative, particularly in children. H_1 blockers may be of some value in the treatment of allergic lesions on the face and lips.

Antihistamines have been evaluated in the control of pain, swelling, and other sequelae of oral surgery, but appear to be of little value in this application.

Key facts
Antihistamines

- These drugs competitively antagonize histamine at receptor sites and can be classified as either H_1 or H_2 receptor antagonists.

- H_1 receptor antagonists are mainly used in the management of allergic conditions and they can be administered topically or systemically; sedation is the main unwanted effect associated with these drugs.

- H_2 receptor antagonists are used in the treatment of peptic ulceration and other inflammatory conditions of the upper gastrointestinal tract; cimetidine inhibits the cytochrome P450 enzyme and thus will have an inhibitory effect on other drugs metabolized by this enzyme.

5-HT agonists/antagonists

The ergot alkaloids are a group of compounds that can act as either agonists or antagonists at 5-HT receptors. Drugs which are active at 5-HT receptors are used as anxiolytics and in the treatment of migraine (see Chapter 15) as well as antiemetics (see Chapter 18).

Corticosteroids

Corticosteroids and synthetic steroids have potent anti-inflammatory properties. Their general pharmacology and physiology is discussed in Chapter 20.

Anti-inflammatory and immunosuppressive properties

Steroids inhibit many of the processes associated with inflammation and the immune responses. In its early stages they reduce the capillary permeability caused by histamine and bradykinin, which in turn reduces oedema. They also inhibit both bradykinin formation and the migration of white blood cells into the site of inflammation. In its later stages, steroids reduce granulation-tissue formation by inhibiting the proliferation of fibroblasts and blood vessels. It is now established that steroids can affect eicosanoid synthesis by several possible mechanisms. These include:

1. Inhibition of the cyclo-oxygenase enzyme COX-2 by inhibiting transcription of the relevant gene.

2. Inhibition of the transcription of the gene for the enzyme phospholipase A_2. This enzyme acts on cell-membrane phospholipids and converts them to arachidonic acid (see p 51).

3. Corticosteroids also induce the formation of an anti-inflammatory protein known as lipocortin-1, which also has an inhibitory effect on phospholipase A_2.

Other mediators of inflammation and the immune response whose synthesis, or release, or both, is inhibited by corticosteroids include platelet-activating factor, interleukins, and tumour necrosis factor. Tumour necrosis factor (TNF) is released from phagocytic cells after stimulation with either bacterial toxins or interleukin-1. In lymphoid tissue, corticosteroids decrease the clonal expansion of T and B lymphocytes and decrease the action of cytokine-secreting T lymphocytes.

Using steroids to suppress inflammation is only palliative, for the underlying cause of the inflammation remains. Steroids should not be used where an infection is suspected.

Topical corticosteroid therapy

Topical corticosteroids are extensively used in the treatment of many dermatological conditions. However, they are not without unwanted effects, the most common of which—atrophy of the skin—can occur as early as 3–4 weeks after treatment begins. Atrophy is especially common on the face where the skin is normally thin. Both the epidermis and dermis are affected: in the epidermis there is a reduction in cell size and number; and in the dermis there is decreased fibroblast activity and collagen synthesis, which reduces dermal support. This in turn leads to dilatation of small blood vessels and to telangiectasia; the telangiectactic vessels rupture easily and produce ecchymosis.

Absorption of topical corticosteroids may lead to adrenal suppression (see Chapter 20). The extent of suppression is dependent upon the steroid potency, the duration of treatment, the amount used, and the skin area treated. Although isolated cases of severe adrenocortical suppression have been reported, the suppressive effect of topical steroids on cortisol levels is of little clinical significance with normal usage. As a general rule, little adverse effect on cortisol production is likely to occur with the application of a potent steroid ointment of up to 50 g weekly for an adult or 15 g weekly for a child.

The dental use of topical corticosteroids (for example hydrocortisone sodium succinate 2.5 mg, triamcinolone acetonide 0.1 per cent and betamethasone sodium phosphate 0.1 per cent) does not result in significant adrenocortical suppression.

Allergic contact dermatitis due to topical steroids is very rare and is more commonly due to a constituent of the base (for example lanolin).

Use of steroids in dentistry

Oral ulceration and oral mucosal lesions

Steroids are widely used in the treatment of recurrent oral ulceration and other oral mucosal lesions such as erosive lichen planus, erythema multiforme, and pemphigus. Many of these conditions are treated by topical applications and best results are achieved when the period of contact between steroid and lesion is maximal. Severe oral ulceration may require systemic steroids. In some instances, injection of a steroid into the lesion may be of benefit. Topical steroid preparations include triamcinolone acetonide 0.1 per cent; hydrocortisone sodium succinate 2.5 mg; betamethasone sodium phosphate 0.1 per cent (topical spray). Intralesional steroids are triamcinolone hexacetonide and hydrocortisone acetate. Prednisolone is the most widely used systemic steroid.

Pulpal inflammation

Steroids are often applied over a carious exposure of the dental pulp. One such preparation, Ledermix—contains triamcinolone and a tetracycline (demeclocycline hydrochloride). However, its efficacy is not established.

Temperomandibular-joint pain

Intra-articular injections of hydrocortisone or prednisolone are of value in certain inflammatory joint conditions. However, their use can cause deterioration of the articular surface of the joint and it is unwise to repeat the procedure more than twice.

Bell's palsy

This is a unilateral facial paralysis affecting one or more branches of the facial nerve. It is of unknown aetiology but may be subsequent to a viral infection. Prednisolone is the treatment of choice and therapy must be started within 5–6 days of onset of the paralysis. It is usual to start off steroid administration with a high dose, tailing this off over 10 days.

Postoperative pain and swelling after dental surgery

There has been much interest in the use of steroids to reduce pain, swelling, and other sequelae after removal of impacted lower third molars and after orthognathic surgery. For this, a course of steroids is usually short so unwanted effects are minimized. Methylprednisolone and betamethasone are used and are usually given intramuscularly just before surgery. The efficacy of steroids for reducing postoperative pain remains equivocal, and such pain is best treated with an NSAID.

Emergency uses

The use of steroids in the treatment of an adrenal crisis as well as anaphylactic and allergic reactions is dealt with in Chapters 20, 23, and 26.

Key facts
Corticosteroids

- The anti-inflammatory and immunosuppressive properties of the corticosteroids reside mainly with their inhibitory actions on eicosanoid synthesis and cytokine production from lymphocytes. The inhibition of these compounds also has further 'knock-on' effects for other mediators of inflammation and the immune responses.

- The anti-inflammatory properties of corticosteroids are extensively employed in dermatology, however they are not without unwanted effects on the skin and can cause atrophy of both the dermis and epidermis.

- The immunosuppressive properties of corticosteroids are used post-transplant to prevent graft rejection and in certain autoimmune diseases.

- Corticosteroids are used in dentistry for their anti-inflammatory properties: they are mainly used in the treatment of oral mucosal lesions.

The immune system

The immune system is one of the body's defence mechanisms against infection. It consists of a complex network of cells (macrophages as well as T and B lymphocytes) and macromolecules (immunoglobulins, interferons, cytokines), which interact to eliminate pathogenic micro-organisms, foreign proteins, and other 'non-self' substances. The immune system can therefore be said to have a dual function, namely to distinguish between 'self' and 'non-self', and to eliminate 'non-self'.

The branches of the immune system can be categorized as non-specific and specific accordingly. The non-specific system provides the first line of defence and is often regarded as innate or inborn. Specific immunity is often acquired during an infection, when there is considerable interaction between both systems.

Non-specific defence mechanisms

The non-specific defence system involves cellular activity and the production of endogenous proteins. Polymorphonuclear leucocytes (PMNs), monocytes, eosinophils, and basophils are the cellular components, whereas complement proteins and interferons contribute to the chemical component.

Polymorphonuclear leucocytes

PMNs are the predominant type of white blood cell with phagocytic activity. They play a major role in inflammation, migrating from the circulation in response to various chemotactic stimuli. At the site of injury, PMNs phagocytose bacteria and other foreign proteins, and release lysosomal enzymes and free oxygen radicals.

Monocytes

Monocytes, like most white blood cells, are produced in the bone marrow. They account for 5% of the total WBC count. When monocytes migrate from the circulation and enter the tissues, they are referred to as macrophages. Although macrophages are distributed throughout most tissues, they are most abundant in the reticuloendothelial system. Macrophages have phagocytic activity and are essential for the recognition and processing of antigen for subsequent presentation to lymphocytes. The cells also release a variety of chemical mediators (cytokines and prostaglandins) which act as vital signals between other immunocompetent cells.

Eosinophils

These cells constitute less than 2% of the WBC count, but numbers are raised in patients with parasitic infections and in some allergies, such as hay fever and asthma.

Basophils

These WBCs contain prominent cytoplasmic granules which release numerous pharmacologically active substances including histamine and heparin. In the tissues, basophils are referred to as mast cells.

Chemokines

These are a group of polypeptides that are chemotactic to PMNs and regulate the expression of integrins (proteins that facilitate the adherence of PMNs to vascular endothelium). The chemokines induce the adherence of various leucocytes to the vascular endothelium. Following migration of these WBCs into tissues, the cells are attracted towards high localized concentrations of chemokines. Thus these mediators play a very significant role in the inflammatory response, especially WBC migration and chemotaxis.

Interferons

Interferons are glycoproteins that have a variety of biological activities. Essentially, they afford a degree of resistance to further viral infections (see Chapter 11). The interferons have been classified into three types: interferon-α (IFN-α) is secreted by all nucleated cells following an infection with a virus; interferon-β (IFN-β) is secreted by fibroblasts infected with a virus; and interferon-γ (IFN-γ) is produced by T cells following stimulation by antigen or mitogen. IFN-γ has multiple effects on the cellular components of the immune system (Table 4.3).

The specific immune response

This response forms the basis of immunity, and either involves the production of specific proteins (antibodies or humoral response) or

Table 4.3 Biological properties of interferon-gamma

1.	Inhibits viral replication in nucleated cells
2.	Inhibits growth of normal cells and tumour cells *in vitro*
3.	Promotes cell differentiation
4.	Increases phagocytosis of macrophages
5.	Increases cytotoxicity of macrophages and natural killer cells
6.	Increases antibody production by plasma cells
7.	Inhibits proliferation of B cells

cytotoxic cells (cell-mediated response). Antibodies bind to antigens (such as pathogens), whereas cytotoxic cells destroy other cells infected with pathogens.

The humoral response

B lymphocytes are the essential cellular component of the humoral response. They have surface-bound membrane receptors (antibody or immunoglobulin molecules) that bind with antigen. The antigen is then internalized, processed, and presented on the cell surface. Helper T lymphocytes (see below) then interact with the processed antigen, leading to the proliferation and differentiation of B lymphocytes into antibody-secreting plasma cells. IL-1 secreted by macrophages is also involved in this interaction. In addition, B lymphocytes can also respond directly to antigens without involving the helper T lymphocyte.

IMMUNOGLOBULINS

These are chains of peptides—two light chains and two heavy chains—joined together by disulfide bridges. In humans, there are five classes of immunoglobulins, commonly abbreviated to IgG, IgA, IgM, IgD, and IgE.

IMMUNOGLOBULIN G

This is the main immunoglobulin formed during the secondary response. It can cross the placenta and is essential for the early protection against infection in newborn children. Immunoglobulin G is found in all cavities of the body where its main function is to neutralize bacterial toxins, thus activating the complement system. The activated complement products are chemotactic for white blood cells and cause an increase in capillary permeability. IgG can be subdivided into four subclasses, referred to as IgG1, IgG2, IgG3, and IgG4.

IMMUNOGLOBULIN A

This is referred to as the secretory immunoglobulin, for it appears in all secretions produced by the body. Its function is the defence of exposed external body surfaces against infection. IgA is synthesized locally by plasma cells, and coats micro-organisms thus inhibiting their adherence to the surfaces of mucosal cells and preventing entry into the body. IgA is an important constituent of breast milk and therefore helps to protect the newborn baby against infection during the first month of life.

IMMUNOGLOBULIN M

This is a high molecular weight immunoglobulin found on the surface of lymphocytes. It appears early in the response to infection and is very efficient at agglutinating bacteria. Hence high concentrations of IgM are associated with bacteraemias.

IMMUNOGLOBULIN D

IgD is very susceptible to proteolytic degradation and has a short plasma half-life. Like IgM, IgD is found on the surface of lymphocytes, and it seems that IgM and IgD are antigen receptors that interact with each other to control lymphocyte activation and suppression.

IMMUNOGLOBULIN E

Only small amounts of IgE are found in serum as this immunoglobulin is firmly fixed to the surface of mast cells. Combination between antigen and IgE results in mast-cell degranulation, with the release of histamine and other potent chemicals. This is the underlying mechanism for hay fever, asthma, and anaphylaxis. Immunoglobulin E also protects the mucosal surfaces of the body by activating plasma factors and effector cells.

The cell-mediated immune response

T lymphocytes are responsible for cell-mediated immunity. When stimulated, they proliferate and develop into cytotoxic T lymphocytes (CTL). These cells can destroy other cells infected with the pathogen against which they were induced. Another population of T lymphocytes—helper T cells (T_H)—is involved in B-cell activation (see above) and these play an important role in the induction of the cell-mediated response. Cytokines produced by these cells during an immune response facilitate the differentiation of both B and T lymphocytes as well as macrophages.

Helper T cells and cytotoxic T lymphocytes can be distinguished by cell-differentiation antigens, which are integral membrane glycoproteins. Helper T cells express the CD3 and CD4 markers, whilst CTLs express the CD3 and CD8 markers.

FUNCTIONS OF T LYMPHOCYTES

CTLs specifically destroy virus-infected cells and so prevent viral replication. The cells produce a variety of cytokines, including interleukins, interferon-γ (see above), and tumour necrosis factor. These molecules modulate a range of immunological activities which are discussed later.

Some CTLs suppress the immune response. It is not clear whether these suppressor cells are a different or overlapping population of CTL cells.

INTERLEUKINS

Interleukins are produced by various blood cells during immune as well as inflammatory responses. Their properties are summarized in Table 4.4.

TUMOUR NECROSIS FACTOR

The supernatant of endotoxin-treated macrophages contains a protein which can destroy tumour tissue in a tumour-bearing ani-

Table 4.4 Properties of the interleukins produced during the immune and inflammatory responses

Interleukin	Source	Properties
Interleukin-1	Macrophages, B cells, and endothelial cells	Stimulates T cells; induces syntheses of acute phase proteins; induces fever; induces PGE_2 and collagenase release; promotes maturation and clonal expansion of B cells and stimulates production of immunoglobulin; chemotactic for macrophages and PMNs; stimulates release of interleukin-2 and interferon-γ.
Interleukin-2	Helper T lymphocyte (T_H) cells	Supports the proliferation and differentiation of T- and B-lymphocytes; increases cytotoxic activity of natural killer cells.
Interleukin-3	Helper T lymphocytes	Haemopoietic growth factor which stimulates the growth and differentiation of bone marrow stem cells; also growth factor for mast cells and stimulates release of histamine.
Interleukin-4	Helper T lymphocytes	Growth factor for mast cells and T lymphocytes; causes differentiation and growth of B cells; stimulates production of immunoglobulins.
Interleukin-5	Helper T lymphocytes; mast cells	Promotes growth and differentiation of eosinophils and B cells; stimulates production of IgA.
Interleukin-6	Macrophages, bone marrow stromal cells; fibroblasts and endothelial after stimulation with interleukin-1	Differentiation of B cells; stimulates proliferation of T lymphocytes; promotes interleukin-3-induced haemopoiresis; stimulates production of acute phase proteins.
Interleukin-7	Bone marrow cells; thymic stromal cells	Induces differentiation of lymphoid stem cells into progenitor B and T cells.
Interleukin-8	Macrophages and endothelial cells	Chemotactic to PMNs induces adherence of PMNs to vascular endothelium and extravasation into tissues.
Interleukin-9	Helper T lymphocytes	Supports proliferation of T cell.
Interleukin-10	Helper T lymphocytes	Suppresses macrophage cytokine production.
Interleukin-11	Bone marrow stromal cells	Promotes differentiation of progenitor B cells and megakaryocytes. Induces synthesis of acute phase proteins.
Interleukin-12	Macrophages and B cells	Activates T lymphocytes
Interleukin-13	Helper T lymphocytes	Inhibits activation and release of inflammatory cytokines from macrophages; important regulator of the inflammatory response.
Interleukin-15	T cells	Supports growth of intestinal epithelium and T cell proliferation.
Interleukin-16	T cells and eosinophils	Induces expression of class II MHC. Chemotactic for monocytes and eosinophils.

mal. This protein is known as tumour necrosis factor (TNF). *In vivo*, it is produced by macrophages which have phagocytosed bacterial products. This cytokine shares many of the properties associated with interleukin-1, including acute-phase inflammatory reactions, inducing the production of acute-phase proteins, potentiation of fever, stimulation of collagenase, osteoclastic activity, and prostaglandin production.

TNF also causes haemorrhagic necrosis of tumours *in vivo* and has both cytostatic and cytotoxic effects on tumour cells *in vitro*. These properties suggested that the compound would be valuable in the treatment of malignant diseases. However, its use as a chemotherapeutic agent is limited by the fact that it is also responsible for cachexia (general debility of the body) and septic shock.

Other properties of TNF include activation of polymorphonuclear leucocytes (PMNs) and an increase in the adhesiveness of endothelial cells.

Key facts
Immune system

- The immune system is the body's main defence system and comprises both a cellular and chemical component.

- The immune response can be further divided into non-specific and specific; the latter also involves a humoral and a cell-mediated response.

- Cells that have a significant role in the immune system include PMNs, T and B lymphocytes, monocytes, eosinophils, and basophils.

- Endogenous substances secreted by those cells that contribute to the immune responses are interferons, chemokines, immunoglobulins, interleukins, and tumour necrosis factor.

Immunosuppressants

When foreign tissue or cells are introduced into the body, the immune system is activated and the foreign material eliminated. This is an essential protective role, but in some circumstances it may need to be suppressed. For example, immunosuppression is required to prevent rejection in organ transplants. The main immunosuppressants used clinically are corticosteroids (see above), cyclosporin, and azathioprine. Cytotoxic drugs also suppress the immune system and these are discussed in Chapter 18.

Cyclosporin

Cyclosporin is a hydrophobic cyclic endecapeptide derived from the metabolic products of two fungal species, *Tolypocladium inflatum* and *Cylindrocarpon lucidum*. It was originally developed as an antifungal agent, but its activity was weak. Early investigations showed that it had an inhibitory effect on lymphocyte proliferation.

Since the discovery of its immunosuppressant properties, several studies have shown that cyclosporin acts selectively on the T-lymphocyte response, and has little or no action on B lymphocytes. Its main use is to prevent graft rejection in organ transplantation. The drug is also used in disorders involving autoimmunity, such as psoriasis, type 1 diabetes mellitus, rheumatoid arthritis, and severe oral ulceration.

Cyclosporin pharmacokinetics

Cyclosporin can be administered orally, intramuscularly, or intravenously. After oral administration it is absorbed from the gastrointestinal tract, but there are marked variations in absorption in different people. Peak plasma concentrations occur 3–4 hours after dosage, and the drug has a serum half-life of 17–40 hours. Cyclosporin is extensively metabolized in the liver, mainly through the cytochrome P450 mono-oxygenase system. Its metabolism involves *N*-demethylation, hydroxylation, and cyclization. Most of the metabolites are excreted in the faeces, via the bile.

To maintain immunosuppression, an oral therapeutic dose of 10–20 mg kg body weight^{-1} day^{-1} is required, which produces a serum concentration of 100–400 ng mL^{-1}. A new cyclosporin preparation (Neoral) is now available which possess greater bioavailability than previous cyclosporin preparations. Thus patients can be placed on lower doses of cyclosporin when given this preparation.

Cyclosporin pharmacodynamics

Cyclosporin acts on the T-lymphocyte response, and the role of this response in graft rejection can be summarized as follows:

(1) recognition of graft-tissue antigen as foreign material;

(2) processing of antigen by macrophages, with the subsequent production and release of IL-1;

(3) activation by IL-1 of precursor CTLs, which acquire receptors for IL-2;

(4) activation of T-helper lymphocytes, with the production and release of IL-2, which is accentuated by IL-1;

(5) the clonal amplification of activated CTLs, leading to cell-mediated lysis and graft rejection;

(6) the activation of suppressor T lymphocytes which can modulate these responses.

Cyclosporin inhibits many of these stages, acting at both a cellular and molecular level. At concentrations of 10–20 ng mL^{-1}, it inhibits IL-2 synthesis so limiting clonal amplification of CTLs. At a higher concentration (100 ng mL^{-1}), cyclosporin inhibits the ability of CTLs to respond to IL-2. The mechanism of this inhibition is uncertain, but the drug may block the induction of IL-2 receptors on these cells. By contrast, cyclosporin spares suppressor T lymphocytes.

Thus cyclosporin appears to be selective in its actions on T lymphocytes. Suppressor T lymphocytes seem to be resistant to cyclosporin, whereas CTLs and helper T lymphocytes are sensitive to it. These differential effects of cyclosporin on the various subsets of T lymphocytes may be due to different binding properties between the drug and different cell types, and subsequent internalization of the cyclosporin molecules into the cell structure.

Unwanted effects

Cyclosporin has many unwanted effects. Of concern to dentists is the fact that it can cause gingival overgrowth (see below). Nephrotoxicity is another well-documented and frequently observed unwanted effect, which is of particular significance in renal transplant patients. This toxicity appears to be related to serum levels and is accompanied by a hyperuricaemia and hypercalcaemia. Many transplant patients are concurrently taking nifedipine (a calcium-channel blocker) which reduces cyclosporin-induced renal toxicity.

Other unwanted effects of cyclosporin include hypertension, hepatotoxicity, neurotoxicity, increased risk of neoplasia, anaemia, and hypertrichosis.

CYCLOSPORIN-INDUCED GINGIVAL OVERGROWTH

Cyclosporin, along with phenytoin and the calcium-channel blockers, is implicated as a cause of gingival overgrowth. Approximately 30% of dentate transplant patients experience significant gingival changes that warrant surgical excision. This incidence increases to 50% if the patient is concurrently taking nifedipine.

The pathogenesis of cyclosporin-induced gingival overgrowth is uncertain. The relationships of the incidence and severity of gingival overgrowth to pharmacokinetic variables of the drug are equivocal. Most studies have shown a positive relationship between gingival overgrowth and poor oral hygiene. However, subjecting renal transplant patients to an intensive plaque control programme fails to prevent the occurrence of gingival overgrowth. Genetic factors do appear to be important in the expression of drug-induced gingival overgrowth. Indeed, some patients are particularly sensitive to the drug and rapidly develop gingival changes. Genetic factors could determine the populations of specific phenotype fibroblasts within the gingival tissues, or affect the pharmacokinetics of cyclosporin. Identifying cyclosporin-gingival responders is fairly straightforward, however their management presents a very difficult problem.

The histological appearance of cyclosporin-induced gingival overgrowth is comparable to that resulting from phenytoin therapy. The overgrowth has been described as consisting primarily of connective tissue with an overlying irregular multilayered, parakeratinized epithelium of varying thickness. The connective tissue is highly vascular with focal accumulations of infiltrating inflammatory cells (mainly polymorphonuclear leucocytes and plasma cells).

Cyclosporin-induced gingival overgrowth is treated by gingivectomy and thorough plaque control, together with the removal of plaque-retentive factors.

Although cyclosporin-induced gingival overgrowth is a serious unwanted effect of the drug, even more significant is the potential for malignant change to occur within the hyperplastic gingival tissues. Squamous cell carcinoma has been reported in the gingival tissues from patients with overgrowth. Also, the incidence of Kaposi's sarcoma is increased in immunosuppressed patients, (see later). The risk of such malignant changes suggests the need for biopsy in cases of severe cyclosporin-induced gingival overgrowth.

Azathioprine

This is a purine derivative with selective immunosuppressant activity against the cell-mediated system. Azathioprine is metabolized in the liver to mercaptopurine, a purine analogue that inhibits DNA synthesis. The drug appears to increase suppressor T-lymphocyte activity and reduce helper T-lymphocyte activity. Azathioprine can be given orally or parenterally.

Unwanted effects

There are many of these and, because of these risks, the use of this drug should be balanced against the severity of the patient's condition and the expected clinical effect. The most serious unwanted effect of azathioprine therapy is depression of bone-marrow function causing a leucopenia and thrombocytopenia. Routine haematological screening is required for all patients taking azathioprine. Other unwanted effects include gastrointestinal intolerance, allergic reactions, and skin rashes.

Uses

Azathioprine is mainly used to prevent the rejection of organ transplants, but it is also used as an alternative to corticosteroids in pemphigus, systemic lupus erythematosus, severe rheumatoid arthritis, and thrombocytopenic purpura.

Other immunosuppressants

New drugs that suppress the immune system include FK 506 and fujimycin. These are currently being evaluated, particularly in organ transplant patients, and evidence to date suggests that they are comparable to cyclosporin yet have fewer unwanted effects.

Dental problems of the immunocompromised patient

The increases in organ transplant surgery and HIV infections have produced a large cohort of patients with a compromised immune system. The main consequence of immunodeficiency is the increased risk of infection, particularly those of fungal and viral origin, and malignancy.

Candidiasis remains the most frequent fungal infection in these patients. The incidence and severity of fungal infections is dependent upon the degree of immunosuppression (either disease- or drug-induced). The more severe the immunosuppression, the greater the incidence of fungal infections. Oral candidal infections in immunosuppressed patients show a variable response to topical antifungal therapy (i.e. nystatin pastilles or miconazole oral gel). For recurrent infections and those that appear resistant to topical antifungals, systemic fluconazole is the drug of choice (see Chapter 11). This antifungal agent has a greater volume of distribution, more reliable oral absorption, and a longer half-life (30 h) when compared to other systemic antifungals. However, fluconazole does inhibit the hepatic metabolism of cyclosporin, which can result in a raised plasma concentration of the latter. This can give rise to an increased risk of nephrotoxicity: thus it is advisable to monitor cyclosporin concentrations whilst the patient is being treated with fluconazole.

The herpes group of viruses, in particular cytomegalovirus (CMV) and herpes simplex virus (HSV), are those most frequently associated with immunosuppressed patients. The antiviral agents aciclovir and ganciclovir are effective agents against the herpesviruses (see Chapter 11). Other virus-related lesions that occur in immunosuppressed patients include hairy leukoplakia, which is thought to be related to the Epstein–Barr virus.

Immunosuppressed patients appear to be more susceptible to the development of malignant neoplasms. Malignancies that are more common in these patients include lymphomas, skin and lip cancers, and Kaposi's sarcoma. It is also recognized that the various malignant neoplasms occur 20–30 years earlier in such patients than expected in non-immunosuppressed individuals. Squamous cell carcinoma appears to be a particular problem in organ transplant patients, and often the dental surgeon is the first to recognize such malignancy. Any suspicious lesion should be biopsied together with advice on limiting exposure to sunlight and smoking.

Key facts
Immunosuppressants

- Corticosteroids, cyclosporin, and azathioprine all possess immunosuppressant properties by mainly targeting the cell-mediated immune response or cytokines released as a consequence of this response.

- Immunosuppressive agents are used in a variety of diseases where there is an underlying defect in the immune response (e.g. autoimmune diseases). They are also used extensively in organ transplant patients to prevent graft rejection.

- Many of the unwanted effects of these drugs are related to immunosuppression *per se*, and include an increased susceptibility to infection and malignant change.

- Cyclosporin is of particular concern to the dental surgeon since it is associated with the unwanted effect of gingival overgrowth.

Further reading

Nicod, L. P. (1993). Cytokines, an overview. *Thorax*, 48, 660–7.

Samuelson, B. (1983). Leukotrienes: mediators of immediate hypersensitivity reactions and inflammation. *Science*, 220, 568–75.

Seymour, R. A., Thomason, J. M., and Nolan, A. (1997). Oral lesions in organ transplant patients. *Journal of Oral Pathology and Medicine*, 26, 297–304.

Thornbury, N. A. (1994). Inflammation: key mediator takes shape. *Nature*, 370, 251–2.

5

The pharmacology of pain

The pharmacology of pain

Dentistry and pain are often synonymous. Indeed, fear of dental treatment is an important contributory factor to the extensive dental neglect in the UK. It is an everyday occurrence for the dental surgeon to diagnose and treat pain arising from the teeth and associated structures. This topic is thus very relevant for dentists and it is essential that they have a thorough understanding of the mechanisms of pain. This chapter describes those mechanisms that form the basis for appropriate pain control, which is dealt with in subsequent chapters. The first section deals with the neuroanatomy and neurophysiology of pain, including theories of pain. The remainder of the chapter considers the neuropharmacology of pain, at a peripheral and a central level. Table 5.1 lists definitions and terms associated with pain.

Neuroanatomy of pain: nociceptive pathways

This section gives an outline of the peripheral and central pathways involved in pain. The second part deals with pathways specifically related to the trigeminal nerve, which are of particular importance to the dental practitioner.

Peripheral and central pathways: general aspects

There is no single nerve pathway that is devoted exclusively to transmitting and processing information concerned with pain. The detection and signalling of tissue damage or nociception (from the Greek *nocere*, to damage) plays a primary role in protecting the organism. It is hardly surprising that such a system is elaborate and uses complex neural pathways, both excitatory and inhibitory. Some of the inhibitory pathways include feedback loops which can reduce pain.

The four main systems comprising the nociceptive pathways are shown diagrammatically in Figs 5.1(a) and (b).

Nociceptors

A nociceptor can be defined as a receptor preferentially sensitive to a noxious or potentially noxious stimulus (see Table 5.1). It is important to realize that the stimulation of nociceptors may, but need not necessarily, lead to the subjective phenomenon of pain,

which is the result of higher functions of the nervous system carried out particularly at thalamic and cortical levels. There are two main types of nociceptor:

1. High-threshold mechanoreceptors connected to A delta (A-δ) axons conducting at 5–10 m s^{-1}: These mechanoreceptors are distributed only to skin and mucous membranes in a punctate fashion, areas in between being unresponsive. As their name suggests, they are activated by high-intensity mechanical stimulation, including pinprick, and possibly also by noxious thermal stimuli above 45 °C. This accounts for the severe pricking sensation that accompanies the withdrawal reflex triggered by the sudden application of heat to the skin.

2. Polymodal nociceptors consisting of bare nerve endings connected to unmyelinated C fibres that conduct at 0.5–2 m s^{-1}: These are distributed widely in skin and also in deep tissues and are activated by high-intensity mechanical, chemical, and thermal (above 45 °C) stimuli. Stimulation of polymodal nociceptors results in a tonic contraction of muscles related to the area concerned (in contrast to the stimulation of high-threshold mechanoreceptors that elicits a withdrawal reflex; see above and also Table 5.2). It seems probable that these polymodal nociceptors are stimulated by one or more substances released during inflammation (see later).

Nociceptive information, which arises as a result of stimulating the high-threshold mechanoreceptors and polymodal nociceptors, is transmitted via the A-δ and C peripheral nerve fibres, respectively, to the spinal cord. These two sets of nerve fibres enter the spinal cord via the dorsal root (Fig. 5.1(a)) where they branch profusely. They end in the marginal zone and substantia gelatinosa, forming synapses with cells of the second-order neurones.

In addition, large A-β fibres connected to touch receptors also enter the dorsal horn. From here they travel up in the dorsal columns of the spinal cord, but they also give off collaterals that synapse with the cell bodies of the second-order neurones. In addition, collaterals from both the small fibres (A-δ and C) and large fibres (A-β) synapse with the cell bodies of local short interneurones, the axons of these interneurones terminate close to

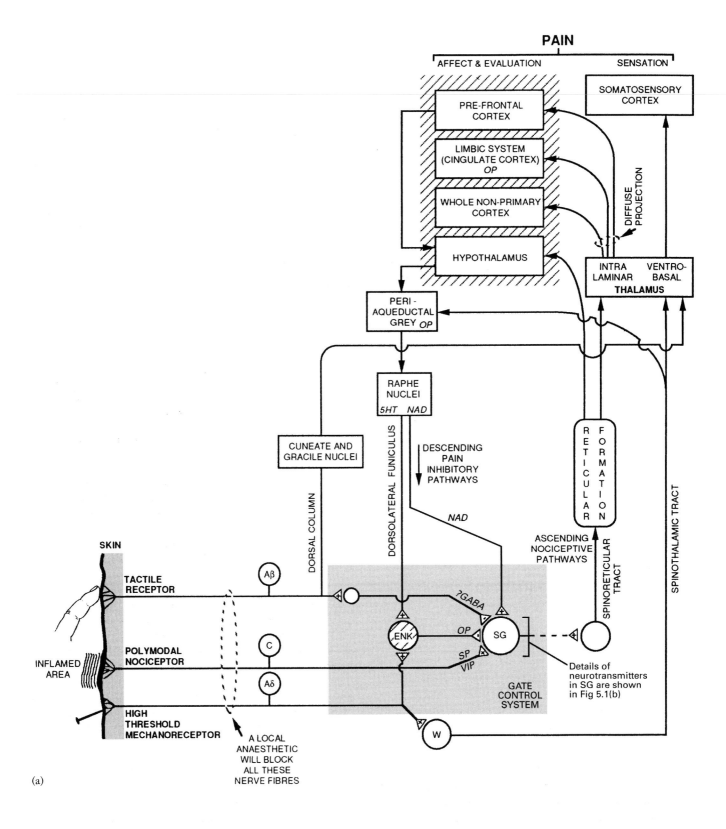

(a)

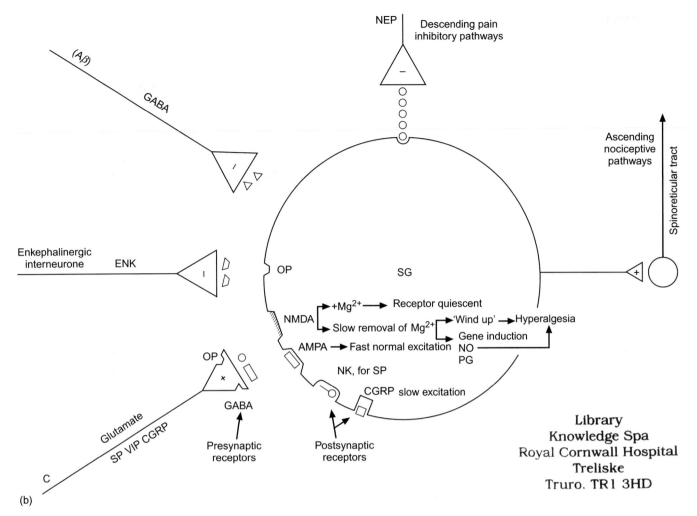

Fig. 5.1(a) The principal neuronal circuits involved in the sensory and emotional (affect and evaluation) components of nociception. The afferent pathways involved in transmitting nociceptive information from an inflamed area of skin to the higher centres via the dorsal horn, the gate-control system, the ascending tracts, and the thalamus are shown. The sensory component of nociception is somatotopically projected to the somatosensory cortex where it is analysed. The emotional (affective and evaluative) components of nociception undergo diffuse projection from the thalamus to other parts of the cortex, in particular the prefrontal cortex and the cingulate cortex of the limbic system, which contains opioid receptors. Note the connections of the tactile receptor responding to a finger stroking the skin and those of the high-threshold mechanoreceptor responding to the prick of a pin.

The descending pain-inhibitory pathway, which passes via the dorsolateral funiculus, is also shown. This pathway starts from the periaqueductal grey, and receives inputs from the hypothalamus and the ascending spinothalamic tract. It then descends via the raphe nuclei that give rise to neurones releasing 5-HT and norepinephrine (noradrenaline); the endings of these fibres synapse with the enkephalinergic neurones in the dorsal horn. This completes a long feedback loop and is an essential part of the gate-control system. The descending pathway from the prefrontal cortex via the hypothalamus to the periaqueductal grey allows higher cortical processes (cognitive processes) to modify the appreciation of pain.

Fig. 5.1(b) Enlarged and more detailed view of the right-handed part of the shaded area (gate-control system) in Fig. 5.1(a). This diagram shows the neurotransmitters and postsynaptic receptors which are now believed to be important in the transmission of nociceptive information. The ending of the C-fibre co-releases glutamate (excitatory amino acid, EAA), substance P (or vasoactive intestinal peptide, VIP), and calcitonin gene-related peptide (CGRP), which act respectively on AMPA, NK and CGRP receptors. The NMDA (N-methyl-D-aspartate) receptor is normally held in a quiescent state by Mg^{2+} ions, but under abnormal conditions there is a slow removal of Mg^{2+} ions resulting in activation of this receptor by glutamate. This in turn leads to important secondary effects, including the release of NO and PG and the phenomenon of 'wind up' that causes hyperalgesia. The latter occurs in certain chronic neuropathic pain states including orofacial pain. Abbreviations: Aβ, C, and Aδ, the posterior root ganglion cells of these three types of fibre; SP, substance P; VIP, vasoactive intestinal polypeptide; GABA, γ-aminobutyric acid; OP, opioid peptides; SG, cell in the substantia gelatinosa (lamina 2); ENK, enkephalinergic neurone; T, transmission cell; W, Waldeyer cells; 5-HT, 5-hydroxytryptamine; NEP, norepinephrine (noradrenaline); NK1, neurokinin-1; NMDA, N-methyl-D-aspartate; NO, nitric oxide; PG, prostaglandin. A + or − sign indicates whether the neurotransmitter released from a nerve ending excites or inhibits the postsynaptic nerve cell.

Table 5.1 Pain terms: a list of definitions as recommended by the International Association for the Study of Pain Subcommittee on Taxonomy (1986)

Pain	An unpleasant sensory and emotional experience associated with actual or potential tissue damage, or described in terms of such damage
Allodynia	Pain due to a stimulus that normally does not provoke pain
Analgesia	Absence of pain in response to stimulation that would normally be painful
Causalgia	A syndrome of sustained burning pain, allodynia, and hyperathia after a traumatic nerve lesion, often combined with vasomotor and sudomotor dysfunction and later trophic changes
Dyaesthesia	An unpleasant abnormal sensation, whether spontaneous or evoked
Hyperaesthesia	Increased sensitivity to stimulation, excluding special senses
Hyperalgesia	An increased response to a normally painful stimulus
Hyperpathia	A painful syndrome, characterized by increased reaction to a stimulus, especially a repetitive stimulus, as well as an increased threshold
Neuralgia	Pain in the distribution of a nerve or nerves
Neuritis	Inflammation of a nerve or nerves
Neuropathy	A disturbance of function or pathological change in a nerve; in one nerve, mononeuropathy; in several nerves, mononeuropathy multiplex; if diffuse and bilateral, polyneuropathy
Nociception	Activity in a nerve fibre, which arises as the result of the stimulation of nociceptors. If nociception reaches consciousness it is perceived as pain
Nociceptor	A receptor preferentially sensitive to a noxious stimulus or to a stimulus that would become noxious if prolonged
Pain threshold	The least stimulus intensity at which a subject perceives pain
Pain tolerance level	The greatest stimulus intensity causing pain that a subject is prepared to tolerate

the endings of the small and large fibres as these synapse with the cell body of the second-order neurone (see Fig. 5.1 (a)). It is thought that these short interneurones release enkephalins that presynaptically inhibit the endings of the primary afferent neurones. However, the collaterals from the primary afferent neurones control the enkephalinergic neurones in opposite ways: activation of the large fibres increases, whereas activity in the small fibres (A-δ and C) decreases, their activity. This provides a neuropharmacological basis for the gate-control theory of pain. These neural connections mean that increasing the amount of activity in the large A-β fibres tends to reduce the probability of onward transmission from the first-order to the second-order neurones; whereas increasing the activity in the small fibres (A-δ and C fibres) has the opposite effect, increasing the probability of onward transmission. Since, in practice, there is likely to be simultaneous activity in both the large (A-β) and small (A-δ and C) fibres, the probability of onward transmission of nociceptive information (from A-δ and C fibres) depends on the *ratio* of the activities of the large and small fibres. This prediction is in accord with the well-known effect that rubbing an injured part (i.e. stimulating the large A-β fibres) reduces pain due to activation of small A-δ and C fibres.

Spinothalamic tract

The nociceptive peripheral afferents synapse with marginal cells. These send axons across to the other side of the cord which then ascend as the spinothalamic tract to the ventroposterior nucleus of the thalamus. The spinothalamic tract contains about 1500 fibres,

of which about 30% carry nociceptive information, 60% tactile information, and the remaining 10% carry information about the movement of joints. From the thalamus, a third set of neurones relays the information to the postcentral gyrus, from where it is projected in a discrete and somatotopic way (Fig. 5.1).

Spinoreticular tract

This crossed multisynaptic pathway extends from the spinal cord to the intralaminar nuclei of the thalamus and includes connections to the hypothalamus (responsible for the autonomic concomitants of pain) and to the limbic system (responsible for the emotional component of pain). The spinoreticular tract is larger than the spinothalamic tract and contains about 25 000 axons. Further sets of neurones relay nociceptive information from the thalamus to the whole of the cerebral cortex. Experimental and clinical evidence suggests that the spinoreticular tract is more important for true pain sensation than the spinothalamic tract, which is mainly concerned with pricking pain.

Descending pathways for the inhibition of pain

In addition to ascending pathways, the spinal cord contains important descending inhibitory pathways that form part of a much larger descending inhibitory system. Those concerned with pain extend from the periventricular grey matter via the periaqueductal grey matter and nucleus raphe magnus to the spinal cord where they impinge upon the endings of the primary afferent neurones. This forms an inhibitory (negative feedback) descending pathway that contributes to the pain-gate mechanism at the spinal cord level, where it assists in the control of the nociceptive input to supraspinal level.

Neuroanatomy of dental pain

The sensory supply to the teeth, jaws, and oral mucosae is derived from the maxillary and mandibular divisions of the trigeminal nerve whose cell bodies are found in the Gasserian ganglion. The pain-receptor system innervated by the trigeminal nerve consists of both myelinated and unmyelinated nerve fibres. In the teeth, each nerve fibre supplies approximately eight terminal filaments to the subodontoblastic plexus of Rashkow. Afferent fibres pass centripetally towards the apex of the tooth root as pulpal nerves, to join the individual dental branches of the maxillary and mandibular divisions of the trigeminal nerve.

There are two groups of nerve fibres present in the dental pulp: C fibres and A-δ fibres. The C fibres are unmyelinated and have diameters of 0.25–2.5 μm, whereas the A-δ fibres are myelinated, and have slightly larger diameters of 2–5 μm. The human dental pulp is richly innervated compared with the skin or cornea. It has been estimated that the pulp of a human upper incisor tooth contains approximately 500 myelinated nerve fibres and 40–150 unmyelinated fibres. The area of the pulpodentinal junction in a human upper incisor is approximately 40 mm^2, so there is enormous overlap of the receptive fields of the individual fibres.

The trigeminal nucleus

The primary sensory afferent fibres of the trigeminal nerve enter the brainstem at the level of the mid-pons and terminate in the trigeminal nuclear complex of the brainstem. The complex comprises four nuclei—the motor nucleus and three sensory nuclei (mesencephalic, principal, and spinal). The mesencephalic nucleus probably has a proprioceptive function and receives fibres from the muscles of mastication, tongue and face, as well as the periodontal ligament. The principal sensory nucleus is found in the pons, and receives the ascending sensory fibres from all three divisions of the nerve. The descending fibres form the spinal tract of the trigeminal nerve, which descends through the medulla oblongata into the upper cervical part of the spinal cord. As the tract descends, terminals and collaterals are given off to synapse with cells of the spinal nucleus. The arrangement of nerve fibres in the spinal tract from the three divisions of the trigeminal nerve is constant, so selective cutting is possible in patients suffering from intractable facial pain.

The spinal nucleus is itself subdivided, from above downwards, into oral, interpolar, and caudal parts (Fig. 5.2). Clinical experience suggests that the caudal part of the spinal nucleus and the upper cervical segments of the dorsal horn are especially important in the conduction of impulses mediating pain from the teeth, jaws, and face.

There are three layers of cells that can be identified in the caudal division of the spinal nucleus—the marginal, gelatinosal, and magnocellular layers (Fig. 5.3). Nociceptive C fibres from the face, jaws, and teeth terminate mainly in the marginal and gelatinosal layers, whilst A-δ fibres terminate both in the marginal layer of the caudal subdivision and more densely in the oral subdivision.

Projections from the trigeminal nuclei

Neurones in the marginal, gelatinosal, and magnocellular layers of the spinal nucleus are interconnected; local circuits extend to incorporate the subjacent lateral reticular formation (Fig. 5.4), whose neurones are activated by painful stimulation in the

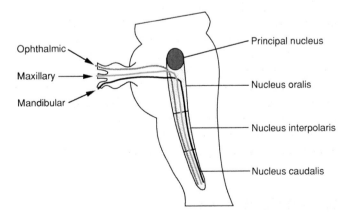

Fig. 5.2 Spinal nucleus of the trigeminal nerve. This is immediately below the principal nucleus and is in three parts – nucleus oralis (oral), nucleus interpolaris (interpolar), and nucleus caudalis (caudal).

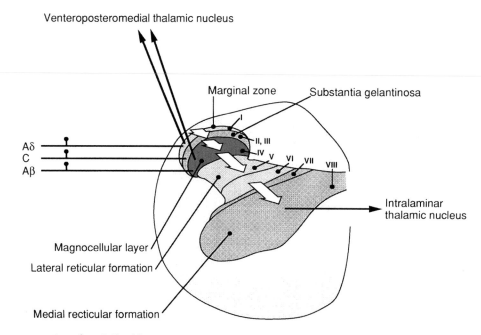

Fig. 5.3 Transverse section of medulla oblongata. Roman numerals identify the layers – The caudal division of the spinal nucleus has three layers: marginal zone, substantia gelatinosa, and magnocellular layer. (Based on Bowsher 1980.)

trigeminal region. Efferent fibres from the lateral reticular formation appear to follow one of two courses. Most of the efferents project further medially to converge on neurones of the medial reticular formation. However, some of the efferent axons from the lateral reticular formation join together with those of the magnocellular layer and marginal zone of the spinal nucleus to form the trigeminal lemniscus, projecting to the ventroposteromedial thalamic nucleus.

Information from all over the body converges on the medial reticular formation and is transmitted to the intralaminar thalamic nucleus. The reticular system probably acts as a centre controlling what information is passed on and what is rejected. It therefore has an important role in mediating and modulating information relating to nociception.

Thalamus

All information concerning nociception reaches the thalamus. Peripheral A-δ fibres project mainly to the ventroposteromedial thalamic nucleus, whereas impulses that originate in the peripheral C fibres seem mainly to reach the intralaminar nuclei (Fig. 5.4).

Efferent projections from the ventroposteromedial thalamic nucleus end in the orofacial region of the primary somatosensory area in the lower part of the postcentral gyrus. In this site there is somatotopic representation of the body surface, the lips being especially well represented. The teeth and jaws, by comparison,

are poorly represented at the cortex and this is probably related to the fact that nerves from several teeth converge on the trigeminal nuclei. This may also explain why patients with pulpal pain are frequently uncertain as to which tooth is involved. If part of the cortex in the postcentral gyrus is destroyed, there is loss of conscious, thermal, and mechanical sensation (including pinprick) in the appropriate part of the body. However, such destruction does not lead to the loss of true pain sensation. The intralaminar nuclei give rise to the diffuse thalamocortical projections whereby the whole of the cerebral cortex, but particularly the frontal region, is activated. Here, the information is recognized and interpreted as being painful.

Although the ventroposteromedial nucleus and intralaminar nuclei are very different in structure and function, there are many connections between the two systems. Clinical evidence suggests that the ventroposteromedial nucleus and its projections into the postcentral gyrus are involved in the localization and discrimination of pain. The intralaminar nuclei and their projections to the frontal region may be responsible for the emotional suffering and psychological components of pain. Evidence for the latter comes from patients who have undergone a frontal leucotomy operation. Postoperatively, patients who had suffered from chronic pain no longer complained much of their pain and they behaved as if they were indifferent to it, showing that the sensation of pain and its unpleasant emotions can be separated by neurosurgery. Patients would, however, still feel pain when a noxious stimulus was applied.

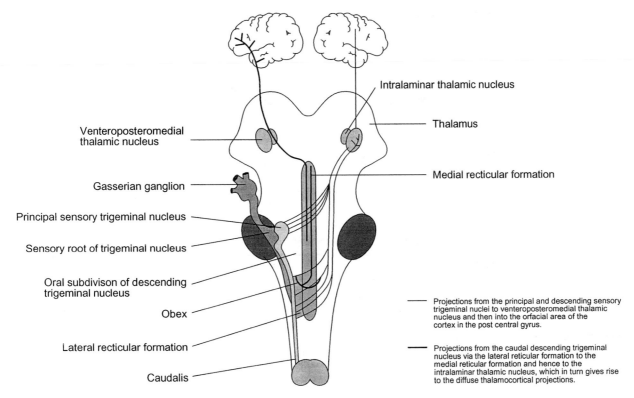

Venteroposteromedial thalamic nucleus

Gasserian ganglion

Principal sensory trigeminal nucleus

Sensory root of trigeminal nucleus

Oral subdivison of descending trigeminal nucleus

Obex

Lateral recticular formation

Caudalis

Intralaminar thalamic nucleus

Thalamus

Medial recticular formation

— Projections from the principal and descending sensory trigeminal nuclei to venteroposteromedial thalamic nucleus and then into the orfacial area of the cortex in the post central gyrus.

— Projections from the caudal descending trigeminal nucleus via the lateral reticular formation to the medial reticular formation and hence to the intralaminar thalamic nucleus, which in turn gives rise to the diffuse thalamocortical projections.

Fig. 5.4 The brainstem and thalamus, to show sensory trigeminal nuclei and their connections. (Based on Bowsher 1980.)

Key points
Neuroanatomy of dental pain

- The sensory supply to the teeth, jaws, and oral mucosa is derived from the maxillary and mandibular divisions of the trigeminal nerve.

- The trigeminal nucleus is located in the brainstem and consists of four nuclei – motor, mesencephalic, principal, and spinal.

- The spinal nucleus is further divided in oral, interpolar, and caudal parts, with the latter being particularly important in mediating nociception from the teeth, jaws, and face.

- Three layers of cells can be identified in the caudal division of the spinal nucleus – marginal, gelatinosal, and magnocellular layers: C-fibres terminate in the marginal and gelatinosal layers, whilst A-δ terminate in the marginal layer.

- Efferent fibres from the trigeminal nuclei form circuits with fibres from the reticular formation and pass via the trigeminal lemniscus to the thalamus.

Neurophysiology of pain
First and second pain

The two sets of primary afferent neurones conveying nociceptive information from nociceptors to the dorsal horn of the spinal cord have very different characteristics (Table 5.2). The high-threshold mechanoreceptors are connected to A-δ axons conducting at $5-10 \, \text{m s}^{-1}$, whereas the polymodal nociceptors are connected to unmyelinated C fibres conducting at $0.5-2 \, \text{m s}^{-1}$. Stimulation of the A-δ system is characterized by first, fast, pricking pain accompanied by a flexion reflex. By contrast, stimulation of the C system is associated with second, slow, aching pain probably accompanied by a tonic reflex response, particularly if the pain is chronic. Both systems can be blocked by the suitable application of a local anaesthetic. In contrast, appropriate amounts of an opioid can block slow pain but they do not affect fast pain. In a mixed nerve trunk, which contains all sizes of A fibres as well as C fibres, appropriate concentrations of a local anaesthetic will block conduction in all these fibres (see Chapter 8), although in practice the aim is to use concentrations sufficient to block only A-δ and C fibres.

Table 5.2 Features of first and second pain

Feature	First, rapid or ? acute pain	Second, slow or ? chronic pain
Adequate stimulus	Pinprick, heat	Tissue damage
Nerve fibres	A-δ fibres (small myelinated)	C fibres (unmyelinated)
Conduction velocity	5–15 metres s^{-1} (11–33.5 m.p.h.)	0.5–2 metres s^{-1} (1–4.5 m.p.h.)
Distribution	Body surface, including mouth and anus	All tissues except brain and spinal cord
Reflex response	Withdrawal (flexion), phasic muscle contraction	Spasm, rigidity, tonic muscle contraction*
Biological value	Causes organism to avoid possible tissue damage	Brings about enforced rest of damaged part, so promoting natural healing
Effect of morphine	Very little	Suppression of pain sensation, abolition of spasm

* This reflex reaction involves both agonists and antagonists, which is part of the definition of spasm or rigidity; it is a pathological rather than a physiological reaction.

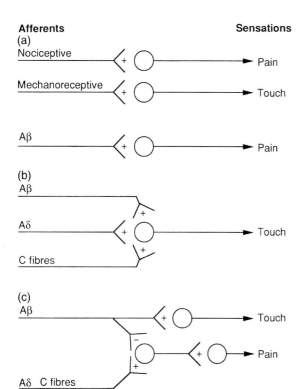

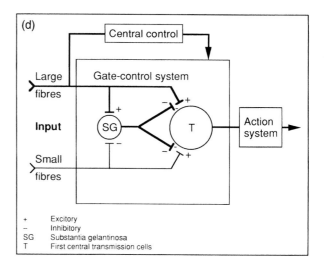

Fig. 5.5 Diagrammatic representation of the various pain theory: (a) Von Frey's specificity theory; (b) Goldscheider's sensory summation theory; (c) Noordenbos' sensory interaction theory; (d) Melzack and Wall's gate-control theory.

Theories of pain

Various theories have been put forward on how nerve impulses give rise to the sensation of pain. There is no generally accepted pain theory; in the following discussion, each of the theories described has evolved from the previous one.

Specificity theory

This theory (see Fig. 5.5(a)), which originates from Descartes, is based on the existence of a specific pain system, relaying messages from nociceptors in the skin to a pain centre in the brain. A major expansion to the specificity theory came from von Frey in 1895, who postulated that certain nerve endings in the skin were activated by tissue damage, giving rise to pain sensations. His theory was based on the distribution of 'sensory spots' (touch, cold, warmth, and pain) on the skin. 'Pain spots' were the most numerous, and free nerve endings were the most abundant histologically identifiable structures. Von Frey based his hypothesis on Muller's 'doctrine of specific nerve energies', which stated that specific sensory fibres carry information related to specific sensations (light, sound, and so on). Von Frey proposed that stimulation of free nerve endings gave rise to pain sensations in brain. The specificity theory is concerned primarily with the sensory discriminative aspects of pain and its quality, location on the skin, intensity, and duration.

It has since been shown that the theory has defects based on anatomical, psychological, and physiological grounds. Perhaps the major defect is its inability to explain some of the characteristics of clinical pain, in particular, phantom limb pain, post-herpetic neuralgia, and trigeminal neuralgia. Such pains do not support the concept of a direct-line nervous system. Furthermore, surgical intervention is unsuccessful in abolishing these pains permanently, which suggests that central control plays a major role in pain sensation. Similarly, the specificity theory does not explain referred pain that can be triggered by stimulating normal skin. A mechanism of referred pain based on this theory would require convergence of noxious input from different sites on neurones responding exclusively to pain. The theory also fails to explain the paroxysmal episodes of pain produced by mild stimulation of trigger zones in trigeminal neuralgia.

Central summation (pattern) theory

Dissatisfaction with the specificity theory led to the central summation theory (see Fig. 5.5(b)), which proposed that the intensity of the stimulus and central summation were the critical determinants of pain. This theory proposes that pain is not a separate entity, but results from overstimulation of other primary sensations (touch, light, sound, and so on). Goldscheider, in 1894, proposed this theory after observing the excessive reaction of patients with tabes dorsalis (tertiary syphilis) to mild repeated skin stimulation. He proposed that nerve impulses that evoke pain are produced by the summation of the skin sensory input at the dorsal horn cells. Pain results when the total output of the cells exceeds a critical level due to excessive activation of receptors (normally responsive to non-painful stimuli) or when pathological conditions enhanced summation produced by such stimuli.

A major deficit of this theory is its failure to recognize receptor specialization in response to painful stimuli. However, the emphasis on central summation and convergence was an important advance in the understanding of pain mechanisms.

Sensory interaction theory

An important addition to the summation theory was the concept of sensory interaction, which proposes that rapidly conducting, large-fibre pathways inhibit or suppress activity in slow conducting, small-fibre pathways that convey painful or other noxious information (see Fig. 5.5(c)). A shift in the ratio of large to small fibres in favour of the small fibres would result in increased neural transmission, summation, and excessive pathological pain. This theory stresses the importance of multisynaptic afferent systems in the spinal cord, and stands in marked contrast to the idea of a straight-through system. Its strength is the recognition of considerable interaction between pain pathways and other sensory pathways.

This theory helps to explain different pathological pain states. For example, hyperalgesia following peripheral nerve injury can be explained by a greater loss of large nerve fibres than of smaller fibres. A reduction in large-fibre activity would decrease the ratio of large- to small-fibre activity resulting in more central summation and an increase in pain. Burning pain in post-herpetic neuralgia can be explained on the basis of large-fibre destruction, a release of inhibitory mechanisms, and central summation. Finally, the ineffectiveness of various surgical lesions that attempt to interrupt the 'pain pathways' in permanently abolishing pain may be due to the diffuse, extensive connections within the ascending multisynaptic pathways. The sensory interaction theory stresses inhibition as an important physiological mechanism in pain transmission.

Gate-control theory

The gate-control theory was proposed by Melzack and Wall in 1965. It combines the strengths of the previous pain theories and adds some of its own. Although some of the detailed physiological mechanisms and anatomical connections have been added to or amended, the theory provides a general framework for viewing the many aspects of the pain experience (Fig. 5.5(d)).

For the trigeminal nerve, the gate-control system is located in the caudal division of the spinal nucleus. Activity in the very fast A-β fibres exercises an inhibitory effect on the relay nerve impulses in the slower conducting A-δ and C fibres (nerve fibres associated with the nociception). Therefore, the level of activity in the gate is regulated, at least in part, by the activity in the A-β fibres. If there is a high level of activity in these fibres, few nociceptive impulses in the A-δ and C fibres are allowed to pass through the gate-control system.

A further influence on the level of activity in the gate-control system is activity in the higher centres of the brain. Such activity passes down from the cortex as efferent impulses travelling along the corticofugal pathway to the spinal nucleus. It is postulated that incoming (afferent) nociceptive impulses from the periphery can be blocked at the gate as a result of descending (efferent) impulses originating from higher centre activity such as thought, memory, emotions, or even by pain originating from other parts of the body (see Fig. 5.1).

As described above, afferent fibres from the trigeminal spinal nucleus travel to the reticular formation. The ascending fibres of the reticular formation constitute the reticular activating system, which is constantly bombarded by a variety of incoming impulses. Nerve impulses from the reticular activating system ascend via the thalamus to the cerebral cortex. The level of activity in the reticular activating system determines the level of consciousness: it exercises both a facilitatory and inhibitory effect on the cerebral cortex.

The reticular activating system is connected with the limbic system, which is regarded as being the emotional centre, and the origin of fear and anxiety. The limbic system exercises considerable control over the hypothalamus and pituitary gland: nociception can influence the central regulation of the autonomic nervous system and therefore accounts for various visceral manifestations of pain, such as perspiration, salivation, hypertension, and the release of catecholamines into the blood.

The gate-control theory and its recent modifications have stressed the importance of both descending control mechanisms and activity in large sensory fibres in modulating the pain experience. The theory may explain why the toothache sufferer often obtains relief by applying heat to the appropriate part of the face. The heat would excite additional nerve fibres, so closing the 'gate' mechanism and reducing further transmission of painful impulses from the offending tooth.

Dental electroanalgesia is another technique that uses the gate mechanism for controlling pain arising from dental procedures. It may be useful in patients where conventional local anaesthetics may be a problem, such as haemophiliacs and patients who are allergic to the drugs.

Key facts
Neurophysiology of pain

- First and second pain are recognized entities and are associated with A-delta and C-fibres, respectively.

- Several theories of pain have been postulated over the years, including the specificity theory, central summation theory, sensory interaction theory, and the gate-control theory.

- The gate-control theory remains the most acceptable, and suggests a gating mechanism that can modulate nociception reaching the cortex.

- The gating mechanism appears to be influenced by activity in A-beta fibres and also by descending control mechanisms.

Peripheral mediators of pain

When tissue is damaged either as a result of an infection, trauma, or an operative procedure, an inflammatory response is initiated. As a consequence, various cytokines and other inflammatory mediators are released from circulating leucocytes and platelets, by vascular endothelial cells, from mast cells, and other immune cells present in the tissues and from the nerve fibres themselves. The various mediators considered to be hyperalgesic include metabolites of arachidonic acid, serotonin, adenosine, histamine, bradykinin, interleukins, nerve growth factor, and substance P.

Metabolites of arachidonic acid

Arachidonic acid is derived from cell-membrane phospholipids by the action of the enzyme phospholipase A_2. This enzyme is activated by trauma or infection. Once released, arachidonic acid is acted on by two further enzyme systems. Cyclo-oxygenase activity results in the formation of prostaglandins, thromboxane, and prostacyclin, whereas lipo-oxygenase activity results in the production of the leukotrienes.

Prostaglandins

Prostaglandins of the E series (e.g. PGE_2) are particularly associated with the production of pain that accompanies trauma, infection, and injury. Intravenous and intramuscular injections of prostaglandins of the E series cause headache and long-lasting pain, respectively. The intradermal administration of histamine, bradykinin, or PGE_2 produces pain of short duration, but only PGE_2 causes hyperalgesia. Histamine, bradykinin, or PGE_2 do not produce pain when given singly via the subcutaneous route. However, the addition of PGE_2 to bradykinin or to histamine is overtly painful, whereas the further addition of bradykinin or histamine is not. In areas already sensitized by prostaglandins, subsequent infusions of bradykinin or histamine cause pain. These findings suggest that prostaglandins, particularly of the E series, are able to sensitize nociceptors to both chemical and mechanical stimulation.

Initially, it was thought that prostaglandins lowered the threshold of the polymodal nociceptors of C fibres. However, it is now speculated that distinct prostaglandin receptors may exist in a variety of tissues. The interaction between PGE_2 and polymodal nociceptors on C fibres may be due to a direct binding of these agonists to receptors on the free nerve fibre. Such binding may alter the sensitivity of the nerve ending to other mediators of pain and inflammation, notably histamine and bradykinin.

Leukotrienes

An intradermal injection of leukotriene B_4 (LTB_4) decreases the mechanical and thermal thresholds for nociception. The mode of action of LTB_4 in sensitizing nerve fibres appears to be similar to that produced by PGE_2. LTB_4 causes the release from polymorphonuclear leucocytes of a compound identified as 8R, 155-dihydroxyeicosatetraenoic acid. This compound also decreases the mechanical and thermal thresholds of C-fibre mechanonociceptors and produces mechanical hyperalgesia. A further leukotriene, LTD_4, can also sensitize sensory neurones indirectly by stimulating the synthesis and release of other leukotrienes and prostaglandins.

5-Hydroxytryptamine (5-HT; serotonin)

5-HT is an amine that is released from platelets and mast cells during tissue damage. When 5-HT is applied to raw skin (e.g. a blister base) is causes a mild and transient pain. This is due to activation of $5-HT_3$ receptors found on some small-diameter neurones. Pain produced by 5-HT can be inhibited by a specific $5-HT_3$ antagonist. In addition, 5-HT also sensitizes free nerve endings to the nociceptive actions of bradykinin.

Adenosine triphosphate (ATP) and adenosine

ATP is present in all cells and when released by tissue damage it can act on the surrounding cells including the sensory neurones.

An intradermal injection of micromolar concentrations of ATP produces a sharp, transient pain. This action is thought to be due to an opening of ion channels permeable to both Na^+ and Ca^{2+}. Adenosine, the breakdown product of ATP, also provokes pain when administered to a human blister base, and can produce hyperalgesia. The mechanisms of action of adenosine are not well understood, but are thought to be due to a direct effect on sensory neurones.

Histamine

This is a vasoactive amine released from mast cells when subjected to either mechanical or chemical trauma. In general, low concentrations of histamine induce itch, whereas higher concentrations produce pain. The mechanism of histamine-induced pain is uncertain. Some sensory neurones possess histamine H_1 receptors. Activation of these receptors increases membrane calcium permeability.

Bradykinin

Bradykinin is a polypeptide formed from plasma α_2-globulins by a complex series of proteolytic reactions. It is one of the most potent endogenous pain-producing (algogenic) substances released during inflammation. Bradykinin directly stimulates nociceptive nerve terminals and also sensitizes them to other stimuli including those of a mechanical and chemical nature. There is also synergism between the excitatory action of bradykinin and other endogenous mediators associated with pain (e.g. prostaglandins and 5-HT). The pharmacological effects of bradykinin are mediated via two main classes of bradykinin receptor, B_1 and B_2. The B_2 receptors are the most pharmacologically active. When bradykinin activates a B_2 receptor on nerve fibres, an inward (depolarizing) current is generated which results in an increase in membrane conductance to sodium ions.

Interleukins

A variety of cytokines (interleukins, interferons, tumour necrosis factor) are released by phagocytic and various immunocompetent cells. These molecules have a variety of fundamental functions in the inflammatory responses. They can also influence the activity of sensory neurones, probably by indirect routes. For example, interleukin-1β (IL-1β) and interleukin-6 (IL-6) can stimulate the release of prostaglandins. Thus, these cytokines enhance the important relationship between pain and inflammation.

Nerve growth factor (NGF)

This is a neurotrophic factor, produced in limited amounts by a range of cell types (e.g. fibroblasts and Schwann cells). NGF may be of considerable importance in inflammatory pain. Animal studies have shown that an injection of NGF leads to increased sensitivity to noxious stimuli, whereas animals exposed to antibodies to NGF have a reduced response to painful and inflammatory stimuli. It also stimulates the release of histamine and

leukotriene C_4 from human basophils. In inflammatory-induced hyperalgesia, there is likely to be a subtle interplay between the nerves, inflammatory cells, and resident tissue cells at sites of tissue damage. NGF may have a significant role in co-ordinating such interplay.

Substance P

This neurotransmitter (so-called because it is a powder) is located in 10–33% of dorsal root ganglion neurones and is transported to the peripheral primary afferent terminals. When released, it contributes to the inflammatory response by causing vasodilatation, increased vascular permeability, increased production and release of lysosomal enzymes, release of PGE_2, interleukins 1 and 6 (IL-1, and IL-6). Substance P does not have a direct effect on cutaneous nociceptors, but due to its proinflammatory effect it makes a significant contribution to hyperalgesia.

Key points
Peripheral mediators of pain

- The so-called peripheral mediators of pain are produced or released as a consequence of tissue damage and are intimately associated with inflammation.

- Many of the substances implicated in peripheral pain (nociception) stimulate free nerve endings to produce nociceptive impulses.

- Prostaglandins of the E series, bradykinin, and histamine are the most significant substances involved in nociception and hyperalgesia.

- Other substances that may play a role in inflammatory pain include 5-HT, ATP, nerve growth factor, and substance P.

Central mediators of pain

Transmission of nociceptive information from the primary afferent neurone to secondary, tertiary, and higher order neurones is achieved by chemical transmitters called neurotransmitters. Knowledge of central neurotransmitters is still relatively sparse and they are under intense study; consequently the picture is in a state of flux. It has become clear that, at any particular synapse, two or more transmitters may be simultaneously released (corelease), each performing a particular role. The resultant effect is due to the blend of the pharmacological soup released from the nerve endings that act on the nerve membrane of the neurone with which the neurotransmitter is communicating. This may be the postsynaptic membrane of the nerve cell of the next order (for example, transmission from primary to secondary neurone) or it may be the adjacent presynaptic endings of a neurone whose nerve cell is in a remote site. The former is an example of a neurotransmitter acting as a direct link between two neurones; the latter is an example of a neurotransmitter modulating transmission at an adjacent synapse by altering the release of neurotransmitter(s) from its presynaptic endings.

The central neurotransmitters involved in nociception can be classified by chemical type and also according to pharmacological action.

Amino acids

Aspartate and glutamate are ubiquitous and excite most nerve cells in the dorsal horn. Therefore, they are unlikely to be involved exclusively in the transmission of nociceptive information; presumably they operate in conjunction with other neurotransmitters and neuromodulators (see above). There is now strong evidence that these amino acids act on receptors specific for the exogenous chemical substance N-methyl-D-aspartate (NMDA) and which are therefore called NMDA receptors. These are now thought to play an important role in chronic neuropathic pain including some forms of chronic orofacial pain, for example post-herpetic neuralgia of the face.

By contrast, γ-aminobutyric acid (GABA) and glycine are endogenous inhibitory amino acids. GABA probably acts as an important postsynaptic inhibitor of the cell bodies of second-order neurones in the substantia gelatinosa (see Fig. 5.1). This explains the well-known phenomenon where rubbing a painful part of the body relieves the local pain. Rubbing stimulates tactile receptors and hence A nerve fibres. In turn, these probably activate an interneurone in the dorsal horn (Fig. 5.1), which releases GABA. GABA inhibits firing of the second-order neurone, thereby blocking the onward transmission of nociceptive information to the brain. The elegant experimental work of Duggan and Foong (1985) provides strong evidence for this mechanism.

Peptides

With the aid of modern microchemical techniques, a large number of neuropeptides have been isolated from the dorsal horn of the spinal cord. Unfortunately, the precise role played by each these agents is far from clear and it will take a great deal of study before a complete picture can be assembled. The neuropeptides can be divided into two main groups:

(1) the opioid peptides—the endorphins and enkephalins;
(2) the non-opioid peptides—which include substance P (one of the tachykinins), vasoactive intestinal peptide (VIP), cholecystokinin (CCK), somatostatin, bombesin, neurotensin, and calcitonin gene-related peptide (CGRP).

Only the opioid peptides and substance P will be discussed in this chapter.

Opioid peptides (see Table 5.3)

The term 'opioid' means opiate-like and is used to refer to any substance possessing pharmacological actions like those of an opiate such as morphine, but which is chemically unrelated to an opiate. The actions of opioids are blocked by specific opioid antagonists such as naloxone.

Enkephalins

These peptides were originally identified in pig brain extracts by Hughes et al. (1975). Two structurally similar peptides were found—methionine enkephalin (Met-enkephalin) and leucine enkephalin (Leu-enkephalin)—each of which is derived by enzymatic cleavage from a larger and independent precursor, proenkephalin A. It was then discovered that the Met-enkephalin amino-acid sequence is present in pituitary peptide, β-lipotropin, as residues 61–65. Soon afterwards, it was shown that the C-fragment of β-lipotropin (residues 61–91) interacts specifically with opioid receptors: it is now known as β-endorphin (see below).

All these peptides have properties in common with morphine, such as production of analgesia, physical dependence and tolerance, and the contraction of smooth muscle. Their actions can be reversed or blocked by the specific opioid antagonist naloxone. There is now evidence that the enkephalins are neurotransmitters of specific (enkephalinergic) nerve fibres in the brain that modulate sensory information pertaining to pain and emotional behaviour. Regional variations in enkephalin levels parallel the distribution of opioid receptors. The levels of enkephalins are highest in brain fractions that contain nerve terminals, and their concentration profile is similar to the distribution of opioid receptors (Akil et al. 1984).

The dynorphins

These may act as neurotransmitters or neurohormones; they are produced by enzymatic cleavage from the precursor, prodynorphin. The dynorphins are larger peptides than the enkephalins but their physiological role is uncertain.

The endorphins

There are at least four endorphins—peptides designated α-, β-, γ-, and δ-endorphins—of which β-endorphin is the most significant. All are derived by enzymatic cleavage from the precursor pro-opiomelanocortin, which is also the precursor for β-lipotropin and corticotropin.

The endorphins are neurohormones that are released into the bloodstream and have a variable duration of action. They are found mainly in the anterior pituitary gland, in the same cells as corticotropin and β-lipotropin. All these hormones are secreted in parallel during stress, possibly as an adaptive mechanism: the endorphins may help to relieve any pain which the individual might then incur.

The discovery that β-endorphin has potent and long-lasting analgesic activity (Omaya et al. 1980), which can be reversed by the opioid antagonist naloxone, suggested it was the long-sought, non-addictive analgesic. It seemed a reasonable assumption that humans are unlikely to become addicted to an

Table 5.3 Classification of opioid peptides and their receptors

	Mu (μ)	Delta (δ)	Kappa (κ)	Sigma (σ)*
Putative endogenous agonists (opioid peptides)	β-endorphin	Met-enkephalin; Leu-enkephalin	Dynorphin A1–13 Dynorphin A1–8; Dynorphin B	?
Distribution of peptidergic neurones	Anterior pituitary; hypothalamus	Striatum; preoptic hypothalamus; limbic system; raphe nuclei; spinal cord; adrenal medulla; sympathetic ganglia; myenteric ganglia	Posterior pituitary; hypothalamus; spinal cord; submucus plexus of GI tract	?
Potency order of endogenous agonists	β-end > dyn A > Met > Leu	Met = Leu–β-end > dyn A	dyn A >> β-end >> Leu = Met	
Synthetic agonist	Morphine	DPDPE (experimental)	Pentazocine	Phencyclidine; Pentazocine
Antagonist	Naloxone	Naloxone; but less potent than at μ	Naloxone; but less potent than at μ	Naloxone; but less potent than at μ
Effector pathways	cAMP →	cAMP →	?	?
Ion-channel actions	K^+ channel activator	K^+ channel activator	Ca^{2+} channel inhibitor	?
Effects:				
– Analgesia	Supraspinal analgesia	Analgesia	Spinal analgesia	No analgesia
– Psychotropic	Euphoria[†]	Euphoria[†]	Sedation	Dysphoria ± hallucinations
– Respiration	Respiratory depression	Respiratory depression	Respiratory depression	Respiratory and motor stimulation
– GI tract	Constipation (central)	Constipation (peripheral)	—	—
– Pupil	Miosis	—	Miosis	Mydriasis
– Dependence	Physical dependence	—	Physical dependence (nalorphine type)	—

* Sigma receptors are not considered to belong to the family of opioid receptors. However, they are important because some of the side-effects produced by opioids are probably due to the stimulation of sigma receptors.

† With clinical opioid analgesia 'euphoria' implies a sense of peaceful well-being that accompanies the relief of pain. By contrast with opioid abuse (especially intravenous administration or 'mainlining') the word 'euphoria' implies a state of temporary ecstasy.

DPDPE is D-penicillamine, D-penicillamine enkephalin. (Thompson 1990.)

endogenous substance. However, in experimental animals, repeated injections of β-endorphin have produced tolerance and dependence.

If there is a pain-suppressing system, why do people feel pain? The answer may be connected with the fact that a painful stimulus activates both A-δ and C fibres. Pain transmitted by A-δ fibres (first pain) acts as a warning system; this type of pain is hardly affected by morphine or other opioids. C-fibre-induced pain is perhaps more clinically relevant, and is affected by morphine. It may be inferred that pain of a protracted nature (suffering) is more likely to be modulated by endorphin release than warning pain: suppression of protracted post-traumatic pain may serve a useful purpose.

The human placenta produces β-endorphin (Houck *et al.* 1980), which may be distributed to the fetus, so exposing it to high perinatal endorphin levels. However, the significance of this is unclear. Behavioural investigations have shown that pain sensitivity in newborn babies is relatively low when compared with adults, although pain reactions can be evoked. Sensitivity becomes much greater after a few days of life. This pattern of reaction to pain may be related to residual maternal levels of β-endorphin in the central nervous system.

Pain sensitivity varies between ethnic groups, and there are correlations between experimental measures of pain and β-endorphin levels in the cerebrospinal fluid (CSF). Patients with high endorphin levels have high pain thresholds and high pain tolerance levels. At the risk of oversimplification, it seems that constitutional differences in response to pain, and differences in attitude to potentially painful or other noxious stimuli, may be related to endorphin activity (von Knorring *et al.* 1978).

Certain pathological conditions are characterized by abnormal insensitivity to pain. One such is congenital analgesia, in which there may be a central defect. However, two cases have been reported of patients who responded to naloxone, with a lowering of pain threshold and a return to pain responsiveness (Dehen *et al.* 1978; Yanagida 1978). This response suggests that these patients may have excessive endorphin production and activity. Patients with schizophrenia seldom complain during venepuncture, lumbar puncture, or other painful diagnostic procedures, and their pain sensitivity also increases after they have received naloxone. Schizophrenics and patients with endogenous depression frequently have elevated CSF levels of endorphins (Bellenger *et al.* 1979; Geschwind 1975).

Opioid receptors

These were first isolated in 1973 (Pert and Snyder 1973), and four types have been described—μ (mu), κ (kappa), δ (delta), and σ (sigma). Strictly speaking, the σ-receptor is not a pure opioid receptor but it is included in this group because it is activated by some opioids, and accounts for certain unwanted effects. Subtypes of μ-receptors (for example μ_1 and μ_2) have also been described. The effects of stimulating the different opioid receptors together with the sources of the endogenous ligands are summarized in Table 5.3.

Morphine and related compounds appear to have different affinities for the various opioid receptors, which may account for many of their differing pharmacological properties. Opioid receptors are found throughout the central nervous system: there are high concentrations in the limbic system, the substantia gelatinosa, the spinal nucleus of the fifth cranial nerve (V), and the thalamus. The receptors appear to be the site of action of the endogenous opioid peptides—the enkephalins, dynorphins, and endorphins (Chang and Cuatrecasas 1981; Martin 1983).

Substance P

Substance P (so-called because it was a powder) is a polypeptide, discovered by von Euler and Gaddum (1931). Evidence suggests that substance P is a neurotransmitter in small-diameter fibres, particularly C fibres. Staining techniques have shown that substance P is found in the following areas related to pain:

(1) cell bodies of posterior root ganglia projecting to the substantia gelatinosa of the spinal cord;
(2) caudal division of the trigeminal (V) spinal nucleus;
(3) nucleus raphe pallidus and magnus;
(4) periaqueductal grey area.

That substance P is specifically related to pain is indicated by the disappearance of nerve endings containing it (sited in the caudal division of the trigeminal nerve) after removal of tooth pulps in cats. The tooth pulp is innervated almost exclusively by pain fibres.

In general, endogenous opioid peptides suppress pain, whereas substance P promotes it (Sweet 1980). However, application of substance P to exposed tooth pulp does not excite sensory neurones and its role in the pulp is still obscure (Gazelius *et al.* 1977). Substance P and enkephalins do interact: the release of substance P is inhibited not only by Met-enkephalin, but also by β-endorphin and morphine.

The role of substance P and enkephalins in pain transmission

The discovery of the interaction between substance P, enkephalins, and opioid receptors (Jessel and Iversen 1977) helps to explain some neuropharmacological aspects of the gate-control theory of pain (Melzack and Wall 1965).

Within the substantia gelatinosa, a nociceptive impulse transmitted via small C fibres causes the release of substance P at the synapse (Fig. 5.1(a)). Substance P binds to specific postsynaptic receptors, and the impulse is transmitted onwards. Synapsing with the small C-fibre terminal is an enkephalinergic fibre that releases Met-enkephalin on excitation. Met-enkephalin binds to opioid receptors on the terminal of the C fibre, hyperpolarizes the membrane, and so inhibits the release of substance P. If this happens, the nerve impulse carrying nociceptive information does not progress beyond the synapse.

The enkephalinergic fibres are, in turn, connected to the cortex via the nucleus raphe magnus. The transmitter substance in raphe neurones is not enkephalin, but 5-hydroxytryptamine (5-HT). Their terminals synapse with and activate enkephalinergic interneurones in the substantia gelatinosa (Fig. 5.6). Activity in the nucleus raphe magnus is under the descending control of the cortex.

In addition to the enkephalinergic pain-suppressing system, activity in the large sensory A-β fibres can cause presynaptic inhibition (depolarization) of activity in small-fibre (C-fibre) terminals. This mechanism constitutes the gate control. Clinically, the gate control can be activated by transcutaneous electrical nerve stimulation (TENS) in which high-frequency, low-intensity electrical pulses pass through pad electrodes. Analgesia produced by this stimulation is not naloxone-reversible (Thompson and Filshie 1993).

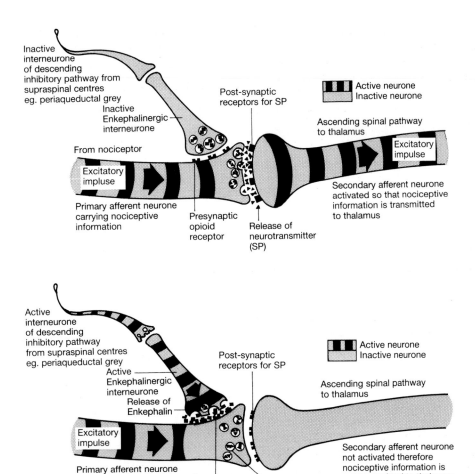

Fig. 5.6 The interaction between an enkephalinergic fibre and a C fibre.

Key points
Central mediators of pain

- A variety of substances have a role as central mediators in nociception and pain. Of the many substances identified, the most significant are the opioid peptides and substance P.

- The family of opioid peptides can be further categorized into enkephalins, dynorphins, and endorphins.

- The enkephalins (met- and leu-enkephalin) are neurotransmitters found in enkephalinergic fibres that modulate nociception and emotional behaviour.

- Dynorphins may act as either neurotransmitters or neurohormones.

- Endorphins are neurohormones released from the anterior pituitary (along with β-lipotropin and corticotropin).

- Activity of the various opioid peptides can be reversed by naloxone, which suggests that these endogenous compounds exert their pharmacological actions via the opioid receptors.

- Four types of opioid receptors have been described: μ(mu), κ (kappa), δ (delta), and σ (sigma). Mu and kappa receptors are mainly involved with nociception.

- Substance P is a neurotransmitter specifically related to pain and nociception.

- In general, substance P promotes pain, whereas opioid peptides suppress pain.

Central processing of pain and its control by therapeutic agents

The earlier sections of this chapter have presented an account of the anatomical, physiological, and pharmacological basis of pain, or to be more accurate, of nociception. Nociceptive information may or may not reach the higher centres of the brain, where it is interpreted as a painful response. This section aims to draw together and summarize the different systems and mechanisms. It should be read in conjunction with Fig. 5.1.

Sensory receptors

For the purpose of this account only three sensory modalities need be considered:

1. *Tactile or touch receptors* connected to A-β nerve fibres, which conduct tactile information, for example rubbing the skin.

2. *High-threshold mechanoreceptors* connected to A-δ nerve fibres, which conduct nociceptive information of the type induced by a strong mechanical stimulus, for example a pinprick. Activation of this pathway gives rise to 'first', 'rapid', or 'aversive' pain (see Table 5.2).

3. *Polymodal nociceptors* connected to unmyelinated C nerve fibres, which conduct nociceptive information of the type induced by physical, chemical, or mechanical stimulation. Activation of this pathway (probably with activation of some A-δ fibres) gives rise to 'second,' 'slow', or 'tissue-damage' pain (see Table 5.2).

Connections of primary afferent neurones in the spinal cord

The A-β, A-δ, and C-fibre pathways pass through the dorsal root to the spinal cord, where they connect with the dorsal columns and the spinothalamic, and spinoreticular tracts.

C nerve fibres

In an inflamed area of skin, polymodal nociceptors connected to C fibres are excited by chemical, physical, and mechanical stimulation. Nociceptive impulses pass from the peripheral to the central end of the fibre, which synapses with second-order neurones in the substantia gelatinosa (lamina 2) in the dorsal horn of the spinal cord. The axons of the second-order neurones cross to the opposite side of the spinal cord where they synapse with other neurones which then form the spinoreticular tract. This is a polysynaptic tract that eventually becomes the reticular formation and from where fibres ascend to end in the intralaminar nucleus of the thalamus and also in the hypothalamus. From the intralaminar nucleus of the thalamus, other neurones arise to form a diffuse projection system that passes to the prefrontal cortex, the limbic system, and the whole non-primary cortex. The emotional experience of pain, which has affective and evaluative components, is believed to be represented in these areas of the brain.

A-β nerve fibres

Stroking the skin excites tactile receptors and generates impulses in A-β fibres that travel to the dorsal horn and up the dorsal columns to end in the cuneate and gracile nuclei. From here the information ascends via second-order neurones that decussate to reach the contralateral sensory cortex after relaying in the thalamus. However, the A-β fibre gives off an important collateral which is thought to synapse with a short interneurone, the ending of which forms an inhibitory synapse with the cells of the substantia gelatinosa (see Fig. 5.1). When the tactile receptors are stimulated, this neuronal pathway is activated via the interneurone, and causes the release of an inhibitory transmitter, possibly GABA. This prevents the stimulation of the substantia gelatinosa cell by excitatory transmitters such as those released from the central endings of the C fibres on stimulation of polymodal nociceptors, thus blocking transmission of this nociceptive information to the higher centres. This antagonism between the inputs of the A-β and C fibres forms the basis of the gate-control system (Melzack and Wall 1965). It explains how rubbing or stroking a sore part of the body relieves the pain, and how this can be done more precisely using TENS.

A-δ nerve fibres

Stimulation of high-threshold mechanoreceptors has two important effects. The first is activation of primary afferent A-δ neurones, which excite the second-order Waldeyer cells whose axons then cross to the other side of the spinal cord and ascend as the spinothalamic tract. This terminates in the ventrobasal nucleus of the thalamus to synapse with third-order neurones, which are somatotopically projected to the sensory cortex where the sensory component of pain is analysed. *En route*, the spinothalamic tract gives off important collaterals to the periaqueductal grey (see below).

The second important consequence of activating A-δ fibres by stimulation of high-threshold mechanoreceptors is to activate short enkephalinergic neurones in the dorsal horn which synapse with the substantia gelatinosa cells. This dual connection of A-δ fibres, activation of high-threshold mechanoreceptors by a stimulus such as a pinprick, leads both to accurately localized pain and to inhibition of transmission of nociceptive information from polymodal nociceptors. This phenomenon forms the basis of segmental analgesia induced by acupuncture (Thompson and Filshie 1993).

Descending pathways

An important function of the descending inhibitory pathways in the spinal cord is to inhibit the onward transmission of nociceptive information as it enters the dorsal horn. The inhibitory pathway descends from the periaqueductal grey area to the raphe nuclei, from where it descends in the dorsolateral funiculus of the spinal cord (see Fig. 5.1(a)). At each segmental level (only one segment is shown in the diagram), axons from the dorsolateral funiculus peal off to synapse with the enkephalinergic neurones.

The periaqueductal grey area contains a complex of neurones that respond to opioid peptides (and hence also to opiates such as morphine) by activating the descending pain-inhibitory pathways. These include neurones that release 5-HT and norepinephrine (noradrenaline) where they synapse with the enkephalinergic neurones in the dorsal horn. Drugs that facilitate transmission at synapses where 5-HT and/or norepinephrine are neurotransmitters can produce useful analgesic effects in certain chronic pain conditions. For example, low doses of tricyclic antidepressant drugs (for example amitriptyline) are used widely (see below).

The periaqueductal grey area receives important inputs from the spinothalamic tract, from the hypothalamus, and, via the hypothalamus, from the prefrontal cortex (see Fig. 5.1(a)). A long feedback loop is formed through the following connections: enkephalinergic neurone in the dorsal horn–Waldeyer cells and spinothalamic tract–periaqueductal grey–raphe nuclei–dorsolateral funiculus–enkephalinergic neurone.

This loop is activated when high-threshold mechanoreceptors are stimulated, and this is thought to be the mechanism involved in the extrasegmental effect of acupuncture The descending pain-inhibitory pathway is also thought to be activated by cognitive processing in the prefrontal cortex, which influences the periaqueductal grey via connections in the hypothalamus (via the arcuate nucleus which is not shown in Fig. 5.1). It seems likely that this connection allows the emotional component of pain to be influenced by higher psychological processing such as occurs with cognitive therapy, behavioural therapy, relaxation therapy, and hypnosis.

This summary has stressed the modern concept that pain has both sensory and emotional components; that the neuronal connection between the periphery and centre is highly selective; and that there is no single part of the brain which is the 'pain centre'. Many different areas of the central nervous system are involved in processing nociception and pain, so the experience of pain can be modified by many different physical and psychological factors. As a consequence, clinical pain conditions can be treated by different methods, sometimes used in combination.

Methods to relieve pain

The many methods used to relieve pain may at first sight seem to form a heterogeneous collection. In fact, if the principles of neuroanatomy, neurophysiology, and neuropharmacology of nociception and pain are applied to the therapeutic control of pain, the apparent wide variety of approaches can be condensed into the five basic methods summarized in Table 5.4 and described below.

1 REMOVE PERIPHERAL STIMULUS: To remove the causative factor by, for example, extracting a carious tooth is simple in theory, but may not be so easy to carry out in practice. Alternatively, the peripheral stimulus can be detached by

Table 5.4 Methods to relieve pain

	Method	Examples
1.	Remove peripheral stimulus	Surgical, e.g. ablation Cryotherapy Neurolytic, e.g. phenol, ethanol Radiotherapy, to shrink neoplasm Pharmacological, e.g. NSAID, corticosteroid; antiepileptic for neuroma
2.	Interrupt nociceptive input	Pharmacological: non-invasive, e.g. NSAID; invasive, e.g. local anaesthetic Surgical: e.g. neurectomy
3.	Stimulate nociceptive inhibitory mechanisms	Massage and spinal mobilization; TENS; vibration (A-β fibres) Heat thermoreceptors, A-β fibres Cold thermoreceptors, A-β fibres Electro/acupuncture nociceptors, A-β fibres Counterirritants nociceptors, ?C fibres
4.	Modulate central appreciation of pain and/or emotional concomitants	Pharmacological, e.g. opioid analgesics, Psychotropic drugs, general Anaesthetics Psychological, e.g. school for bravery, cognitive/behavioural therapy, counselling, relaxation, biofeedback, hypnosis
5.	Block or remove secondary factors maintaining pain	Sympathetic nerve block: Pharmacological, e.g. adrenoceptor blocker; Physical, e.g. chemical, surgical Vasodilators for pain associated with vascular spasm Antiseptics for pain associated with spasm of skeletal muscle Other, e.g. pituitary ablation for widespread cancer pain

surgery or destroyed by cryotherapy (freezing), neurolysis (with phenol or ethanol), or radiotherapy. A more selective method is to use a pharmacological agent such as a non-steroidal anti-inflammatory drug (NSAID), which, possibly through suppression of superoxide formation, can help to bring about physical resolution of the inflamed area evoking pain. Another method is to use a corticosteroid to reduce the raised tissue pressure associated with local inflammation. In a neuroma, nociceptive impulse generators may be silenced by an anticonvulsant drug.

2 INTERRUPT NOCICEPTIVE INPUT: At the periphery, nociceptive input can be interrupted by blocking the production of the prostaglandins that sensitize the polymodal nociceptors to pain-inducing agents such as bradykinin. Alternatively, a local anaesthetic can be applied to sensory nerve endings or to a main nerve trunk. A radical, but irreversible, approach is to cut the nerve trunk transmitting nociceptive information to the spinal cord. However, this may trigger the development of neuropathic (neurogenic) pain, which is severe, unpleasant (allodynia and dyaesthesia), and can be exceedingly difficult to control. For this reason, neurectomy is now used only to control the pain of a patient whose life expectancy is short.

3 STIMULATE NOCICEPTIVE INHIBITORY MECHANISMS: It has always been known that when a part of the body is hurt it is often helpful to stimulate it gently by stroking, rubbing, massage, and applying heat or cold. More sophisticated methods include acupuncture, electroacupuncture, TENS, and, most recently, transcutaneous spinal electroanalgesia (TSE). All these methods stimulate tactile or thermal receptors or high-threshold mechanoreceptors connected to the larger groups of sensory nerve fibres (A-β and A-δ) in skin and also some in underlying muscle (group III), except TSE, the mechanism of which is unknown (see Fig. 5.1).

TENS is the most readily controlled method of stimulating A-β fibres connected to the tactile receptors. However, for it to be effective, the electrical stimulation must be strong enough to produce tingling ('pins and needles') in the stimulated area. Although TENS can be used to produce dental analgesia, it is uncomfortable for the patient and newer forms of electroanalgesia are being developed that are more comfortable and effective, for example Cedeta (cell demodulated electronic targeted anaesthesia).

4 MODULATE CENTRAL APPRECIATION OF PAIN AND/OR EMOTIONAL CONCOMITANTS: Because pain is an unpleasant sensory and emotional experience, it is not surprising that it can be relieved by modulating the emotional component even when the sensory component cannot be attenuated.

The emotional component of pain is a combination of affect and evaluation, and one or both can be modulated by pharmacological and/or psychological methods. For example, opioid analgesics, such as morphine, produce a profound change in both the affective and the evaluative components of severe pain. Patients taking morphine often comment that, although they can still feel their pain, it no longer troubles them. This effect is thought to be due to morphine stimulating opioid receptors in the cingulate cortex, which is concerned with the emotional component of pain. Similarly, psychotropic drugs, particularly certain antidepressants, can be used in low doses to modulate the emotional response to pain even in patients who are not clinically depressed. General anaesthetics produce a relatively unselective inhibition of brain function, which can only be achieved at the price of loss of consciousness.

The remarkably potent analgesic effects of psychological manipulation, for instance by suggestion and distraction, have been marshalled for therapeutic use by clinical psychologists. These technique are of particular benefit for patients suffering from chronic pain conditions that have failed to yield to other methods of pain control, and these methods are often used in pain relief clinics. The emotional component of dental pain and a visit to the dental surgery raises the problem of how members of the general public, especially their children, should be educated and counselled before undergoing dental treatment. Techniques such as relaxation therapy, biofeedback therapy, and hypnosis can all be effective in patients who are very anxious before or during dental treatment.

5 BLOCK OR REMOVE SECONDARY FACTORS: Some pain conditions are triggered or maintained by secondary factors, and these need to be treated before the patient can obtain adequate or lasting pain relief. Important examples are: overactivity of the sympathetic nervous system (causing reflex sympathetic dystrophy); vascular spasm (in some forms of peripheral vascular disease); and spasm of skeletal muscle (muscle cramps). These conditions are treated with, respectively, an adrenoceptor blocker, a vasodilator, and an antispastic agent. In the case of overactivity of the sympathetic nervous system, an alternative approach would be surgical sympathectomy of the affected part. In some forms of widespread cancer pain, ablation of the pituitary gland is followed by rapid and dramatic relief of pain, although the mechanism for this is still not clear.

Key points
Methods to relieve pain

- Several methods can be employed to relieve pain by blocking or removing the nociception stimuli at various stages of conduction throughout the CNS.

- Removal of the peripheral stimulus can involve a tooth extraction or pulp extirpation in the case of dental pain. NSAIDs and corticosteroids also have peripheral activity.

- Interrupt nociceptive impulse: this involves the use of NSAIDs and local anaesthetic agents.

- Stimulate nociceptive inhibitory mechanisms: TENS is probably the most useful application of such an approach to control pain at this level.

- Modulate the central appreciation of pain and/or emotional concomitants: opioids and various psychotropic drugs bring about 'pain relief' by such a central action.

- Block or remove secondary factors: drugs that target the sympathetic nervous system, or reduce spasms in blood vessels or muscles, may be useful adjuncts in pain control.

Rational treatment of dental pain

Whatever the pain, it is essential to try to diagnose its cause before attempting treatment. Some pains are simple to diagnose and to treat rationally, but others are very difficult to diagnose and consequently can only be treated empirically. Where more than one pain exists it is essential to try to diagnose and treat each pain separately. A combination of analgesic methods should only be used when single treatments have failed.

Future developments in analgesia

There is enormous scope for improving methods of analgesia but progress will depend on unravelling pain mechanisms. NSAIDs are the analgesics prescribed most commonly for the treatment of dental pain. The development of COX-2 enzyme inhibitors could have a significant impact on dental pain control (see Chapter 4). These compounds are likely to as effective as most NSAIDs (which inhibit both COX-1 and COX-2), but have fewer unwanted effects. A further approach would be to find compounds that interfere with another key step in the stimulation of the nociceptors. This requires a better understanding of nociceptor mechanisms than is yet available, but this approach is being pursued by at least one major pharmaceutical company.

It is also worthwhile to consider developing new methods to tackle the central end of nociception. One technique is to use psychotherapy to modulate activity in areas of the brain where the affective and evaluative components of pain are processed. A simple approach is to counsel patients before dental treatment. This could well represent a good economic investment because of the long-term positive effect it would produce on the dental health of the public and their general well-being. It could also obviate the need for expensive drugs with their potential for producing adverse reactions. Novel drugs with highly selective actions on the emotional and/or evaluative components of pain would still be extremely useful for the control of dental and other pains. Indeed, where necessary, they might be used in conjunction with counselling. Dental pain control has an exciting and rewarding future.

References

Akil, H., Watson, S. J., Young, E., Lewis, M. E., Khachaturian, H., and Walker, J. M. (1984). Endogenous opioids: biology and function. *Annual Review of Neuroscience*, 7, 223–55.

Bellenger, J. C., Post, R. M., Sternberg, D. E., Kammen, D. P., Cowdry, R. W., and Goodwin, F. K. (1979). Headaches after lumbar puncture and insensitivity to pain in psychiatric patients. *New England Journal of Medicine*, 30, 110.

Bowsher, D. (1980). Central mechanisms of orofacial pain. *British Journal of Oral Surgery*, 17, 185–97.

Chang, K. W. and Cuatrecasas, P. (1981). Heterogeneity and properties of opiate receptors. *Federation Proceedings*, 40, 2729–34.

Dehen, H., Willer, J. G., Prier, S., Boureau, F., and Chambier, J. (1978). Congenital insensitivity to pain and the morphine-like analgesic system. *Pain*, 5, 351–8.

Duggan, A. W. and Foong, F. W. (1985). Bicuculline and spinal inhibition produced by dorsal column stimulation in the cat. *Pain*, 22, 249–59.

Gazelius, B., Olgart, L., Edwall, L., and Trowbridge, H. O. (1977). Effects of substance P on sensory nerves and blood flow in the feline dental pulp. In *Pain in the trigeminal region* (ed. D. J. Anderson and B. Matthews) pp. 95–101. Elsevier, Amsterdam.

Geschwind, N. (1975). Insensitivity to pain in psychotic patients. *New England Journal of Medicine*, 296, 1480.

Houck, J. G., Kimball, C., Chang, G., Pedigo, N. W. Y., and Yamamuraz, H. I. (1980). Placental beta-endorphin-like peptides. *Science*, 207, 78–9.

Hughes, J. H., Smith, T. W., Kosterlitz, H. W., Fothergill, I. A., Morgan, B., and Morris, H. R. (1975). Identification of two related pentapeptides from the brain with potent opiate agonist activity. *Nature*, 258, 577–9.

International Association for the Study of Pain: Subcommittee on Taxonomy. Classification of chronic pain; descriptions of chronic pain syndromes and definition of pain terms (1986). *Pain*, Suppl. 3, S1–S225.

Jessel, T. M. and Iversen, L. L. (1977). Opiate analgesics inhibit substance P release from rat trigeminal nucleus. *Nature*, 268, 549–51.

Martin, W. R. (1983). Pharmacology of opioids. *Pharmacology Review*, 35, 283–323.

Melzack, R. and Wall, P. (1965). Pain mechanisms: a new theory. *Science*, 150, 971–9.

Omaya, T., Jin, T., Yamaya, R., Ling, N., and Guillemin, R. (1980). Profound analgesic effects of beta-endorphin in man. *Lancet*, i, 122–6.

Pert, C. B. and Snyder, S. H. (1973). Opiate receptor: demonstration in nervous tissue. *Science*, 179, 101–4.

Sweet, W. H. (1980). Neuropeptides and monoaminergic neurotransmitters: their relation to pain. *Journal of the Royal Society of Medicine*, 73, 482–9.

Thompson, J. W. (1990). Clinical pharmacology of opioid agonists and partial agonists. In *Opioids in the treatment of cancer pain* (ed. D. Doyle), Royal Society of Medicine Services International Congress and Symposium Series, No. 146, pp. 17–38. Royal Society of Medicine Services; London.

Thompson, J. W. and Filshie, J. (1993). Transcutaneous electrical nerve stimulation (TENS) and acupuncture. Chapter 4.2.8. In *Oxford textbook of palliative medicine*, (ed. D. Doyle, G. W. C. Hanks, and N. Macdonald), pp. 229–44. Oxford University Press.

von Euler, U. S., and Gaddum, J. H. (1931). Unidentified depressor substance in certain tissue extracts. *Journal of Physiology*, 72, 74–87.

Von Knorring, L., Almay, B. G. L., Johansson, F., and Terenius, L. (1978). Pain perception and endorphin levels in cerebrospinal fluid. *Pain*, 5, 359–67.

Yanagida, H. (1978). Congenital insensitivity and naloxone. *Lancet*, ii, 520–1.

Further reading

Hockfelt, T. (1991). Neuropeptides in perspective: the last 10 years. *Neuron*, 7, 867–79.

6

Aspirin, other non-steroidal anti-inflammatory drugs, and paracetamol

- Aspirin
- Para-aminophenols
- Other NSAIDs
- Further reading

Aspirin, other non-steroidal anti-inflammatory drugs, and paracetamol

The non-steroidal anti-inflammatory drugs (NSAIDs), or aspirin-like analgesics, interfere with the biochemical mediators of inflammation (Chapter 4), especially those associated with pain. Most of these drugs inhibit the synthesis of the prostaglandins by blocking the cyclo-oxygenase enzyme system at or near the site of injury. Hence these analgesics are sometimes referred to as peripherally acting analgesics. In addition to their analgesic properties, they have anti-inflammatory and central antipyretic activity. All these properties are important in the treatment of dental pain.

The prostaglandins, particularly PGE_2, sensitize free nerve endings to the nociceptive properties of histamine and bradykinin, which produce pain (see Chapter 4). Therefore any analgesic that inhibits the production of prostaglandins will primarily reduce pain occurring at the site of inflammation.

Aspirin

Aspirin (acetylsalicylic acid) is the most widely used medicinal agent in the Western world. It is a weak organic acid structurally related to salacin, a natural product found in willow bark (*Salix alba*). The drug is nearly always taken orally, and soluble preparations are more efficacious than tablet formulations. The normal dose of aspirin is 300 mg.

Pharmacokinetics

Aspirin is rapidly absorbed from the gastrointestinal tract, partly from the stomach, but mainly from the upper small intestine. It is then quickly hydrolysed to salicylate by esterase enzymes (aspirin esterases) in the gut wall, blood, and liver. The half-life of aspirin in humans is 20–30 minutes, whereas that of salicylate is 2–3 hours at low doses, but it is 12 hours at anti-inflammatory doses due to saturation of metabolism.

Salicylate is excreted in the urine mainly as salicyluric acid and glucuronides, with 10% excreted unchanged. In the liver, salicylate is conjugated with glycine and glucuronic acid to form salicyluric acid, and acyl and phenolic glucuronides, respectively (Fig. 6.1). A very small fraction of salicylic acid is converted to gentisic acid.

Pharmacodynamics

There is now convincing evidence that many of aspirin's pharmacological properties come from its ability to inhibit the synthesis of the important chemical mediators—the eicosanoids (in particular, the prostaglandins, prostacyclin, and thromboxane; see Chapter 4). Aspirin irreversibly inhibits both cyclo-oxygenase 1 and 2 (COX-1 and COX-2) by acetylating serine 530, thus preventing the binding of arachidonic acid to the active sites of the enzymes. This action, in turn, prevents the synthesis of the prostaglandins. It is now considered that the analgesic and anti-inflammatory actions of aspirin are attributable to inhibition of COX-2, whereas the unwanted effects of aspirin (see below) are due to inhibition of COX-1. In addition to the effects of aspirin, its metabolite, salicylate, also inhibits cyclo-oxygenases.

Pharmacological properties

Analgesic

Aspirin is usually classified as a mild analgesic. It is effective against pain associated with inflammation, such as dental and rheumatic pain. It is also widely used to relieve headaches, migraines, and dysmenorrhoea. Aspirin's analgesic properties are mainly due to the inhibition of the synthesis of prostaglandins PGE_1 and PGE_2. Suitable dose regimens are 600–1200 mg every 4–6 hours. Other putative analgesic actions of aspirin may partly be related to its anti-inflammatory properties (see below), or due to additional antinociceptive activity at both peripheral and central neurones.

Anti-inflammatory

These properties are also related to aspirin's ability to inhibit the COX-2 enzyme and thus the synthesis of eicosanoids, which are important mediators of inflammation (see Chapter 4). In addition, aspirin and other NSAIDs may inhibit the expression or activity of certain endothelial cell-adhesion molecules. This action will have an inhibitory effect on the migration of polymorphonuclear neutrophils (PMNs) and other white blood cells and, hence, will further suppress the inflammatory response. Similarly, aspirin and NSAIDs can directly inhibit the activation and function of PMNs; this is considered to be an important property in the use of these drugs in the management of rheumatoid arthritis.

Antipyretic

Aspirin effectively and rapidly lowers an elevated body temperature (pyrexia) due to infection, tissue damage, malignancy, or other disease states. It has no effect on normal body temperature

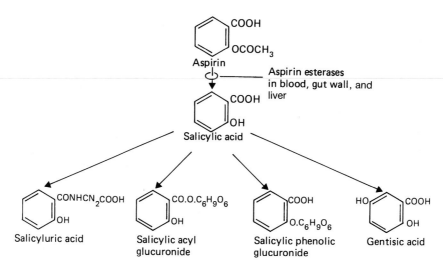

Fig. 6.1 The metabolism of aspirin.

and does not reduce body temperature raised by exercise or ambient heat.

Infection or inflammation is accompanied by the release of cytokines—including interleukin-1β, interleukin-6, interferons, and tumour necrosis factor—from white blood cells. These compounds stimulate the synthesis of prostaglandins of the E series in the hypothalamus, causing a rise in body temperature. The antipyretic properties of aspirin and aspirin-like drugs are due to their inhibition of prostaglandin production in the hypothalamus.

Antithrombotic (Antiplatelet)

These properties are described in Chapter 13.

Unwanted effects

Aspirin has many unwanted effects and they vary markedly between individuals. Some effects are related to dosage and chronic usage.

Gastrointestinal

Aspirin causes a high incidence of gastrointestinal disturbances including epigastric pain, nausea, and gastric erosions leading to blood loss. Faecal blood loss is often related to dose and can be as much as 3–10 mL per day. The blood loss is enhanced by the inhibitory action of aspirin on platelet aggregation (see Chapter 13) The ulcerogenic properties of aspirin are related to its direct irritant effect as well as to prostaglandin inhibition. The gastrointestinal tract is lined with a protective layer of mucus, and prostaglandins (especially PGI_2 and PGE_2) are essential for the synthesis of mucus. In addition, prostaglandins have an inhibitory action on gastric acid production (see Chapter 18). Aspirin and other NSAIDs inhibit prostaglandin synthesis, thus as a consequence there is impaired mucus production and increased gastric

acid production. Both actions makes the gastric mucosa more susceptible to damage. Aspirin should therefore be avoided in patients who suffer from peptic ulceration or inflammatory disease of the gut. If it is essential to use aspirin or similar drugs in such patients, then the prostaglandin analogue, misoprostol, will prevent gastric and duodenal ulceration. Alternatively, enteric-coated aspirin, which is not broken down in the stomach, may cause less gastric irritation.

Haemostatic effects

Aspirin prolongs bleeding time, and this effect can occur after ingestion of a single tablet (300 mg). It is due to impaired platelet aggregation, caused by aspirin inhibiting the synthesis of platelet thromboxane. The increase in bleeding time continues until the platelet population has been replaced (7–10 days)—this is because platelets cannot regenerate cyclo-oxygenase (see Chapter 13).

High doses of aspirin (4–6 g day^{-1}), over a long time, reduce plasma prothrombin levels and cause an increase in clotting time. This effect can be reversed by the administration of fresh-frozen plasma. Aspirin should be avoided by any patient with a haemorrhagic disorder such as haemophilia, liver disease, and by patients taking anticoagulants as it may potentiate their effect.

Tinnitus

High doses of aspirin cause tinnitus and hearing loss due to a rise in labyrinthine pressure. Reducing the dose of aspirin reverses this problem in 2–3 days.

Uricosuric effect

Aspirin at a dosage of 1–2 g per day decreases uric acid secretion, which results in an increase in plasma uric acid concentrations.

Aspirin should not be given to patients suffering from gout, a disorder of uric acid metabolism.

Effects on the kidney

In normal people, aspirin has little effect on the kidney. However, if there is an underlying circulatory problem, such as congestive heart failure, aspirin decreases renal blood flow. This can precipitate acute renal failure. Aspirin also enhances sodium and water retention, which can increase oedema formation in some patients.

Metabolic effects

OXIDATIVE PHOSPHORYLATION

Aspirin causes the uncoupling of oxidative phosphorylation, and so inhibits a number of ATP-dependent reactions. At normal therapeutic doses, this uncoupling has little untoward effect, but it is serious in overdose (see below).

CARBOHYDRATE METABOLISM

Aspirin in high doses (> 5 g per day) may cause hypoglycaemia. Indeed, it was once used as a treatment of diabetes. In even higher doses (> 10 g per day), aspirin depletes the liver of its glycogen stores and causes hyperglycaemia.

Aspirin hypersensitivity

True hypersensitivity is rare, but many patients confuse unwanted effects, such as nausea and tinnitus, with an allergic response. In a true hypersensitivity reaction, clinical manifestations occur within minutes of aspirin ingestion and may range from rhinitis to life-threatening laryngeal oedema. The management of aspirin hypersensitivity and other drug hypersensitivity reactions is discussed in Chapter 23. The underlying mechanism for hypersensitivity to aspirin is unknown. Although the response resembles anaphylaxis, it does not appear to be immunological in nature. However, the incidence of aspirin hypersensitivity is much higher in patients who suffer from general allergic conditions such as asthma and hay fever, so they should avoid taking aspirin. Other drugs that inhibit cyclo-oxygenase (e.g. ibuprofen and mefenamic acid) may cause a hypersensitivity reaction in patients allergic to aspirin.

Drug interactions

Aspirin binds firmly to plasma proteins and so many displace other drugs from the binding sites, especially warfarin, methotrexate, and sulfonylureas. If such drugs are displaced, their pharmacological properties are enhanced. The problem with warfarin can be further compounded by the antihaemostatic properties of aspirin, which can lead to a fatal haemorrhage.

Aspirin overdose

As aspirin is widely used and readily available to the public, it is not surprising that it is one of the most common drugs for attempted suicide and is often a cause of accidental poisoning in children. Doses of 10–30 g can be fatal.

Overdose of aspirin increases CO_2 production in skeletal muscles, due to deranged metabolism. Initially, this increase stimulates respiration and causes some hyperventilation which may produce a respiratory alkalosis. However, CO_2 production then outstrips its alveolar excretion causing a rise in plasma $p(CO_2)$ and hence a fall in blood pH—this is metabolic acidosis. The acidosis is compounded by the high plasma concentrations of aspirin metabolites, which are themselves acidic and also impair renal function, leading to the accumulation of acidic waste products. Hyperthermia and dehydration accompany aspirin intoxication. If left untreated, death occurs from coma and respiratory depression. Treatment is aimed at preventing further absorption of aspirin by gastric lavage, and at restoring blood pH by the intravenous infusion of bicarbonate. Excretion of aspirin is also promoted by bicarbonate infusion since, in the resulting alkaline urine, a greater proportion of aspirin is in the poorly lipid-soluble unionized form which is not reabsorbed in the tubules and is therefore excreted.

Aspirin and Reye's syndrome

Reye's syndrome is a rare disorder, occurring in childhood, that involves an acute encephalopathic illness and fatty degeneration of the viscera, especially the liver. Its main feature is that it arises after an infectious illness, often chickenpox or influenza. The precise aetiology is unknown, but there is accumulating epidemiological evidence of a link between the syndrome and the consumption of aspirin during a viral infection. A proposed mechanism for Reye's syndrome is that an interaction between aspirin and the viral infection leads to damage of cell mitochondria in genetically susceptible individuals. As a result of this association, paediatric aspirin preparations are no longer available to the public.

Aspirin in dentistry

Aspirin is widely used as an analgesic in postoperative dental pain, and many studies support its efficacy. Efficacy is dose-related, with 1000–1200 mg providing greater analgesia than 500–600 mg, and is also related to the rate at which an individual hydrolyses aspirin to salicylate. Postoperative dental pain is of short duration and usually patients only take analgesics for the first 24–48 hours after surgery. As analgesics are only required for a short time, it is unlikely that unwanted effects such as tinnitus will occur.

If a patient has taken even a single dose of aspirin or an aspirin-containing analgesic *before* tooth extraction or other dental surgical procedure, there may be a risk of postoperative haemorrhage. For such patients, it is important to ensure that the socket is filled with a good blood clot before discharge. If this does not occur, then the socket should be packed with Surgicel and sutured. The patient should not be discharged until haemostasis has been achieved. When aspirin is given postoperatively, there is little risk of haemorrhage as the haemostatic mechanism will be well established.

Some toothache sufferers try to relieve their pain by placing an aspirin tablet in the buccal sulcus against the offending tooth.

This practice is of no value for pain relief, but it does cause severe sloughing and ulceration of the buccal mucosa.

Choline salicylate is the active constituent of the proprietary topical gel Bonjela, which is widely used in the management of minor oral ulceration due to ill-fitting dentures, and in infants who are teething.

Other uses of aspirin and the salicylates

Aspirin is used extensively in a variety of painful conditions, ranging from headache to musculoskeletal pain. It is also contained in a variety of proprietary cold and flu remedies. Sulfasalazine, (a combination of a salicylate and sulfapyridine) is used in the treatment of certain inflammatory bowel disorders and rheumatoid arthritis. The use of aspirin in the management of thromboembolic disorders is discussed in Chapter 13.

Key facts
Aspirin

- Aspirin is a peripherally acting analgesic with additional anti-inflammatory, antipyretic, and antithrombotic properties.
- Most of the pharmacological properties of aspirin are related to the drug's ability to inhibit the synthesis of the prostaglandins.
- The drug is rapidly absorbed from the upper part of the gastrointestinal tract (GIT) and metabolized by esterases to salicylate.
- Unwanted effects of aspirin include gastrointestinal tract irritation, an increase in bleeding time, and tinnitus.
- Aspirin should not be prescribed to patients with peptic ulceration, haemostatic defects, asthmatics, and children under the 12 years of age.

Para-aminophenols

These so-called coal-tar analgesics are all analine derivatives. Phenacetin and acetanalid were first introduced in 1887, but in 1949 it was realized that the active metabolite of both these drugs is N-acetyl-p-aminophenol or paracetamol, which is now the most widely used of this group of analgesics.

Pharmacokinetics

Paracetamol is well absorbed from the small intestine after oral ingestion. Peak plasma concentrations usually occur 30–60 minutes after dosage, and the half-life is approximately 2 hours. The drug is uniformly distributed throughout most body fluids. Paracetamol is conjugated in the liver and the conjugates excreted in the urine.

Pharmacodynamics and pharmacological properties

Paracetamol has both analgesic and antipyretic properties similar to those of aspirin; however, the drug has little or no anti-inflammatory action. This may be attributable to the drug's weak inhibitory effects on the cyclo-oxygenase enzyme system. Also, paracetamol does not inhibit PMN activation in the same manner as aspirin. Neither the site nor the mechanisms of the analgesic action of paracetamol have been clearly established. Different workers have concluded that the site of action is purely peripheral, purely central, or both. It is very much less effective than aspirin as a peripheral cyclo-oxygenase inhibitor, but has the same potency as aspirin in inhibiting brain prostaglandin synthetase. The antipyretic property of paracetamol probably has a similar mechanism to that of aspirin.

Unwanted effects and overdose

Paracetamol has remarkably few unwanted effects and at normal therapeutic doses is probably the safest analgesic. Skin rashes and white blood cell disorders have occasionally been reported. However, the most serious problem with paracetamol is hepatotoxicity after overdose. At normal doses, paracetamol is broken down in the liver to metabolites that are normally innocuous. In overdose, one of the metabolites (probably N-acetyl-p-benzoquinone), which is usually reduced by conjugation with glutathione and then eliminated, accumulates and renders liver cells incapable of synthesizing protein. Acute liver damage can occur after a single dose of 10–15 g; a dose of 25 g is invariably fatal. The problem of overdose is compounded by the absence of untoward effects in the first 24 hours after overdose, during which time serious and perhaps fatal liver damage will have occurred. The overdose victim may therefore take further tablets, but their relations or friends will have seen little obvious signs of illness and so may not seek help. Signs and symptoms of liver damage manifest themselves between 2 and 6 days after overdose. Jaundice and coagulation disorders accompany the hepatotoxicity, which leads to coma and death.

Early treatment is essential in paracetamol overdose. Gastric lavage will prevent further absorption, provided it is in the first hour after dosage. If less than 12 hours have elapsed, then N-acetylcysteine is the treatment of choice. This can be given orally and treatment should continue until there is a significant reduction of plasma paracetamol concentrations. Minimal hepatic damage can be anticipated when the plasma concentration is less than $120\,\mu g\,mL^{-1}$ at 4 hours, or $30\,\mu g\,mL^{-1}$ at 12 hours after ingestion. N-acetylcysteine conjugates with the metabolite, protecting the liver cells from further damage.

If the patient is seen after 24 hours, the success of treatment depends on the magnitude of the initial overdose. If large quantities of paracetamol have been consumed, the patient will suffer a slow and distressing death.

In an attempt to reduce the incidence of paracetamol overdose, some preparations contain a combination of paracetamol and methionine, e.g. Paradote®. Methionine increases the conjugation of N-acetyl-p-benzoquinone with glutathione and may therefore prevent liver toxicity if paracetamol is taken in overdose.

Use in dentistry

Paracetamol is a useful analgesic in patients where aspirin is contraindicated (for example, those with a haemorrhagic diathesis). The efficacy of paracetamol in postoperative dental pain has not been shown to be dose-related, so increasing the dosage may not cause an equivalent increase in analgesia.

Paracetamol elixir is extensively used in the treatment of 'teething', although its efficacy in this poorly defined condition has not been established. Teething is often accompanied by systemic disturbances, particularly pyrexia, which may be due to an infection. The combined antipyretic and analgesic properties of paracetamol, together with its few unwanted effects, make it popular for the relief of these problems, although it might simply palliate the symptoms of the underlying infection that requires medical attention. Paracetamol elixir also contains a high proportion of sugar, and its regular use may increase the incidence of dental caries, especially as the medicine is often given last thing at night.

Key facts
Paracetamol

- Paracetamol is an analine derivative with analgesic, antipyretic, and weak anti-inflammatory properties.

- The drug is well absorbed from the GIT and metabolized in the liver.

- Paracetamol has few unwanted effects, but in overdose is very hepatotoxic due to the formation N-acetyl-p-benzoquinone.

- Paracetamol overdose must be treated promptly and the antidote is N-acetylcysteine.

Other NSAIDs

These analgesics share many of aspirin's pharmacological properties. Like aspirin, they are anti-inflammatory and analgesic because they can inhibit the synthesis of eicosanoids (see Chapter 4). Many NSAIDs also produce unwanted effects similar to those of aspirin, but the incidence of unwanted effects varies markedly between the different groups of these analgesics. Patient who are hypersensitive to aspirin often have a similar reaction when given another NSAID. One main advantage of the NSAIDs over aspirin is their action on platelet cyclo-oxygenase. Aspirin is an irreversible inhibitor of platelet cyclo-oxygenase; thus when a population of platelets are exposed to aspirin, they are unable to regenerate cyclo-oxygenase, and platelet function only returns when the population is replaced. This will have a significant effect on bleeding time and its duration. In contrast, most NSAIDs are reversible inhibitors of platelet cyclo-oxygenase; thus when platelets are exposed to these drugs, the effect on bleeding time is much less than when compared to aspirin, since the platelets can regenerate the cyclo-oxygenase enzyme.

These analgesics have been mainly used in rheumatic and other musculoskeletal disorders, but because of their combined analgesic and anti-inflammatory properties, they are becoming widely used for the treatment of dental pain.

Propionic acid derivatives

Examples of these include ibuprofen, naproxen, flurbiprofen, ketoprofen, and fenoprofen. Ibuprofen is the most widely used analgesic in this group and is becoming increasingly popular in dentistry.

Pharmacological properties and unwanted effects

Ibuprofen is rapidly absorbed following oral administration; peak plasma concentrations occur within 1.5 hours after dosage, and the plasma half-life is 2 hours. Like all propionic acid derivatives, ibuprofen binds extensively to plasma proteins (99% is bound). The drug is broken down in the liver and the metabolites excreted in the urine.

Ibuprofen has similar unwanted effects to those of aspirin. About 15% of patients find these effects so severe that they have to discontinue the drug. Ibuprofen and other propionic acid derivatives should be avoided in patients with a gastrointestinal disorder, haemostatic problems, or a history of hypersensitivity to aspirin.

The fenamates

Mefenamic acid (Ponstan) is the only member of this group used in dentistry.

Pharmacological properties and unwanted effects

Mefenamic acid (Ponstan) is rapidly absorbed after oral administration and peak plasma concentrations occur after 2 hours: the half-life is 3–4 hours. The drug is metabolized in the liver; half of the metabolites are excreted in the urine, and the other half in the faeces. Mefenamic acid is about as active as aspirin as an analgesic and anti-inflammatory agent. However, the incidence of unwanted effects, especially gastrointestinal disturbances, is high. Troublesome diarrhoea occurs in 25% of patients on this drug. As with other NSAIDs, mefenamic acid should not be given to a patient for whom aspirin is contraindicated.

Indometacin (indomethacin)

This is an indole derivative and was developed in 1963. Its use in dentistry is limited because of the high incidence of unwanted effects.

Pharmacological properties and unwanted effects

Indometacin (indomethacin) is one of the most potent inhibitors of cyclo-oxygenase, and a powerful anti-inflammatory agent. A high proportion of patients (30–50%) experience unwanted effects, including gastrointestinal complaints as well as central nervous system disturbances such as dizziness, headache, confusion, and vertigo. The mechanism of these central actions is unknown, but they may be due to prostaglandin inhibition within brain tissue, or to salt and water retention. Severe depression of bone-marrow activity and hypersensitivity reactions have been associated with this drug.

Diflunisal

This is a difluorophenyl derivative of salicylic acid with similar pharmacological properties to aspirin. Its main advantage is its long plasma half-life (about 8 hours) so it only has to be taken twice a day. Diflunisal has a low incidence of unwanted effects, but it has not been established whether this low incidence persists with chronic usage.

Ketorolac and diclofenac

These two analgesics are derivatives of phenylacetic acid that share all the pharmacological properties of the other NSAIDs. Both drugs have a high incidence of unwanted effects, mainly involving the gastrointestinal tract. Diclofenac and ketorolac are both available for parenteral administration and are particularly useful in the management of acute postoperative dental pain, such as after the extraction of impacted lower third molars. Intramuscular diclofenac would also be useful for pain relief in patients where swallowing is difficult.

Efficacy of NSAIDs in dental pain

This group of analgesics has been extensively evaluated in postoperative dental pain and many trials support their efficacy. However, the incidence and severity of unwanted effects sometimes outweighs the advantages of analgesia obtained from these drugs. Ibuprofen and diflunisal appear to have the lowest incidence of unwanted effects. It has not been established whether these two analgesics offer any advantage over 1 g aspirin in the treatment of postoperative dental pain. In general, soluble preparations give an earlier onset of analgesia than tablets. Some studies have advocated the use of preoperative analgesia to provide effective postoperative pain control. The rationale for such analgesic usage is that high serum levels of the drug will be present at the time of the surgical procedure, and hence there will be a more effective inhibition of the biochemical mediators of pain (nociception) and early pain relief. Ibuprofen has been used as a so-called pre-emptive analgesic for the control of postoperative pain after third molar surgery.

Key facts
NSAIDs

- NSAIDs are derived from various organic acids and have similar pharmacological properties to aspirin.

- These drugs are particularly useful in the management of postoperative dental pain, or any pain with a significant inflammatory component.

- Unwanted effects of NSAIDs are similar to those of aspirin, but the incidence and severity varies from compound to compound.

Further reading

Mitchell, J. R. (1988). Acetaminophen (paracetamol) toxicity. *New England Journal of Medicine*, **319**, 1601–2.

Seymour, R. A. and Walton, J. G. (1984). Pain control after third molar surgery. *International Journal of Oral Surgery*, **13**, 457–85.

Vane, J. (1994). Towards a better aspirin. *Nature*, **367**, 215–16.

7

Opioid analgesics

- Opioids and opioid antagonists
- Use of opioids in dentistry
- Further reading

Opioid analgesics

Opioids exert their analgesic effect within the central nervous system by modifying neural activity associated with pain, so they are sometimes referred to as centrally acting analgesics.

The therapeutic properties of the milky exudate obtained from the seed pod of the white poppy *Papaver somniferum* have been known since the third century BC. The dried exudate is opium, and contains the alkaloids morphine and codeine. Although these drugs, and related synthetic compounds, are mainly used as analgesics, they also suppress coughing and reduce gastrointestinal motility.

The term opiate is used to designate drugs derived from opium—essentially morphine and codeine—although it has been loosely applied to morphine derivatives. The term opioid refers to any compound that acts as an agonist at opioid receptors, the effects of which are antagonized by the opioid receptor antagonist naloxone. Narcotics and major analgesics are obsolete terms that have been used to describe this group of drugs.

Opioids and opioid antagonists

Morphine

Morphine, named after Morpheus, the Greek god of dreams, was first isolated in 1803. This drug is the most widely used of the opioids and is considered to be the most potent analgesic in use.

Pharmacokinetics

As with most of the opioids, morphine undergoes extensive first-pass metabolism in the liver when given via the oral route. Hence for optimal use, it is given parenterally. Morphine is conjugated in the liver with glucuronic acid to form both active (morphine-6-glucuronide) and inactive (morphine-3-glucuronide) products. Thus morphine may be considered a pro-drug. The conjugates (mainly morphine-3-glucuronide) are excreted via the kidney, and the half-life of morphine in humans is approximately 3 hours.

Pharmacodynamics and pharmacological properties

ANALGESIA

An understanding of how morphine works as an analgesic must be accompanied by more detailed information about the pain experience. This experience comprises the initial sensation together with emotional, psychological, and suffering components that the sensation evokes. Coronary chest pain or cancer pain have differ-ent significances to the sufferer than, say, toothache or pain from a fractured limb. Morphine is particularly effective against pain that has a large suffering component. In addition to its analgesic properties, it produces other central effects, such as drowsiness, sedation, and euphoria, all of which add to the general comfort of a patient in pain. Morphine does not alter other sensations such as touch, pressure, vision, or hearing. Patients feel a pinprick as normal, though it may be less unpleasant. Morphine is also considered to be more effective against continuous, dull pain than against sharp, intermittent pain.

Although the precise mechanism of morphine-induced analgesia is uncertain, there is much evidence to suggest that the drug combines with opioid receptors (μ and κ) in the substantia gelatinosa, the spinal nucleus of the trigeminal nerve, and the periaqueductal and periventricular grey matter. By activating these receptors, morphine alters the central release of neurotransmitters (probably substance P) from nerve fibres transmitting painful stimuli (see Chapter 5). A 10 mg dose of morphine given intramuscularly provides pain relief within 30 minutes, and the effect lasts 4–5 hours.

GASTROINTESTINAL TRACT

Opium has been used for centuries to treat diarrhoea and dysentery. All the opioids produce a degree of constipation and some are used solely for this purpose (e.g. loperamide hydrochloride and diphenoxylate hydrochloride, see Chapter 18). The drugs act on the smooth muscles of the gastrointestinal tract by increasing muscle and sphincter tone—actions that are mediated by activation of μ- and δ-receptors. This results in delayed emptying of the gut, diminished peristalsis, and a decrease in propulsive motility. The constipating properties of the opioids show marked variation between patients. Morphine can produce painful spasm of the colon and particularly of the biliary tract that can result in biliary colic.

Because morphine and other μ-receptor agonists can prolong gastric emptying time, they may delay the absorption of orally administered drugs.

COUGH SUPPRESSION

Morphine and many of the opioids, especially codeine (see below), are effective antitussives. They have a direct effect on the cough centre in the medulla, and act at low doses (see Chapter 17).

CARDIOVASCULAR EFFECTS

Morphine at therapeutic doses has an insignificant effect on blood pressure, cardiac output, and heart rate. However, it does cause the release of histamine, which produces vasodilatation of the peripheral vessels, leading to a sensation of warmth in many people. Cardiovascular effects also arise when morphine is used to treat breathlessness resulting from pulmonary oedema associated with acute left ventricular failure. The mechanism underlying this effect involves a diminished perception of impaired respiratory function, a reduction in anxiety, which decreases cardiac workload, as well as reductions in cardiac preload and afterload due to venous and arterial dilation respectively.

Unwanted effects

RESPIRATORY DEPRESSION

Morphine and many opioids depress respiration by a direct effect on the respiratory centres in the brainstem. Some degree of respiratory depression occurs with normal therapeutic doses, but in overdose it can be life-threatening. Morphine decreases the response of the respiratory centre to the concentration of CO_2 in the blood. It also depresses the pontine and medullary centres that control respiratory rhythm. The result is a reduction in respiratory rate, minute volume, and tidal exchange. These effects are thought to be mediated by μ-receptors, and perhaps by κ- and δ-receptors. All these receptors are widely distributed in the medullary area of the brain.

DEPENDENCE

One of the main drawbacks of the opioids is the development of tolerance and physical dependence with repeated use. The problem of drug abuse is dealt with in more detail in Chapter 25. Tolerance develops to the depressant actions of the opioids—analgesia, euphoria, drowsiness, and respiratory depression. Both physical dependence and tolerance depend on the dose and frequency of administration. Similarly, the degree of physical dependence determines the intensity of the withdrawal syndrome. However, the problems of physical dependence and tolerance should not be a deterrent to the adequate use of opioids in the management of the pain of terminal illness. Sufficient drug should be given to prevent the recurrence of pain as opposed to only administering when the pain becomes distressing. Less drug is required to prevent the return of pain than is necessary for its relief.

NAUSEANT AND EMETIC EFFECTS

Nausea and vomiting are common unwanted effects associated with morphine and many opioids. They are due to direct stimulation of the chemoreceptor trigger zone in the medulla. The incidence of nausea and vomiting is much higher in ambulatory patients, which suggests that a vestibular component is active. The administration of an antiemetic, such as cyclizine tartrate or prochlorperazine, may reduce this problem (see Chapter 18).

EFFECTS ON THE PUPIL

Morphine and many of the more potent opioids cause constriction of the pupil (miosis), due to an excitatory action on the autonomic segment of the nucleus of the oculomotor nerve (Edinger–Westphal nucleus). Because of the miosis, it is unwise to give morphine to patients with a suspected head injury as it will mask the pupillary constriction reflex, which is an important indicator of brain damage.

ACTIONS ON THE BLADDER

Morphine reduces urinary flow by inhibiting the urinary voiding reflex and increasing the tone and amplitude of contractions of the ureters. Both actions are probably mediated via μ- and δ- receptors in the lower segments of the spinal cord. Morphine also increases the release of antidiuretic hormone which further reduces the production of urine.

Overdose

Death from overdose of opioids (especially heroin, diacetylmorphine) is due to respiratory depression. Someone who has taken an overdose, accidentally or intentionally, will be asleep and difficult to arouse; the respiratory rate will be very low; blood pressure will drop; and the pupils will be constricted and show no response to light. The skin will be cold and clammy, and all skeletal muscles will be flaccid, including the tongue, which may fall back and block the airway.

Treatment is to establish and maintain an airway and then administer an opioid antagonist such as naloxone. The usual dose of naloxone is 0.4 mg intravenously, which can be repeated after 2–3 minutes if required. The half-life of naloxone is short (about 1 hour) and further doses may be necessary to avoid a relapse into a coma state.

Uses of morphine

Although morphine is widely used to treat pain after general surgery, its main use is in the relief of pain from cancer and other terminal illnesses. Its combined analgesic, euphoriant, and sedative properties are a considerable advantage in reducing the pain and suffering that often accompany a terminal illness. A variety of other opioids are also used, particularly those that are effective by mouth, thus avoiding repeated injections in frail patients.

As morphine suppresses the cough reflex and respiratory activity, it should not be used indiscriminately in postoperative pain, as such suppression can lead to pneumonia.

Key facts
Morphine

- Morphine is a pure opioid agonist that occurs naturally in opium.

- Parenteral administration of morphine is more effective than oral administration since the drug undergoes extensive first-pass metabolism.

- Morphine is metabolized in the liver to the more active morphine-6-glucuronide, and the drug has a half-life of 3 hours.

- Pharmacological effects of morphine are mainly mediated via the μ- and κ-receptors; these include analgesia, euphoria, and sedation.
- Unwanted effects of morphine include constipation, respiratory depression, dependence, nausea and vomiting, and constriction of the pupil.
- Morphine is used extensively in the management of cancer pain and acute postoperative pain (normal dose = 10 mg). There is little indication for the use of this drug in dentistry.

Use of opioids in patients with suspected head injuries

Morphine and opioids are contraindicated in these patients because they depress respiration, as well as constricting the pupils (see above). Patients with suspected head injuries are likely to have impaired respiration. The respiratory-depressant properties of morphine and associated CO_2 retention cause cerebral vasodilatation and an increase in intracranial pressure, and these effects are markedly exaggerated in patients with head injuries.

Codeine

Codeine, or 3-methylmorphine, is a naturally occurring alkaloid present in opium. Like all the opioids, it binds to opioid receptors in the central nervous system. The drug is metabolized in the liver to form norcodeine and morphine, so the morphine component may account for codeine's analgesic properties. About half the codeine is excreted in the urine unchanged or conjugated with glucuronide, about 10% is excreted as morphine glucuronide, and the remainder is excreted as norcodeine glucuronide.

Pharmacological properties

Codeine is one of the few opioids that is effective when taken by mouth, but it is only useful in treating mild to moderate pain. Peak plasma concentrations occur 1 hour after oral dosage, and analgesia lasts 2–4 hours. On a dose per dose basis, codeine has about 8% the potency of morphine, but it is appreciably more effective than morphine when given by mouth. Many proprietary analgesics contain mixtures of codeine and either paracetamol or aspirin. Combining both a peripherally and a centrally acting analgesic appears to enhance the efficacy of the combination—an effect that is often more than additive.

Codeine is a very effective antitussive, and so is contained in many proprietary cough medicines.

Unwanted effects

Codeine can produce all the unwanted effects of the opioids as a group, such as nausea, vomiting, sedation, and dizziness. As with morphine, these effects are more often observed in ambulatory patients than those in bed. When the drug is administered orally in the usual therapeutic doses (30–60 mg), the incidence of unwanted effects is low, and those that do occur are annoying rather than serious. Codeine can depress respiration, but the degree of depression is of little clinical significance except in overdose. Repeated doses often cause constipation, and so the drug has been used as an antidiarrhoeal.

The risk of dependence or addiction to codeine is small. The usual dose regime of codeine (30–60 mg four times daily), even when given for several months, does not induce significant dependence. Most addicts who have resorted to codeine have done so because nothing better was available.

Key facts
Codeine

- Codeine is a naturally occurring alkaloid found in opium.
- It is effective when given by mouth (normal dose = 30 mg) and is metabolized in the liver to norcodeine and morphine.
- The drug is often used as a constituent of compound analgesics where it is combined with either paracetamol or aspirin.
- Codeine is also used extensively as a cough suppressant (antitussive).
- Unwanted effects of codeine are similar to those of morphine.

Pethidine (meperidine)

This is a synthetic opioid, first manufactured in 1939. It can be given orally, but optimal analgesia is obtained when it is given intramuscularly. Pethidine is hydrolysed in the liver to meperidinic acid, which is conjugated and excreted in the urine. It also undergoes N-demethylation to norpethidine, which may then be hydrolysed to norpethidinic acid, which is also conjugated and excreted in the urine. A small amount of pethidine is excreted unchanged. Its half-life is about 3 hours.

Pharmacological properties

Pethidine provides rapid analgesia when given via the parenteral route, with the maximum analgesic effect occurring 1 hour after dosage. The duration of analgesia obtained from 50 mg is approximately 2–4 hours—slightly less than that obtained from morphine. It has been estimated that 80–100 mg pethidine has the same potency as 10 mg morphine. However, it is not particularly useful in the management of chronic pain (such as cancer pain) because of its short duration of action and its tendency to cause restlessness. Furthermore, repeated high dosage increases the amount available for N-demethylation to form norpethidine, which can cause convulsions.

Unwanted effects

Pethidine has similar unwanted effects to morphine, including respiratory depression, dependence, and pupillary constriction. Its effect on the muscles of the gastrointestinal tract is considerably less than that of morphine or codeine. At normal doses, it has little effect on the cardiovascular system, but intravenous administration causes an alarming increase in heart rate. In overdose, pethidine sometimes produces excitation of the central nervous system resulting in tremors, muscle twitching, seizures, and an atropine-like action causing an increase in heart rate.

Drug interactions

Pethidine should not be given to patients receiving monoamine oxidase inhibitors (MAOI) as this may cause convulsions, hypothermia, hyperpyrexia, and severe respiratory depression. These are type B reactions, as they are unlike the normal pharmacological effects of pethidine (see Chapter 24).

Concurrent administration of pethidine with either tricyclic antidepressants or chlorpromazine enhances its sedative properties.

Key facts
Pethidine

- Pethidine is a synthetic opioid that can be given orally or parenterally (normal dose = 50 mg).

- It is metabolized in the liver to meperidinic acid, norpethidine, and norpethidinic acid.

- Unwanted effects of pethidine are similar to those of morphine, but the drug causes a severe reaction when given to patients taking monoamine oxidase inhibitors.

Pentazocine

This is a benzomorphan derivative that has both agonistic and weak antagonistic activity at opioid receptors. It acts as an antagonist on the μ-receptor, but as an agonist on the κ- and σ-receptors. This agonism accounts for the high incidence of hallucinations associated with pentazocine. Because of its antagonistic action on the μ-receptor, pentazocine should not be used with an opioid agonist. It was originally thought that it would have little or no abuse potential but, with widespread use, physical dependence and abuse have become apparent. Pentazocine can be administered both orally and parenterally. However, repeated injections should be avoided as the drug causes a local irritation and extensive fibrosis. It is well absorbed from the site of administration and undergoes extensive first-pass metabolism (80%). It is metabolized in the liver and the metabolites are excreted in the kidney; the rate of metabolism shows marked individual variation, which may account for interindividual differences in the drug's pharmacological properties Its half-life is 3–4 hours. An intramuscular dose of 30–50 mg pentazocine is approximately equivalent to 10 mg morphine. When given orally, 50 mg pentazocine produces analgesia equivalent to 60 mg codeine.

Unwanted effects

There is a high incidence of unwanted effects—including hallucinations, nightmares, sedation, dizziness, sweating, and nausea—and their frequency increases with dose. High doses increase blood pressure and heart rate. The effect on blood pressure may be due to an increase in the plasma concentration of catecholamines. The effects of pentazocine on the gastrointestinal tract and respiration are similar to those of the other opioids. It raises pulmonary artery pressure and therefore should not be used to reduce chest pain following a myocardial infarction. Although the drug is a μ-receptor antagonist, tolerance and dependence can develop with long-term use, and it is now classified as a *Schedule 2* drug (see Chapter 3).

Key facts
Pentazocine

- Pentazocine is a benzomorphan derivative that is an agonist at the δ- and κ-receptors, but is an antagonist at the μ-receptor.

- The drug undergoes marked interindividual first-pass metabolism.

- The normal dose of pentazocine is 50 mg, which can be given either parenterally or orally.

- Pentazocine has a high incidence of unwanted effects, including hallucinations, nightmares, and dysphoria.

- It causes a rise in pulmonary artery pressure and thus should not be used to relieve the pain associated with an acute myocardial infarction.

Dihydrocodeine

This moderately potent analgesic in relationship to codeine is in wide clinical use. It is derived from codeine and was first manufactured in 1911. Structurally, dihydrocodeine is related to both codeine and morphine and so shares some of the properties of these drugs. It can be given orally or parenterally and has a half-life of 3–4 hours. When given orally, the drug undergoes extensive first-pass metabolism. It is metabolized in the liver to dihydromorphine, which is conjugated with glucuronide and excreted via the kidneys. Dose regimens of dihydrocodeine are 30 mg every 4–6 hours.

Unwanted effects

Dihydrocodeine is associated with a high incidence of unwanted effects, including nausea, dizziness, and constipation. It is estimated that 25% of patients who take dihydrocodeine experience side-effects unpleasant enough to prevent them from taking further doses.

Dextropropoxyphene

This is a tertiary amine ester, both chemically and pharmacologically related to methadone and other opioids. However, its efficacy as an analgesic agent is questionable, and as an individual compound the drug is not used in dentistry. Co-proxamol—a combination of dextropropoxyphene (32.5 mg) and paracetamol (325 mg)—is a widely prescribed analgesic preparation in the UK.

Unwanted effects

The toxicity of co-proxamol presents a serious problem in overdose, and death has been reported from as few as 15 tablets taken with alcohol. The effects of overdose of dextropropoxyphene in co-proxamol are similar to those of other opioids, but a particularly worrying feature is the rapid onset of respiratory depression. Patients surviving the effects of dextropropoxyphene in co-proxamol may develop hepatic necrosis from the paracetamol component. The continuing popularity of preparations containing dextropropoxyphene is difficult to understand; controlled studies have failed to show that dextropropoxyphene is any more effective than paracetamol or aspirin alone.

Fentanyl

Fentanyl is a highly lipid-soluble, quick-acting ($t_{0.5}$ 30 min) synthetic opioid. It is a μ-agonist with an estimated potency 80–100 times that of morphine. Fentanyl and its congeners (alfentanil and sufentanil) have little or no effect on the cardiovascular system, so they are mainly used as intravenous supplements during anaesthesia.

Combination analgesics

Combination analgesics (such as co-proxamol) contain both a peripherally acting analgesic (for example, aspirin or paracetamol) and a centrally acting analgesic (for example, codeine or dextropropoxyphene). The rationale is that they will block pain at the site of the injury as well its transmission in the central nervous system. Such preparations are widely used.

Evidence from clinical trials suggests that combined analgesics are more effective than the individual constituents alone. This effect is often more than additive although, since two drugs are used, the incidence of adverse effects is higher.

Naloxone

This is a competitive opioid antagonist, mainly used to treat opioid overdose, particularly the effects on respiration. It must be given intravenously (0.4–0.8 mg) for immediate effect. If the respiratory depression is not reversed, the dose is repeated after 2 minutes. The half-life of naloxone is only 1 hour and more doses may be required. Naloxone can also be used if there is a problem in diagnosing physical dependence or addiction to the opioids, for it will induce symptoms of withdrawal in people who are dependent.

Buprenorphine

This is a semisynthetic opioid derived from thebaine. An intramuscular dose of 0.4 mg buprenorphine has an analgesic potency equivalent to 10 mg of intramuscular morphine; the duration of analgesia with this dose of buprenorphine is about 6 hours. The drug is particularly well absorbed when given sublingually. It is extensively bound to plasma protein (96%) and has a plasma half-life of about 3 hours. Most of the drug is eliminated unchanged in the faeces following biliary excretion.

Receptor binding studies suggest that buprenorphine is a partial agonist for the μ-receptor but may act as an antagonist at other opioid receptors.

Unwanted effects of buprenorphine are similar to those of morphine and include sedation, nausea, vomiting, dizziness, sweating, and dependence.

Methadone

This is a synthetic opioid, first manufactured during the early 1940s. It is well absorbed from all routes of administration, and is effective when given orally. Methadone is broken down in the liver and the metabolites are excreted in the urine; the plasma half-life is 24–36 hours. It is a μ-agonist, and, on a dose per dose basis, is as effective an analgesic as morphine. However, it has the advantages of a longer duration of action and efficacy when given orally. The main uses of methadone are the relief of pain, treatment of opioid abstinence syndrome, and treatment (by substitution) of heroin addiction.

Use of opioids in dentistry

Although morphine and related analgesics are widely used in relieving pain, their dental application is limited. Most types of dental pain, such as in pulpitis, dry socket, or pericoronitis, can be effectively treated by local measures, so the dental surgeon is unlikely to prescribe opioids for these conditions.

Pain after a dental surgical procedure is the main indication for recommending or prescribing analgesics. However, such pain has a major inflammatory component and, as the opioids possess no anti-inflammatory action, their efficacy is doubtful in this context. Clinical trials to evaluate codeine, dextropropoxyphene, and pentazocine have all shown that they are poor at relieving pain after the removal of impacted lower third molars. One study showed that dihydrocodeine, when given intravenously, increased the severity of postoperative dental pain compared with a placebo.

Critical reappraisal of evidence supporting the efficacy of opioids in dental pain indicates that they are of virtually no value. This may be due to the relative absence of any significant emotional component of the pain, a factor likely to be present after major in-patient surgery. Pain after general surgery has a greater inflammatory element than pain after dental surgery, but patients' reactions to their pain may differ because of their own expectations. For example, people undergoing major abdominal surgery as in-patients are likely to have a different view of their circumstances from people who have impacted lower third molars removed in an out-patient clinic. The patients may have different levels of anxiety, particularly if the surgery has been undertaken for a life-threatening condition.

Thus analgesics with an established anti-inflammatory property (such as aspirin) appear to offer more advantages in the treatment of dental pain than the opioids.

Further reading

Brownstein, M. J. (1993). A brief history of opiates, opioid peptides and opioid receptors. *Proceedings of the National Academy of Sciences USA*, 90, 5391–3.

Hoskins, P. J. and Hanks, G. W. (1991). Opioid agonists–antagonist drugs in acute and chronic pain states. *Drugs*, 41, 326–44.

Parkhouse, J. (1975). Simple analgesics. *Drugs*, 10, 366–93.

Seymour, R. A. and Walton, J. G. (1984). Pain control after third molar surgery—a review. *International Journal of Oral Surgery*, 13, 457–85.

Local anaesthetics (local analgesics) and vasoconstrictors

Local anaesthetics (local analgesics) and vasoconstrictors

Anaesthesia means the loss of all forms of sensation. Thus the term local anaesthesia means a localized loss of pain, temperature, touch, and pressure. In dentistry, under normal circumstances, it is neither necessary nor desirable to block all forms of sensation. Only loss of pain—in other words local analgesia—is needed. In practice, the terms local anaesthesia and local analgesia are used synonymously. This is reasonable because the agents and techniques used are insufficiently precise to make it possible to select at will a local action that is either anaesthetic or analgesic. Local analgesia may be produced by various methods:

(1) by reducing the temperature;

(2) by stimulating large fibre nerve activity, thus blocking the perception of smaller diameter (pain) fibre transmission;

(3) by physically damaging nerve trunks, for example by sectioning a nerve;

(4) by chemically damaging nerve trunks, for example by neurolytic agents;

(5) by rendering the tissues anaemic;

(6) by blocking transmission at sensory nerve endings or along nerve fibres with drugs.

The last of these methods is the most important therapeutically. Method (1) has a limited application but may be employed to produce surface anaesthesia. Method (2) is a potential growth area in dental pain control and includes such techniques as acupuncture and the use of electrical stimulation devices known as TENS (transcutaneous electronic nerve stimulation) machines. Methods (3), (4), and (5) are unsafe for therapeutic use. Many different substances can interfere with the transmission of nerve impulses but, for a drug to be clinically acceptable as a local anaesthetic, it must be able to produce a *fully reversible* block of nerve conduction at concentrations that do not damage the tissues. The properties of the 'ideal' local anaesthetic are shown in Table 8.1. Unfortunately this ideal material does not exist. Not even the first criterion of specificity is satisfied. Local anaesthetics will stabilize any excitable membrane including motor neurones. The central nervous and cardiovascular systems are especially sensitive to the actions of local anaesthetic drugs.

Table 8.1 Properties of an ideal anaesthetic

An ideal local anaesthetic should:
Have a specific and reversible action
Be non-irritant
Produce no permanent damage
Have no systemic toxicity
Have a high therapeutic ratio
Be active topically and by injection
Have a rapid onset
Have a suitable duration of action
Be chemically stable and sterilizable
Be able to be administered with other agents, e.g. vasoconstrictors, without loss of properties
Be non-allergenic
Be non-addictive

Chemistry

Local anaesthetic drugs are weak organic bases and are insoluble in water. However, they can be converted into soluble salts, usually the hydrochlorides, and these are the forms used clinically. Their detailed chemical structures vary, but most local anaesthetics are built on a common plan, composed of three parts:

(1) an aromatic residue with an acidic (lipophilic) group: (R_1);

(2) a connecting intermediate aliphatic chain, with either an ester or amide link, usually an amino-alcohol (R_2);

(3) a terminal substituted amino (hydrophilic) group: (R_3 and R_4).

Thus a general formula may be written as follows:

$$R_1CO—R_2—N \diagdown \begin{matrix} R_3 \\ R_4 \end{matrix}$$

$$(1) \quad (2) \quad (3)$$

The groups R_3 and R_4 may form part of a cyclic system, as in mepivacaine and bupivacaine, two of the agents shown in Fig. 8.1, which shows the structure of some common local anaesthetics according to this plan.

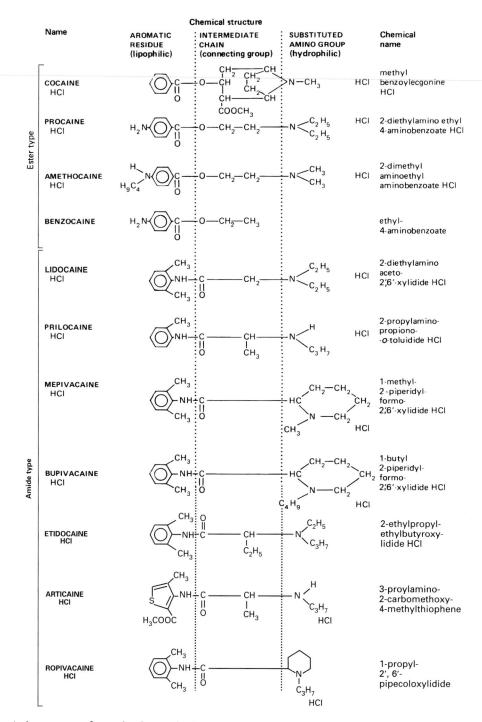

Fig. 8.1 Chemical structures of some local anaesthetics.

Classification of local anaesthetics

Local anaesthetics can be categorized in a number of ways (for example duration of action). However, the major classification is based on their chemical structure and the determining factor is the nature of the intermediate chain. Thus local anaesthetics are classified as either amides or esters. Amides and esters differ in two important respects: (1) they vary in their propensity to produce hypersensitivity reactions and (2) they are metabolized in different ways (see later).

Physicochemical properties

There are four properties that need to be considered in relation to local anaesthetic activity:

(1) ionization;

(2) the partition coefficient;

(3) protein binding; and

(4) vasodilatory ability.

Ionization

As local anaesthetics are weak bases, it follows that they exist partly in an unionized form and partly in an ionized form, the proportion of each depending upon the pK_a or dissociation constant of the particular drug (i.e. the pH at which the ionized and non-ionized forms of the drug are present in equal amounts), and the pH of the surrounding medium (see Table 8.2). For example, procaine (as procaine hydrochloride) has a pK_a of 9.0. The proportion of procaine that is unionized at the physiological pH of 7.4 can be calculated from the Henderson–Hasselbach equation (see Chapter 1):

For procaine, $pK_a = 9.0$

$$pH = 7.4.$$

For bases, $pH = pK_a - \log_{10} \dfrac{\text{ionized base}}{\text{unionized base}}$;

so, $\log_{10} \dfrac{\text{ionized base}}{\text{unionized base}} = pK_a - pH$

$$= 9.0 - 7.4$$

$$= 1.6.$$

Taking antilogs on both sides of the equation:

$$\frac{\text{ionized base}}{\text{unionized base}} = \frac{39.8}{1.0};$$

i.e. approximately $= \dfrac{40.0}{1.0}$.

Therefore, the percentage ratio of ionized to unionized molecules (40) in a total of 41 molecules is:

$$\frac{40}{41} \times 100 = 97.6\%.$$

Expressed the opposite way round, the ratio of unionized:ionized molecules is 1/41 (2.4%). Thus, at pH 7.4 only a small pro-

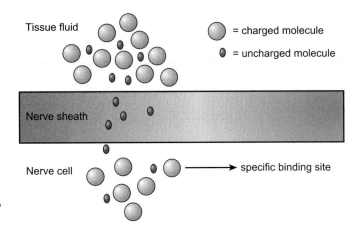

Fig. 8.2 Both charged and uncharged molecules are important in the action of local anaesthetics. The uncharged molecule crosses the lipid nerve sheath and the charged molecule binds to a specific receptor to block the sodium channel (see Figs 8.3 and 8.4).

portion of a dose of injected procaine will be in the lipid-soluble form that readily crosses the lipid-containing sheaths of nerves. Both the unionized and ionized forms are important in producing local anaesthesia (Fig. 8.2). The unionized form is able to cross the fatty sheath of nerves and gain ready access inside the nerve fibres; once the anaesthetic gains entry to the cytoplasm of the nerve cell, the ionized form blocks conduction (see 'Mechanism of action of local anaesthetics' below). As these two forms of a local anaesthetic are in equilibrium, as soon as some unionized molecules arrive inside the cell some will become ionized, the proportion depending upon the pK_a of the drug and the intracellular pH, which is normally lower (pH 7 or less) than the extracellular pH of 7.4.

Table 8.2 lists the pK_as of some local anaesthetics, including those commonly used in dentistry, and indicates the percentage of each drug in the unionized from at pH 7.4. In general, the amide types have a lower pK_a than the ester types (with the exception of benzocaine, which does not form soluble salts and can therefore only be used as a surface local anaesthetic). This means that the proportion of the lipid-soluble (unionized) form present in solution at physiological pH is considerably greater with the amides (for example lidocaine (lignocaine), 25%) than with the ester type (for example procaine, 2.4%). This accounts for the faster onset of action of lidocaine (1–2 min) compared with procaine (2–5 min).

Partition coefficient

The partition coefficient measures lipid solubility (see Chapter 1) or, to be more precise, the relative solubilities of an agent in fat and water—the more fat-soluble and the less water-soluble a compound is, the higher the numerical value (see Table 8.2). All other things being equal, the greater the fat solubility, the greater the ease and rapidity with which a compound will cross a lipid barrier

Table 8.2 Pharmacokinetic data for certain local anaesthetics

Solution	PKa	% base at pH 7.4	Partition coefficient	Protein binding (%)	Half-life (min)	Max dose (mg/kg) [ceiling mg]
Lidocaine	7.9	25	3	64	90	4.4 [300]
Prilocaine	7.9	25	1	50	90	6.0 [400]
Mepivacaine	7.6	33	1	77	120	4.4 [300]
Bupivacaine	8.1	17	28	96	160	1.3 [90]
Etidocaine	7.9	25	141	94	160	8.0 [400]
Articaine	7.8	29	1	67	75	7.0 [500]
Procaine	9.0	2	0.6	6	6	6.0 [400]

such as a nerve sheath. Thus the greater the partition coefficient, the faster the onset of anaesthesia.

Protein binding

Most drugs bind to plasma proteins in varying degrees (see Chapter 1) and local anaesthetics are no exception (see Table 8.2). The two proteins chiefly involved are: (1) α_1-acid glycoprotein, which has high affinity but low capacity and (2) albumin, which has low affinity but high capacity. The binding is a simple reversible one and tends to increase in proportion to the number of side chains of the molecule. For example, lidocaine is 64% bound, and bupivacaine is 96% bound. In general, the degree of protein binding is related to the duration of action of the local anaesthetic, because the bound portion acts as a reservoir from which free drug can be released to replace what has left the site either due to diffusion or metabolism. The duration of action of lidocaine is 15–45 minutes, whereas that of bupivacaine is 6 hours.

Vasodilatory ability

In addition to protein binding, the duration of activity is influenced by the vasodilatory ability of the anaesthetic agent. For example, prilocaine is less protein-bound (50%) than lidocaine (64%) and yet has a slightly longer duration of action because it does not have the strong vasodilator action of lidocaine. Most local anaesthetics (with the exception of cocaine) show some vasodilatory action.

Key facts
Chemistry of local anaesthetics

- Local anaesthetics reversibly inhibit neurotransmission.
- Local anaesthetic molecules consist of hydrophilic and lipophilic terminals separated by an intermediate chain.

- Local anaesthetics are classified as esters or amides: these differ in their mode of biotransformation and allergenicity.
- The physicochemical properties affecting local anaesthetic action are:
  - the dissociation constant;
  - partition coefficient;
  - protein binding;
  - vasodilator ability.

Pharmacological actions of local anaesthetics

These are:

(1) reversible block of conduction in nerve endings and nerve trunks;

(2) direct relaxation of smooth muscle, for example to produce vasodilatation via vascular smooth muscle; and inhibition of neuromuscular transmission in skeletal muscle. Intra-arterial injection of the ester agent procaine is the treatment of choice to reverse arteriospasm produced by inadvertent intra-arterial injection which could occur during intravenous sedation (see Chapter 9).

(3) class I antidysrhythmic-like action on the heart (see Chapter 16);

(4) stimulation and/or depression of the central nervous system.

These apparently different actions of local anaesthetics are due largely, if not entirely, to a common mechanism of action on excitable cell membranes.

Mechanism of action of local anaesthetic drugs

The site of action of local anaesthetics is the nerve cell membrane and there are various sites on this membrane where local anaesthetics could act. Two theories to explain the mechanism of action of local anaesthetics are given some credence. These are:

(1) the membrane expansion theory, and

(2) the specific binding theory.

Before considering these theories it is important to consider the normal mechanism of nerve conduction.

Nerve conduction

The conduction of an impulse along a nerve fibre depends on ion fluxes across the nerve cell membrane. The most important component of the nerve cell membrane, as far as ion movement is concerned, is the sodium channel.

SODIUM CHANNELS

It is useful to consider a simplified model of the sodium channel to explain its function during impulse conduction (see Figure 8.3). This model dictates that the channel can exist in one of three states:

(1) resting

(2) active

(3) refractory.

To explain these different conformations it is proposed that the sodium channel involves at least two 'gates'. One of these is named an 'activation' or 'm' (for make) gate, whereas the other is an 'inactivation' or 'h' (for halt) gate (see Fig 8.3a). In the resting state (i.e. in the absence of a nerve impulse) the nerve cell membrane is permeable to potassium ions but essentially impermeable to sodium ions (Fig 8.3a). The m gate is closed inhibiting sodium entry. The result is a difference of electrical potential, such that the inside of the nerve cell is approximately 80 millivolts negative to the outside. The intracellular concentration of sodium ions is normally kept low by means of an active extrusion process known as the sodium pump.

The depolarization that occurs with the arrival of a nerve impulse during the active phase opens the m gate (Fig. 8.3b). Sodium permeability transiently increases several hundred-fold. As the concentration of sodium ions outside the nerve cell is more than 10 times that inside the fibre, these ions diffuse rapidly into

Fig. 8.3(a) A diagrammatic representation of the sodium channel during the resting phase with the m gate closed.
Fig. 8.3(b) During the firing phase the m gate opens.
Fig. 8.3(c) During the refractory phase the h gate closes.
Fig. 8.3(d) The local anaesthetic receptor site is exposed when the h gate closes.
Fig. 8.3(e) The local anaesthetic (la) binds to the receptor site maintaining and blocking the sodium channel.

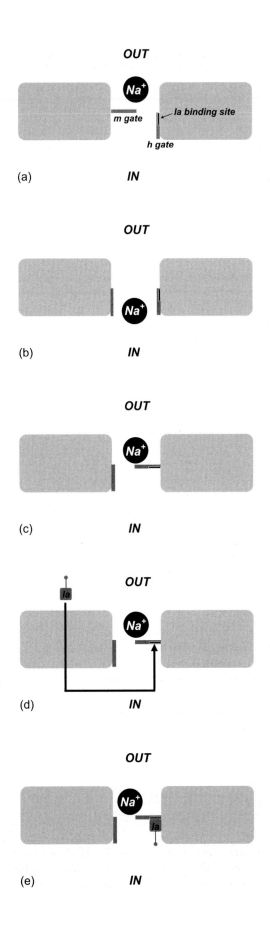

the cell. This sodium influx is soon stopped by the closure of the h gate (Fig. 8.3c). Once closed, the h gate cannot reopen until full repolarization has taken place, thus explaining the phenomenon of the refractory period after excitation. During the refractory period the nerve cannot be excited no matter how large the stimulus. During depolarization there is a temporary reversal of electrical polarity across the cell membrane. This permits an outflow of potassium ions down their concentration gradient (which is opposite to that of sodium). The outward movement of potassium ions brings about a repolarization during which a short-lived hyperpolarization (reversal or overshoot) occurs. The sodium pump, which is temporarily overwhelmed during the inward rush of sodium ions, then extrudes the excess of sodium ions. This is accompanied by a re-entry of potassium ions and recovery of the membrane potential to the resting value.

It is obvious from the above that a crucial step in nerve cell activity is the entry of sodium ions during the firing stage. Local anaesthetics achieve their effect by inhibiting this sodium influx. The model depicted above describes the sodium channel in simple terms, however it is a complex structure. The channel appears to be composed of three subunits (known as α, β_1, and β_2). The α-subunit (Fig. 8.4a) is the major constituent and contains the channel through which sodium ions pass. The other subunits are much smaller. The β_1-subunit maintains the functional stability of the channel. However, the function of the β_2-subunit is unclear as its removal does not appear to affect sodium channel function. The α-subunit is composed of the sodium channel surrounded by four identical or very similar protein domains (I, II, III, and IV). Each domain contains six segments (S1, S2, S3, S4, S5, and S6), each of which is a helix that spans the thickness of the cell membrane (Figs 8.4(a–f)). These helices are interlinked. Segments 1, 2, and 3 are negatively charged. Segment 4 is positively charged and during depolarization this segment twists away from the channel (Fig. 8.4c). Part of the lining of the channel is made up of the linkage between segments 5 and 6; it is this last linkage which appears to provide the binding site for channel blocking drugs (Fig. 8.4d). It is thought that interconnecting loops of protein between domains III and IV can produce physical blockade of the channel due to conformational change (Figure 8.4d). Figure 8.4 relates possible configurational changes within the channel to the simple m and h gate model shown in Figure 8.3.

Membrane expansion theory

This is a non-specific mechanism similar to the action of general anaesthetic agents (see Chapter 9). It relies upon the lipophilic moiety of the local anaesthetic and can explain why non-polarized drugs such as benzocaine achieve conduction blockade. Membrane expansion occurs due to the incorporation of the local anaesthetic molecules into the lipid cell membrane. The resultant swelling produces physical obstruction of the sodium channel, which inhibits entry of the cation thus preventing nerve cell depolarization.

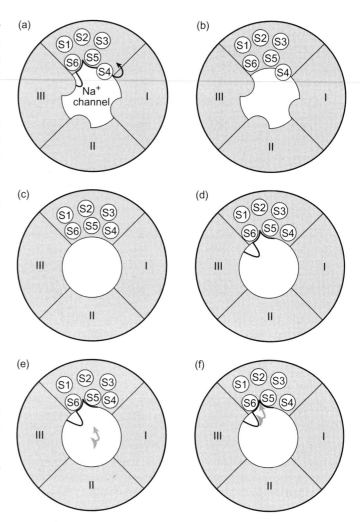

Fig. 8.4 The structure of the α-subunit of the sodium channel. The subunit consists of four protein domains surrounding the channel. Each domain contains six protein segments. Segment 4 is equivalent to the m gate in Fig. 8.3. An interconnecting link of protein between domains III and IV performs the function of the h gate shown in Fig. 8.3. Figs 8.4(b–f) show the conformational changes thought to occur within the channel at different phases equivalent to those shown in Figs 8.3(a–e). Figure 8.4(b) is the channel at the resting phase; Fig. 8.4(c) is the firing phase; Fig. 8.4(d) is the refractory period; Figs 8.4(e) and (f) show the attachment of the local anaesthetic molecule to the exposed receptor site.

Specific receptor theory

This theory dictates that the local anaesthetic binds to a specific receptor within the sodium channel. Strong support for this mechanism is provided by the fact that different isomers of local anaesthetic molecules can vary greatly in their efficacy. The theory requires the presence of a charged local anaesthetic molecule. Binding of the local anaesthetic molecule to a site within the sodium channel is unlikely *per se* to produce physical obstruction to the entry of sodium. However, the act of binding could produce conformational changes within the channel or, if the binding site is related to the h gate, maintain the h gate in the closed position (see Figures 8.3e and 8.4f). This latter scenario explains the phenomenon of frequency-dependent (also known as use-dependent) block. If closure of the h gate is required to expose a binding site for the local anaesthetic then the nerve must fire at least once to enable the h gate to assume the closed position. Importantly, the more rapidly a nerve fires, the more opportunities there will be for the local anaesthetic to attach to the exposed binding site. Pain-transmitting fibres discharge with a greater frequency than motor fibres and this explains why pain transmission is more susceptible to the action of local anaesthetics than motor function.

Role of calcium

Calcium ions regulate the movement of sodium across nerve cell membranes, therefore an adequate extracellular concentration of calcium is essential for normal nerve transmission. Reducing calcium concentration can potentiate the action of a local anaesthetic because both agents compete for the same phospholipid receptor. Nevertheless, it seems that calcium is not involved in the primary nerve-blocking action of local anaesthetics.

Differential sensitivity of nerve fibres to local anaesthetics

The phenomenon of frequency dependence was mentioned above. As a rule the susceptibility of nerve fibres to local anaesthetics is inversely proportional to their diameter, so small nerve fibres are more sensitive than larger fibres. This appears to be related to the greater susceptibility of smaller nerve fibres to a sodium lack. As sensory information is carried by nerve fibres smaller than those that carry motor information, sensation is lost before motor activity is blocked. In general terms, pain is the first sensation to disappear followed by temperature, touch, and pressure.

Myelination also influences the activity of local anaesthetics. In general terms, when everything else is equal, a myelinated fibre is more susceptible to the action of a local anaesthetic than an unmyelinated nerve. This is due to the fact that local anaesthetics may partially block potassium efflux during repolarization, which could sustain depolarizing currents. Myelinated fibres do not rely on potassium loss for repolarization and thus are more susceptible to blockade.

Key facts
Mechanism of action of local anaesthetics

- Local anaesthetics reversibly block the sodium channel by a combination of two mechanisms:
  - membrane expansion;
  - binding to a specific receptor in the sodium channel.

Fate and metabolism of local anaesthetics

Absorption
A number of factors influence the rate of entry of the local anaesthetic into the circulation, including:

(1) the drug itself—local anaesthetics vary in their vasodilatory ability;

(2) the volume and concentration administered;

(3) the route of administration—for example, intraosseous administration is similar to intravenous as far as systemic spread is concerned;

(4) the vascularity of the tissues—the rate of absorption being faster in more vascular tissues. Intraoral injections produce rapid vascular uptake compared to subcutaneous administration. Peak plasma levels occur around 30 minutes after intraoral injection;

(5) whether or not a vasoconstrictor drug has been added to prolong the action of the local anaesthetic (discussed later).

Distribution
Once absorbed into the circulation the local anaesthetic is partially bound to plasma proteins (α_1-glycoprotein and albumin) and red blood cells. The unbound portion, however, is free to enter any organ of the body. Local anaesthetics are not inhibited by any barriers to diffusion. Importantly, they will cross both the blood–brain barrier and the placenta. Highly perfused organs such as the brain, liver, and kidneys are capable of receiving high levels of local anaesthetics.

Metabolism
The manner in which the circulating local anaesthetic is metabolized is governed by its chemical classification.

ESTER METABOLISM
Esters are primarily metabolized in plasma by the enzyme pseudocholinesterase (Figure 8.5). This occurs rapidly, with the elimination half-life of procaine being less than 2 minutes. Approximately 1 in 2800 of the population lack pseudocholinesterase, thus these individuals are at risk of an overdose of ester local anaesthetics (they also suffer from suxamethonium apnoea during general anaesthesia (Chapter 9)). The use of amide local anaesthetics is safe in these patients. Although the majority of ester hydrolysis occurs in plasma some also takes place in the liver. The products of ester hydrolysis have no local anaesthetic action and may undergo further biotransformation in the liver before elimination. Para-aminobenzoic acid (PABA), the major metabolite of the esters, is the agent responsible for most ester allergies.

AMIDE METABOLISM
Amide metabolism (Fig. 8.6) is more complex than that of the esters, with the elimination half-lives of lidocaine and prilocaine

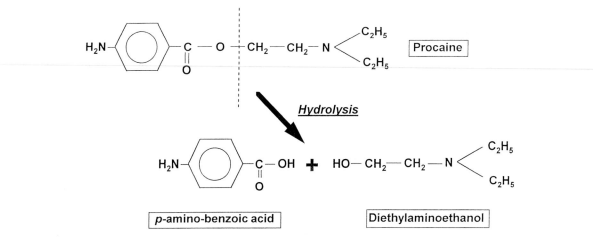

Fig. 8.5 Metabolism of the ester local anaesthetic procaine.

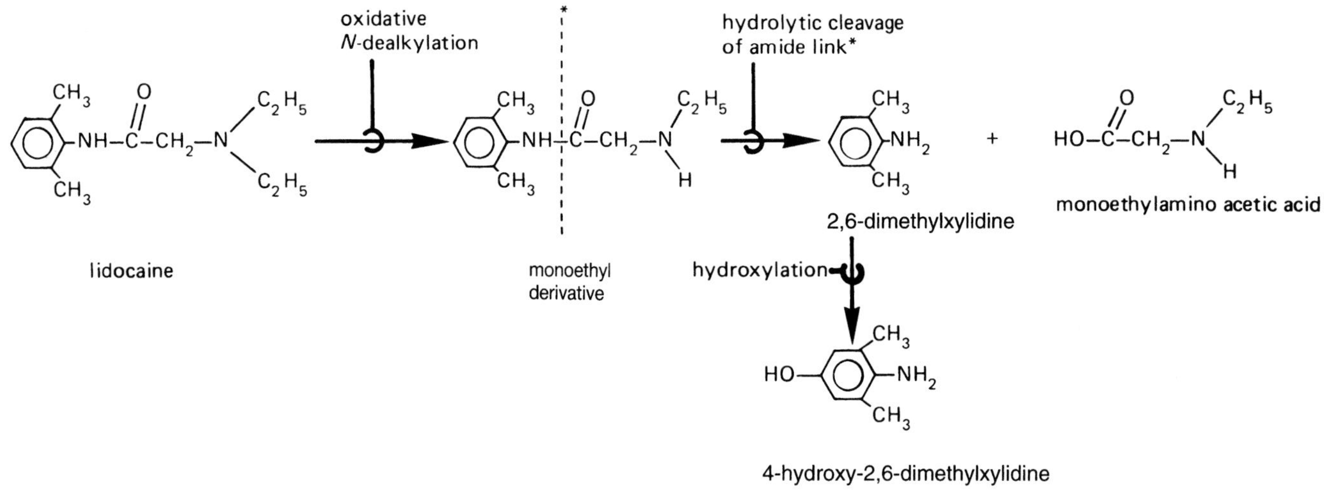

Fig. 8.6 The metabolism of lidocaine (see text for details).

being around 90 minutes. Most amides are metabolized in the liver, although prilocaine undergoes some biotransformation in the lungs and kidneys. Hepatic enzymes dealkylate and hydrolyse the amides. Conjugation with glucuronic acid, hydroxylation of the aromatic ring, and further dealkylation may also occur before excretion. Unlike the esters, some of the products of amide metabolism possess local anaesthetic (and sedative) properties.

Articaine is unusual for an amide in that its structure protects it from the action of hepatic amidases. Although an amide it is metabolized principally by plasma esterases (it has an ester side-chain as part of its thiophene ring which is cleaved).

The liver is of importance in the metabolism of local anaesthetics because it is the major site of metabolism of many of them, and because it is the source of plasma cholinesterase,

which is important in the metabolism of those anaesthetics that contain an ester linkage. For these reasons, a normal dose of local anaesthetic given to a patient suffering from impaired liver function could result in relative overdosage. Dose reduction is often necessary for these patients—where severe liver disease is present, consultation with the supervising physician is essential. Similarly, as liver function decreases with age the absolute ceiling dose (see later) given to elderly patients must be reduced. As a working rule the maximum dose in those over 65 years of age should be 50% of that recommended in healthy young adults.

Excretion

Excretion occurs via the kidney. Normally less than 3% of an administered dose of the commonly used dental local anaesthetic agents is excreted unchanged in urine.

Ester-type local anaesthetics

Throughout this section, see Fig. 8.1 for details of chemistry.

Procaine

This was the archetypal dental local anaesthetic prior to the introduction of lidocaine. Its use has declined for a number of reasons (see below).

Pharmacokinetics

Procaine is rapidly metabolized by the readily available plasma esterases.

Preparations

Procaine is no longer available in dental cartridges in the UK and must be drawn up from an ampoule. The normal presentation is a 2% solution; however, epinephrine (adrenaline) (1:80 000) may be added to this solution to increase efficacy. Procaine is not available as a topical agent.

Recommended uses in dentistry

The only indication for the use of procaine as a local anaesthetic in dentistry is in a patient with a proven allergy to the amide group of local anaesthetics. The other use of procaine relevant to dental practice (specifically intravenous sedation (see Chapter 9)) is that it is part of the recognized regimen to treat arteriospasm. For this indication, procaine is administered intra-arterially. This is due to its excellent vasodilatory properties.

Onset and duration of action

Procaine provides extremely short-lived pulpal anaesthesia of approximately 5 minutes' duration and has a long onset time of around 10 minutes.

Dosages

The maximum dose of procaine is 6 mg kg^{-1} with a ceiling of 400 mg.

Amethocaine

This ester local anaesthetic agent is also known as tetracaine. It was first synthesized in Germany in 1928 and is the most potent of the ester type to be used clinically.

Pharmacokinetics

Amethocaine is hydrolysed by plasma cholinesterase about four times more slowly than procaine. Although its rate of onset is slow, it is rapidly absorbed from mucous membranes because of its very high lipid solubility: its partition coefficient is 80.

Preparations

Although it is effective when given by injection, amethocaine is not used in this manner due to its toxicity. It is available in topical preparations both on its own and in combination with other anaesthetic agents such as lidocaine. A recent formulation (Ametop) is an effective topical dermatological agent.

Benzocaine

Benzocaine is the most commonly used ester local anaesthetic in the UK.

Pharmacokinetics

Benzocaine is hydrolysed very rapidly by plasma esterases to p-aminobenzoic acid, and this presumably accounts for its low toxicity.

Preparations

Due to its extremely poor water solubility this agent is unsuitable for injection and is only provided in topical preparations. It is available in a number of concentrations up to 20%, both alone and in combination with other agents.

Recommended uses in dentistry

Benzocaine is useful as an intraoral topical anaesthetic prior to local anaesthetic injections.

Dosages

Due to its extremely poor solubility in water and poor absorption, toxic reactions to benzocaine are almost unknown.

Cocaine

Cocaine is rarely used these days due to the problems of misuse (see Chapter 25). However, it is mentioned for the sake of completeness. Cocaine is unique among local anaesthetic agents in that it produces vasoconstriction. It has a half-life of 30 minutes.

Pharmacokinetics

Cocaine is metabolized in the liver and also by plasma esterases; the plasma route is probably more important in humans.

Preparations

Cocaine is available as a topical preparation as a 4–10% solution.

Recommended uses in dentistry

The obvious disadvantages of cocaine, particularly its potential for abuse, mean that it should not be considered as a normal part of the dental local anaesthetic armamentarium. It is occasionally used topically (intranasally) during apical surgery on maxillary incisor teeth when the nasal floor is in close proximity.

Dosages

The maximum dose in a healthy adult is 100 mg. This equates to 1 mL of the 10% solution (the maximum dose per kg of body weight is 1.5 mg kg^{-1}).

Key facts
The ester local anaesthetics

- These are:
  - procaine
  - amethocaine
  - benzocaine
  - cocaine.
- Amethocaine and benzocaine are useful topical anaesthetics.

Amide-type local anaesthetics

Lidocaine (lignocaine)

Lidocaine is the most commonly used dental local anaesthetic in the UK. It was synthesized in 1943 and has been in clinical use since 1948. In the UK it has the proprietary names Xylocaine, Lignospan, and Lignostab.

Pharmacokinetics

Lidocaine is highly lipophilic (partition coefficient 3; see Table 8.2) and so is rapidly absorbed. It undergoes virtually complete biotransformation in the liver and has a systemic $t_{0.5}$ of approximately 90 minutes. It is subject to three metabolic transformations—oxidative-N-dealkylation, hydrolysis, and hydroxylation (see Fig. 8.6). It is first dealkylated to the monoethyl derivative, then the amide link is broken by hydrolysis yielding 2,6-dimethylxylidine and monoethyl aminoacetic acid. Finally, the dimethylxylidine undergoes hydroxylation to 4-hydroxy-2, 6-dimethylxylidine. It seems that only the first metabolite (monoethyl aminoacetyl-2,6-xylidide) possesses local anaesthetic properties. All the metabolites have longer half-lives and are less toxic than the parent drug. Negligible amounts of unchanged drug are excreted in the urine.

Preparations

In the UK lidocaine is available in dental local anaesthetic cartridges as a plain 2% solution and as a 2% solution with 1:80 000 epinephrine. Lidocaine is also available in preparations suitable for topical use, i.e.: 4% and 10% sprays, 2% gels, and 5% ointments.

Recommended uses in dentistry

The 'gold standard' dental local anaesthetic in the UK is 2% lidocaine with 1:80 000 epinephrine. The epinephrine-containing solution is ideal for infiltration, intraosseus, intraligamentary, and regional block anaesthesia for the majority of patients. Its use is contraindicated in those allergic to amides and in individuals where increased epinephrine levels may be hazardous. Despite its popularity in the UK, there is no evidence that 1:80 000 epinephrine accords greater efficacy to lidocaine anaesthetics compared to the concentration of 1:100 000 used in other parts of the world.

The plain lidocaine solution is not very effective in obtaining pulpal anaesthesia and its use for soft-tissue procedures is limited due to poor haemorrhage control and reduced duration of action. Lidocaine is an effective topical anaesthetic for use on non-keratinized tissue such as the reflected mucosa. It may be applied topically prior to intraoral injections through reflected mucosa and as a symptomatic treatment for painful mucosal lesions such as ulcers.

Onset and duration of action

Lidocaine has a short onset of action, pulpal anaesthesia being obtained in 2–3 minutes. The plain solution is classified as a short-acting agent and will provide pulpal anaesthesia for about 10 minutes. The epinephrine-containing solution is intermediate in duration providing 45–60 minutes of pulpal anaesthesia.

Dosages

The maximum recommended dose of lidocaine is 4.4 mg kg^{-1} with an absolute ceiling of 300 mg.

Prilocaine

Prilocaine is marketed in the UK under the proprietary name of Citanest. Prilocaine is as potent a local anaesthetic as lidocaine but it is less toxic.

Pharmacokinetics

Prilocaine has a similar profile to that of lidocaine, although it differs in several important ways that account for its lower toxicity. It is less vasodilatory, is distributed more rapidly, and has a larger volume of distribution (see Chapter 1) than lidocaine. Its rate of clearance (2.37 L min^{-1}) is higher than that of all other amide local anaesthetics. This suggests that it may undergo extensive extrahepatic metabolism, resulting in relatively low blood concentrations. This explains why the maximum 'safe' dose of prilocaine (400 mg) is greater than that of lidocaine. It has a half-life of around 90 minutes.

In the liver, prilocaine is cleaved hydrolytically by amidases, to produce α-propyl-aminopropionic acid and o-toluidine. The latter is then oxidized to nitrosotoluidine. The metabolite o-toluidine is capable of causing methaemoglobinaemia (see below), but this is only likely to be significant in adults if more than 600 mg (8.5 mg kg^{-1}) of prilocaine have been administered.

Preparations

In the UK, prilocaine local anaesthetics are provided as plain and vasoconstrictor-containing injectable solutions. The plain solution is 4% prilocaine and the vasoconstrictor-containing version is 3% prilocaine with $0.03\,\text{IU}\,\text{mL}^{-1}$ $(0.54\,\mu\text{g}\,\text{mL}^{-1})$ felypressin. In other parts of the world prilocaine with epinephrine is available.

Prilocaine is combined with lidocaine in the topical anaesthetic agent EMLA (see below), which is used to produce anaesthesia of the skin.

Recommended uses in dentistry

In the UK, 3% prilocaine with $0.03\,\text{IU}\,\text{mL}^{-1}$ felypressin is the usual alternative to lidocaine with epinephrine when a vasoconstrictor-containing solution is required. The main use being in those cases where epinephrine is best avoided. Prilocaine with felypressin is effective when administered as an infiltration or regional block anaesthetic. It is not as effective as lidocaine with epinephrine during intraligamental techniques. The 4% plain solution is more effective than plain 2% lidocaine when a vasoconstrictor-free solution must be employed.

EMLA (eutectic mixture of local anaesthetics) is a 5% mixture of prilocaine and lidocaine. It is an effective topical anaesthetic when applied to skin and therefore is useful prior to venepuncture in children and during dental sedation. At the time of writing a dedicated intraoral formulation of EMLA was being developed by its manufacturers.

Onset and duration of action

Prilocaine has a slightly slower onset of action than lidocaine, pulpal anaesthesia occurring in about 4 minutes.

The plain 4% prilocaine presentation is considered a short-acting agent with pulpal anaesthesia lasting around 10 minutes. 3% prilocaine with $0.03\,\text{IU}\,\text{mL}^{-1}$ felypressin provides duration of anaesthesia similar to that afforded by lidocaine with epinephrine.

Dosages

The maximum recommended dose of prilocaine is $6.0\,\text{mg}\,\text{kg}^{-1}$ with an absolute ceiling of 400 mg.

Mepivacaine

Mepivacaine is the least vasodilatory of the amide local anaesthetics. The proprietary name for mepivacaine in the UK is Scandonest.

Pharmacokinetics

Mepivacaine, like lidocaine, is metabolized in the liver where the amide link is cleaved to yield pipecolylxylidine and monoethylaminoacetic acid. Some unchanged drug is excreted in the urine. However, unlike lidocaine, in neonates it is not metabolized but eliminated by the kidneys. It has a half-life of 120 minutes.

Preparations

In the UK, mepivacaine is available as a 3% plain solution and as a 2% solution with 1:100 000 epinephrine.

Mepivacaine is not available in a topical preparation.

Recommended uses in dentistry

Mepivacaine with epinephrine has identical indications for use as lidocaine with epinephrine, although it has a shorter duration of action. The prime indication for the use of mepivacaine is when a vasoconstrictor-free solution must be employed, as 3% mepivacaine is more effective than plain lidocaine and prilocaine solutions.

Onset and duration of action

Mepivacaine has a rapid onset of action, pulpal anaesthesia being obtained in around 2 minutes. The plain solution provides much longer pulpal anaesthesia than plain lidocaine or prilocaine; pulpal anaesthesia of around 30 minutes being possible. Mepivacaine with epinephrine provides anaesthesia of similar depth as lidocaine with epinephrine, but of slightly shorter duration.

Dosages

The maximum recommended dose for mepivacaine is identical to that for lidocaine, namely $4.4\,\text{mg}\,\text{kg}^{-1}$ with an absolute ceiling of 300 mg.

Bupivacaine

Bupivacaine is provided in the UK under the proprietary name of Marcain. Bupivacaine is classed as a long-lasting local anaesthetic.

Pharmacokinetics

The major part of a dose of bupivacaine is metabolized in the liver. It has a half-life of 160 minutes. After dealkylation and cleavage of the amide link, the metabolite pipecolylxylidine is excreted in the urine. Bupivacaine is absorbed into the systemic circulation from the site of injection more slowly than the shorter-acting amide local anaesthetics lidocaine, prilocaine, and mepivacaine. An important factor here is the greater binding of bupivacaine to plasma and tissue proteins. One useful consequence of this is that less of it passes across the placenta than all the other dental anaesthetics. On the other hand, it has the greatest depressant effect on fetal oxygen saturation.

Preparations

At present, bupivacaine is not supplied in dental local anaesthetic cartridges in the UK although it is available in ampoule form for drawing up into ordinary syringes. The anaesthetic is available in concentrations of 0.25%, 0.375%, 0.5%, and 0.75%. The 0.25% and 0.5% formulations are available with or without 1:200 000 epinephrine. Bupivacaine is not supplied as a topical agent.

Recommended uses in dentistry

Bupivacaine has few indications in routine restorative dentistry. The main uses are in oral surgery. When administered as a regional block bupivacaine confers long-lasting anaesthesia. This is useful for postoperative pain control following procedures such as the surgical removal of impacted third molars. However, some patients find the prolonged soft-tissue anaesthesia somewhat uncomfortable.

Onset and duration of action

The onset time of anaesthesia is slower than that obtained with lidocaine. It may take longer than 5 minutes to obtain pulpal anaesthesia. However, bupivacaine can provide pulpal anaesthesia for 1.5–2 hours. When used as a regional block, soft-tissue anaesthesia of 6–8 hours is possible.

Dosages

The maximum dose of bupivacaine is 1.3 mg kg^{-1} with a ceiling of 90 mg.

Etidocaine

Etidocaine is a long-lasting local anaesthetic first synthesized in the 1970s. It has a similar duration of action to bupivacaine but with a quicker onset.

Pharmacokinetics

Etidocaine is highly lipophilic. Its hepatic clearance is as fast as lidocaine; however, it has a much larger volume of distribution and thus its $t_{0.5}$ is similar to bupivacaine. Etidocaine is dealkylated and hydroxylated in the liver. It is not hydrolysed to the same extent as lidocaine. It has a half-life of 160 minutes.

Preparations

It is not available in dental cartridges in the UK, but is supplied in North America under the trade name Duranest as a 1.5% solution with 1:200 000 epinephrine.

Recommended uses in dentistry

Etidocaine is a long-acting local anaesthetic. Its main indications for use are similar to those mentioned for bupivacaine, namely as a regional block anaesthetic. When used in infiltration techniques for surgical procedures 1.5% etidocaine with 1:200 000 epinephrine is not as effective as 2% lidocaine with 1:80 000 epinephrine.

Onset and duration of action

The duration of action of etidocaine is similar to that of bupivacaine; however, the former drug has a faster onset of action, providing pulpal anaesthesia in 2–3 minutes.

Dosages

The maximum dose of etidocaine is 8 mg kg^{-1} with an absolute ceiling of 400 mg.

Articaine

Articaine is unique among the clinically useful local anaesthetics in that its lipophilic moiety is a thiophene ring. It was introduced in the mid-1970s.

Pharmacokinetics

Unlike the other amides articaine undergoes some biotransformation in plasma. Inactivation by hydrolysis of the ester side-chain

of the thiophene ring is performed by both plasma and liver esterases. It has a half-life of around 75 minutes.

Preparations

Articaine is available in Europe and Canada as a 4% solution with either 1:100 000 or 1:200 000 epinephrine. It was introduced into the UK in late 1998.

Recommended uses in dentistry

The major advantage claimed for articaine is that it has the ability to diffuse widely. It is suggested that palatal anaesthesia can be obtained following maxillary buccal infiltration and that pulpal anaesthesia of mandibular teeth is possible after infiltration anaesthesia in the mandible.

Onset and duration of action

Articaine provides pulpal anaesthesia within 2 minutes of injection. The duration of activity of 4% articaine with 1:200 000 epinephrine is similar to that of 2% lidocaine with 1:100 000 epinephrine.

Dosages

The maximum dose of articaine is 7 mg kg^{-1}.

Ropivacaine

Ropivacaine is a new drug which had just been launched in the UK at the time of writing. It has not been used in clinical dentistry as yet. It is a long-acting agent similar to bupivacaine but is reported to have less cardiotoxicity. It is available in various concentrations: 0.2%, 0.75%; and 1%. The addition of vasoconstrictors does not seem to increase its efficacy in surgical practice.

Pharmacokinetics

Ropivacaine is 94% protein-bound. It has a half-life of around 100 minutes. It is metabolized in the liver where it is hydroxylated and conjugated. Around 4% is excreted unchanged in urine.

Key facts
Amide local anaesthetics

- These include:
  - lidocaine
  - prilocaine
  - mepivacaine
  - bupivacaine
  - etidocaine
  - articaine
  - ropivacaine.

- Lidocaine is the most commonly used local anaesthetic in dentistry. It is employed both topically and by injection. The usual injected formulation is a 2% solution with or without epinephrine. The maximum dose of lidocaine is 4.4 mg kg^{-1}.

- Prilocaine is used as an anaesthetic at a dose of 3% with felypressin, or as a 4% plain solution. It is also a constituent of the topically active EMLA cream. The maximum dose of prilocaine is $6.0 \, mg \, kg^{-1}$.

- Mepivacaine is used as a 2% solution with epinephrine, or as a 3% plain solution. The maximum dose of mepivacaine is $4.4 \, mg \, kg^{-1}$.

- Bupivacaine, etidocaine, and ropivacaine are long-acting amides.

Vasoconstrictors

Vasoconstrictors were originally added to dental local anaesthetic solutions to reduce the systemic uptake of the anaesthetic agent in an attempt to limit toxicity. Although vasoconstrictors influence the entry of anaesthetic agents into the bloodstream this effect is not dramatic. However, the addition of a vasoconstrictor to a dental local anaesthetic solution confers a number of advantages, including:

- longer lasting anaesthesia;
- more profound anaesthesia;
- reduced operative haemorrhage.

On the other hand vasoconstrictors can increase unwanted effects (see below).

The vasoconstrictors added to dental local anaesthetic solutions are either sympathomimetic amines or synthetic polypeptides. Examples of the former group include epinephrine, norepinephrine, levonordefrin, and phenylephrine. At present, the only sympathomimetic amine added to local anaesthetic solutions used in the UK is epinephrine, although others in this group are available elsewhere. Ornipressin, vasopressin, and felypressin are examples of synthetic polypeptides that have been included in dental local anaesthetic formulations. Felypressin is the only one of this group available in solutions marketed in the UK.

Epinephrine (adrenaline)

In addition to its use in dental local anaesthetic solutions, epinephrine has other uses in dentistry. It is available in gingival retraction cord to reduce gingival bleeding during restorative procedures such as impression-taking during the construction of crowns. It is also present in the emergency drug box for the treatment of anaphylactic shock and life-threatening asthmatic attacks (see Chapters 14 and 26).

Mechanism of action of epinephrine (adrenaline)

Epinephrine produces vasoconstriction by interacting with adrenoceptors in blood vessels. A number of receptors are important; α_1- and α_2-adrenoreceptors produce vasoconstriction in the skin and mucous membranes, β_2-receptor stimulation results in vasodilatation in skeletal muscle.

Metabolism of epinephrine (adrenaline)

Notwithstanding the fact that epinephrine is a vasoconstrictor, its appearance in the systemic circulation is rapid, peak plasma levels occurring a few minutes after an intraoral injection. The fact that it is usually injected in combination with a vasodilatory anaesthetic such as lidocaine will contribute to this phenomenon.

Most of the injected dose is absorbed and distributed throughout the body. Metabolism of exogenously administered epinephrine is mostly extraneuronal, it is first methylated by the enzyme catechol-*o*-methyl transferase (COMT) (see Chapter 14). This enzyme is widely distributed throughout the body. Following methylation epinephrine is transported to the liver for deamination (by monoamine oxidase), and may also be conjugated mainly with sulfate prior to excretion in urine. About 1% of an administered dose of epinephrine is excreted unchanged in urine.

Dental local anaesthetic solutions in the UK contain epinephrine in a concentration of 1:80 000 (12.5 $\mu g \, mL^{-1}$). In other countries epinephrine concentrations of 1:50 000, 1:100 000, and 1:200 000 are available in dental local anaesthetic solutions. A 1:80 000 solution is a potent concentration of epinephrine. A 2.2 mL dental local anaesthetic cartridge with epinephrine at this concentration will contain 27.5 μg of the catecholamine. This is a large dose when one considers the circulating epinephrine levels measured in dental patients (Table 8.3).

Systemic effects of epinephrine (adrenaline)

Epinephrine, being a naturally occurring hormone, exerts a number of physiological responses. A number of systems are affected, including:

- the heart
- blood vessels
- haemostasis
- the lungs
- gastrointestinal tract
- genitourinary system
- biological membranes
- metabolism
- wound healing.

EFFECTS ON THE HEART

Epinephrine has both direct and indirect actions on the heart. Direct cardiac effects are due to the activation of β_1-adrenoceptors. This increases the rate and force of contraction of the heart, thus raising cardiac output. In addition to an increase in

Table 8.3 Plasma epinephrine (adrenaline) levels

Patients awaiting dental local anaesthesia	0.027 $\mu g \, L^{-1}$
Patients awaiting third molar surgery	0.034–0.144 $\mu g \, L^{-1}$
Phobic dental patients during dental local anaesthesia	0.86 $\mu g \, L^{-1}$

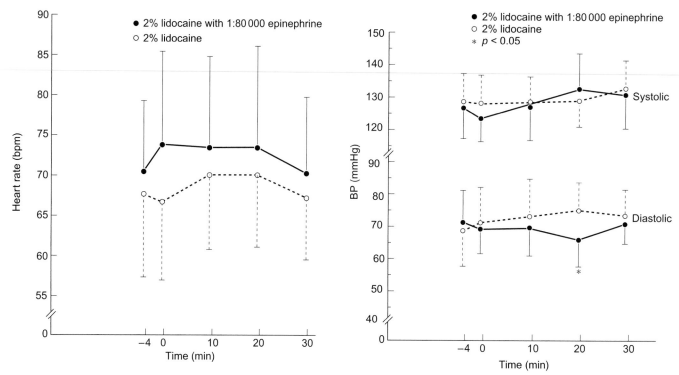

Fig. 8.7 Changes in heart rate 10, 20, and 30 minutes after the injection of two cartridges of either plain lidocaine or lidocaine with epinephrine into the maxillary buccal sulcus of volunteers. The point −4 is the preinjection heart rate. bpm, beats per minute.

Fig. 8.8 Changes in blood pressure (BP) 10, 20, and 30 minutes after the injection of two cartridges of either plain lidocaine or lidocaine with epinephrine into the maxillary buccal sulcus of volunteers. The point −4 is the preinjection blood pressure.

the pulse rate, the cardiac effects may lead to a rise in systolic blood pressure. Standard dental doses of epinephrine have little effect on pulse and systolic blood pressure (Figs 8.7 and 8.8).

EFFECTS ON BLOOD VESSELS

Epinephrine has the greatest vasoconstrictive potency of the sympathomimetic amines. Blood vessels are under the influence of α_1-, α_2-, and β_2-adrenoreceptors. In the skin and mucous membranes α-adrenoceptor agonism causes vasoconstriction. The α_1-receptors are intimately associated with sympathetic nerve terminals and are therefore susceptible to the actions of both endogenous norepinephrine release and exogenous epinephrine. In contrast, α_2-receptors are not so intimately associated with sympathetic synapses and are more susceptible to the effects of circulating epinephrine.

Blood vessels containing β_2-receptors are found principally in skeletal muscle, they are uncommon in skin and mucous membrane. Stimulation of β_2-adrenoreceptors produces vasodilatation through the activation of adenylyl cyclase. This opens up vascular pools in skeletal muscle, resulting in a lowering of the peripheral resistance and thus a fall in diastolic blood pressure. Slight falls in diastolic blood pressure may occur following standard doses of epinephrine-containing dental local anaesthetics (Figure 8.8).

The peripheral vasoconstriction produced by epinephrine is, of course, an advantage when performing surgery as operative blood loss is reduced. Epinephrine-containing local anaesthetics provide much better haemostasis than felypressin-containing solutions and, unless there are medical contraindications, should be used for surgical procedures.

HAEMOSTASIS

The vasoconstrictive effects mentioned above are not the only contribution to haemostasis provided by epinephrine. This catecholamine promotes platelet aggregation. Platelet aggregating effects have been noted after intraoral injections of epinephrine-containing local anaesthetics. Contrary to these promoting effects during the early stages of haemostasis, epinephrine can compromise the stability of formed blood clot because it is a fibrinolytic agent (see below).

EFFECTS ON LUNGS

Stimulation of β_2-adrenoceptors in the lungs leads to bronchiolar muscle relaxation. This is an important feature of the use of epinephrine in the reversal of the life-threatening bronchoconstriction that occurs during the severe allergic reaction of anaphylactic shock. No changes in lung function have been reported following the administration of normal doses of dental local anaesthetics.

EFFECT ON THE GASTROINTESTINAL TRACT

Epinephrine reduces gut-wall contractions and stimulates sphincter closure. These effects have never been demonstrated at dental doses. Salivary secretion is decreased by epinephrine at large doses, but the effect of epinephrine-containing local anaesthetics on salivary flow in dental patients has not been demonstrated.

EFFECT ON THE GENITOURINARY SYSTEM

Epinephrine inhibits urination by causing sphincter contraction and detrussor relaxation. Epinephrine inhibits uterine contraction. These effects are merely of academic interest during dental use.

EFFECTS ON BIOLOGICAL MEMBRANES

Epinephrine, by activating a membrane-bound, sodium–potassium pump, produces hyperpolarization of excitable biological membranes. In animal models this epinephrine-induced hyperpolarization has been shown to induce analgesia following spinal administration. Such an effect has never been demonstrated in humans.

EFFECTS ON METABOLISM

Epinephrine is involved in the control of a number of metabolic processes and also influences the concentrations of a number of plasma constituents including glucose and potassium. Glucose concentration is increased due to an α-adrenoceptor inhibition of insulin release. Plasma potassium levels fall due to β_2-adrenoceptor activation of a membrane-bound, sodium–potassium pump pushing potassium intracellularly. The amounts of epinephrine injected during dental local anaesthesia have been shown to raise circulating glucose levels and reduce plasma potassium concentration (Figs 8.9 and 8.10, respectively).

EFFECTS ON WOUND HEALING

Epinephrine interferes with wound healing by two mechanisms. First, the catecholamine reduces local tissue oxygen tension. Second, as mentioned above, epinephrine produces fibrinolysis.

Felypressin

Felypressin (Fig. 8.11) reduces local blood flow by causing vascular smooth muscle to contract. Felypressin is an analogue of the naturally occurring peptide vasopressin (Figure 8.11), differing only by two amino-acid components. It binds to the vasopressin V_1 receptor and produces vasoconstriction by a phospholipase C-dependent release of intracellular calcium. The vasoconstrictive potency of the polypeptides is less than that of the catecholamines. Unlike the catecholamines, felypressin's activity is more marked on the venous compared to the arteriole side of the circulation. Felypressin-containing local anaesthetics provide poorer control of haemorrhage than epinephrine-containing solutions during operative procedures.

The concentration of felypressin in dental local anaesthetic cartridges in the UK is 0.03 IU mL^{-1} (0.54 µg mL^{-1}).

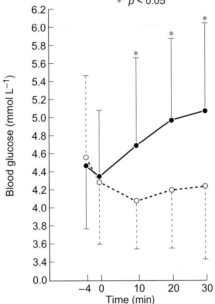

- ● 2% lidocaine with 1:80 000 epinephrine
- ○ 3% prilocaine with 0.03 IU ml^{-1} felypressin
- * $p < 0.05$

Fig. 8.9 Changes in blood glucose concentration 10, 20, and 30 minutes after the injection of two cartridges of either lidocaine with epinephrine or prilocine with felypressin into the maxillary buccal sulcus of volunteers. The point −4 is the preinjection blood glucose

Key facts
Vasoconstrictors

- Vasoconstrictors used in local anaesthetics in the UK are epinephrine and felypressin.

- Epinephrine is present at concentrations of 1:80 000, 1:100 000 and 1:200 000.

- Felypressin is present at a concentration of 0.03 IU mL^{-1}.

- Vasoconstrictors increase the depth and duration of action of local anaesthetics.

- Vasoconstrictors reduce haemorrhage during surgical procedures.

- Vasoconstrictors, especially epinephrine, produce systemic effects.

Other constituents of dental local anaesthetic solutions

In addition to the local anaesthetic agent and a vasoconstrictor, dental local anaesthetic solutions contain other components. These may include the following:

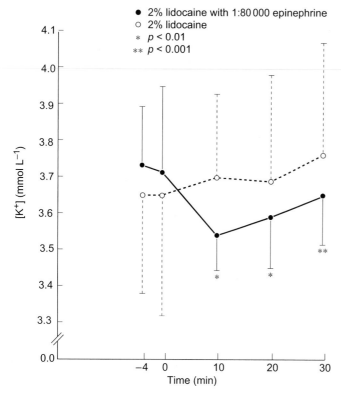

concentration.

Fig. 8.10 Changes in plasma potassium concentration $[K^+]$10, 20, and 30 minutes after the injection of two cartridges of either plain lidocaine or lidocaine with epinephrine into the maxillary buccal sulcus of volunteers. The point −4 is the preinjection plasma potas-

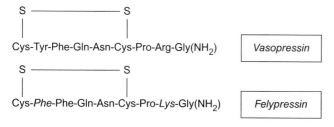

sium concentration.

- a reducing agent;
- a preservative;
- a fungicide (for example thymol);
- Ringer's solution (the vehicle).

A reducing agent such as sodium metabisulfite is added to prevent oxidation of epinephrine when it is present as a vasoconstrictor.

Many modern local anaesthetic solutions are preservative-free, although some contain methylparaben as the preserving agent.

Methylparaben is a derivative of PABA, which is the product of ester local anaesthetic metabolism responsible for allergy to the esters. Thus preservative-free amide solutions should be employed when treating a patient with an ester allergy.

Unwanted effects of dental local anaesthesia

Some unwanted effects are due to apprehension about the injection and are therefore unrelated to the agent employed. Other effects are due to the anaesthetic agent, while others are due to the vasoconstrictor or other additive.

Effects unrelated to the solution

Psychogenic effects

The most common psychogenic complication of local anaesthesia is fainting. The chances of this happening are reduced by sympathetic management and administration of the anaesthetic to patients in the semisupine position.

Infection

The introduction of agents capable of producing generalized infections such as HIV and hepatitis is a complication that should not occur when appropriate cross-infection control measures are employed.

Unwanted effects of local anaesthetic agents

Hypersensitivity

Drug allergy due to a local anaesthetic is rare but important, the main features and underlying mechanism of which are dealt with in Chapter 23. A number of allergic reactions to dental local anaesthetics, ranging from localized sloughing of mucosa to anaphylaxis, have been reported. The ester group of local anaesthetics are more likely to produce allergic reactions compared to the amides. Indeed, the topical ester agent benzocaine has been shown to produce contact sensitivity in around 5% of patients with eczema. Fortunately, hypersensitivity reactions to the amides are extremely rare and most patients who report themselves to be allergic are usually found not to be so when investigated. Other side-effects such as syncope or panic attacks are often mistakenly interpreted as hypersensitivity reactions.

If a patient is known to be hypersensitive to a local anaesthetic with a formula based on p-aminobenzoic acid (for example, procaine) it is almost certain that they will show cross-hypersensitivity to any other local anaesthetic based on that acid (for example, amethocaine). On the other hand, they might well not show cross-hypersensitivity to lidocaine or prilocaine because these compounds are not derivatives of p-aminobenzoic acid (see Fig. 8.1). Nevertheless, it would be unwise to make this assumption in the absence of specific tests for hypersensitivity to lidocaine or prilocaine. These tests are not without their own risks and should be carried out by a specialist in this field. If an allergy is confirmed by such tests it is important to examine other local anaesthetics at the same time to determine which agents can be used safely on that patient.

It should be pointed out that the preservatives found in some local anaesthetic solutions may be a more likely cause of allergy than the anaesthetic agent (see below).

Toxicity

Although concentrations in excess of toxic levels may be achieved during accidental intravascular injection, overdosage of local anaesthetics is unlikely in most adults. However, this can occur in small children with as little as two or three cartridges (Table 8.4). The ester type of local anaesthetic may produce prolonged systemic toxic effects in individuals with atypical forms of pseudocholinesterase. Similarly, systemic reactions to the amide group of anaesthetics may be more likely in patients with liver disease.

Central nervous system toxicity

Central nervous tissue is particularly sensitive to local anaesthetics, and plasma concentrations incapable of influencing peripheral neurone activity may profoundly affect central nervous system function. The plasma concentration of lidocaine at which central nervous system toxicity occurs in humans is around $5\,\mu g\,mL^{-1}$. The effect on the central nervous system at low doses may be excitatory, such as involuntary muscle activity (as a result of the anaesthetic blocking inhibitory activity). At high concentrations the effect is depressant, which may eventually lead to unconsciousness and ultimately respiratory arrest. Fatalities attributable to local anaesthetic overdose are generally due to the depressant effect on the central nervous system.

Cardiovascular toxicity

Effects on the cardiovascular system can be due to the direct action of the local anaesthetic on cardiac tissue and the peripheral vasculature, and also indirectly via inhibition of the autonomic nerve fibres that regulate cardiac and peripheral vascular function. Most local anaesthetic agents have a depressant action on the heart, although cocaine increases heart rate and myocardial excitability. The fact that local anaesthetics affect the cardiovascular system is used therapeutically. Lidocaine is employed in the treatment of cardiac dysrhythmias (see Chapter 16). However, not all effects are beneficial. At low concentrations, via disinhibition of sympathetic activity, heart rate and cardiac output may be increased; at toxic levels, cardiac output may be reduced leading to circulatory collapse. The most cardiotoxic local anaesthetic agent used in dentistry is bupivacaine.

Methaemoglobinaemia

The main toxic effect of prilocaine is cyanosis due to methaemoglobinaemia. Methaemoglobin is haemoglobin that contains iron in the ferric rather than the ferrous state. This reduces the red blood cell's oxygen-carrying capacity. Clinically, the condition presents as cyanosis associated with lethargy and respiratory distress which does not respond to oxygen therapy. Treatment is intravenous administration of 1% methylene blue at a dose of 1.5 $mg\,kg^{-1}$. The methaemoglobinaemia is due to one of prilocaine's metabolites, namely *o*-toluidine, which oxidizes ferrous ions to ferric ions. Methaemoglobinaemia has also been produced by other local anaesthetic agents, for example articaine and benzocaine.

Treatment of toxicity

The best treatment of toxicity is prevention. Prevention is aided by:

(1) aspiration to avoid intravascular injection;

(2) slow injection;

(3) dose limitation (see Table 8.4).

When a toxic reaction occurs then the procedure is:

1. Stop the dental treatment.

2. Provide basic life support.

3. Call for medical assistance.

4. Protect the patient from injury.

5. Monitor vital signs.

Drug interactions

Interactions may occur between local anaesthetic agents and other drugs which the patient may be prescribed.

Table 8.4

Solution	Maximum dose $(mg^{-1}kg)$ (absolute ceiling (mg))	Maximum number of 1.8 ml cartridges in a 70 kg adult	Maximum number of 1.8 ml cartridges in a 5-year-old child weighing 20 kg	Maximum number of 2.2 ml cartridges in 70 kg adult	Maximum number of 2.2 ml cartridges in a 5-year-old child weighing 20 kg
2% Lidocaine	4.4 (300)	8.3	2.4	6.8	2
2% Mepivacaine	4.4 (300)	8.3	2.4	6.8	2
3% Mepivacaine	4.4 (300)	5.6	1.6	4.5	1.3
3% Prilocaine	6.0 (400)	7.4	2.2	6	1.8
4% Prilocaine	6.0 (400)	5.5	1.7	4.5	1.4

Procaine inhibits the antibacterial activity of sulfonamides, and it is theoretically possible that some oral hypoglycaemic agents that are structurally related to the sulfonamides may interfere with the action of procaine.

Local anaesthetic agents may enhance the action of neuromuscular blocking agents, for example lidocaine has been shown to enhance the period of apnoea produced by suxamethonium.

As mentioned above, lidocaine is used as an anti-arrhythmic agent in cardiology. The minimum therapeutic level of lidocaine for cardiac treatment ($1\,\mu g\,mL^{-1}$ of plasma) can be obtained during dental local anaesthesia. It has thus been suggested that care should be taken when using lidocaine with other membrane-stabilizing agents.

A theoretical interaction which can increase local anaesthetic toxicity is that produced by β-adrenoceptor blockers (beta-blockers). These drugs interfere with the metabolism of local anaesthetics by affecting hepatic activity. First, they compete with the local anaesthetics for hepatic enzymes and, second, they reduce hepatic blood flow. These interactions may be important when approaching the maximum doses permissible in healthy patients (see Chapter 1).

Apparently innocuous drug combinations can interact and cause significant problems especially in children. Methaemoglobinaemia has been reported in a child following the application of the topical anaesthetic EMLA. It was concluded from that case that prilocaine (in the EMLA) had interacted with a sulfonamide (which can also produce methaemoglobinaemia) that the child was already receiving.

Unwanted effects of vasoconstrictors

As well as conferring advantages to local anaesthetic solutions, the addition of vasoconstrictors can produce unwanted effects. This is not surprising as epinephrine is a naturally occurring agent and felypressin is similar to endogenous vasopressin. Adverse effects attributable to the vasoconstrictors are more likely with epinephrine-containing solutions as the catecholamine is present in such a potent concentration in dental local anaesthetic solutions (see Table 8.3).

Unwanted effects of epinephrine (adrenaline)

TOXICITY
Epinephrine toxicity presents with the following symptoms:

- anxiety
- restlessness
- trembling
- pounding headache
- palpitations
- sweating with pallor
- weakness
- dizziness
- respiratory distress.

The treatment of an epinephrine overdose is:

1. Stop the treatment.
2. Reduce cerebral blood pressure by sitting the patient upright.
3. Administer oxygen.

CARDIOVASCULAR EFFECTS
Epinephrine may increase cardiac output by raising stroke volume and heart rate, although such changes are not readily demonstrated at dental doses. Mean arterial pressure, however, may be lowered as peripheral resistance is reduced due to the dilator effect on skeletal muscle arterioles (Fig. 8.8).

It would appear sensible to limit the amount of epinephrine used in patients suffering from cardiac disease, but the maximum quantities recommended for such patients vary. A maximum of three cartridges of a 1:80000 ($75\,\mu g$ epinephrine) solution in adult patients is sensible. The use of epinephrine is best avoided in the presence of certain cardiovascular disorders, such as unstable angina, recent myocardial infarct, and refractory cardiac dysrhythmias.

Epinephrine should also be avoided in patients suffering from the rare disease phaeochromocytoma (a tumour of the adrenal glands which produces excess catecholamines).

Patients who are hyperthyroid may be at risk of a crisis when given exogenous epinephrine; however, in patients receiving thyroid replacement therapy there is no need for concern.

METABOLIC EFFECTS
In addition to cardiovascular effects epinephrine has an influence on metabolism. There is a decrease in circulating plasma potassium following the intraoral injection of clinical doses of lidocaine with 1:80000 epinephrine (see Fig. 8.10). Such fluctuations in plasma potassium concentration might affect myocardial stability in susceptible patients.

Similarly, the blood glucose concentration increases significantly following buccal infiltrations of clinical doses of epinephrine-containing dental local anaesthetics, although this is unlikely to represent a hazard (Figure 8.9).

Drug interactions
A number of drugs could interact with the epinephrine contained in dental local anaesthetic solutions. Theoretical interactions could occur with the following:

(1) monoamine-oxidase inhibitors;
(2) tricyclic antidepressants;
(3) phenothiazines;
(4) beta-blockers;
(5) thyroid hormones;
(6) non-potassium sparing diuretics;
(7) drugs of abuse.

MONOAMINE-OXIDASE INHIBITORS

Although exogenous epinephrine is a substrate for monoamine-oxidase, termination of its action is mainly due to extraneuronal uptake and metabolism is principally via catechol-*o*-methyl transferase. Monoamine-oxidase is relatively unimportant in the metabolism of exogenously administered epinephrine, and thus concurrent use of monoamine oxidase inhibitors is *not* a contraindication to the use of epinephrine-containing local anaesthetics.

TRICYCLIC ANTIDEPRESSANTS

Tricyclic antidepressants inhibit the uptake of catecholamines at sympathetic nerve terminals. Neuronal uptake is the prime mechanism for the inactivation of norepinephrine released from noradrenergic nerve terminals. The carrier protein has a lower affinity for epinephrine, although blockade of neuronal uptake with tricyclic antidepressant drugs could lead to increased pressor effects of epinephrine. However, there is *no* clinical evidence that the amount of epinephrine used in dental local anaesthetics has any significant interaction with tricyclics; however, it is probably wise to limit the amount of epinephrine administered to such adult patients to around 50 μg (2 cartridges of a 1:80 000 solution).

PHENOTHIAZINES

Epinephrine may potentiate the hypotension produced by large doses of phenothiazines. This is because phenothiazines produce α-adrenoceptor blockade, thus only the β-adrenoceptor agonist effects of epinephrine are produced. However, within the normal dose range of phenothiazines this is *not* a problem and the use of epinephrine in the quantities employed during dental local anaesthesia is not contraindicated in patients taking phenothiazines.

β-BLOCKERS

The pressor effects of epinephrine are enhanced by β-adrenoceptor antagonists because the vasodilatory β_2-adrenoceptors are blocked. Hypertensive crises have been reported in dental patients taking β-blockers. The same mechanism may prolong, even further, the duration of pulpal anaesthesia afforded by epinephrine-containing local anaesthetics in those receiving β-blockers. This latter phenomenon would not be considered a contraindication for the use of such local anaesthetics in patients medicated with β-blockers.

THYROID HORMONES

Thyroid hormones do not cause any drug interaction problems if used at normal replacement doses.

NON-POTASSIUM SPARING DIURETICS

The decrease in circulating potassium levels attributable to epinephrine in dental local anaesthetic solutions (see above) has been shown to be exacerbated by therapeutic doses of non-potassium sparing diuretics (thiazide and loop diuretics) in oral surgery patients. The dose limitation described above for patients with cardiac disease is recommended for individuals taking these drugs.

DRUGS OF ABUSE

In addition to interactions with prescribed medications, epinephrine will interact with drugs of abuse such as cocaine. Cocaine is a sympathomimetic agent and it can produce catecholamine hypersensitivity and increased adrenergic responses. It would be wise to avoid epinephrine-containing local anaesthetics in cocaine abusers if the illicit drug has been taken within the previous 24 hours.

Other drugs of abuse that can exacerbate the effects of epinephrine include cannabis and inhalants. The performance-enhancing drugs clenbuterol and ephedrine are also sympathomimetic agents, and additive effects with these could be a cause of concern (see Chapter 25).

Unwanted effects of felypressin

Felypressin at high concentrations may cause coronary vasoconstriction, so it is wise to limit the amounts of felypressin-containing solutions to no more than three cartridges in adult patients with cardiac disease.

Felypressin contains some oxytocic activity and thus it might be considered unwise to use this drug in pregnant patients. However, the amount of oxytocic activity contained in a standard dental local anaesthetic cartridge is around 100-fold less than that needed to stimulate uterine contraction.

Unwanted effects of other constituents of dental local anaesthetic solutions

The preservatives used in some local anaesthetic solutions may be allergenic, and these are more likely than the amide anaesthetic agent to be the cause of allergic reactions to local anaesthetic solutions. Methylparaben, a preservative structurally related to *p*-aminobenzoic acid (from which most of the commonly used ester local anaesthetics are derived), is present in some amide local anaesthetic solutions. It is better to avoid the use of methylparaben-containing solutions in patients allergic to the ester local anaesthetics in case cross-reactivity occurs. In addition, methylparaben can act as the initial antigenic stimulant as it is available in many other compounds such as toothpaste and suntan oils.

Sulfites are present in some local anaesthetics to prevent the breakdown of the vasoconstrictor component, and these chemicals are known allergens especially in asthmatic patients.

Key facts
Unwanted effects of local anaesthesia

- These can be due to:
  - psychogenic effects;
  - the local anaesthetic agent;
  - the vasoconstrictor;
  - preservatives.

(cont.)

- Hypersensitivity reactions can be caused by the local anaesthetic agent or the preservative.

- Toxicity can de due to the anaesthetic agent or epinephrine.

- Drug interactions may occur between the anaesthetic agent or epinephrine and the patient's medication.

Further reading

Jastak, J. T., Yagiela, J. A., and Donaldson, D. (1995). *Local anesthesia of the oral cavity*. Saunders, Philadelphia.

Malamed, S. F. (1997). *Handbook of local anesthesia* (4th edn). Mosby, St Louis.

Meechan, J. G., Robb, N. D., and Seymour, R. A. (1998). *Pain and anxiety control for the conscious dental patient*. Oxford University Press, Oxford.

9

General anaesthesia and sedation

General anaesthesia and sedation

General anaesthesia

General anaesthesia is the drug-induced absence of the perception of all sensation, allowing surgery or other painful procedures to be carried out. A general anaesthetic comprises three component parts known as the 'triad of anaesthesia':

(1) narcosis (sleep);

(2) muscle relaxation;

(3) reflex suppression (analgesia).

General anaesthesia is usually induced by intravenous agents and maintained by inhalation agents. Several other drugs are used in conjunction with general anaesthetic agents to ensure a safe, smooth, and uneventful operative procedure. These include drugs used to premedicate the patient and neuromuscular blocking agents.

Mode of action of anaesthetic agents

It is the physicochemical properties of anaesthetic agents that are responsible for their mode of action rather than the chemical configuration of the drug itself. Most anaesthetic agents do not act via specific receptors but instead exert their effects by interacting with components of the cell membrane, especially lipids and proteins. The interface of anaesthetic agents with lipids in the cell membrane is thought to cause a functional disturbance in the cell, either by producing an expansion in cell volume or by increasing the fluidity of the cell membrane. In addition, it is believed that anaesthetic molecules can bind to functional proteins in the cell membrane. These proteins may represent receptors or ion channels, which are subsequently altered as a result of attachment of the anaesthetic molecule. The interaction of anaesthetic agents with both membrane lipids and proteins produces sufficient alteration in cell function so that neural transmission is inhibited.

Clinically, there is a close correlation between anaesthetic potency and lipid solubility (or oil:water partition coefficient, see Chapter 8). Inhalational agents with a low solubility, such as nitrous oxide, are poor anaesthetic agents. Conversely, other agents with a high solubility (e.g. halothane) are potent anaesthetic agents. Lipid solubility is inversely related to the minimum alveolar concentration (MAC) of an anaesthetic gas. The MAC value is the minimum inhaled concentration of the drug required to prevent a response to a surgical stimulus. The MAC for nitrous oxide is very high (105%) which means that it is very difficult to use nitrous oxide alone to produce general anaesthesia.

Premedication agents

Premedication may be defined as the administration of drugs before an anaesthetic with a view to facilitating the operation and anaesthetic. Drugs used for this purpose are divided into those used for their sedative effects, and those used for their anticholinergic effects. The properties required of an ideal premedication agent are the ability:

(1) to alleviate preoperative anxiety;

(2) to provide some degree of postoperative amnesia, especially in children; so that a possibly unpleasant experience is not remembered;

(3) to make the induction and maintenance of anaesthesia smoother;

(4) to reduce the amount of anaesthetic agents required by enhancing their effects;

(5) to provide additional analgesia during surgery and in the postoperative period;

(6) to reduce salivary and bronchial secretions;

(7) to reduce activity in the parasympathetic nervous system, especially in the vagal plexus.

Opioids, anxiolytics, antipsychotics, and anticholinergic drugs are used as premedication agents.

Opioids

Morphine, pethidine, and papaveretum (a mixture of opium alkaloids) are the main opioids used in this way. The pharmacological properties and mode of action of the opioids have been discussed in Chapter 7. Their analgesic, sedative, and euphoriant properties make them popular as premedication agents, although administration inevitably requires an intramuscular injection. The dose regimens are shown in Table 9.1. Morphine does produce certain unwanted effects, in particular, nausea and vomiting. The incidence of post-operative vomiting with morphine is about 20%, but is higher in ambulatory patients. Postoperative vomiting and

Table 9.1 Dosage and routes of administration of opioids used as premedication agents

Drug	Route	Adult dose (mg)	Child dose (mg kg^{-1})	Times of administration
Pethidine hydrochloride	IM	50–150	1–2	1 hour before operation
Morphine sulfate	IM	10–15	0.2	1–1.5 hours before operation
Papaveretum	IM	10–20	0.3	45–60 min before operation

Table 9.2 Dosages and routes of administration of neuroleptic drugs used as premedication agents

Drug	Route	Adult dose	Child dose	Times of administration
Promethazine hydrochloride	Oral		2–5 years 15–20 mg 5–10 years: 20–25 mg	1–2 hours before operation
	IM	25–50 mg	6.25–12.5 mg	1 hour before operation
Trimeprazine tartrate	IM	3–4.5 mg kg^{-1}	2–4 mg kg^{-1}	1–2 hours before operation

nausea can be reduced by use of an antiemetic such as cyclizine, prochlorperazine, or ondansetron. The incidence of these effects is less after papaveretum. Pethidine is a less powerful analgesic than either morphine or papaveretum, but has a lower incidence of unwanted effects.

All the opioids produce a degree of respiratory depression and suppression of the cough reflex; however, it is important to avoid this suppression after abdominal and chest surgery where coughing is essential to clear the lungs of excessive secretions, and reduce the risk of pneumonia.

Anxiolytics

The benzodiazepines (diazepam, lorazepam, and temazepam) are used orally to provide preoperative sedation. Their use is discussed below in the section 'Oral sedation'. There is an increasing trend to use benzodiazepines rather than opioids as premedication agents. Certainly, for in-patient dental surgical procedures, premedication with an oral benzodiazepine such as temazepam is preferred to one of the opioids.

Antipsychotics (neuroleptics)

Phenothiazine derivatives, such as promethazine and trimeprazine, are sometimes used as premedication agents. These drugs are effective as preanaesthetic sedatives and they have a powerful potentiating effect on general anaesthetics. Phenothiazine derivatives also have important antiemetic properties and are valuable in patients who fear or who have a predisposition to postoperative vomiting. They also depress respiration, but not as markedly as the opioids, and cause a varying amount of hypotension. Dose regimens are shown in Table 9.2.

Anticholinergics

Most gaseous anaesthetic agents cause an increase in salivary and bronchial secretions during induction and light anaesthesia. This excessive production of saliva and mucus may cause respiratory obstruction, which will interfere with the smooth course of the anaesthetic and, more seriously, may put the patient's life at risk. It is thus essential that every patient, except those having the briefest of anaesthetics, should receive a drug that reduces these secretions. The need to depress salivary secretion during anaesthesia is even more important in children than in adults: the larynx and trachea are so small that a minimal quantity of secretion may cause laryngospasm. Anticholinergic drugs reduce secretions and prevent overactivity of the parasympathetic nervous system especially in the vagus nerve. Drugs used to reduce salivary and bronchial secretions are atropine sulfate, hyoscine, and glycopyrrolate.

Atropine sulfate

Atropine is the archetypal anticholinergic agent that was used extensively to reduce salivary and bronchial secretions during anaesthesia. It produces these effects by antagonizing the actions of acetylcholine at muscarinic receptors (see Chapter 14). Atropine can be given intravenously immediately before anaesthesia, the adult dose being 300–600 μg. The same dose can be given intramuscularly 30–60 minutes before induction. For children the dose is 20 μg kg^{-1}. The use of atropine has now been superseded by new anticholinergic agents (see later).

HYOSCINE

Like atropine, this antagonizes the effect of endogenous acetylcholine at muscarinic receptors. The adult dose of hyoscine needed to dry up secretions is 200–600 μg given intramuscularly 30–60 minutes before induction of anaesthesia. Unlike atropine, hyoscine is a central nervous system depressant and causes a varying amount of drowsiness. It also depresses the vomiting centre and as such is an antiemetic. At high doses, atropine may act as a stimulant of the central nervous system. Elderly people are sometimes confused by hyoscine and it is therefore best avoided in their premedication.

Both atropine and hyoscine block the action of acetylcholine released from vagal nerve endings in the heart. This gives some protection against the vagal stimulation.

GLYCOPYRROLATE

This is a quaternary ammonium anticholinergic agent. It is highly ionized at physiological pH and thus poorly penetrates the blood–brain barrier and the placenta. Glycopyrrolate produces prolonged and good control of salivary and pharyngeal secretions at doses that do not produce marked changes in heart rate. It has less effect on the cardiovascular system than atropine.

Glycopyrrolate is also used as a preoperative or intraoperative antimuscarinic agent to attenuate or prevent the intraoperative bradycardia sometimes associated with the use of suxamethonium, or due to cardiac vagal reflexes. The usual adult does of glycopyrrolate is 0.2–0.4 mg intravenously or intramuscularly before the induction of anaesthesia. For children, the dose is 4–8 μg kg^{-1} up to a maximum of 0.2 mg. Glycopyrrolate and atropine are used to prevent the muscarinic side-effects of cholinesterase inhibitors such as neostigmine, which are used to antagonize the activity of non-depolarizing muscle relaxants.

Key facts
Premedication agents

- Premedication agents are administered preoperatively to facilitate the anaesthetic and operation.

- Premedication aims to produce anxiolysis, analgesia, and amnesia.

- Oral benzodiazepines are used to provide anxiolysis prior to oral surgical procedures.

- Anticholinergic agents are used in premedication to reduce salivary and bronchial secretions.

- The use of premedication will smooth the induction of anaesthesia and may reduce the amount of drug required to maintain the anaesthetic.

Neuromuscular blocking agents

These are widely used in anaesthetic practice because, by specifically blocking the neuromuscular junction, they enable light levels of anaesthesia to be used with adequate relaxation of the muscles of the abdomen and diaphragm. Neuromuscular blocking agents produce relaxation of abdominal muscles (which allows surgical access) and paralysis of respiratory muscles. Prior to their introduction into anaesthetic practice, anaesthesia had to be very deep indeed to achieve the same degree of relaxation. They also relax the vocal cords, so allowing the passage of an endotracheal tube.

There are two types of neuromuscular blocking agents, with different mechanisms of action: non-depolarizing (competitive) muscle relaxants and depolarizing muscle relaxants. To understand their action it is necessary to review the events of muscle contraction.

Muscle contraction

Acetylcholine bridges the gap between a motor nerve terminal and the motor/muscle end-plate or postsynaptic membrane. The sequence of events leading to muscle contraction is as follows:

1. An action potential travels down the motor nerve and causes the release of packets or 'quanta' of acetylcholine. Each quantum consists of many millions of acetylcholine molecules.

2. The released acetylcholine crosses the synaptic cleft and interacts with nicotinic receptors on the end-plate of a muscle fibre (See Chapter 14).

3. In the resting phase the muscle cell membrane is polarized, the interior being electronegative to the exterior. The surge of released acetylcholine impinging upon the end-plate receptor of the muscle brings about a massive increase in the permeability of the postsynaptic membrane to sodium ions. Sodium ions enter and generate a local end-plate potential. When this depolarization of the end-plate potential reaches a critical threshold, this triggers off a muscle action potential that is propagated along the muscle fibre, causing it to contract.

4. Acetylcholine is very rapidly broken down by cholinesterases in the neuromuscular junction; the motor end-plate repolarizes and is then ready to be stimulated again.

Non-depolarizing muscle relaxants

TUBOCURARINE

Natives of South America used to smear their arrows with curare to paralyse their victims. The active component of curare is D-tubocurarine, and although this drug is now rarely used as a neuromuscular blocking agent, it was the first compound to be used for this purpose.

Tubocurarine is highly ionized and ineffective by mouth, so it is given intravenously. In humans it produces paralysis of all voluntary muscles, including those of respiration, so patients should always have their respiration controlled until the drug has been inactivated. Its action commences about 3–4 minutes after injection and lasts up to 40 minutes. Thus the dose needs to be repeated every 40 minutes to maintain muscle relaxation.

Tubocurarine produces its action by occupying nicotinic receptors on a muscle end-plate. It competes with acetylcholine for the motor end-plate and prevents access of acetylcholine to the receptor so that the depolarization necessary for muscular contraction does not occur. Tubocurarine is therefore a competitive neuromuscular blocking agent.

Tubocurarine is largely used as an adjunct to general anaesthesia. To produce deep muscular relaxation by means of a general anaesthetic substance, the depth of anaesthesia has to be profound, and this may cause serious depression of the medullary centres of respiration and circulation. Tubocurarine will produce a profound muscular relaxation so that only a minimal amount of the general anaesthetic agent will be required. It does not in itself affect consciousness.

The actions of tubocurarine can be reversed by the administration of neostigmine, which is an anticholinesterase agent (see Chapter 14). The competition between acetylcholine and tubocurarine for the same receptor sites is a quantitative phenomenon. Neostigmine prevents the destruction of acetylcholine by cholinesterases and so prolongs its effects, with the result that the activity of tubocurarine is overcome. When tubocurarine has been used as an adjunct to general anaesthetic agents it is customary to assist recovery by the intravenous injection of neostigmine. However, before giving neostigmine, it is essential to administer atropine sulfate or glycopyrrolate intravenously to prevent the muscarinic actions of accumulated acetylcholine (for example, slowing the heart).

In addition to producing neuromuscular blockade, tubocurarine is a weak ganglion blocker, and it also causes the release of histamine. Peripheral vasodilatation caused by the histamine release, together with the sympathetic ganglia blockade, will lower the blood pressure. If tubocurarine is rapidly injected intravenously, there is likely to be a severe drop in blood pressure. The release of histamine may also cause flushing of the skin and bronchospasm.

Tubocurarine does not cross the blood–brain barrier or the placenta.

PANCURONIUM

This is more potent than tubocurarine but has a shorter period of action. It acts in the same way by competitive block but, unlike tubocurarine, it does not normally block transmission in autonomic ganglia and so does not significantly alter the blood pressure. However, if rapidly injected intravenously, the drug may cause a rise in blood pressure as a consequence of vagal blockade and tachycardia. Pancuronium does not cause histamine to be released from mast cells and so is unlikely to induce bronchospasm. It thus has obvious advantages and is widely used to produce relaxation in clinical anaesthesia.

In addition to producing muscular relaxation during anaesthesia, drugs like pancuronium may be used to produce relaxation in a number of pathological conditions, for example tetanus.

ATRACURIUM AND VECURONIUM

These are the neuromuscular blocking agents most often used at the present time. They have little effect on the cardiovascular system, so there is relatively little change in blood pressure. Atracurium (but not vecuronium) may produce histamine release but this is much less marked than with tubocurarine. Neither drug produces sympathetic blockade. Atracurium has an advantage over other non-depolarizing muscle relaxants in patients with renal or hepatic impairment, in that it is degraded by non-enzymatic Hofmann elimination, which is independent of renal and hepatic function.

Depolarizing muscle relaxants

SUXAMETHONIUM

This depolarizes the postsynaptic membrane and maintains this state so that the adjacent muscle fibres are electrically inexcitable. Although suxamethonium is fairly quickly hydrolysed by plasma cholinesterase, its action is long enough (5 minutes) to be clinically useful. It is the ideal agent for use when passing an endotracheal tube. It is injected intravenously and within half a minute it produces complete muscular relaxation. Its short duration of action makes it useful in preventing muscular movements during electroconvulsive therapy (sometimes used in the treatment of severe or drug-resistant depression). If longer procedures are required then the drug can be used in repeated dosage.

The action of suxamethonium may be prolonged in patients with low plasma cholinesterase levels due to liver disease. However, the prolonged apnoea that occasionally follows the administration of suxamethonium could be due to the presence of an abnormal cholinesterase. It has been estimated that about 1 in 2800 people have this atypical esterase, which hydrolyses suxamethonium more slowly than plasma cholinesterase so that the duration of neuromuscular block is prolonged. This is an example of an unwanted effect—idiosyncrasy (see Chapter 23). This condition is inherited and is treated by positive-pressure artificial respiration with oxygen and maintenance of a patent airway until recovery of normal respiration. Neostigmine 0.5–2 mg IV or edrophonium 10 mg IV will facilitate normal respiratory function, but atropine or glycopyrrolate is administered to counteract the muscarinic effects of neostigmine and edrophonium.

Suxamethonium promotes the release of intracellular potassium and this may be important in patients taking digoxin and/or diuretics. Digoxin may itself promote the intracellular depletion of potassium, and many diuretics increase the excretion of potassium. This property is also important in patients with renal failure, therefore suxamethonium is contraindicated in patients with kidney disease. The drug has a number of muscarinic actions, including increased salivary secretion. Muscle injury may occasionally occur with suxamethonium: this may be due to a direct action of the drug on muscle or may follow potassium depletion from muscles. A significant loss of potassium can produce dangerous cardiac dysrhythmias.

Occasionally, malignant hyperpyrexia has followed the use of halothane with suxamethonium. This condition is familial with an incidence of between 1 in 15 000 and 1 in 50 000. It is characterized by a severe, rapid rise in temperature, muscle rigidity, a massive rise in oxygen consumption, and carbon dioxide production. Malignant hyperpyrexia is treated by rapid cooling, inhalation of 100% oxygen, and the intravenous administration of dantrolene $1\,mg\,kg^{-1}$ body weight. Dantrolene blocks the release of calcium ions from the sarcoplasmic reticulum, so reducing muscle tone and heat production.

Key facts
Neuromuscular blocking agents

- Neuromuscular blocking agents are primarily used in anaesthesia to produce relaxation of the vocal cords to allow endotracheal intubation, and relaxation of the abdominal muscles to allow surgical access.

- There are two types of muscle relaxants: non-depolarizing and depolarizing.

- Non-depolarizing muscle relaxants block acetylcholine receptors on the motor end-plate. They are used where abdominal muscle paralysis is required.

- Depolarizing muscle relaxants act by depolarizing the post-synaptic membrane thereby preventing muscle contraction. They are used mainly to relax the vocal cords prior to endotracheal intubation.

- The action of non-depolarizing muscle relaxants can be reversed using the anticholinesterase, neostigmine.

Intravenous anaesthetic agents

These are widely used to induce anaesthesia. They are very potent drugs and, once injected, little can be done to terminate their action. All can also be used to maintain anaesthesia during short, painful operations such as the reduction of a dislocation. The most widely used intravenous anaesthetic agents are sodium thiopental (thiopentone), methohexital (methohexitone), etomidate, and propofol. Ketamine is sometimes used for intravenous induction.

Sodium thiopental (thiopentone)

Sodium thiopental is an ultrashort-acting barbiturate (ethyl thiobarbiturate). The sodium salt is water-soluble and the anaesthetic dose is 3–5 mg kg^{-1} body weight.

PHARMACOKINETICS

Sodium thiopental (thiopentone) is given intravenously and produces loss of consciousness in 10–20 seconds. The maximum depth of anaesthesia occurs 40 seconds after dosage and the patient becomes conscious 2–3 minutes after administration. The drug rapidly enters the brain because of its high lipid solubility. Its short action is attributable to the rapid fall in plasma concentration that occurs when it is distributed into the tissues, especially into the muscles, then adipose tissue. About 85% of sodium thiopental is bound to plasma proteins, and the drug is metabolized in the liver, the metabolites being excreted via the kidney. The final metabolism of thiopental is slow—it has a $t_{0.5}$ of approximately 400 minutes.

PHARMACOLOGICAL PROPERTIES

Sodium thiopental (thiopentone) depresses many of the functions of the central nervous system (see Chapter 15), resulting in sedation, anaesthesia, and a dose-related respiratory depression. Like other barbiturates, it has no analgesic properties and low doses may even increase sensitivity to pain. It is also an anticonvulsant and can be used in an emergency for status epilepticus.

Anaesthetic doses of sodium thiopental produce a reduction in cardiac output and in the force of cardiac contraction. There is also a transient drop in blood pressure. Administration of thiopental is often associated with laryngospasm and even bronchospasm, but the mechanism of these reactions is unknown. It has no effect on the uterus, but it does cross the placenta and can depress the fetal cardiovascular system.

USES

Sodium thiopental (thiopentone) is widely used to induce unconsciousness prior to inhalation anaesthesia, and to provide anaesthesia for short operative procedures, such as the reduction of a dislocation, and in electroconvulsive therapy.

UNWANTED EFFECTS

Cough, laryngospasm, and bronchospasm are reported unwanted effects of thiopental (thiopentone), but these are rare. Because of the incidence of laryngospasm and bronchospasm, thiopental should not be used in asthmatics. An extravascular injection of sodium thiopental will cause pain and tissue necrosis may occur if the concentration of the solution is greater than 2.5%. If it is inadvertently injected into an artery, the endothelial and deeper layers are immediately damaged, then an endarteritis and sometimes thrombosis may occur. This damage is caused by both the drug crystallizing out of solution due to reduced dilution in blood, and a change in pH. If untreated, ischaemia and even gangrene may result. Damage to the arterial wall is instantaneous and treatment should be rapid. The needle should be left *in situ* and the artery infused with 5–10 mL of 1% procaine, which will reduce the pain and arteriospasm. Heparin should then be administered to inhibit thrombus formation, and a regional block of the sympathetic nerves performed, to cause arterial dilatation. The damage from intra-arterial injections of sodium thiopental is much less when the concentration of the solution is 2.5% or less.

Sodium thiopental, together with other barbiturates, must not be given to patients with porphyria—a condition which has a high incidence in South Africans of Afrikaner descent. In patients with porphyria barbiturates cause widespread demyelination of the peripheral and cranial nerves and disseminated lesions throughout the central nervous system, resulting in pain, weakness, and paralysis; these may be life-threatening.

Methohexital (methohexitone)

Like sodium thiopental (thiopentone), this is also an ultrashort-acting barbiturate (sodium oxybarbiturate), and consequently both drugs have similar pharmacological properties. However, the terminal half-life of methohexital (methohexitone) is much shorter (240 minutes) than that of thiopental, so it is more suited for use in day-case surgery. Anaesthesia is induced with a dose of

$1 \, \text{mg} \, \text{kg}^{-1}$ body weight, and recovery is rapid. Unwanted effects include pain on injection, involuntary movements, cough, and laryngospasm. Methohexital (methohexitone) has convulsant properties and can induce fits during anaesthesia. Because of this property, it is contraindicated in patients with a history of epilepsy or other convulsive disorders and, unlike sodium thiopental, must not be used to treat status epilepticus.

Etomidate

Chemically, etomidate is a carboxylated imidazole derivative. For induction purposes, it is used at a dose of $0.2–0.3 \, \text{mg} \, \text{kg}^{-1}$ body weight. Its main advantages over the short-acting barbiturates are rapid recovery and lack of 'hangover' effect for the patient. Both these properties may be due to the short plasma half-life (about 1 hour). Intravenous injections of etomidate are painful and cause extraneous muscle movements. Because it does not cause histamine release, it can be used as an induction agent in asthmatics and in patients with a history of drug hypersensitivity. Etomidate has little or no effect on the cardiovascular system and is therefore mainly used for patients with cardiac disease. Prolonged use of etomidate can cause adrenocortical suppression. However, such use would only occur in intensive care units.

Ketamine

This soluble anaesthetic induction agent is usually given intravenously, but can be given intramuscularly. It is used as a 1%, 5%, or 10% solution. Ketamine has high lipid solubility and rapidly passes the blood–brain barrier. An intravenous dose of $10 \, \text{mg} \, \text{kg}^{-1}$ body weight produces anaesthesia within 30 seconds that lasts for 5–10 minutes. Unlike the short-acting barbiturates, ketamine is associated with profound sedation and analgesia. It produces dissociation but not unconsciousness, so airway reflexes are maintained. The fact that it can be administered intramuscularly is useful where there are poor veins.

The main unwanted effects of ketamine are vivid hallucinations and nightmares. The drug also raises blood pressure and pulse rate, and so should not be used in hypertensive patients. Ketamine is particularly useful in the management of mass casualties, especially in anaesthetizing trapped patients so that amputations can be performed.

Propofol

This is a relatively new phenolic (di-isopropylphenol), intravenous, anaesthetic-induction agent. The drug is also licensed for use in the maintenance of anaesthesia, provided the surgical procedure does not exceed 1 hour. The use of propofol is increasing, and it is fast becoming the agent of choice for the induction of anaesthesia and for maintenance in day-case surgery. The dose needed for induction is $2–2.5 \, \text{mg} \, \text{kg}^{-1}$ body weight. Light general anaesthesia can be maintained by repeated bolus injections of 25–50 mg or by a continuous infusion. Recovery from such an anaesthetic is usually rapid, and is often accompanied by euphoria.

PHARMACOKINETICS

Propofol is highly lipophilic and, following an intravenous dose, there is a rapid decline in blood concentrations, indicating a swift distribution into the tissues. The pharmacokinetic profile is best described as a three-phase sequence:

(1) a very rapid distribution from blood ($t_{0.5}$ about 2–4 minutes);

(2) a rapid intermediate phase reflecting metabolic clearance ($t_{0.5}$ 35–45 minutes);

(3) a slower final phase, representing the slow return of drug to the blood from a poorly perfused deep compartment, probably body fat ($t_{0.5}$ 200–300 minutes).

The drug is mainly metabolized in the liver, and the metabolites are excreted via the kidney.

UNWANTED EFFECTS

Cardiorespiratory depression is the main unwanted effect; apnoea can occur on induction and the drug has a marked hypotensive effect. Another unwanted effect is pain on injection, and this is particularly marked when propofol is injected into a small vein. Accidental extravasation does not produce any tissue damage.

Propofol is more expensive than other intravenous induction agents, but its recovery characteristics and low incidence of unwanted effects make it particularly suitable for day-case procedures.

Key facts
Induction agents

- Induction agents are used to obtain an adequate depth of anaesthesia as rapidly and safely as possible.

- The ultrashort-acting barbiturate sodium thiopental (thiopentone) is the induction agent most widely used in modern anaesthesia.

- Thiopental (thiopentone) rapidly induces surgical anaesthesia but has a short duration of action. Its side-effects include respiratory depression and hypotension.

- Propofol is a more recent intravenous anaesthetic agent, which is being increasingly used as an induction agent and for maintenance of anaesthesia in day-case surgery.

Inhalational anaesthetic agents

Inhalational anaesthesia is the most widely used form of maintenance anaesthesia in the UK. The various stages of anaesthesia were first described by Guedel in 1937. The stages listed below were originally described with reference to ether and are subject to modification when considering their applicability to modern anaesthetic techniques and agents. Many of the widely used anaesthetic agents bring the patient to Stage III very rapidly, and the subtle differences between the stages of anaesthesia may not be distinguishable. Furthermore, the depth of anaesthesia cannot be judged by the degree of muscular relaxation if a neuromuscular blocking agent has been used. In the classical description, inhalation anaesthesia occurs in four stages:

STAGE I—ANALGESIA STAGE: During this stage, the patient is still conscious and can talk, but feels giddy and sleepy. There is a progressive decrease in reaction to painful stimuli, and an increase in respiratory and pulse rate. The eyelash reflex is gradually lost. This stage is obtained during relative analgesia sedation.

STAGE II—EXCITEMENT STAGE: Although patients are unconscious during this stage, it is known as the excitement stage because they may be agitated and struggle. Alternatively, they may be quiet. Their response may depend on the type of patient, the presence or absence of stimuli, and the skill of the anaesthetist. During the excitement stage, conscious control is removed, and patients may struggle from a fear that has been concealed during Stage I or because they are being subjected to some stimulus, such as a premature attempt to extract teeth. In Stage II, the pupils dilate, the pulse is rapid and strong, but respiration is irregular.

STAGE III—SURGICAL ANAESTHESIA: The characteristic features of surgical anaesthesia concern eye signs and the muscles of respiration. There is a decrease in the range and activity of the movements of the eyeballs until eventually the eye comes to rest in the central position and remains there. In the early phase of surgical anaesthesia there is complete functioning of the intercostal muscles and diaphragm.

STAGE IV—RESPIRATORY PARALYSIS: At the stage of respiratory paralysis, the heart still beats and the patient may be kept alive if adequately oxygenated by artificial means. If such support is not given, the pulse will be rapid, there will be a drop in blood pressure, and the pupils will dilate. This will be followed by complete respiratory and circulatory collapse, and the patient will die.

The depth of anaesthesia needed depends upon the type of operation. Most dental procedures can be carried out during the early phases of Stage III.

Inhalation anaesthetic agents

The properties of an ideal inhalation anaesthetic agent are:

(1) a rapid and pleasant induction of, and recovery from, anaesthesia;

(2) the ability to produce rapid changes in the depth of anaesthesia;

(3) the ability to produce adequate relaxation of skeletal muscles;

(4) the production of analgesia;

(5) a wide margin of safety;

(6) no unwanted effects or other adverse properties in normal use.

Inhalation anaesthetic agents can be classified into two groups: gaseous agents (nitrous oxide); and volatile liquids (halothane, enflurane, and isoflurane).

Nitrous oxide

This colourless, odourless gas was the first agent to be used as an anaesthetic. It is stored as a liquid and gas under pressure at 750 pounds per square inch (52 bar) in metal cylinders. The gas is not flammable but supports combustion. Nitrous oxide has a very low solubility in blood (but not as low as nitrogen), and a state of equilibrium between alveolar and arterial tension is quickly reached. It is not significantly metabolized and is excreted unchanged in the expired gases.

PHARMACOLOGICAL PROPERTIES
Nitrous oxide is a weak anaesthetic agent with an MAC of 105%. In high concentrations—80% or more—nitrous oxide produces anaesthesia and severe hypoxia, so it is unsuitable for use as a sole anaesthetic agent. Is therefore used as an adjunct to other gaseous inhalation agents. The mechanism for nitrous oxide-induced anaesthesia remains uncertain. It is an excellent analgesic agent, and may exert its analgesic properties by initiating the release of the endogenous opioids (see Chapter 7). When nitrous oxide is mixed with an adequate amount of oxygen (30%), the mixture has little or no effect on the cardiovascular or respiratory system. However, it is a direct myocardial depressant and also stimulates the sympathetic nervous system. As a result of these two actions, cardiac output remains unchanged.

UNWANTED EFFECTS
The incidence of nausea and vomiting after the administration of nitrous oxide alone is approximately 15%, which compares unfavourably with halothane. *In-vitro* studies have shown that nitrous oxide interrupts cell division in the presynthetic (G_1) phase of the DNA synthesis cycle (see Chapter 19). Excessive use of nitrous oxide may suppress spermatogenesis and the production of white and red blood cells in the bone marrow. However, this problem does not appear to arise in normal clinical use.

In experimental animals, nitrous oxide can cause megaloblastic anaemia and neuropathy through oxidation of the cobalt ion of vitamin B_{12}. This finding may be significant to personnel repeatedly exposed to nitrous oxide, such as anaesthetic, dental, and operating-theatre staff. Scavenger systems should be fitted to all systems where nitrous oxide is used to ensure that the atmosphere does not contain more than 100 p.p.m. A neuropathy similar to that of vitamin B_{12} deficiency has been observed in dental surgeons who regularly abuse nitrous oxide. Nitrous oxide may have a deleterious effect if used in patients who have an air-containing closed space in their bodies as the gas diffuses into such a space with a resulting build-up of pressure. This effect may be dangerous in cases of pneumothorax, because the lesion may enlarge and so compromise respiration.

Uses

Nitrous oxide is used as an adjunct to other inhalation anaesthetic agents such as halothane or enflurane. Low doses are used in sedation and are discussed later. Entonox is a commercially available mixture of 50% nitrous oxide and 50% oxygen: it is widely used to produce analgesia without loss of consciousness, and is especially useful in obstetric practice, for changing painful dressings, as an aid to postoperative physiotherapy, and in emergency ambulances. In ambulance emergencies, the mixture is very efficacious at reducing the pain of myocardial infarction. Cylinders containing Entonox must always be stored in a warm room because at low temperatures nitrous oxide becomes a liquid, separates out from the mixture, and falls to the bottom of the cylinder. If this occurs, the patient will be exposed to 100% oxygen until this has been used up. He or she will then be exposed to 100% nitrous oxide.

Halothane

This halogenated hydrocarbon is the most widely used anaesthetic agent. At room temperature, it is a colourless liquid that decomposes on contact with light. The liquid has a pleasant smell and readily vaporizes with a boiling point of 50 °C. It is not inflammable and is non-explosive. Halothane can be used to induce anaesthesia at a concentration of 2–4%, and anaesthesia can be maintained with a concentration of 1–2%. Although intravenous anaesthetic agents are commonly used to induce anaesthesia (see above), induction can be achieved with halothane. The vapour does not irritate the larynx so induction is smooth and a deep anaesthesia can be achieved rapidly.

Pharmacokinetics

About 60–80% of halothane is eliminated unchanged in the expired gases. The portion absorbed is biotransformed in the liver, and the metabolites excreted via the kidney.

Pharmacological properties

Halothane has a marked effect on the cardiovascular system, causing a dose-related reduction in blood pressure. The hypotension is due to a reduction both in cardiac output and in the baroreceptor response. Halothane also causes a slowing of the heart rate mediated by the vagus nerve and, more importantly, sensitizes the myocardium to catecholamines, which can provoke severe dysrhythmia. Such sensitization can be a problem in certain dental surgical procedures where injections of a local anaesthetic solution containing epinephrine (adrenaline) may be used to maintain a relatively bloodless field. It is recommended that the amount of epinephrine should not exceed 0.1 mg in 10 minutes or 0.3 mg in 1 hour. The sensitization of the myocardium to catecholamines is enhanced by an increase in carbon dioxide levels. This can arise as a result of respiratory depression or obstruction.

Halothane depresses respiration, causing a reduction in gaseous exchange. However, it also produces bronchodilatation, making it a suitable agent for use in asthmatic and bronchitic patients. Halothane has no analgesic properties. It does produce a degree of muscle relaxation, although this is rarely enough for most types of surgery.

Unwanted effects

Hepatic necrosis has been associated with halothane anaesthesia at an incidence of 1 in 10 000 anaesthetic administrations. However, the incidence increases with repeated halothane anaesthesia, especially a previous exposure in the past 3–6 months. Clinical signs and symptoms of a halothane-induced hepatic necrosis usually arise 2–5 days after administration. The patient becomes pyrexic, and complains of nausea and vomiting. Death occurs in half of these patients. The mechanism of hepatic necrosis is uncertain. Any residual halothane that is not expired is likely to be metabolized in the liver; however, a metabolite may induce an immune response resulting in hepatitis. Although halothane hepatitis is serious, other complications of general anaesthesia occur with much greater frequency. A rare unwanted effect of halothane is the syndrome of malignant hyperpyrexia.

Enflurane

This is a halogenated ether. At room temperature it is a colourless, non-flammable liquid with a mild, sweet odour. Anaesthesia can be smoothly induced with enflurane 4%, and maintained with concentrations of 1.5–3%. Induction is associated with a mild stimulation of salivary flow and tracheobronchial secretions, but these are not usually troublesome. Enflurane also alters certain types of electrical activity in the brain that may be epileptogenic, so it should not be used in patients with a history of epilepsy.

Pharmacokinetics

About 80% of enflurane is excreted unchanged in the expired gases. Of the remainder, only 2–5% is metabolized in the liver; metabolites are excreted via the kidney.

Pharmacological properties

Enflurane produces a dose-dependent reduction in blood pressure in a manner similar to halothane. Its effect on the heart is also similar to that produced by halothane, but there is a smaller incidence of dysrhythmias. Epinephrine- (adrenaline) containing local anaesthetic solutions can be used safely with enflurane.

Enflurane causes respiratory depression, and patients are usually ventilated when this agent is being used. Deep anaesthesia with enflurane is associated with muscle twitching of the limbs, jaw, face, and neck. These muscular movements are usually self-limiting, and are prevented by reducing the depth of anaesthesia. Because of this unwanted effect, enflurane should be avoided in epileptic patients. It has no significant effect on the liver and is often used in preference to halothane when repeated anaesthesia is required.

Isoflurane

This is an isomer of enflurane: chemically, it is halogenated methylethyl ether. Its physical properties are similar to those of enflurane. Induction of anaesthesia with isoflurane is smooth and rapid, and can be achieved with a concentration of 3%; maintenance is achieved with 1.5–2.5%.

PHARMACOLOGICAL PROPERTIES

Like the other halogenated volatile liquids, isoflurane causes a reduction in blood pressure, but has little or no effect on cardiac output. Administration is associated with an increase in heart rate but no arrhythmias. It does not sensitize the heart to catecholamines so epinephrine- (adrenaline) containing local anaesthetic solutions can be used safely with this agent. Respiration is depressed with isoflurane, and it may also stimulate airway reflexes, causing increased secretion, coughing, and laryngospasm. The incidence of nausea and vomiting is similar to that produced by the other halogenated compounds, and hepatotoxicity does not appear to be a problem.

Desflurane

This is another volatile anaesthetic agent, which is similar to isoflurane, but has the lowest blood solubility of any of the inhalation agents. The low solubility allows rapid alteration of the depth of anaesthesia and quick recovery. Both aspects of this inhalation agent make it very useful for day-stay anaesthesia. The cardiovascular effects of desflurane are similar to those of isoflurane.

Sevoflurane

This is the newest inhalational anaesthetic agent, a fluorinated methyl-isopropyl ether, which is extremely non-irritant and highly insoluble. It produces very smooth induction of anaesthesia and rapid recovery with few unwanted effects. It is expensive but is rapidly becoming the modern inhalational anaesthetic agent of choice, especially for day-case anaesthesia.

Key facts
Inhalational anaesthesia

- Inhalational agents are used primarily to maintain general anaesthesia.

- Nitrous oxide is a weak anaesthetic agent but has a useful analgesia effect. It is used as an adjunct to other inhalational anaesthetic agents and it is a useful sedation agent.

- The halogenated hydrocarbons are the traditional inhalational anaesthetic agents. Halothane can cause hepatic necrosis.

- Sevoflurane is a new inhalational agent, which is non-irritant and produces rapid and smooth recovery.

Assessment of patients for anaesthesia

Before any general anaesthetic is administered it is essential to check that the patient has had nothing to eat or drink for a period of 4–6 hours before induction. Children are allowed water up to 2 hours before the anaesthetic. If possible, the patient's bladder should be empty. Where anaesthetics are being administered to out-patients, the patient must be accompanied by a responsible adult.

The medical conditions listed below can cause complications during anaesthesia and where possible patients should be treated under local anaesthesia. If a general anaesthetic has to be used, patients should be referred to hospital, and the anaesthetic should always be administered by an experienced anaesthetist.

Pregnancy

During the first trimester, drugs employed in anaesthetic practice could impair the development of the fetus and placenta. The middle trimester is probably the optimal time for a general anaesthetic if this is definitely required. In the final trimester, the bulky uterus will cause a reduction in gastric emptying; it may also impair venous return from the lower extremities, which will cause a reduction in cardiac output. These effects are more pronounced if the patient lies flat.

Cardiovascular problems

Any disorders of this, the body's main transport system, will have serious implications during general anaesthesia.

Patients with angina pectoris should have a percutaneous preparation of glyceryl trinitrate applied to their skin before an anaesthetic. Those with ischaemic heart disease are already suffering from some degree of oxygen deprivation and any additional deprivation may produce an infarct.

All antihypertensive drugs are potentiated by general anaesthetic agents, especially the barbiturates and halothane, and a severe hypotensive attack could result from this interaction. Halothane may have some ganglion-blocking activity, and could also enhance the antihypertensive effects of other drugs.

Respiratory disorders

General anaesthesia should be postponed in patients with acute diseases of the upper respiratory tract such as the common cold. Those with disease of the lower respiratory tract are prone to excessive mucus production, and should be referred for a medical opinion before a general anaesthetic is administered.

Haematological disorders

All types of anaemia can affect the course of a general anaesthetic, but the two most serious forms are sickle cell disease and thalassaemia.

Sickle cell disease is an inherited disease found in about 10% of people of Afro-Caribbean origin. In homozygous sickle-cell disease, the red blood cells contain an abnormal haemoglobin (Hb_s). When such cells are exposed to a reduced oxygen tension or a rise in blood pH they become sickle-shaped (sickling) and haemolysis occurs. Dehydration, stasis of the circulation, and pyrexia also predispose to sickling. Patients with the heterozygous sickle-cell trait may have some Hb_s in their red blood cells and the amount needs to be determined before a general anaesthetic is administered. It is essential that patients from these ethnic backgrounds have their sickle-cell status determined before having a general anaesthetic.

Thalassaemia is a rare inherited anaemia that occurs mainly in mid- and southern Europeans. The red blood cells in thalassaemia have a short life-span and contain fetal haemoglobin. Sufferers usually have a severe hypochromic anaemia.

Endocrine disorders

The problem of administering a general anaesthetic to patients suffering from diabetes or adrenocortical suppression is discussed in Chapter 20.

Hyperthyroidism causes tachycardia, and disturbances such as dysrhythmias or even cardiac failure. Therefore the hyperthyroid patient is at risk when a general anaesthetic is administered because of the possible precipitation of dangerous dysrhythmias.

Neurological disorders

Methohexital (methohexitone) should not be used as an intravenous anaesthetic agent in patients with a history of epilepsy, as this could result in status epilepticus. Similarly enflurane should also be avoided in these patients.

Patients with a history of spasticity, myasthenia gravis, and multiple sclerosis are a special anaesthetic risk and should be anaesthetized in hospital.

Drug therapy

Patients taking monoamine oxidase inhibitors should not be given pethidine as a premedication, as severe and life-threatening interactions occur (see Chapter 24).

Key facts
Assessment of patients for anaesthesia

- Assessment of medical fitness for anaesthesia is essential.

- Cardiorespiratory, haematological, endocrine, and neurological conditions as well as pregnancy can cause complications during anaesthesia. Patients with significant systemic disease should be treated in hospital.

- A full drug history is required prior to anaesthesia as dangerous interactions can occur between prescribed drugs and anaesthetic agents.

Anaesthetic emergencies

The two emergencies to be discussed in this section are respiratory obstruction and anaphylaxis. Other emergencies can occur at any phase of general anaesthesia. These include cardiac arrest and syncope, and are discussed in Chapter 26.

Respiratory obstruction

Obstruction of the airway during anaesthesia can be caused by several factors:

(1) *anatomical*—large tongue, retrognathic mandible, enlarged adenoids and tonsils;

(2) *operative problems*—obstructing the airway by applying too much back pressure during dental extractions, or too much flexion of the head;

(3) *pathological problems*—upper respiratory tract infection, blocked nasal airway;

(4) *laryngeal spasm*—caused by blood, saliva, mucus, pus, vomitus, or foreign bodies touching the vocal cords;

(5) *obstruction below vocal cords*—caused by inhaled foreign body, or bronchospasm.

Signs and symptoms

If respiratory sounds can still be heard, this is an indication of only *partial* blockage of the airway; no respiratory sounds means *total obstruction*. With complete obstruction there is alternate indentation of the intercostal spaces and jerking movements of the abdominal wall because of the efforts of the diaphragm, which is the most powerful muscle of respiration. Respiratory obstruction leads to circulatory collapse if not urgently treated.

Treatment

In the first instance, try and find the cause of the obstruction. The cervical spine should be extended to open the pharynx, and the mandible lifted forward. With a laryngoscope, inspect the larynx for foreign material such as blood, saliva, and mucus, and remove it with suction. This, however, can be an extremely difficult procedure even for an experienced anaesthetist. Foreign bodies such as tooth fragments should be removed with McGill's forceps. Respiratory obstruction in small children can usually be cleared by holding them upside down and thumping their back. If these measures fail to dislodge the obstruction, an attempt should be made to intubate the patient. This can be a difficult procedure, but respiratory depression is an emergency.

If the patient cannot be intubated, a cricothyrotomy should be carried out. For this technique, the neck is extended and a cricothyroid cannula inserted through the cricothyroid membrane. If a cricothyroid needle is not available, a large venepuncture needle could allow sufficient air (200 mL) to pass into the lungs. Oxygen should be administered through the cannula. If circulatory collapse has occurred, resuscitation techniques described in Chapter 26 should be employed.

Anaphylaxis

An anaphylactic reaction can occur with any of the drugs used during anaesthesia. Anaphylaxis is an immediate (Type I) hypersensitivity reaction caused by the release of histamine following exposure to an antigen in a previously sensitized individual.

Signs and symptoms

The patient will have acute breathing difficulties caused by bronchospasm and laryngospasm. Oedema of the face and neck will develop and the patient will appear very pale. There will be severe hypotension followed by cyanosis and circulatory collapse if left untreated.

TREATMENT

The management of anaphylactic reactions is described in Chapter 24.

Key facts
Anaesthetic emergencies

- Respiratory obstruction is a life-threatening anaesthetic emergency. Early recognition and immediate intervention to restore a patent airway are essential.

- Anaphylactic reactions to drugs used during anaesthesia are rare but when they do occur they can be serious. Management is aimed at reversing bronchial and laryngeal spasm and maintaining the circulation.

Sedation

Fear of dentistry affects nearly half of the adult population and is the most common reason why people fail to seek regular dental care. Historically, dentistry has always been closely associated with pain, and it is this fear of pain that produces a disproportionate level of anxiety in dental patients. Such individuals are unable to undergo treatment while they are fully conscious but can usually be successfully managed using pharmacological methods of sedation.

The General Dental Council (1998) defines sedation as, 'A technique in which the use of a drug, or drugs, produces a state of depression of the central nervous system enabling treatment to be carried out, but during which communication can be maintained and the modification of the patient's state of mind is such that the patient will respond to command throughout the period of sedation. Techniques used should carry a margin of safety wide enough to render the unintended loss of consciousness unlikely'. The aim of sedation is to produce anxiolysis so that treatment can be performed with minimal psychological and physiological stress.

Sedation is indicated for the management of anxious adults and children, for medically compromised and handicapped patients, and for patients undergoing extensive oral surgery. Patients undergoing sedation are conscious and their protective reflexes are intact. Accordingly, sedation has been promoted as a safer alternative to general anaesthesia. Indeed, a Department of Health (UK) report stated that, in dental practice, 'Sedation should be used in preference to general anaesthesia wherever possible'.

The properties of an 'ideal' sedation agent should be:

(1) to alleviate fear and anxiety;

(2) to produce amnesia and analgesia;

(3) to suppress the pharyngeal (gag) reflex, but not protective laryngeal reflexes;

(4) to produce a rapid onset of sedation and rapid recovery;

(5) to have a wide margin of safety with no side-effects;

(6) to require no special procedures or equipment to administer;

(7) to be inexpensive.

Sedation techniques used in dentistry in the UK can be categorized into three types according to the route of administration—inhalation, oral, and intravenous. Whichever sedation technique is used, local anaesthesia must be also employed. Sedation techniques on their own are not sufficient to reduce painful impulses arising from dental procedures. It should be emphasized that the difference between sedation and anaesthesia is a question of degree. Excessive administration of a sedative agent will ultimately result in general anaesthesia and the subsequent of loss of protective reflexes.

Inhalational sedation

Nitrous oxide is the main inhalation agent used to provide sedation in dentistry, although the efficacy of low concentrations of isoflurane, enflurane, and sevoflurane is also being evaluated. After the introduction of nitrous oxide as an anaesthetic agent in the 1840s it was soon recognized that low concentrations, in combination with oxygen, could produce effective sedation.

Nitrous oxide is a very safe sedation agent. The high MAC value gives a wide margin of safety between sedation and general anaesthesia. Provided that patients undergoing nitrous oxide sedation receive at least 30% oxygen then it is virtually impossible to accidentally produce anaesthesia, unless the patient has an idiosyncratic sensitivity to the gas. Nitrous oxide does not undergo any significant metabolism and thus produces very little systemic disturbance. Its low blood/gas solubility produces a rapid onset of sedation and rapid recovery. The gaseous mixture can be rapidly cleared from the bloodstream in the lungs within 5 minutes of breathing normal air.

There are two methods of inhalational sedation using nitrous oxide in current use. The first employs a fixed concentration of 50% nitrous oxide and 50% oxygen in the form of Entonox gas. This is used primarily in obstetrics and accident medicine and has little role in sedation for dental purposes. The second method, known as 'relative analgesia', uses variable mixtures of nitrous oxide in oxygen to produce a level of sedation that is titrated according to the individual patient's needs.

Relative analgesia

This method of sedation was introduced by Langa in the 1940s. It is a form of inhalational sedation that uses a dedicated machine to deliver a variable mixture of nitrous oxide and oxygen to the patient via a small nose mask. The machine can deliver nitrous oxide concentrations to a maximum of 70%, with a minimum of 30% oxygen being administered to the patient at all times. The concentration of nitrous oxide is increased in an incremental fashion and is titrated to produce a variable level of sedation according to the patient's response. The technique must be accompanied by semi-hypnotic suggestion and psychological reassurance. It is essentially a psychopharmacological method of sedation and is used primarily in the management of paediatric dental patients.

PATIENT PREPARATION

Each patient should be carefully assessed as to their suitability for relative analgesia sedation. A certain level of understanding and co-operation is required and the minimum age at which this form of sedation can be used is generally 3–4 years. The patient should have a light meal approximately 2 hours before the appointment but does not need to starve as for general anaesthesia. Child patients must be accompanied by a responsible adult, although adult patients undergoing relative analgesia sedation as the only type of anxiolysis can be discharged afterwards without an escort. Prior to the appointment, patients should be given full written details of the sedative technique and its likely effects and written consent *must* be obtained.

RELATIVE ANALGESIA TECHNIQUE

At the appointment, the technique should be explained and an appropriately sized nosepiece is selected and placed on the nose. The gas delivery tubing is attached to the nosepiece and 100% oxygen is administered at a flow rate of 4–$6 \, \text{L min}^{-1}$. The patient is instructed to breathe slowly and regularly. Once they are breathing comfortably nitrous oxide is gradually added to the oxygen in 10% increments. The level of nitrous oxide is increased until appropriate signs of sedation become evident and the patient feels sufficiently relaxed and ready to commence treatment. During induction, quiet and reassuring verbal contact should be maintained between the operator and the patient. This continuous reassurance and encouragement produces a state of semi-hypnosis.

SIGNS OF SEDATION

The signs of inhalation sedation produced by nitrous oxide are categorized as either objective or subjective.

OBJECTIVE SIGNS

The patient remains awake, follows instructions, and responds to questions. There is a reduced response to painful stimuli, and the patient appears drowsy and relaxed. The respiratory rate is normal and smooth with little or no gagging or coughing. There is no excessive movement of the limbs; the pupil size, eye reactions, pulse, and blood pressure are normal.

SUBJECTIVE SIGNS

These are:

(1) mental and physical relaxation, and relief of anxiety;

(2) euphoria, headiness, and a feeling of floating;

(3) an indifference to surroundings and to the passage of time;

(4) feelings of warmth and tingling of extremities;

(5) buzzing or ringing in ears;

(6) sounds seeming distant.

Once the patient is adequately sedated, a topical analgesic is applied, followed by an injection of a local anaesthetic. The oper-

ative procedure is performed whilst maintaining the flow of nitrous oxide/oxygen and continuous verbal encouragement. On completion of treatment, the nitrous oxide flow is switched off and the patient breathes 100% oxygen for 2 minutes. Oxygen is administered to prevent diffusion hypoxia. This condition might theoretically occur when nitrous oxide passes rapidly down its concentration gradient from the blood into the alveoli, flooding the lungs with nitrous oxide and displacing oxygen. Asking the patient to breath 100% oxygen ensures that the possibility of hypoxia is minimized. After 10–15 minutes the patient should be fit to leave the surgery.

Contraindications to relative analgesia

Although nitrous oxide (Entonox) is widely used in maternity units, it should not be used for dental purposes during pregnancy. In the early stages of pregnancy there is the possibility of teratogenicity and miscarriage. In the later stages, there is a risk of relaxation of the uterus leading to premature labour, although this is most unlikely if the concentration of nitrous oxide stays below 25%. Inhalation sedation techniques are unsuitable for patients with acute or chronic nasal obstruction, including upper respiratory tract infections, chronic bronchitis, or an attack of hay fever. The obese patient may be intolerant of the supine position because of difficulties in breathing due to diaphragm compression. Mentally handicapped patients may not have sufficient understanding and tolerance to cope with relative analgesia.

HAZARDS OF RELATIVE ANALGESIA

Nitrous oxide can produce occupational disease in dental staff who are exposed to high levels of the gas on a daily basis. During relative analgesia some nitrous oxide escapes into the dental surgery atmosphere every time the patient exhales. The level of pollution in the surgery should be minimized by actively scavenging the exhaust gas and ensuring that the room is well ventilated.

Key facts
Inhalational sedation

- Nitrous oxide approaches the properties of an ideal sedation agent.

- Relative analgesia using variable mixtures of nitrous oxide in oxygen is a safe and effective form of inhalational sedation for use in dentistry.

- Relative analgesia is used mainly for child dental patients as it is non-invasive.

- Relative analgesia is a form of psychopharmacological sedation, which relies jointly on the sedation agent and on semi-hypnotic suggestion by the operator.

- Nitrous oxide can cause occupational disease in dentists and dental nurses who are chronically exposed to high levels of nitrous oxide pollution.

Oral sedation

The oral administration of drugs to produce sedation has the advantages of relative safety and acceptability. The disadvantages of the oral route are the delayed onset of action, unreliable drug absorption, inability to easily regulate the intensity of the drug effect, and often a prolonged duration of action. For these reasons, oral sedative agents are mainly used to ensure that patients have a restful night before a dental procedure and to provide some degree of sedation in the period before the appointment. Drugs used for this purpose include the benzodiazepines, antihistamines, and triclofos sodium.

Oral sedation can be particularly useful in children. However, a reduction of anxiety can make some children hyperactive and difficult to control. Thus, it is important to distinguish between anxiolysis and sedation. Benzodiazepines will reduce anxiety in children but may not necessarily produce sedation. Antihistamine (H_1-receptor blockers) and triclofos sodium are more suited for children (see Chapter 15).

Benzodiazepines

Diazepam, temazepam, and lorazepam are the main benzodiazepines used for oral sedation. The general pharmacology of these drugs is dealt with in Chapter 15, and dose regimens are shown in Table 9.3. Elderly patients are unusually sensitive to diazepam and if this drug is used the normal adult dose should be halved. Conversely, children show a degree of resistance to diazepam and should be prescribed a dose regimen of $0.2–0.5 \, \text{mg} \, \text{kg}^{-1}$ body weight. Unwanted effects of diazepam include dizziness, an increased awareness of painful stimuli, ataxia, and prolonged postoperative drowsiness.

Temazepam and lorazepam are both classified as sedative–hypnotics. They are especially useful in the anxious patient for ensuring undisturbed sleep before a dental appointment. Both drugs have a short half-life and there is little 'hangover' effect.

Antihistamines

Some antihistamines (H_1-antagonists; see Chapter 4) cause drowsiness and sedation as unwanted effects, but they can also be used therapeutically for this purpose. Trimeprazine and promethazine are widely used as sedative agents especially in children (Table 9.2). Both drugs also have antiemetic properties. Trimeprazine is especially useful for out-patient sedation, but unwanted effects include persistent drowsiness, disturbed dreams, nasal stuffiness, and headache. Promethazine is less effective than trimeprazine as a sedative agent and may produce restlessness, irritability, and hallucinations.

Triclofos sodium

Triclofos is chemically related to chloral hydrate, and both drugs are discussed in Chapter 15. It is mainly used as a sedative/hypnotic in children, and dosages are shown in Table 9.3. Unwanted effects from triclofos sodium include drowsiness, dizziness, headache, and gastrointestinal disturbances.

Key facts
Oral sedation

- Oral sedation has the advantages of being relatively safe and acceptable to patients.
- Its use is limited by the unpredictability of absorption and effect.
- Oral sedation is used for anxiolysis prior to a dental appointment and is especially useful in children.

Intravenous sedation

The administration of sedative agents via the intravenous route is probably the most reliable and effective method of producing

Table 9.3 Dose regimes of drugs used for oral sedation

Drug	Adult dose	Child dose	Times of administration
Diazepam	5 mg	2–5 mg*	5 mg at night 5 mg on wakening 5 mg, 2 hours before dental procedure
Temazepam	10–30 mg	—	40–60 minutes prior to dental procedure
Lorazepam	1–5 mg	—	1–3 mg at night 1–5 mg, 2–6 hours before dental procedure
Trimeprazine tartrate	$3–4.5 \, \text{mg} \, \text{kg}^{-1}$	$2–4 \, \text{mg} \, \text{kg}^{-1}$	1–2 hours before dental procedure
Promethazine hydrochloride	—	2–5 years: 15–20 mg	1–2 hours before dental procedure
Triclofos sodium	1–2 g	1 year: 100–250 mg 1–5 years: 250–500 mg 6–12 years: 0.5–1 g	30 min before retiring to bed

* See comments above.

sedation. Furthermore, this route provides a rapid onset of action, and the dose of the agent used can be titrated to each patient's needs. The disadvantage of intravenous sedation is the inability to reverse the actions of the drug once administered, although for benzodiazepine sedation the effects can be completely reversed using the antagonist flumazenil. The technique also requires a certain level of patient co-operation to allow venepuncture and venous cannulation. Intravenous sedation is particularly useful for the moderately to severely anxious patient, and for medically compromised and handicapped patients. It is not recommended for use in children where titration of the sedation agent is difficult and the effects are unpredictable.

Early pioneers of intravenous sedation were Jorgenson and Drummond-Jackson (1940s–1960s). Jorgenson's technique involved the intravenous administration of an incremental dose of pentobarbital (pentobarbitone), followed by pethidine and hyoscine. Not only did the patients become sedated, but many accidentally slipped into general anaesthesia with loss of the airway and laryngeal reflexes. This technique is no longer used in the UK because of the narrow margin of safety between sedation and anaesthesia.

Drummond-Jackson advocated the intravenous administration of incremental doses of methohexital (methohexitone) so producing ultralight anaesthesia. Much controversy surrounded the safety and efficacy of this technique, especially the use of the same person as both operator and anaesthetist. This technique is condemned by anaesthetists as dangerous, and has been replaced with the advent of the benzodiazepines.

The benzodiazepines are the most widely used intravenous sedation agents used in dentistry today. Diazepam was the first intravenous benzodiazepine to be manufactured but it has largely been superseded by midazolam, which has more favourable properties. As well as producing sedation, both drugs produce amnesia, which is especially useful for certain dental procedures.

Diazepam

Diazepam is available as a $5\,mg\,mL^{-1}$ emulsion preparation (Diazemuls) for intravenous sedation. The drug is administered into a vein on the dorsum of the hand or antecubital fossa. The solution should be injected slowly in an incremental manner and the dose titrated until the required level of sedation is achieved. During the period of injection, the patient's speech becomes slurred and there is ptosis of the upper eyelid (Verril's sign). Apnoea may occur during the onset of sedation, and oxygen must always be available. Normal adults usually require 5–20 mg and the duration of sedation is usually 45–60 minutes. Most patients can leave the dental surgery about 1–1.5 hours after administration, but there is a rebound effect and the patient may feel drowsy for 6–8 hours after dosage. This is probably due to the redistribution of an active metabolite, desmethyl diazepam. Patients must always be accompanied and escorted home. They should not be allowed to drive or operate machinery for 24 hours after intravenous diazepam.

Another unwanted effect arising from intravenous diazepam is pain at the site of injection. This occurred in the old formulation of diazepam which contained propylene glycol. The solution was irritant to veins and produced painful thrombosis. This problem was overcome by the introduction of the emulsified oil preparation of diazepam (Diazemuls).

Midazolam

This is a potent, water-soluble imidazobenzodiazepine. It is the agent of choice for intravenous sedation, having a shorter half-life (about 2 hours) than diazepam and a shorter duration of action. It is metabolized in the liver to an active metabolite α-hydroxymidazolam. For dental sedation, 5 mL ampoules of midazolam at a concentration of $2\,mg\,mL^{-1}$ are used. Midazolam is administered slowly intravenously at the rate of 1 mg (0.5 mL) per minute, with the total dose being titrated according to the patient's response. Midazolam has twice the potency of diazepam and the sedative end-point is reached much more abruptly than with diazepam. Administration of midazolam too rapidly can produce significant respiratory depression and an acute reduction in arterial oxygen saturation. This is particularly true in the elderly, who often demonstrate extreme sensitivity to the benzodiazepines and a rather slow circulation time.

Unwanted effects of midazolam are few. The drug is water-soluble and thus there is no pain on injection. Although the metabolism of midazolam is faster than that of diazepam, there is still a prolonged amnesic effect. Patients must always be accompanied by a responsible adult and abstain from driving or operating machinery for 24 hours after final dosage.

One unwanted effect following the intravenous usage of midazolam (and diazepam) is sexual fantasy. The popular press and case reports seem to imply that young women are most susceptible. Seemingly, various dental procedures carried out under sedation can have sexual connotations for some patients. As a consequence claims of assault have been made against dental practitioners. To avoid such litigation it is imperative that there should always be a chaperone present throughout the sedation period and recovery.

Combined intravenous preparations

Over the years, it has become the practice of some operators to supplement intravenous sedation with benzodiazepines by adding a centrally acting analgesic such as pentazocine or pethidine. The rationale for this procedure is twofold. First, the opioids potentiate the sedative properties of the benzodiazepines and the patient therefore requires a reduced dose of the latter. Second, when this sedation mixture is used for dental surgical procedures, the opioids may provide some degree of postoperative pain relief.

Opioids and benzodiazepines produce respiratory depression, and deaths have occurred following the use of this sedation technique. It should also be noted that the efficacy of the opioids in postoperative dental pain is uncertain and their use for this purpose is very questionable. Supplementing benzodiazepine sedation with other drugs is unsafe and is not recommended.

Flumazenil

Flumazenil is an imidazobenzodiazepine that acts as a specific antagonist at the benzodiazepine receptor, thereby blocking the central actions of this group of drugs. The drug is given intravenously since it undergoes extensive first-pass metabolism. It has a short half-life (less than 1 hour) and should not be used for the routine reversal of benzodiazepine sedation in ambulatory patients. Flumazenil is mainly used as an emergency drug for the reversal of respiratory depression following the intravenous administration of either diazepam or midazolam and for the management of benzodiazepine overdose.

The usual dosage for benzodiazepine reversal is two increments of 200 µg given intravenously over 15 seconds. If the desired level of consciousness is not obtained within 60 seconds, a further dose of 100 µg can be injected. This can be repeated at 60-second intervals up to a maximum dose of 1 g. If there is still no improvement then another cause for the respiratory depression should be sought whilst instituting basic life-support measures.

Propofol

In small doses propofol can be used to induce and maintain sedation. Its principal advantage as a sedative agent is that the level of sedation can be altered intraoperatively and there is a short recovery period following cessation of sedation, which allows earlier discharge of the patient. The disadvantage of propofol is that the drug must be administered by continuous infusion which requires an expensive infusion pump. The use of propofol sedation in dentistry is still being developed and at the present time propofol sedation should only be used by experienced dental sedationists.

Recommendations on general anaesthesia and sedation in dentistry

There has been considerable concern over the use of general anaesthesia in dental practice, following a number of death in otherwise healthy children undergoing general anaesthesia for dental procedures. In 1990 the UK Department of Health published an expert working party report (otherwise known as the Poswillo report) which gave recommendations on the use of general anaesthesia, sedation, and resuscitation in dentistry. The aim of this report was to enhance the safety of general anaesthesia in dental practice by ensuring that standards of equipment, monitoring, and recovery were equivalent to those in a hospital environment. This has now been superseded by guidelines from the UK General Dental Council (1998) and the UK Royal College of Anaesthetists (1999). The key elements of the new GDC guidelines are that dentists are no longer permitted to administer general anaesthetics. All general anaesthetics for dental procedures must be administered by specialist anaesthetists. The use of general anaesthesia for dental treatment has been restricted to patients where other methods of pain and anxiety control are not suitable.

The above reports have all recommended the use of conscious sedation as a safe and effective alternative to general anaesthesia for dental patients. This has led to an increased demand on sedation services. Conscious sedation techniques are now being widely taught and practised. Sedation is having a tremendous impact on dentistry by improving the acceptability of treatment for many adult and paediatric dental patients, including those who are anxious, medically compromised, or handicapped. It should be remembered that although sedation has an excellent safety record, the drugs being used are potentially dangerous and dentists require formal postgraduate training before they can undertake sedation in dental practice.

Key facts
Intravenous sedation

- Intravenous sedation is the most reliable and effective form of sedation for dental purposes but it is restricted to use in adult patients.

- Sedation via the intravenous route has a rapid onset and the dose is easily titratable but the technique requires venepuncture for drug administration.

- The benzodiazepines have the advantage of producing sedation and amnesia but can induce respiratory depression.

- Flumazenil reverses the effects of benzodiazepine sedation and is useful in the management of overdose.

References

General Dental Council (1998). *Maintaining standards: Guidance to dentists on personal & professional conduct*. Sections on general anaesthesia, conscious sedation and resuscitation. London.

Poswillo, D. E. (1990). *General anaesthesia, sedation and resuscitation in dentistry*. Report of an expert working party. Department of Health, London.

Royal College of Anaesthetists (1999). Standards and guidelines for general anaesthesia for dentistry. London.

Further reading

Girdler, N. M. and Hill, C. M. (1998). *Sedation in dentistry*. Butterworth Heinemann, Oxford.

Hill, C. M. and Morris, P. J. (1991). *General anaesthesia and sedation in dentistry* (2nd edn). Wright, Bristol.

Malamed, S. F. (1995). *Sedation: a guide to patient management*. Mosby, St Louis.

Meechan, J. G., Robb, N. D., and Seymour, R. A. (1998). *Pain and anxiety control for the conscious dental patient*. Oxford University Press, Oxford.

Ryder, W. and Wright, P. A (1988). Dental sedation: a review. *British Dental Journal*, 165, 207–16.

10

Antiseptics and disinfectants

Antiseptics and disinfectants

The elimination of cross-infection is a major responsibility for all health care workers. Transmission of conditions such as viral hepatitis and human immunodeficiency virus (HIV) should never occur when rigorous cross-infection control is practised. In dentistry this is achieved by a number of methods, such as employing single-use disposable items (for example, dental local anaesthetic needles) and ensuring that all non-disposable instruments are properly sterilized, preferably by autoclaving (the physical methods of sterilization are beyond the scope of this text and readers are referred elsewhere). However, certain areas within the dental surgery, which are non-disposable and which are unsuitable for autoclaving, will be subjected to contamination by blood or saliva. Such areas include the dentist's and assistant's hands, work surfaces, and the handles of operating lights. Infective organisms found on these sites are treated by chemicals known as antiseptics and disinfectants. Although it is possible to render a site sterile by the use of antiseptics and disinfectants (if the time of exposure is long enough), it is often the case that these substances merely reduce the number of viable micro-organisms to a population size that is not a threat to most individuals. Many chemical substances are disinfectants; however, at the concentrations used to destroy micro-organisms, they may also damage host tissue. It should not be forgotten that, in addition to the use of chemicals, dentists must also employ appropriate physical protection (such as gloves, masks and visors) as part of their cross-infection control measures.

Terminology

Antiseptics are substances used to destroy micro-organisms on living tissue, such as the dentist's hands. Disinfectants are used to destroy micro-organisms on inanimate objects such as work surfaces. An antiseptic thus has to be more selective in its toxicity.

Mechanism of action of antiseptics and disinfectants

There are a number of ways that antiseptics and disinfectants can affect micro-organisms. These include:

(1) protein denaturation (usually bactericidal);

(2) cell osmolysis (bactericidal);

(3) interference with metabolism (normally bacteriostatic).

Individual antiseptics and disinfectants

These will be considered in groups of agents with similar chemical structures. More detailed information relating to some of these compounds is given in Chapter 12 (antiplaque agents).

Alcohols

The alcohols most commonly used as disinfectants are ethyl alcohol and isopropyl alcohol. They are used for disinfecting the skin but are ineffective when applied to the oral mucosa. The usefulness of alcohols is limited because they do not kill bacterial spores. Similarly, many viruses resist treatment with alcohols. Alcohols achieve antisepsis by denaturing and precipitating proteins. Unfortunately, the precipitated salivary and plasma proteins can form a protective coat around the micro-organisms. Thus, as much of these biological fluids as possible should be removed before applying alcohol to surfaces. In addition to being a disinfectant in its own right alcohol is also used as a vehicle for other antiseptic agents. The activity of these other antiseptics, such as chlorhexidine and iodine (see later), is increased in the presence of alcohol.

It is curious that alcohols are effective in concentrations of 50–70%%, but higher concentrations are useless.

Surgical spirit, which is a mixture of ethyl and methyl alcohols, is used for cleaning surgical surfaces.

Aldehydes

Aldehydes produce their antimicrobial effects through the alkylation of proteins.

Formaldehyde

This has bactericidal activity against bacteria, fungi, and viruses. However, its action is very slow—in 0.5% concentrations it would take about 12 hours to kill bacteria. In addition, it is fairly toxic. Formaldehyde is usually used in 2–8% concentrations to disinfect inanimate objects.

Glutaraldehyde

This aldehyde is much superior to formaldehyde as a disinfectant and acts against all micro-organisms, including bacterial spores and viruses. It is much less volatile than formaldehyde and causes less odour. Unlike alcohol, glutaraldehyde is not inactivated by the presence of biological fluids. It is marketed as a useful preparation in a 2% concentration. This is used for 'cold sterilization' of instruments and is recommended for the treatment of articles that cannot be autoclaved but have been contaminated by viruses. Contaminated surfaces should be exposed to glutaraldehyde for at least 1 hour, and preferably for longer, for example up to 12 hours. Glutaraldehyde has irritant and sensitizing properties and must be handled with great care.

Bis-biguanides

Bis-biguanides are active against a wide range of organisms. They are cationic surface-acting agents that interfere with cell-membrane permeability. The bis-biguanide most commonly used in dentistry is chlorhexidine.

Chlorhexidine

Chlorhexidine (Hibitane) finds extensive use in medicine and in dentistry as an antiseptic and disinfectant. Many preparations are available.

Skin preparation

Chlorhexidine gluconate, as a 1% and 4% solution, is used for the preparation of surgical sites and surgeon's hands. A 0.5% solution in isopropyl alcohol is also available for these functions.

Intraoral use

There are chlorhexidine-containing toothpastes (a 1% chlorhexidine gluconate gel), oral rinses (0.2% chlorhexidine gluconate solution), and a slow-release device for use in periodontal pockets. More information on these presentations is given in Chapter 12.

General purpose antiseptic

A 5% chlorhexidine gluconate solution is available as a general purpose antiseptic. Chlorhexidine solutions are also useful as storage media for sterile instruments.

Chlorhexidine is highly effective against a wide variety of organisms, both Gram-positive and Gram-negative, but more particularly Gram-positive. It is especially effective in alcoholic solution. It is non-irritant to the tissues in the recommended concentration, and is non-toxic.

Halogens

Halogens achieve antisepsis by reacting chemically with microbial proteins, therefore leading to the inactivation of enzymes. They are widely used as disinfectants, not only in the health-care environment but also in the home (domestic bleaches are halogens).

Chlorine

Chlorine is an oxidizing agent that has a rapid, potent, and brief action. It is effective against most bacteria (including spores), some fungi, yeasts, and viruses. It is commonly used in the form of hypochlorites, organic chloramines, chlorinated isocyanurates, and similar compounds which are capable of liberating chlorine.

Chlorine is inactivated by organic matter: it combines with the proteins of the tissues as well as with those of bacteria, with consequent rapid loss of its activity.

In dentistry, a 2% solution of sodium hypochlorite is used as an antiseptic irrigant of root canals, and is an effective solvent of necrotic tissues such as a dead pulp. Syringing should be undertaken under rubber dam. In the past this syringing was alternated with 5–10 volumes hydrogen peroxide and the final irrigation performed with saline solution. Care had to be exercised to ensure that neither the hypochlorite solution nor the hydrogen peroxide got through the root apex where they would cause irritation, and to ensure that hydrogen peroxide was not sealed into a canal. Today, irrigation is generally performed by sodium hypochlorite alone. Uses of hypochlorite solutions include the rapid disinfection of hard surfaces and babies' feeding bottles.

Sodium dichloroisocyanurate is a chlorine preparation used in dentistry. It contains about 62% available chlorine and is a stable source of chlorine. Its actions and uses are similar to chlorine and sodium hypochlorite. For instance, it is used for disinfecting babies' feeding bottles and for the treatment of water in swimming pools.

Iodine

This acts as an antiseptic in much the same way as chlorine. It is bactericidal and is also a fungicide, but one difference is that it is not readily inactivated by organic matter. It is applied to skin before surgery, when it is used in the form of a weak iodine solution—2.5% iodine in potassium iodine, water, and alcohol. When painted on the skin this solution is said to produce a sterile area in about 5 minutes, that lasts some time. Unfortunately, it does discolour the skin and very occasionally causes hypersensitivity reactions. A weak solution of iodine was sometimes painted on inflamed gingivae, where it was supposed to act as a counterirritant.

Iodoform

This is mildly antiseptic due to the slow liberation of iodine when applied to tissues. Preparations containing iodoform are used in dentistry. All have a strong, persistent, and characteristic smell. One such preparation is Whitehead's Varnish, which contains 10% iodoform with benzoin, storax, and balsam of Tolu in solvent ether. Whitehead's Varnish, usually incorporated into ribbon gauge, is used in the management of 'dry socket', and as a dressing after the surgical removal of third molars and cysts. Another iodoform preparation, once very popular in dentistry, is Kri-Paste, which consists of Kri Liquid (40%) and iodoform (60%). Kri Liquid contains (approximately) 45% parachlorphenol; 49% camphor; and 6% methanol. It was frequently used to sterilize root canals, and the paste was used as a root-canal filler.

Iodophors

Iodophors are combinations of iodine and surface-active detergents, an example of which is povidone–iodine. These combinations do not irritate or stain the skin. Povidone is a water-soluble polymer that seems to prolong the activity of many drugs, and does so with iodine by liberating it slowly from the complex. Such combinations are probably effective against most Gram-positive and Gram-negative organisms after about 15 seconds contact; prolonged exposure kills bacterial spores, and some viruses and fungi are also susceptible to this compound. Povidone–iodine mouthwash (povidone–iodine, 1%) is available, and may be used either undiluted or diluted with an equal volume of warm water as a mouthwash for mucosal infections.

Oxidizing agents

These act by liberating oxygen, which oxidizes bacterial protein. All the available oxygen is soon used up and the antiseptic action quickly exhausted. They have the advantage that their products are non-toxic.

Hydrogen peroxide

This oxidizing agent is a weak antiseptic. When brought into contact with living tissue it is decomposed into water and oxygen, but it gives off its oxygen rapidly and so its germicidal action is limited. It has been used as a mild antiseptic mouthwash in the treatment of acute ulcerative gingivitis (15 mL of the 20 volume solution—approximately 6%—to a half a tumbler of warm water). Its use in this form of gingivitis was advocated because of the anaerobic nature of the infection. Apart from its antiseptic properties, hydrogen peroxide exerts a mechanical cleansing action through the effervescence produced by the liberation of the oxygen. A stronger solution of hydrogen peroxide (30% aqueous solution) is used to bleach discoloured, root-filled teeth.

Sodium perborate

In solution this may also be used in the treatment of acute ulcerative gingivitis, for it too liberates oxygen when in contact with organic matter. 'Bocasan' (buffered sodium peroxyborate monohydrate) is said by the manufacturers to release far more effervescent oxygen than ordinary sodium perborate.

Phenols, cresols, and their derivatives

Phenol itself is rarely used these days; however, its derivatives are sometimes employed. They achieve their effect by all the methods described earlier, namely cell-wall disruption, precipitation of proteins, and enzyme inactivation.

Phenol

Phenol is associated with Lister's pioneering work in the field of antiseptics. As an antiseptic it has now been largely superseded by less toxic chemicals. It was often used as liquefied phenol, which is 80% phenol in water. Its action on micro-organisms is largely due to the fact that it is more soluble in lipids and proteins than in water. Consequently, it ignores a watery medium and concentrates on the lipid- and protein-rich microbial bodies. There is significance in this differential solubility, for oily phenolic preparations are virtually valueless as antiseptics.

When applied to the skin or mucous membranes in weak or moderately weak solutions, phenol produces some feeling of anaesthesia as it does have a depolarizing local anaesthetic action. It is this property that made it popular as an ingredient of mouthwashes (see Chapter 12). If a strong solution is applied to the skin it is irritant and caustic, producing a burning pain. The area of skin will show a white slough if the application of the strong phenol is prolonged: this local action is due to the precipitation of proteins. Phenol is not firmly held in the protein precipitate and is thus capable of quite deep percutaneous penetration.

Camphorated paramonochlorphenol (CMCP)

This is a 35% solution of parachlorphenol in camphor and has been widely used as a medicament in root canals. Its pronounced disinfectant property depends on the liberation of chlorine in the presence of phenol, the chlorine replacing one of the hydrogen atoms in phenol. It is comparatively non-irritant. A commonly used antiseptic today is a 1% aqueous parachlorphenol solution.

Cresol

This has about three times the bactericidal potency of phenol and is about as toxic. However, metacresyl acetate (Cresatin) is a cresol derivative that is used as a chemical antiseptic for the irrigation of root canals. It is not irritant to the periapical tissues and has an analgesic effect on residual pulp tissue.

Chloroxylenols

These are less effective against microbes than other phenolic agents and what activity they do have is considerably reduced in the presence of organic matter. Dettol (about 5% chloroxylenol) is a well-known preparation. Solutions of chloroxylenol are often so ineffective that they are liable to be contaminated by *Pseudomonas pyocyanea*: indeed the growth of this organism may be encouraged by such solutions.

Hexachlorophene (hexachlorophane)

This is very effective against Gram-positive cocci and is an excellent surface disinfectant. Preparations containing hexachlorophene are used on the skin before surgery, and as a presurgical hand cream. Hexachlorophene is not very irritant to the tissues, but neurotoxic effects have been reported in babies as a result of absorption following application in dusting powders. This problem may be related to the widespread application of the powder, particularly on raw skin surfaces.

Triclosan

Triclosan is a phenol that has been incorporated into soaps, mouthrinses, and toothpastes. In addition to having an antimicrobial action, triclosan appears to possess some anti-inflammatory activity.

Surface-acting agents

These agents act as detergents by interacting with membrane proteins and lipids; they have both fat- and water-soluble groups in the same molecule. They are classified according to the electric charge on the water-soluble group—cationic, positive charge; anionic, negative charge; amphoteric, positive and negative charges; and non-ionic, that is unionized. Non-ionic forms have little activity, but the others all have some degree of antibacterial activity, the cationic agents being the most effective. These substances are very active detergents, but are only weak antiseptics.

Some cationic surface-active agents have attracted interest: these are the quaternary ammonium compounds, which include:

(1) *cetrimide* (Cetavlon)—used as an aqueous or alcoholic solution for skin disinfection and wound cleansing;

(2) *benzalkonium chloride* (Roccal)—used as a 1% solution for preoperative skin preparation.

The quaternary ammonium compounds are incompatible with soaps and are inhibited by organic matter. Sometimes these agents are combined with other substances; for instance, chlorhexidine gluconate 1.5% and cetrimide 15% in a solution called Savlon Concentrate, which is used for general antisepsis. They are poor antiseptics, but are used as antiplaque agents in dentistry (see Chapter 12).

Dyes

These are complex organic substances, which are all derived in some way from coal tar. They include the aniline dyes, gentian violet, brilliant green, and the acridine dyes: acriflavin and proflavine.

Gentian violet and brilliant green are effective against some Gram-positive organisms, but Gram-negative organisms are very resistant. Their effectiveness is decreased by the presence of pus and serum. Gentian violet is a fungicide and, before the introduction of the antifungal antimicrobials, was used in the treatment of oral thrush (acute candidiasis). It stains the tissues blue, and is messy: with newer agents now available, it is no longer used. In fact, gentian violet is now only licensed for topical application on unbroken skin.

Heavy metals

Heavy metals (such as mercury and silver) have been used in the past as antiseptics, but have been superseded. Tin (as stannous fluoride) has been used as an antiseptic in toothpaste (see Chapter 12).

Disinfection against hepatitis and HIV

Hepatitis and HIV transmission in the dental surgery will not occur when using sterile instruments, and appropriate physical protection will shield the dentist. Hepatitis viruses are highly transmissible and any area exposed to infected biological fluid should be treated as a matter of urgency. Fortunately, simple disinfectant measures will clear these viruses from inanimate areas in the surgery; for example, a sodium hypochlorite solution applied for 10 minutes is effective. HIV is susceptible to the measures used to combat hepatitis viruses.

The dental uses of antiseptics

These can be summarized as follows:

(1) skin preparation before surgery;

(2) preoperative preparation of the oral mucosa;

(3) sometimes as an ingredient of dentifrices;

(4) inhibition of dental plaque;

(5) cleaning operating areas;

(6) the cold sterilization of instruments and equipment (where heat sterilization is impractical);

(7) storage of sterilized surgical equipment;

(8) preparation of the surgeon's and assistants' hands;

(9) irrigation of root canals in endodontics.

Key facts

- Antiseptics and disinfectants achieve their effect by:
  - denaturing protein;
  - affecting cell walls and producing osmolysis;
  - inhibiting micro-organism metabolism.

- Antiseptics are used in dentistry:
  - as components of mouthwashes;
  - as components of toothpastes;
  - as disinfectants;
  - as an aid to sterilization;
  - for skin and mucosal cleansing prior to surgery.

Astringents

These substances are said to precipitate proteins in superficial cells and thereby form a protective layer against irritants and bacterial invasion. This layer is also supposed to inhibit the exudation of leucocytes and serum. There is much doubt concerning the efficacy of astringents: their effect is mainly subjective, merely causing the mucous membranes to feel shrunken and shrivelled. Astringents are classified into two groups:

(1) the soluble salts of heavy metals, for example iron, lead, zinc, copper, aluminium, silver, and mercury.

(2) the vegetable astringents.

Metallic astringents

The zinc salts are the main components of this group. For example, zinc sulfate and zinc chloride are used as mouthwashes. It has been suggested that although the so-called astringent action of zinc mouthwashes may have little or no value, perhaps zinc salts themselves are helpful in promoting healing. Although such mouthwashes have been used in the healing of ulcers, their value is doubtful.

Silver nitrate is an astringent antiseptic that found much favour in dentistry at one time. Its astringent action is powerful but superficial: concentrated solutions are caustic but not penetrating. A 10% solution of silver nitrate has been used to reduce the sensitivity of dentine exposed at the necks of teeth. The solution is burnished into the exposed tissue using a plastic instrument. Even if this is effective, the solution stains and is unsuitable for anterior teeth.

Vegetable astringents

Tannic acid is an example of a vegetable astringent. At one time it was used in dentistry in powder form as a haemostatic, the powder being applied to the bleeding tooth socket and covered with a gauze pack. It was also a constituent of some mouthwashes, but no longer finds favour in dentistry as it is ineffective.

Caustics

A caustic is a chemical cauterizing (burning) agent. A number of substances act as caustics when concentrated, including zinc chloride, zinc sulfate, silver nitrate, phenol, and chromic acid. Trichloracetic acid is still perhaps of some interest in dentistry as a caustic agent. Sometimes a small amount of a 10% solution placed beneath an operculum will relieve the discomfort of a mild pericoronitis—it does so by simply destroying sensory nerve endings.

Further reading

British Dental Association (1996). *Infection control in dentistry.* Advice sheet *A12.* BDA Advisory service. British Dental Association, London.

Scully, C., Cawson, R. A., and Griffiths, M. J. (1990). Occupational hazards to dental staff. *British Dental Journal*, London.

11

Antimicrobial chemotherapy

- Antibacterial drugs
- Antifungal drugs
- Antiviral agents
- Infections due to prions
- Further reading

Antimicrobial chemotherapy

Chemotherapy is the use of chemicals to destroy or inhibit the growth of cells. Two broad classes of chemotherapeutic agents are used pharmacologically: antimicrobials and anticancer drugs, the latter are discussed in Chapter 19. This chapter is concerned with antimicrobial chemotherapeutic drugs. The basis of antimicrobial chemotherapy is a differential sensitivity of host (patient) and target (microbe) cells to the action of the drug. The drug may affect a structural component of the target cell which is not found in the host, for example the bacterial cell wall. Alternatively, the chemotherapeutic agent may inhibit a metabolic pathway peculiar to the target cell, such as the synthesis of folate.

Along with analgesics, antimicrobials are one of the few systemically active drugs commonly prescribed in dentistry. Therefore it is important that dentists have an understanding of this group of drugs. In this chapter the pharmacology of the different antimicrobials will be discussed. In addition, their use in dentistry will be described. Antimicrobials can be classified as being:

- antibacterial
- antifungal
- antiviral
- antiprotozoal
- antihelminthic
- antitrematodal.

The only member of the last three groups of relevance to dental practice in the UK is the antiprotozoal drug metronidazole as it also possesses antibacterial activity. The most commonly prescribed agents are the antibacterials, although antiviral and antifungal agents are widely used in the practice of oral medicine.

Strictly speaking, the term antibiotic refers to an antimicrobial agent produced by a micro-organism; however, the term has slipped into common usage as a synonym for an antibacterial agent.

Routes of administration

Antimicrobial drugs can be administered;

- topically;
- orally;
- by intramuscular injection;
- by intravenous injection or infusion.

Antibacterial drugs

There are many different antibacterials and they have no common structure. Some (such as penicillin) are produced by micro-organisms to destroy other microbes, others (for example sulfonamides) are entirely synthetic. Antibacterial drugs can be classified as:

- bactericidal (kill bacteria);
- bacteriostatic (prevent growth of the bacterial population—adequate host defences are required to eliminate bacterial infection).

Combination therapy with antimicrobials

Antimicrobial agents may be used in combination, for example in the treatment of polymicrobial infections or in the empirical management of serious infections. Synergism can occur by a number of mechanisms such as the sequential inhibition of a metabolic process (see co-trimoxazole later). However, not all combinations are helpful since bacteriostatic agents can inhibit the action of bactericidal drugs.

Mechanism of action of antibacterial drugs

Antibiotics can affect bacteria in a number of ways, i.e.:

(1) by inhibiting bacterial cell-wall synthesis (e.g. penicillins);

(2) by inhibiting protein synthesis (e.g. tetracyclines);

(3) by interfering with bacterial nucleic acid (e.g. metronidazole);

(4) by antimetabolic actions (e.g. sulfonamides).

Antifungal drugs affect membrane permeability and most antiviral agents affect nucleic acid or protein synthesis.

Resistance

Some species of bacteria are protected against the actions of certain antibiotics by virtue of the fact that the drug will not reach the target site (for example the cell wall may be impermeable). On the other hand, bacteria that would normally be expected to be susceptible to a particular antibiotic can develop resistance. Resistance to antimicrobials can be produced by a number of mechanisms (Figs 11.1(a–c)):

(1) by the decreased permeability of the cell membrane to the drug (resistance to ampicillin);

(2) by inactivation of the drug by enzymes (e.g. beta-lactamase inactivates some penicillins);

(3) by alteration of the drug receptor site (the mechanism of erythromycin resistance is a change in the ribosomal binding site);

(4) by the development of an alternative metabolic pathway unaffected by the drug (e.g. in sulfonamide resistance);

(5) by increased elimination of the drug from the cell (fluoroquinolones may be actively expelled from the cell).

Resistance can develop from one bacterial generation to the next by mutation (vertical transfer) (Fig. 11.2). Mutation is not a result of exposure to antibiotics, there are spontaneous mutations occurring continually in the bacterial population (in an infection this population is large) and some of these will co-incidentally confer resistance. In an established infection the resistant organisms will preferentially survive. However, due to the small number obtained by mutation, host factors will usually succeed in their destruction. Clinically important drug resistance is mainly due to the transfer of genetic material by means other than mutation (Fig. 11.2). This genetic material is contained in extrachromosomal elements known as plasmids. Plasmids containing DNA which encodes for antibiotic resistance are known as R plasmids. Movement of R plasmids allows the transfer of resistance horizontally between bacteria, which may be of different species. This horizontal transmission can be achieved by conjugation (transfer via a sex pilus), transduction (via a bacteriophage), or transformation (appropriation of free DNA from the same or a similar species from the environment).

Key facts
Antibacterial drugs

- Antibacterial drugs are either bacteriocidal or bacteriostatic.

- Antibacterial drugs act by one of the following mechanisms:
  - inhibition of cell-wall synthesis;
  - inhibition of protein synthesis;
  - interference with bacterial nucleic acid synthesis;
  - inhibition of bacterial cell metabolism.

Antimicrobials that interfere with bacterial cell-wall synthesis

Antimicrobials that interfere with bacterial cell-wall synthesis are the beta-lactams, the glycopeptides, and bacitracin.

The bacterial cell wall is a rigid structure composed of

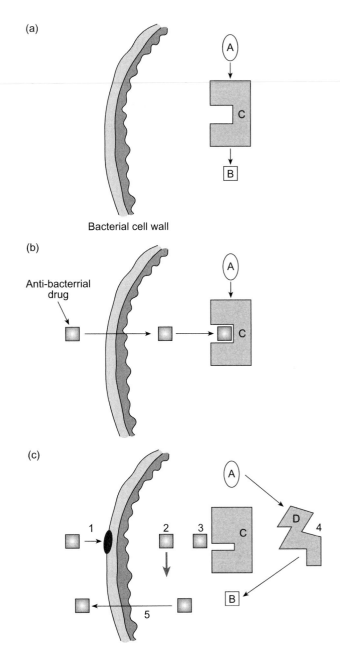

Fig. 11.1 A diagrammatic representation of how resistance can develop to an antibacterial drug. (a) Shows an essential bacterial process where component A is converted to component B via the pathway C (C could be an enzyme). (b) Shows the antibacterial drug (the shaded square) blocking the function of C. (c) Shows the points of the possible mechanisms of resistance. 1, inhibition of drug uptake; 2, inactivation of the drug by the bacterium; 3, alteration of the drug receptor site on pathway C by the bacterium; 4, development of a new pathway D by the bacterium; 5, increased elimination of the drug by the bacterium.

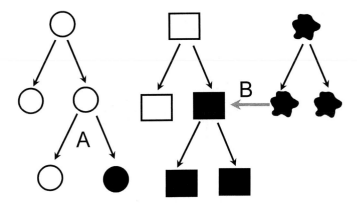

Fig. 11.2 Mechanisms of development of bacterial resistance. A, vertical transfer within species via mutation; B, horizontal transfer between species via transfer of extrachromosomal DNA such as plasmids.

peptidoglycan that surrounds the cell membrane. In Gram-positive bacteria the cell wall is made up of multiple layers of peptidoglycan, whereas in Gram-negative organisms it is only one layer thick. Peptidoglycan consists of chains of alternating amino-sugars (N-acetylglucosamine and N-acetylmuramic acid) crosslinked via the peptide side-chains of N-acetylmuramic acid (Fig. 11.3(a)). Peptidoglycan is synthesized in stages. The acetylglucosamine–acetylmuramic acid complex forms a glycan unit, which is the building brick of the wall. The glycan units are then carried across the cytoplasmic membrane of the bacterial cell by means of a lipid carrier and incorporated into the cell wall.

The final stage involves joining the peptides of one layer to the peptides of the next via a peptide link, a process known as transpeptidation. Cell-wall synthesis can be inhibited at various stages by antimicrobials. If the cell wall is not intact, the bacterium is destroyed and therefore those antimicrobials that interfere with cell-wall production are bactericidal.

Beta-lactam antimicrobials—penicillins

The antibacterial properties of penicillin were discovered in 1928 when Alexander Fleming noted that the growth of staphylococci was inhibited by a substance derived from the genus *Penicillium*. There are a number of penicillin derivatives in clinical use, all are bactericidal.

MECHANISM OF ACTION There are specific binding sites on bacteria for penicillins (and the other beta-lactam antimicrobials). After binding, the penicillins jeopardize bacterial cell-wall integrity by two mechanisms. The main one is a repression of cell-wall synthesis by inhibition of the enzyme responsible for creating the crosslinks between the peptide chains (see Fig. 11.3(b)). The second mechanism relies upon the fact that bacteria produce enzymes called autolysins, which can create defects in their cell walls. These enzymes are normally inhibited. Penicillin inactivates the autolysin inhibitors.

PENICILLIN RESISTANCE Penicillin resistance is produced by one of three methods:

1. Some bacteria can produce beta-lactamase (penicillinase). There are more than 100 varieties of beta-lactamase, some of which are very specific and will only inactivate penicillins; others will inactivate other beta-lactam drugs such as the cefalosporins (cephalosporins) (see below) as well as the penicillins. *Staphylococcus aureus* resistance is mainly due to the production of beta-lactamase.

2. The bacteria may alter the structure of penicillin binding proteins. This is the mechanism responsible for the production of methicillin-resistant staphylococci (see below).

3. The bacterial cell membrane can be impermeable to some bacteria. This is the mechanism by which many Gram-negative bacteria are resistant to penicillin.

Many types of penicillin are now available. Of those originally isolated, benzylpenicillin was found to be the most suitable for use and its basic properties will now be described, together with the general pharmacodynamics of the group.

BENZYLPENICILLIN (PENICILLIN G)

SPECTRUM OF ACTIVITY Benzylpenicillin has a relatively narrow spectrum of antibacterial activity. It is effective against most Gram-positive cocci, and also against some Gram-negative bacteria such as *Bacteroides melaninogenicus*.

Naturally occurring resistant strains are found amongst susceptible organisms. Such resistant strains of viridans streptococci may occur in the mouth together with a majority of sensitive strains, and this poses a hazard for patients with valvular defects of the heart (see later).

Resistant strains of *Staphylococcus aureus* existed before the era of antimicrobials but, in the early days of penicillin, were probably few compared with those staphylococci sensitive to the antibiotic. Today the position is different: the sensitivity of *Staph. aureus* to benzylpenicillin is very variable, with most strains being resistant. In some hospitals there is a high proportion of *Staph. aureus* which is resistant to many antibacterial agents and this has caused a serious problem. These are termed MRSA which stands for methicillin-resistant *Staph. aureus*.

PHARMACOKINETICS Benzylpenicillin is unstable in acidic conditions. Therefore it cannot be relied upon to produce satisfactory clinical results if given by mouth, because a high proportion of the original drug is rendered inactive by the acid contents of the stomach. When given by intramuscular injection, it is quickly absorbed: the maximum concentration is reached within 30 minutes and then rapidly falls. To maintain a satisfactory plasma concentration, at least 300 mg of benzylpenicillin should be administered intramuscularly every 4–6 hours. It should also be remembered that tissue concentrations take time to equilibrate with those of plasma.

The drug is partially bound to plasma proteins (46–58%) and, although it passes into serous cavities, the concentration is low,

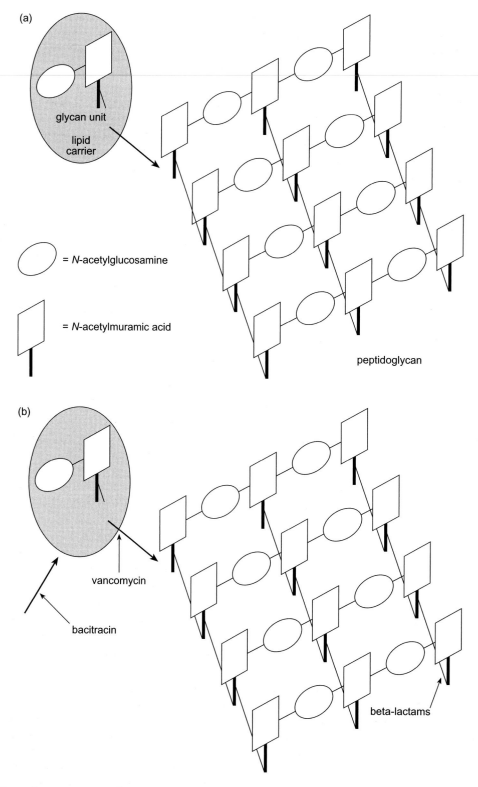

Fig. 11.3(a) Shows the construction of the peptidoglycan cell wall of bacteria. (b) Shows the stages affected by antibacterial drugs.

especially in the cerebrospinal fluid and joint cavities. When the meninges are inflamed there is increased penetration of the penicillin into the cerebrospinal fluid, providing adequate concentrations. The half-life of benzylpenicillin is less than 1 hour.

The major part (80%) of any dose is excreted rapidly by the kidney through extensive tubular secretion. The remaining 20% is excreted via glomerular filtration. Excretion can be delayed by the administration of substances that compete with penicillin for active tubular secretion. Such a drug is probenecid; by delaying excretion, it prolongs therapeutic plasma concentrations. Benzylpenicillin readily diffuses from the maternal to the fetal circulation.

Less soluble compounds of penicillin delay absorption from the site of injection. An example is procaine penicillin, prepared by the interaction of procaine hydrochloride and benzylpenicillin. The peak concentration of procaine penicillin is reached in 4 hours and thereafter falls over the next 24 hours. Even less soluble compounds are available, such as benethamine penicillin and benzathine penicillin, the effects of which last up to days or weeks. Unfortunately, the less soluble compounds produce lower plasma concentrations than benzylpenicillin.

Phenoxymethylpenicillin (penicillin V)

Spectrum of activity The range of antibacterial activity is similar to that of benzylpenicillin, but it is somewhat less active against streptococci.

Pharmacokinetics This is an oral penicillin that resists destruction in gastric juice and is absorbed from the upper part of the small intestine, although incompletely. Maximum blood concentration is reached in 1 hour and excretion is as rapid as benzylpenicillin. Administration every 4–6 hours is necessary to maintain therapeutic concentrations.

Other acid-resistant penicillins

Other acid-resistant penicillins have been introduced, such as phenethicillin. Although more completely absorbed than phenoxymethylpenicillin, they do not seem to offer any real advantages. Phenoxymethylpenicillin is less protein-bound than these later penicillins and consequently there is more antibiotic freely available to diffuse to the site of infection. Phenoxymethylpenicillin remains the acid-resistant penicillin of choice.

Penicillinase-resistant penicillins

These drugs, which include methicillin, cloxacillin, flucloxacillin, and temocillin, are reserved for the treatment of staphylococcal infections. Treatment of such infections should be started with one of these drugs, unless the antibiotic sensitivity of the strain is known. Staphylococcal infection in dental practice is rare, but is likely to be serious, calling for supervision in a hospital.

Methicillin was the first of the penicillinase-resistant penicillins, and it must be administered by injection as it is not acid-resistant. It is probably less active against staphylococci than are cloxacillin and flucloxacillin, and it has been implicated in a number of unwanted effects, including granulocytopenia. It finds little use in clinical practice today, having been superseded by the other penicillinase-resistant penicillins. Flucloxacillin is better absorbed from the gut and is to be preferred to cloxacillin for oral therapy.

Broad-spectrum penicillins

Examples of these drugs include ampicillin, amoxicillin (amoxycillin), bacampicillin, pivampicillin, and talampicillin (the last three are pro-drugs for ampicillin). The broad-spectrum penicillins possess activity against Gram-negative organisms as they have the ability to penetrate the lipid barrier of Gram-negative cell walls.

- Ampicillin

Spectrum of activity Ampicillin is effective against Gram-positive organisms, although slightly less so than benzylpenicillin. However, it has much greater activity against Gram-negative bacteria. It is destroyed by penicillinases and should not, therefore, be used to treat resistant staphylococcal infections.

Pharmacokinetics Ampicillin is acid-resistant and can be administered orally, but for maximal effect it should be given parenterally.

- Amoxicillin (amoxycillin)

Spectrum of activity Amoxicillin has the same spectrum of antibacterial activity as ampicillin.

Pharmacokinetics It is related to ampicillin but is more rapidly and completely absorbed from the gastrointestinal tract. Peak concentrations in plasma are about twice as high as those attained by ampicillin after oral administration of the same dose. Another advantage is that absorption does not appear to be affected by food. The half-life of the drug is in the region of 6 hours.

Beta-lactamase inhibitors

Beta-lactamase inhibitors may be added to drug formulations to confer resistance to many beta-lactamase producing bacteria. They are not themselves antimicrobial. There are two such agents used in formulations available in the UK. Clavulanic acid is combined with amoxicillin in the preparation co-amoxiclav and tazobactam is combined with piperacillin in Tazocin®.

Extended-spectrum and reversed-spectrum penicillins

Ticarcillin, carbenicillin, piperacillin, and azlocillin are known as extended-spectrum penicillins and are used in infections caused by *Pseudomonas aeruginosa*. Others, such as mecillinam and pivmecillinam, are active against a wide variety of Gram-negative bacilli, such as *Escherichia coli*, *Proteus mirabilis*, and salmonellae. These have no activity against *P. aeruginosa*, penicillinase-producing staphylococci, or enterococci, and much less activity against Gram-positive organisms. They are known as reversed-spectrum penicillins. Mecillinam must be given by injection. Pivmecillinam is an ester of mecillinam and is well absorbed when given orally. After absorption it is hydrolysed to the active agent mecillinam. Pivmecillinam has a local irritant effect on the oesophageal mucosa and occasionally causes oesophagitis. These drugs may be indicated in severe infections due to enterobacteria such as *E. coli*, which account for a high proportion of urinary tract infections.

None of these drugs has a place in dentistry

UNWANTED EFFECTS OF THE PENICILLINS

Penicillin therapy is remarkably free from unwanted effects except for the production of hypersensitivity reactions. Sensitization is often produced by previous treatment, but sometimes a history of such contact cannot be established. However, previous exposure to penicillin may not be obvious; an example of occult exposure is drinking milk from cows treated with the drug. Penicillin is thought to be the most common cause of drug allergy, but this must be considered against the background of its extensive usage. The allergic reactions range from a mild urticaria to a serious anaphylactic shock, which, although rare, may be fatal. The estimated incidence of allergic reactions to penicillin in various areas of the world ranges from 0.7 to 10%.

All preparations of penicillin can bring about hypersensitivity reactions. Although oral preparations are thought to produce reactions much less frequently than parenterally administered penicillin, it must be emphasized that serious reactions have occurred following oral administration. Procaine penicillin is probably the most common offender. All patients who are to receive penicillin, by whatever route, should be questioned as to any previous untoward experience with this drug and offered an alternative antibiotic when necessary.

The penicillins have minimal toxicity. However, intrathecal injection of penicillin G (benzylpenicillin) may produce a severe encephalopathy. Skin rashes appear to be more common with ampicillin than with other penicillins, with an incidence of about 7%. Most of these rashes are of the maculopapular type and seem unrelated to those of true penicillin allergy. The rashes may develop during the course of treatment or sometimes days after treatment has stopped. Ampicillin rashes tend to occur more frequently in patients suffering from infectious mononucleosis, and the drug should not be administered to such patients. Cross-hypersensitivity probably exists between all penicillins in the susceptible patient. However, the maculopapular rash of ampicillin does not necessarily contraindicate later treatment with other penicillins

USES

Penicillins are the most useful antibacterials in the practice of dentistry. They are employed both in the treatment of established infection and in prophylaxis (see below).

Key facts
Penicillins

- Penicillins are bactericidal antibiotics that interfere with cell-wall synthesis.

- Benzylpenicillin has a narrow spectrum of activity; however, there are members of the group such as ampicillin and amoxicillin which have a broad spectrum of bactericidal action.

- Penicillinase-resistant penicillins include flucloxacillin and methicillin.

- Penicillins produce hypersensitivity reactions.

- Penicillins are the first-choice drugs for the treatment of many dental infections.

Beta-lactam antimicrobials–cefalosporins (cephalosporins)

Cefalosporins are closely related chemically to penicillin. The cefalosporins have been divided into four generations, as follows:

(1) first generation—cefalotin (cephalothin), cefalexin (cephalexin), cefazolin (cephazolin), cefradine (cephradine);

(2) second generation—cefuroxime, cefamandole (cephamandole), cefoxitin, cefaclor;

(3) third generation—cefotaxime, ceftazidime, ceftizomine, and cefixime.

(4) fourth generation—cefepime.

SPECTRUM OF ACTIVITY

These are broad-spectrum antimicrobials with activity against a wide range of Gram-positive and Gram-negative bacteria.

The first generation has good activity against Gram-positive but a moderate effect on Gram-negative bacteria. They are active against many streptococci, *Neisseria gonorrhoeae*, and *Corynebacterium diphtheriae*. They have no activity against *Pseudomonas aeruginosa*, *Streptococcus faecalis*, *Bacteroides fragilis*, and most of the enterobacteria.

The second generation of cefalosporins is largely resistant to beta-lactamase, and they are much more active against almost all Gram-negative bacilli. Cefamandole is very active against the enterobacteria and staphylococci.

The third generation of cefalosporins is more active than either of the other two generations against certain Gram-negative bacteria.

The fourth generation is similar to the third but is more resistant to some beta-lactamase producing species.

MECHANISM OF ACTION The mechanism of action of the cefalosporins is exactly the same as that described above for the penicillins (Fig. 11.3(b)).

PHARMACOKINETICS The first cefalosporins, cefaloridine and cefalothin, both had to be administered parenterally. Cefalexin is an orally administered first-generation drug. Later preparations include: cefradine (oral and parenteral administration); cefazolin (parenteral); cefuroxime (parenteral); cefamandole (parenteral). Cefadroxil is an oral cefalosporin. Once absorbed into the circulation, the cefalosporins exhibit variable binding to plasma proteins from 20 to 90% (for example cefaloridine, 20%; cefalotin, 70%). The cefalosporins are mainly excreted by the kidney, some unchanged and others as metabolites.

UNWANTED EFFECTS

It seems that the incidence of allergic reactions to cefalosporins is lower than that of the penicillins, the reactions that do occur being similar to those caused by penicillins.

In penicillin-sensitive patients, the use of cefalosporins should be viewed with caution as it seems that patients with a history of penicillin allergy are predisposed to accelerated reactions to cefalosporins: such reactions suggest that the underlying mechanism is likely to be due to partial cross-allergenicity, rather than to a generalized and unspecific tendency to drug hypersensitivity. Patients with a history of mild urticaria to penicillins do not seem to be at a great risk of an allergic reaction when given cefalosporins, but a patient with a severe immediate reaction to penicillin should not be given a cefalosporin. About 10% of patients who are allergic to penicillins react in some way to the cefalosporins.

Cefalosporins have been implicated in renal damage, but this was most commonly due to the original cefaloridine.

Some of the later generation cefalosporins, such as cefamandole can produce a disulfiram-like reaction if taken with alcohol (see Chapter 24).

USES

In general terms there appear to be few absolute indications for the use of the cefalosporins in dentistry, although they are much used in other branches of medicine especially orthopaedic surgery.

Key facts
Cefalosporins

- Cefalosporins inhibit cell-wall synthesis in the same way as penicillins.
- Cefalosporins are bactericidal.
- Cefalosporins show cross-allergenicity with penicillins.
- Cefalosporins have few indications for use in dentistry.

Glycopeptide antimicrobials

These include vancomycin and teicoplanin.

VANCOMYCIN

SPECTRUM OF ACTIVITY Vancomycin is mainly active against Gram-positive bacteria. It inhibits *Clostridia* species and is active against MRSA.

MECHANISM OF ACTION Vancomycin inhibits cell-wall synthesis, but by a different mechanism from that used by the beta-lactams.

The glycopeptides inhibit the release of the basic disaccharide building block of peptidoglycan from the lipid carrier that transports the glycan units across the cell membrane to the cell wall (Fig. 11.3(b)).

PHARMACOKINETICS Vancomycin is available for intravenous use and also in capsules for oral administration. It is not absorbed from the gut, so when given orally its use is really as a topical application.

USES

Vancomycin is only used to treat serious infections, such as certain staphylococcal infections (for example septicaemia, endocarditis), where the patient is allergic to penicillinase-resistant penicillins. Oral administration is used to treat antibiotic-associated colitis (125 mg every 6 hours for 7–10 days). The glycopeptide antimicrobials are not prescribed routinely to treat infections in dental practice; however, vancomycin and teicoplanin may be used prophylactically in the prevention of infective endocarditis (see below).

Bacitracin

Bacitracin is a topical antimicrobial used in dermatology. It is too toxic for systemic administration. It is mentioned here as it inhibits bacterial cell-wall synthesis by a mechanism that differs from those already described. Bacitracin interferes with the production of the lipid carrier used to transport the basic glycan units of peptidoglycan across the bacterial cell membrane to the cell wall (Fig. 11.3(b)).

Antimicrobials that inhibit protein synthesis

Drugs used in dental and oral surgical practice that interfere with the synthesis of bacterial proteins include erythromycin, the tetracyclines, clindamycin, the aminoglycosides, fusidic acid, and chloramphenicol.

In order to describe the various ways in which different antimicrobials interfere with protein synthesis, it is necessary to review briefly the normal mechanisms of bacterial protein synthesis (Figs 11.4(a), (b)).

The primary information for protein synthesis is stored by DNA, and is transmitted to mRNA (messenger RNA) during transcription. The process of protein synthesis takes place on ribosomes, these consist of rRNA (ribosomal RNA) and protein, and lie either free in the cytoplasm or attached to the cytoplasmic membrane. The cytoplasmic membrane of bacteria corresponds to the membrane of mammalian cells. Bacterial ribosomes consist of a 30S and a 50S component (the 'S' refers to Svedberg unit, a measure of relative density as determined by the speed of centrifugation). They thread themselves on to the end of a strand of mRNA, and contain two attachment sites for amino acids. At the same time, the available amino acids become temporarily attached to tRNA (transfer RNA), each amino acid having its own specific tRNA. mRNA consists of a long chain made up of four nucleotides grouped into codon triplets, each of which represents a code for a specific amino acid. Similarly, each amino acid is 'recognized' by its specific anticodon triplet on a tRNA molecule, this couples to it and transports it to the appropriate codon triplet site on mRNA when the acceptor site on the ribosome becomes available. Transpeptidation then takes place, whereby the peptide chain already attached (by means of tRNA) is transferred to the amino acid attached to tRNA at the acceptor site, thus freeing the tRNA originally carrying the peptide chain. Translocation of the ribosome now takes place and it moves along mRNA and opens up a new acceptor site, which contains another codon for the next amino acid in the chain. The whole process is then repeated.

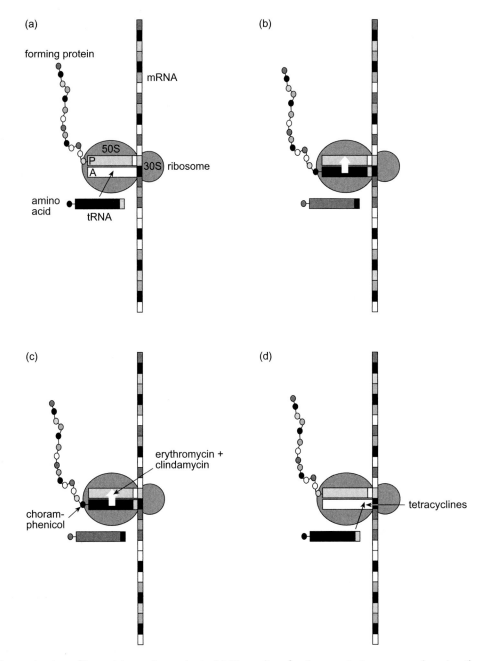

Fig. 11.4 The mechanism of bacterial protein synthesis. (a) The coding for the protein is transported to the ribosome by mRNA. The amino-acid building blocks are carried to the ribosome by tRNa which binds to the A site of the 50S subunit (the other site known as the P site is filled by the preceding tRNA molecule which is now attached to the developing protein. (b) Shows transpeptidation where the growing protein is linked to the tRNA molecule at the A site; the tRNA at the A site then tranlocates to the P site and the ribosome moves on a codon and awaits entry of further tRNA at the A site. (c–e) Show the site of action of different antibacterial drugs.

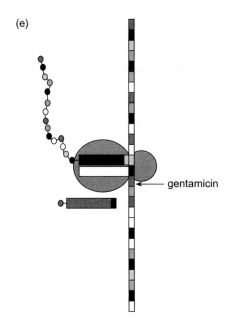

(e)

gentamicin

Fig. 11.4 (*cont.*)

Erythromycin

Erythromycin belongs to that group of drugs known as the macrolides. It is a bacteriostatic drug but bactericidal in high concentrations. Other macrolides include azithromycin and clarithromycin. The latter drug being useful in the management of gastrointestinal ulcers caused by *Helicobacter pylori* (see Chapter 18).

SPECTRUM OF ACTIVITY Erythromycin has a narrow spectrum of activity, similar to that of benzylpenicillin, but is more active against *Staph. aureus*. Gram-negative enterobacteria, such as *E. coli* and salmonella, are resistant to erythromycin. On the other hand, some of the Parvobacteria, such as *Haemophilus influenzae* and *Bordetella pertussis* are sensitive to erythromycin. The Gram-negative *Legionella pneumophilia* is also sensitive.

MECHANISM OF ACTION Erythromycin binds to the 50S ribosomal subunit and interferes with the translocation stage of protein synthesis (Fig. 11.4(c)). Drugs that affect translocation are, for some reason, liable to give rise to resistant mutants.

PHARMACOKINETICS Erythromycin base is destroyed by acid gastric juices and so is administered in enteric-coated tablets. It is absorbed from the upper part of the small intestine. Peak plasma concentrations are reached in about 4 hours and, to achieve this, the tablets should be taken in the absence of food. However, erythromycin estolate is more acid-stable and is usually given in the form of capsules. It is absorbed to a greater extent than any other oral preparation of erythromycin, and gives peak plasma concentrations within about 2 hours. Higher concentrations of erythromycin can be achieved by intravenous administration, although this has a tendency to produce thrombophlebitis. The half-life of erythromycin is in the order of 1.5–2 hours.

Erythromycin is widely distributed throughout the body tissues, and 2–5% of the orally administered drug is excreted in its active form in urine. Although a proportion of the drug is also excreted in the bile, some of which is reabsorbed, the greater part of it seems to be broken down in the body.

UNWANTED EFFECTS
All preparations of erythromycin can cause gastrointestinal upsets such as nausea, vomiting, and diarrhoea; epigastric discomfort is not infrequent and is likely to be very marked if large doses are given.

Hypersensitivity reactions are rare with the base, but the estolate produces a high incidence of cholestatic hepatitis, which is thought to be due to hypersensitivity. This condition starts about 10–12 days after the commencement of treatment and presents with abdominal pain, jaundice, and fever. On stopping the drug the symptoms and signs disappear, but re-exposure to the preparation may cause an immediate recurrence of the hepatitis.

Although erythromycin has been regarded as a relatively innocuous antimicrobial, it has a number of interactions that need to be taken into account. It may potentiate the effects of digoxin, warfarin, carbamazepine, and high doses of theophylline. This problem may be due to reduced metabolism of the drugs in question, because erythromycin acts as an hepatic enzyme inhibitor. More recently, the concomitant administration of erythromycin with the antihistamines astemizole and terfenadine has been contraindicated. Astemizole and terfenadine are newer H_1-receptor antagonists, causing less sedation than the older antihistamines. Erythromycin inhibits the metabolism of these drugs and there is a potential risk of cardiac dysrhythmia in patients who receive these antihistamines together with erythromycin.

USES
Erythromycin is a useful alternative to penicillin in dentistry when the patient is known to be hypersensitive to the latter. It can be regarded as a second-choice antimicrobial to penicillin for the treatment of dental infections. It is not, however, the alternative in the prevention of infective endocarditis (see below).

An important use for erythromycin in medicine is the treatment of infections caused by *Legionella pneumophilia* (legionnaire's disease).

Key facts
Erythromycin

- Erythromycin interferes with the translocation stage of protein synthesis by binding to the 50S ribosomal subunit.
- Erythromycin is bacteriostatic (bactericidal at high doses).
- Erythromycin has a similar antibacterial spectrum to penicillin.
- Erythromycin is an alternative to penicillin in the treatment of dental infections.

Tetracyclines

The tetracyclines are a closely related group of broad spectrum bacteriostatic antimicrobials. This group includes tetracycline, chlortetracycline, demeclocycline, doxycycline, lymecycline, minocycline, and oxytetracycline The early agents were derived from micro-organisms, the modern drugs are synthetic.

SPECTRUM OF ACTIVITY Tetracyclines have a broad spectrum of activity against micro-organisms. Susceptible species include Gram-positive organisms, which are also sensitive to penicillin, and many Gram-negative organisms resistant to penicillin. Tetracyclines are also active against rickettsia (for example, typhus), brucella, and diseases due to *Chlamydia trachomatis*, causing lymphogranuloma venereum. They are also effective against *H. influenzae*, treponemata, and some protozoa. Initially the tetracyclines were effective against aerobic Gram-negative bacilli, but now many species are resistant.

MECHANISM OF ACTION Tetracyclines bind to a receptor in the 30S subunit and this blocks the entry of incoming amino acetyl tRNA complexes to their functional location in the ribosome (Fig. 11.4(d)). The non-antibacterial properties of the tetracyclines are described in Chapter 12.

PHARMACOKINETICS The tetracyclines are generally administered orally, but occasionally are given by intravenous infusion. They are also used in controlled-release devices for the management of periodontal disease (see Chapter 12).

Absorption from the gastrointestinal tract is fairly rapid, but significant amounts are retained in the bowel. Absorption is reduced if the drug is taken with milk or with substances containing calcium, magnesium, iron, or aluminium, all of which chelate with tetracyclines. The chelate formed between metallic ions and tetracyclines is not absorbed.

The original tetracyclines (tetracycline, chlortetracycline, and oxytetracycline) produce adequate and maintained plasma concentrations by the administration of 250 mg at 6-hourly intervals. They have a half-life of about 6–10 hours; the maximal concentration in the plasma is reached in 2–4 hours after oral administration, and gradually falls to about half this amount in 9–12 hours, and to a very low concentration at 24 hours.

Demeclocycline, on the other hand, has a half-life of about 16 hours, and satisfactory plasma concentrations may persist for 24 hours or more.

Doxycycline and minocycline have longer half-lives, in the region of 16–18 hours. They are more lipid-soluble than oxytetracycline and hence penetrate bacterial cell walls more readily. Doxycycline, for instance, is given in an initial dose of 200 mg—maximum plasma concentration being reached in 2 hours—and this is followed by a daily dose of 100 mg.

Tetracyclines are widely distributed in the tissues and also enter the cerebrospinal fluid. As they chelate with calcium ions, they are localized in bone and teeth. Excretion of the tetracyclines is in both the urine and the faeces, but mainly via the kidneys. Clearly, excretion is affected by the state of renal function (see later). The exceptions are doxycycline and minocycline, where elimination is in the faeces, following biliary excretion.

UNWANTED EFFECTS

Hypersensitivity reactions are rarely encountered with the tetracyclines but, where they are, cross-hypersensitivity between the various members of the group will be present. Large doses of tetracyclines given parenterally can damage the liver; pregnant women appear to be particularly susceptible. Photosensitivity is a recognized side-effect, especially with demeclocycline.

Immediately after absorption, tetracyclines are incorporated into calcifying tissues and become a permanent, discolouring feature in the teeth. The use of tetracyclines should be avoided during the formative period of the crowns of the teeth. There is a clear linear relationship between the number of courses of treatment with tetracyclines and the discoloration of developing teeth in children under 12 years of age. Of the original tetracyclines, chlortetracycline produced a grey–brown discoloration; yellow staining of varying intensity occurred in patients who had taken tetracycline, oxytetracycline, or demethylchlortetracycline. The third type, a brownish-yellow discoloration, was of mixed origin. Of the earlier tetracyclines the least objectionable staining was produced by oxytetracycline. Minocycline stains the pellicle and can cause oral pigmentation.

In infants, increased intracranial pressure with bulging fontanelles has been observed with tetracycline therapy. This is not a common occurrence and all signs clear up on cessation of treatment.

Gastrointestinal disturbances may complicate therapy with tetracyclines: some patients complain of abdominal discomfort or a feeling of nausea, and there may even be vomiting or diarrhoea. These effects may result from the direct irritant action of the drug on the intestinal mucosa, or may occur because of an alteration of the gut flora. All antimicrobials have the ability to alter the normal microbial flora of the upper respiratory tract, intestinal tract, and genitourinary tract, and probably do so to some extent in every individual. Pseudomembranous colitis is a rare, but serious, complication of tetracycline therapy. It is characterized by severe diarrhoea and mucus-containing stools, caused by the colonization and multiplication of the organism *Clostridium difficile* in the colon, a process encouraged by the alteration of the normal gut flora by the antimicrobial. *Cl. difficile* produces a toxin that damages the gastrointestinal mucosa. Tetracyclines are not the only antimicrobials capable of producing this serious condition; it may occur with others, including ampicillin, amoxicillin, and clindamycin (see below). The treatment of the colitis is to stop the drug immediately and to administer oral vancomycin or metronidazole, to which *Cl. difficile* is sensitive.

Candida albicans is a normal commensal of mucous membranes. The fungus may cause disease in certain predisposed patients, such as diabetics, those with leukaemias or AIDS, and those who have received lengthy treatment with cytotoxic drugs, immunosuppressive drugs, or broad-spectrum antimicrobials.

Patients who have received a long course of treatment with broad-spectrum antimicrobials such as tetracyclines may develop an oral candidal infection that has been named 'antibiotic stomatitis'. This may follow the use of topical antimicrobials in the mouth. The surface proliferation of *C. albicans*, which is known to occur with the administration of broad-spectrum antimicrobials, increases the chances of it invading the tissues and causing infection.

Tetracyclines may cause end-stage renal failure when administered to patients with chronic renal disease. They cause a rise in blood urea, which is often accompanied by deterioration in renal function. While the normal half-life of the original tetracyclines is in the region of 6–10 hours, this may be increased to 57–108 hours in patients with renal failure. Tetracyclines should not, therefore, be given to patients with impaired renal function. Doxycycline and minocycline are possible exceptions to this general statement. Their serum half-life is in the region of 18 hours and is not significantly changed in patients with chronic renal failure.

Severe liver damage can occur after very large doses, and may follow the accumulation of tetracyclines in renal failure. It is also likely to occur following parenteral administration in the third trimester of pregnancy.

USES

There are few indications for the use of tetracyclines in the treatment of dental infections, although doxycycline is sometimes recommended for treating sinusitis. However, they are important in the management of periodontal disease (see Chapter 12).

A tetracycline rinse may be useful in the management of intra-oral herpes infection and also for recurrent aphthous ulceration to prevent secondary bacterial infection. This can be prepared by stirring the contents of a 250-mg tetracycline capsule into a small amount of water. This should be held in the mouth for 2–3 minutes, three times daily for not more than 3 days at a time. Continuous usage may promote oral thrush. The rinse should not be swallowed.

Key facts
Tetracyclines

- Tetracyclines are broad-spectrum antibacterials.

- Tetracyclines block the entry of acetyl tRNA complexes into the ribosome thus interfering with protein synthesis.

- Tetracyclines are bacteriostatic antibacterials.

- Tetracyclines produce intrinsic staining of the teeth and thus should be avoided during the period of dental development.

- Tetracyclines are useful in the management of periodontal disease.

Clindamycin

Clindamycin is one of the lincosamide group of antimicrobials. It is a derivative of lincomycin, which is no longer available.

SPECTRUM OF ACTIVITY Clindamycin is active against Gram-positive bacteria, including penicillinase-producing strains of staphylococci. It is bactericidal at the doses used clinically. Aerobic Gram-negative bacilli are resistant; however, some Gram-negative anaerobic bacteria such as *Bacteroides* species are sensitive.

MECHANISM OF ACTION Clindamycin binds to the 50S ribosomal subunit at the same site as erythromycin and inhibits protein synthesis in the same manner as the latter drug (Fig. 11.4c).

PHARMACOKINETICS Clindamycin is available for intramuscular injection or slow intravenous infusion; it is also presented as capsules and as a paediatric mixture. It is rapidly and almost completely absorbed after oral administration, and its absorption does not seem to be significantly affected by the presence of food in the gut. It produces peak blood concentrations in about 45 minutes and has a half-life of approximately 3 hours. After intramuscular injection of the phosphate form, peak plasma concentrations are only achieved after 3 hours in adults, and somewhat more swiftly in children. Clindamycin is widely distributed throughout the body and penetrates well into bone.

Most of the drug is metabolized and is excreted as metabolites in the urine and bile. A small amount (10%) is excreted unchanged in the urine and an even smaller amount is found in the faeces.

UNWANTED EFFECTS

Diarrhoea is the most common unwanted effect, the incidence being anything from 2% to well over 20%. Unfortunately, some patients have developed pseudomembranous colitis (see above), which can be a very serious problem. Although this condition, often referred to as antibiotic-associated colitis, can occur with other antimicrobials, it seems particularly associated with clindamycin, whether used orally or parenterally. Its occurrence seems to be unrelated to dosage, and it can arise any time during treatment or even after discontinuation of treatment. If it does occur, then the drug should be stopped and the condition treated with oral vancomycin or metronidazole to which *Clostridium difficile*, the causative organism, is sensitive.

Allergic reactions may occur, and skin rashes are observed in a number of patients. There are rare serious reactions, such as the Stevens–Johnson syndrome (severe, febrile erythema multiforme: see sulfonamides below). Interestingly, clindamycin inhibits neuromuscular transmission and could, therefore, potentiate the effect of neuromuscular blocking agents such as tubocurarine.

USES

Clindamycin is a very effective drug in many infections, but the high incidence of diarrhoea and the possible occurrence of colitis must limit its use. It is especially useful in the treatment of infections caused by *Bacteroides* species, and in particular those due to

Bact. fragilis. It should be reserved for infections caused by such organisms and only occasionally used for staphylococcal bone infections after bacteriological identification. The drug of first choice for such bone infections is likely to be flucloxacillin, and there appears to be very little indication for using clindamycin to treat dental infections in patients who are not hypersensitive to penicillin. The importance of clindamycin in dentistry is that it is the alternative to amoxicillin for use as a prophylactic agent against infective endocarditis in those allergic to the latter drug (see later).

Key facts
Clindamycin

- Clindamycin inhibits protein synthesis by interfering with translocation.
- Clindamycin can produce pseudomembranous colitis after prolonged use.
- Clindamycin is an alternative to amoxicillin in the prophylaxis of endocarditis in dentistry.

Aminoglycosides
The aminoglycosides are a group of bactericidal antimicrobials. They include gentamicin, tobramycin, amikacin, netilmicin, the antituberculous drug streptomycin, and the topical agent neomycin.

GENTAMICIN
SPECTRUM OF ACTIVITY Gentamicin has a broad spectrum of activity against many Gram-positive and Gram-negative organisms.

MECHANISM OF ACTION The aminoglycosides bind to the 30S subunit of the bacterial ribosome causing a misreading of mRNA. This results in the production of defective proteins (Fig. 11.4(e)).

PHARMACOKINETICS Gentamicin, as with other aminoglycosides, is not absorbed from the gastrointestinal tract, although there may be some absorption in patients with gastrointestinal disease, for example inflammatory bowel disease. Like other aminoglycosides, gentamicin is rapidly absorbed after intramuscular injection. Intravenous injection should be slow, over a period of 3 minutes. The aminoglycosides can also be given intrathecally.

UNWANTED EFFECTS
Gentamicin is ototoxic, and its unwanted effects include vestibular and auditory dysfunction, although it tends to affect vestibular function more than hearing. The drug is also nephrotoxic but such effects are normally reversible. The aminoglycosides may inhibit transmission at the neuromuscular junction and therefore should not be prescribed to patients suffering from myasthenia gravis.

USES
Gentamicin may be used for treating a variety of infections, including septicaemia, meningitis caused by Gram-negative organisms, and endocarditis caused by *Streptococcus viridans* or *Streptococcus faecalis*. The importance of the drug in dentistry is that it forms part of the regimen for the prophylaxis of infective endocarditis for some patient groups (see below).

Neomycin
Neomycin is not a drug that is used parenterally because it may cause renal damage and is liable to produce deafness: auditory changes may even occur after topical administration. Nevertheless, neomycin alone or in combination with other drugs, such as chlorhexidine, are available for topical use in the ears and nose. Neomycin eye drops or eye ointment are used to treat eye infections.

Sodium fusidate (fusidic acid)
SPECTRUM OF ACTIVITY This bactericidal agent is effective against staphylococci, although resistant strains do emerge *in vivo*, if rather slowly.

MECHANISM OF ACTION Fusidic acid interferes with protein synthesis by the same mechanism as erythromycin.

USES
Sodium fusidate ointment is listed in the *Dental practitioners' formulary*, and may be applied to the fissures of angular cheilitis where *Staph. aureus* has been isolated

Chloramphenicol
SPECTRUM OF ACTIVITY Chloramphenicol is bacteriostatic with a broad spectrum of activity against both aerobic and anaerobic Gram-positive and Gram-negative species.

MECHANISM OF ACTION Chloramphenicol binds to the 50S subunit of the bacterial ribosome at the erythromycin and clindamycin binding site where it interferes with the transpeptidation stage of protein synthesis (Fig. 11.4(c)).

UNWANTED EFFECTS
It creates gastrointestinal disturbance and can produce superinfection with *Candida* spp. However, most important of all it causes an aplastic anaemia. This last complication has rendered chloramphenicol almost obsolete as a systemic drug.

USES
Maxillofacial surgeons use chloramphenicol as a topical application to the eyes in patients with mid-face trauma. It is used to prevent local infection in patients whose eyelids are nonfunctional due to swelling.

Antimicrobials that interfere with bacterial nucleic acid

There are two groups of antimicrobial drugs that interfere directly with bacterial DNA (others, such as the sulfonamides, have an indirect effect on DNA synthesis). These drugs are metronidazole (and related compounds) and the quinolones.

Metronidazole

Metronidazole was originally introduced as an antiprotozoal drug and belongs to the nitroimidazole group of antimicrobial agents.

SPECTRUM OF ACTIVITY Metronidazole is selective for anaerobic organisms. It exhibits bactericidal activity against anaerobic cocci and anaerobic Gram-negative bacilli, including *Bacteroides* and *Clostridium* species.

MECHANISM OF ACTION Strictly speaking, metronidazole is a pro-drug in that it has to be metabolized to an active form (hydroxymetabolite). Once it has diffused into the cell, metronidazole accepts electrons and the nitro group is reduced to a hydroxylamine moiety. It is thought that labile reactive intermediates formed during this reduction are the active antimicrobial compounds. The antimicrobial action involves both inhibition of DNA synthesis and degradation of formed DNA.

PHARMACOKINETICS Metronidazole is available as tablets and for intravenous infusion, it is also available in a controlled-release form for use in periodontal disease (see Chapter 12). The drug is well absorbed after oral administration and a mean peak plasma concentration is produced in 1–2 hours; the plasma half-life is about 8 hours. The drug penetrates into body tissues and fluids, and is metabolized in the liver. Unchanged drug and metabolites are excreted in the urine.

UNWANTED EFFECTS

Numerous unwanted effects have been recorded. These are commonly related to the gastrointestinal tract, for example, nausea, vomiting, indigestion, diarrhoea, and constipation. Dizziness and headaches have also been reported. It is not unusual for the patient to complain of a bitter, metallic taste in the mouth. Occasionally, skin rashes have occurred. Fortunately, the drug is well tolerated and the untoward effects are not often serious. When metronidazole is prescribed, patients should be instructed not to take alcohol as the drug may produce similar reactions to that of disulfiram (Antabuse) when combined with alcohol, it inhibits alcohol metabolism. Metronidazole also potentiates the effects of warfarin and the other coumarin anticoagulants. It seems that metronidazole inhibits an enzyme responsible for the metabolism of warfarin and may enhance warfarin's hypoprothrombinaemic effect. If these drugs are used concurrently, it may be necessary to monitor the patient's INR (International Normalized Ratio).

Metronidazole has been shown to be carcinogenic in rodents fed on high doses for a prolonged period, but there does not seem to be evidence that there is such a risk in man. Although there appears to be no risk in administering metronidazole in pregnancy, as with all other drugs, it should be avoided if possible, especially in the first trimester.

USES

In medical practice, metronidazole is used in the treatment of genital infections with *Trichomonas vaginalis*. It is also effective in the treatment of *Giardia lamblia* infections (giardiasis). Additionally, it is used in the treatment of amoebic infections,

and of anaerobic infections due to *Bacteroides* species, including *Bacteroides fragilis*. *Helicobacter pylori*, which is implicated in the aetiology of peptic ulcers, is also susceptible to metronidazole (see Chapter 18).

Metronidazole is widely used as an antibacterial in dentistry. It is the first-choice treatment for some conditions. The efficacy of metronidazole in the treatment of acute ulcerative gingivitis is well established. One 200 mg tablet is swallowed thrice daily for 3 days. Discomfort usually decreases after 24 hours and ulcerations begin to heal after 48 hours.

Metronidazole is probably as effective as penicillin in the treatment of acute pericoronitis, and it may also have wider uses in dentistry. A variety of bacterial species are found in dental abscesses, including a high proportion of obligate anaerobes of which *Bacteroides melaninogenicus* may well be important. This organism is known to produce tissue-active toxins such as collagenase, hyaluronidase, proteinase, and heparinase. It is possible that these may be concerned in the extensive inflammatory response which characterizes some acute dental infections. Obligate anaerobes are sensitive to both penicillin and metronidazole, and a rapid response to either of these antimicrobial agents would be expected. There is evidence that both are equally effective. Perhaps the true nature of many dental infections has not been appreciated because of the problems associated in the past with the isolation of anaerobes. Metronidazole may be a satisfactory alternative to penicillin in patients with acute dental infections. In acute apical infections, 400 mg tablets two to three times daily should be considered, rather than the 200 mg tablets. Metronidazole is as effective as penicillin, but may be preferred since it produces fewer hypersensitivity reactions and, in addition, there is a lack of bacterial resistance to metronidazole. A further advantage of metronidazole over penicillin is in the treatment of infections due to *Bact. fragilis*. The latter micro-organism is penicillin-resistant, but is not found in dental infections.

Key facts
Metronidazole

- Metronidazole is a pro-drug.
- Once activated metronidazole inhibits bacterial DNA synthesis and promotes the degradation of formed DNA.
- Metronidazole is active against anaerobic organisms.
- Metronidazole is the first-choice treatment for some oral infections such as acute ulcerative gingivitis.

Tinidazole

Tinidazole is an antimicrobial drug closely related to metronidazole. It has been used to treat dental infections but is not used routinely, its advantage over metronidazole is that it has a longer duration of action and thus longer dose interval.

The quinolones

These older bactericidal antimicrobials, which include nalidixic acid and cinoxacin, are not used in dental practice. However, the recently developed fluoroquinolones such as ciprofloxacin are broad-spectrum agents that have proved valuable in medicine.

SPECTRUM OF ACTIVITY The quinolones are active against Gram-negative bacteria but not *P. aeruginosa*. Gram-positive bacteria are predominantly resistant. The fluoroquinolones are effective against both Gram-positive and Gram-negative bacteria, but especially against Gram-negative bacteria.

MECHANISM OF ACTION The fluoroquinolones interfere with the action of DNA gyrase, a bacterial enzyme important in controlling the structure of the individual DNA strands during replication and transcription. When the gyrase is inhibited the DNA strands coil to such an extent that they produce a mechanical obstruction to satisfactory replication.

UNWANTED EFFECTS

The most common adverse effects are nausea, abdominal discomfort, and headache. Concomitant administration of ciprofloxacin or enoxacin with theophylline may lead to elevated plasma concentrations of the latter, with an increased risk of the CNS-stimulant adverse reactions to theophylline. Quinolones may induce convulsions both in patients with a history of epilepsy and in those with no such history. It also appears that convulsions may be produced by interaction between the quinolones and non-steroidal anti-inflammatory drugs (NSAIDs). The CSM advises that the quinolones should be viewed with caution for use in patients with a history of epilepsy or in those taking an NSAID.

USES

Ciprofloxacin is used to treat infections of the respiratory and urinary tracts and is best reserved for those caused by organisms resistant to standard drugs.

Antimicrobials with an antimetabolic action

The earliest of all antibacterial drugs, namely the sulfonamides, have an antimetabolic action on micro-organisms. They are bacteriostatic and they interfere with folate metabolism. Others that act in this way include trimethoprim. These drugs are not widely used in dentistry.

Sulfonamides (sulphonamides)

These were discovered in Germany in 1935, where it was shown that a red dye, prontosil, would cure streptococcal infections in mice. Within a short period, researchers in France and England found that this substance was broken down in the body to two components, one of which—sulfanilimide—was therapeutically active. This was the real beginning of antibacterial chemotherapy and since that time many improvements have been made.

SPECTRUM OF ACTIVITY The sulfonamides are bacteriostatic drugs. They have a wide range of activity against both Gram-positive and Gram-negative organisms, for example streptococci, pneu-mococci, *H. influenzae*, *Vibrio cholerae*, *Neisseria meningitidis*, *E. coli*, and *Neisseria gonorrhoeae*.

MECHANISM OF ACTION Para-aminobenzoic acid (PABA) is an essential metabolite of bacterial cells and is required for the synthesis of folic acid. The sulfonamides competitively inhibit the enzyme dihydropteroate reductase, which is responsible for the incorporation of PABA into the precursor of folic acid (Fig. 11.5). The organisms affected by sulfonamides are those that synthesize their own folic acid; those that use preformed folic acid are unaffected. Fortunately, mammalian cells, that also require folic acid, use preformed folic acid which is obtained from the diet.

Local anaesthetics that are derivatives of PABA, such as procaine and amethocaine, could in theory interfere with the antibacterial action of the sulfonamides. The presence of such local anaesthetics could make PABA available and so redress the balance in favour of the bacteria. However, the injectable dental local anaesthetics used at present (see Chapter 8) are not PABA derivatives and do not antagonize the sulfonamides.

PHARMACOKINETICS Most sulfonamides are readily absorbed from the gastrointestinal tract after oral administration, the small intestine being the main site of absorption. There are exceptions: some sulfonamides are not absorbed and were once used topically in the bowel.

The sulfonamides are widely distributed throughout the body and they cross the blood–brain barrier to enter the cerebrospinal fluid, more so when the meninges are inflamed. They also readily cross the placenta and enter the fetal circulation. The sulfonamides are mainly metabolized in the liver to acetylated forms. The drug is excreted in the urine unchanged or as metabolites.

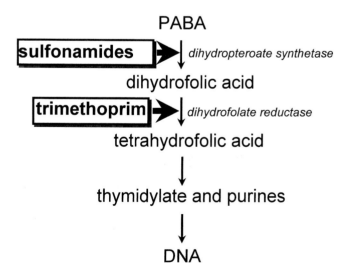

Fig. 11.5 The mechanism of action of sulfonamides and trimethoprim.

UNWANTED EFFECTS

The sulfonamides produce a high incidence of unwanted effects, and this was especially marked with the earlier products. Nausea, with or without vomiting, headache, and malaise were all quite common with the earlier sulfonamides but are rarely seen today.

The most serious effects of the sulfonamides are on the bone marrow. A degree of polymorphonuclear leucopenia does occur but is of little importance in itself. However, agranulocytosis does occasionally arise and, very rarely, haemolytic anaemia occurs. The mechanism of these is not fully understood; they may be manifestations of hypersensitivity. Probably there is very little danger if the treatment is not continued for more than 10 days, although this is not an absolute. After withdrawal of the drug, it may take weeks or months for the granulocytes to return to normal levels; nevertheless, recovery normally ensues. Aplastic anaemia, where all functions of the bone marrow are depressed, is a very rare occurrence indeed.

There are hypersensitivity reactions with the sulfonamides, and their incidence tends to vary with the preparation used: the long-acting sulfonamides are particularly implicated. Skin rashes of various sorts may appear—urticarial, pemphigoid, purpuric, and petechial rashes are all possibilities. Serum sickness-type syndrome may appear after some days of treatment, with fever, joint pains, and rashes. The Stevens–Johnson syndrome—a severe form of erythema multiforme—may occur and may present with blisters in the mouth, genitalia, and skin (Fig. 11.6). The long-acting sulfonamides such as sulfametopyrazine are most likely to be implicated. In addition, there may be ocular involvement. Although an extremely unpleasant condition, it is rarely fatal.

Renal damage from sulfonamides is likely to be rare these days, but this was not so in the past when preparations, particularly the acetylated forms, tended to be less soluble than those used today. These insoluble forms appeared as crystals in the urine (crystalluria), and deposition of crystals in the kidney, ureters, or bladder could lead to obstruction and renal failure.

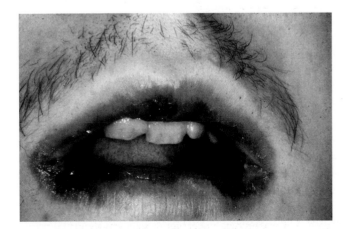

Fig. 11.6 Stevens–Johnson syndrome.

USES

The use of sulfonamides has decreased considerably, mainly because other drugs are available that have fewer adverse effects and are more effective. Sulfamethoxazole is combined with trimethoprim to form the preparation called co-trimoxazole and this is discussed below.

Sulfadimidine is indicated for urinary tract infections and meningococcal meningitis. Sulfadiazine is indicated for meningococcal meningitis, and sulfametopyrazine for urinary tract infections and chronic bronchitis. Many strains of meningococci are now resistant to the sulfonamides.

Trimethoprim–sulfamethoxazole (co-trimoxazole)

SPECTRUM OF ACTIVITY Trimethoprim is an antibacterial agent and has a range of activity similar to that of the sulfonamides. When trimethoprim is combined with a sulfonamide (sulfamethoxazole), as in the preparation co-trimoxazole, it exerts a bactericidal effect.

MECHANISM OF ACTION Like the sulfonamides, trimethoprim inhibits bacteria by metabolic deprivation but at a later stage in their metabolism, by inhibiting the action of the enzyme dihydrofolate reductase (Fig. 11.5). Mammalian cells also possess this enzyme, which is essential for the synthesis of thymidylate and purines required for the production of DNA. However, mammalian dihydrofolate reductase is approximately 50 000 times less sensitive to the inhibitory action of trimethoprim compared to the bacterial enzyme, and this accounts for trimethoprim's selective toxic action on bacteria.

UNWANTED EFFECTS

A high proportion of the unwanted effects that occur with this combination are due to the sulfonamide element and the majority affect skin. Nevertheless, there may be various haematological reactions, such as aplastic or haemolytic anaemias. Theoretically, co-trimoxazole could cause folic-acid deficiency with consequent anaemia, but this is most unlikely to occur in the normal healthy patient given therapeutic doses.

USES

Trimethoprim–sulfamethoxazole is used to treat lower urinary tract infections and is very effective. The combination appears to be particularly useful in the management of chronic and recurrent infections. It is also used for the treatment of exacerbations of chronic bronchitis. It is one of the drugs of choice for the treatment of dysentery (shigellosis) as many of the causative organisms are now resistant to the broad-spectrum penicillins. The combination is useful in the treatment of typhoid and paratyphoid fevers because it seems to be as active as chloramphenicol but with less risk of producing such serious unwanted effects. It may also be useful in the management of the *Salmonella-typhi* carrier state.

Co-trimoxazole may be used occasionally in the treatment of severe dental infections, and in sinusitis and sialadenitis. It is available in tablet form (480 mg), and the dose is 960 mg every

12 hours, although this may be increased to 1.44 g in severe infections. Although the risk of crystalluria is slight, it is desirable when taking this preparation to increase the fluid intake (water).

Because of the incidence of unwanted effects with trimethoprim–sulfamethoxazole, trimethoprim is often used alone. There have been reports of deaths in patients over 65 years of age when the combination drug has been used. Co-trimoxazole should, therefore, be avoided in the elderly and only used if there is no real alternative. Trimethoprim, by itself, has been found to be effective in the treatment of urinary and respiratory tract infections and its use carries less risk of unpleasant unwanted effects.

Sulfasalazine (sulphasalazine)

This preparation is worthy of mention as it is used in the treatment of mild ulcerative colitis, and is a useful prophylactic agent in that condition, maintaining clinical remissions for many patients. Sulfasalazine is broken down in the gut to sulfapyridine and 5-aminosalicylate. It is the salicylate that seems to act as an anti-inflammatory agent in both ulcerative colitis and Crohn's disease. It must not be given to patients with salicylate hypersensitivity.

Use of systemic antibacterials in dentistry

Systemic antibacterials are used in dentistry for two purposes:

1. *therapeutically*: in the management of an established infection. This can be as a definitive treatment, for example in the management of postoperative infection. Antibiotics may also be used as a supportive treatment to the surgical management of infection, such as in the treatment of large collections of pus or in the management of salivary gland infection secondary to a salivary calculus.

2. *prophylactically*: to prevent the occurrence of infection.

Therapeutic use of antibacterials

Antibiotics should not be prescribed without due thought and careful consideration of the advantages over the disadvantages of their use. Although commonly prescribed they are not without their side-effects, around 10 people per year die in the UK as a result of penicillin allergy. Another point worth stressing is that antimicrobials are not analgesics; patients in pain require painkilling medication. Before prescribing an antibacterial to treat a condition the following factors must be considered.

1. Is the condition the result of a bacterial infection?

2. Is the condition serious enough to warrant the administration of systemic chemotherapy? Minor infections may be self-limiting in healthy patients.

The reasons why control must be kept over the prescription of antibacterials include:

(1) the possibility of hypersensitivity reactions;

(2) the possibility of developing resistant organisms (this may affect subjects other than the patient);

(3) the development of 'superinfection' (such as candidiasis) due to disruption of normal bacterial flora.

Hypersensitivity is an absolute contraindication to the use of a specific agent. Other contraindications include the presence of significant liver disease when drugs such as erythromycin should be avoided and the dose of metronidazole reduced. Similarly, high doses of metronidazole should be avoided in pregnancy.

The drugs most commonly used to treat dental infection are the penicillins and metronidazole. The use of antimicrobials in the management of periodontal disease is discussed in Chapter 12. Penicillin G and penicillin V are effective against many of the causative agents of dental infection. Simple dental infections can be treated with 250 mg penicillin V four times daily for 5 days. However, the penicillin-derivative used most effectively at present is the broad-spectrum agent amoxicillin. The use of this drug is mainly due to the fact that most treatments are started empirically, and the condition usually resolves quickly with this broad-spectrum agent. In an ideal world the antibacterial sensitivity of the invading organism would be established before treatment is commenced, but this is time-consuming and impractical for most dental infections. In dental practice, amoxicillin may prescribed orally at a dose of 250–500 mg three times a day for 5 days for adult patients. Alternatively, and this is useful where compliance may be poor, a short course of high-dose amoxicillin can prove effective in controlling dental abscesses. A 3 g dose is administered orally, this may be repeated at 8 hours. When the infection is severe and the patient is hospitalized, the drug is given intravenously at a dose of 0.5–1 g every 8 hours for adult patients.

Patients allergic to penicillin may be treated with either erythromycin or clindamycin. Prolonged use of the latter drug is not advised due to the risk of developing life-threatening pseudomembranous colitis. Any patient developing diarrhoea while taking clindamycin should stop taking the drug immediately. Clindamycin, however, may be used as an acute measure in the treatment of severe dental infection as an intravenous drug at a dose of 300–600 mg. Erythromycin is administered at a dose of 250–500 mg four times a day orally in adults.

It was mentioned above that metronidazole is effective against the causative agents in many dental infections and this may be prescribed at the dose of 400 mg two to three times daily for 5 days (the intravenous dose is 500 mg twice daily). The combination of amoxicillin and metronidazole is useful in the management of severe dental infection.

Prophylactic use of antibiotics

There are two quite different prophylactic uses for antimicrobials in dental practice. First, in the prevention of wound infection. Second, in the prevention of distant infection (such as infective endocarditis) in medically compromised patients following a bacteraemia caused by dental treatment.

PREVENTION OF WOUND INFECTION

When used appropriately antibiotics are valuable in the prevention of wound infection. Unfortunately, they are often misused and this can lead to problems, not only for the patient, but also globally as the number of resistant organisms may increase. There are a number of important principles in the prophylaxis of wound infection and these are discussed below. In addition to the use of sterile instruments, adherence to strict cross-infection control and good surgical technique are extremely important factors in preventing wound infection, but these are outside the scope of this text.

PRINCIPLES OF THE USE OF ANTIBIOTICS TO PREVENT WOUND INFECTION The dental practitioner must:

(1) believe that the probability of wound infection is high;

(2) select the appropriate antibiotic;

(3) begin therapy at the correct time;

(4) use the appropriate dose;

(5) use for the appropriate length of time.

1. **THE PROBABILITY OF WOUND INFECTION MUST BE HIGH:** Some surgical procedure lend themselves to wound infection even in healthy patients. Good examples are surgery to the lower gastrointestinal tract. Such procedures should be 'covered' by appropriate prophylactic antibiotics. There is no type of wound produced in routine dental practice which falls into this category. Even minor oral surgery procedures such as the removal of impacted third molars have a very low incidence of postoperative wound infection and do not merit the use of prophylactic antimicrobials as standard practice in healthy patients. Major maxillofacial operations, however, may necessitate prophylaxis as the incidence of wound infection is related to the duration of surgery. There is a significant increase in the incidence of infection in procedures that last longer than 2 hours, therefore even 'clean' prolonged operations need cover. Other 'clean' procedures which merit prophylaxis are the implantation of prostheses (such as dental implants) and the transplantation of teeth. On the other hand, uncomplicated surgical wounds may become infected in patients with reduced resistance. This may be due to local effects (such as a poor blood supply following therapeutic irradiation) or systemic disease (such as uncontrolled diabetes). Decreased resistance is a more likely cause of wound infection in routine dental practice and simple treatments such as dental extractions may need 'cover' in patients with reduced resistance.

2. **SELECT THE APPROPRIATE ANTIBIOTIC:** It is paramount that the patient is not allergic to the antibiotic chosen. The antibiotic should be bactericidal and be active against the organisms that would normally be expected to infect the wound. In dental practice the first-choice drug is usually a penicillin, amoxicillin being popular.

3. **BEGIN THERAPY AT THE CORRECT TIME:** The objective in the prevention of wound infection is to achieve optimum blood levels within the blood clot formed at the end of the procedure. Therefore if oral administration is used, sufficient time must be allowed to achieve peak plasma levels as the clot is forming. Thus, if it takes 1 hour to reach peak plasma levels the antibiotic would be given at the start of the procedure if the surgery was going to last an hour: if it was a short procedure such as an extraction in a compromised patient, the antibiotic should be administered orally 1 hour before surgery. Alternatively, if the intravenous route is chosen the drug can be delivered during the procedure. When a lengthy major surgical procedure is being performed under general anaesthesia and multiple wounds are being produced then more than one intravenous dose will be required, in such circumstances the dose interval is twice the plasma half-life (this is half the normal therapeutic dose interval).

4. **USE THE APPROPRIATE DOSE:** It is important that bactericidal plasma levels are achieved when administering antibiotics prophylactically. At least twice the normal therapeutic dose is administered. For example, when using amoxicillin prophylactically in adults, the usual dose is 3 g orally (the usual therapeutic dose level is 250–500 mg).

5. **USE FOR THE APPROPRIATE LENGTH OF TIME:** The shortest effective exposure should be used. There are two reasons for this. First, once the blood clot has formed there is a decreased opportunity for the administered drug to be incorporated, indeed after a period of around 3 hours no antibiotic will enter a formed blood clot. Thus late administration is useless. Second, the longer the antibiotic is administered the greater are the chances of resistant organisms developing.

The use of antibiotics prophylactically to prevent wound infection in dental practice can be summed up in the expression 'hit them once and hit them hard'.

PREVENTION OF DISTANT INFECTION

The use of prophylactic antibiotics to prevent infection at a distant site is important in dental practice. Patients susceptible to distant infection include:

(1) patients with congenital abnormalities of the endocardium (such as mitral stenosis);

(2) patients with cardiac prostheses (artificial heart valves).

Patients with non-cardiac (orthopaedic) prostheses such as artificial hips are not considered at risk from late infection from a dental source and do not require antibiotic prophylaxis. Indeed, the chance of a severe adverse reaction to the prescribed antibiotic outweighs the probability of a dentally derived infection of the prosthesis in these patients.

The reason for the use of prophylactic antibiotics in patients with endocardial defects or prostheses is to prevent the life-threatening condition of infective endocarditis. Manipulation of the gingival margin produces a significant transient bacteraemia and the blood-borne bacteria can settle on damaged endocardium thereby producing infective endocarditis. Any dental procedure that involves gingival manipulation (scaling, extractions, matrix band application, and intraligamentary anaesthesia) must be covered by prophylactic antibiotics in susceptible patients. Most of the principles enumerated above for the prevention of wound infection also apply here. A bactericidal antibiotic should be chosen, the appropriate dose must be given at the optimum time, and the shortest effective exposure should be used. However, there is an important difference in relation to the time of administration. In this case, optimum plasma levels of the antibiotic are required at the time of gingival manipulation, this is usually at the start of the procedure. Thus if an oral dose is given, it must be administered 1 hour before the start of the procedure; if the intravenous route is chosen, the drug is delivered just prior to commencement.

At the time of writing, the accepted regimen for the prevention of infective endocarditis following dental treatment is that described below. However, these recommendations are continually under review and it is important that dentists keep informed of current guidelines. Current recommendations can be found in the *British national formulary* and any major changes are reported in professional journals.

ANTIBACTERIAL PROPHYLAXIS FOR THE PREVENTION OF INFECTIVE ENDOCARDITIS FOLLOWING DENTAL TREATMENT

1. Dental treatment under local anaesthesia

    (a) Patients not allergic to penicillin and who have not received a penicillin more than once in the previous month:

    Adults—amoxicillin 3 g orally 1 hour before the operation. The drug should be given with either the dentist or the dental nurse present to ensure that the patient takes it.

    Children—for children under 10 years of age, half the adult dose; and for children under 5 years, a quarter of the adult dose. For children over 10 years, the dosage is the same as for the adult.

    This regimen applies to patients with prosthetic heart valves as well as those with natural valvular disease. A patient who has a properly functioning prosthetic valve is no more likely to get infective endocarditis after dental procedures than one with damaged natural valves. However, if a patient with prosthetic valves does have an attack of infective endocarditis then it is likely to be severe with a poorer prognosis, and treatment may be surgical rather than medical.

    The regimen described above is not suitable for patients who have had endocarditis. Amoxicillin plus gentamicin are advocated for them (see point 3 below).

    (b) Patients who are allergic to penicillin or who have received a penicillin more than once in the previous month:

Adults—oral clindamycin 600 mg 1 hour before the dental procedure.
Children—those under 5 years of age, a quarter of the adult dose; 5–10 years, half the adult dose.

These regimens will cover most problems faced in general dental practice. The dosages recommended seem to provide adequate plasma concentrations for the critical period of 10 hours following the dental procedure.

2. Dental treatment under general anaesthesia

    (a) Patients not allergic to penicillin and who have not received penicillin more than once in the previous month:

    Adults—1 g amoxicillin intramuscularly or intravenously at induction, and 500 mg of oral amoxicillin 6 hours later.
    Children—those under 5 years of age, a quarter of the adult dose; children between 5 and 10 years, half the adult dose.

    An alternative is to give oral amoxicillin 3 g four hours before induction then 3 g oral amoxicillin as soon as possible after the dental treatment. The dose for children under 5 years of age is a quarter of the adult dose; and for those between 5 and 10 years, the dose is half the adult dose.

    These regimens are not suitable for patients with prosthetic heart valves or for those who have had endocarditis (see point 3 below).

    (b) Patients who are allergic to penicillin or who have received a penicillin more than once in the previous month

    Intravenous vancomycin 1 g over a period of at least 100 minutes, then intravenous gentamicin 120 mg at induction or 15 minutes before the treatment. The dose for a child under 10 years is vancomycin 20 mg kg^{-1}, gentamicin 2 mg kg^{-1}.

    or

    Intravenous teicoplanin 400 mg plus gentamicin 120 mg at induction or 15 minutes preoperatively. The dose for children under 14 years of age is teicoplanin 6 mg kg^{-1} intravenously plus gentamicin 2 mg kg^{-1} intravenously.

    or

    Intravenous clindamycin 300 mg over a period of 10 minutes at induction followed by oral or intravenous clindamycin 150 mg, 6 hours later. The dose for children under 5 years of age is a quarter of the adult dose; and for children between 5 and 10 years it is half the adult dose.

3. Patients at special risk: For patients with prosthetic heart valves who require a general anaesthetic, and for patients

who have had endocarditis, the regimen involves intramuscular or intravenous amoxicillin 1 g plus intramuscular or intravenous gentamicin 120 mg at induction, followed by oral amoxicillin 500 mg, 6 hours later. The dose for children under 5 years of age is a quarter of the adult dose of amoxicillin plus gentamicin 2 mg kg^{-1}; the dose for children between 5 and 10 years is half the adult dose of amoxicillin plus gentamicin 2 mg kg^{-1}. These regimens are suitable for special-risk patients who are not allergic to penicillin. If the patient is allergic to penicillin or has received a penicillin more than once within the previous month, the regimens are as indicated above.

Patients classified as at special risk are: (1) those who have had infective endocarditis previously; (2) those who have prosthetic heart valves and require a general anaesthetic; and (3) those who are allergic to penicillin or who have had a penicillin more than once in the previous month, and require a general anaesthetic. Special-risk patients should be referred to hospital for dental treatment.

It should be re-emphasized that patients who have had infective endocarditis are regarded as at-risk whether they are to receive treatment under local anaesthesia, without local anaesthesia, or with general anaesthesia.

Key facts
Use of systemic antibacterials in dentistry

- Antibacterials are used in dentistry to:
  - treat established bacterial infections;
  - prevent wound infection;
  - prevent distant infections such as endocarditis.

- When used to prevent wound infection a high concentration of antibacterial is required in the formed blood clot, thus the drug is administered preoperatively.

- The first-choice drug in the prophylaxis of endocarditis is amoxicillin. In patients allergic to penicillin clindamycin is the drug of choice.

Antifungal drugs

Antifungal medications are frequently prescribed in the practice of oral medicine. Both topical and systemic (oral) administration are used. As there are fungal organisms resident in the oral cavity, fungal infection is usually the result of a decrease in host resistance (such as HIV infection) or an alteration in the host flora (for example caused by a broad-spectrum antimicrobial such as a tetracycline). An underlying cause should always be sought if an apparently healthy individual presents with an oral fungal infection.

MECHANISM OF ACTION The antifungals used in dentistry exert their effect by interfering with the structure of the mycelial cell membrane and altering its fluidity. This affects permeability, transmembrane transport, and the activity of membrane-bound enzymes.

Nystatin

This is effective against *C. albicans* and some other fungi.

MECHANISM OF ACTION Nystatin is active against yeasts and fungi but inactive against bacteria. This selective toxicity is due to the presence of ergosterol in the cytoplasmic membrane of fungi and yeasts, but not in bacterial membranes. A hydrophobic interaction between nystatin and the membrane ergosterol molecule creates a pore with a hydrophilic ion-channel in the membrane. This allows the loss of intracellular ions and disrupts the osmotic function of the membrane, with consequent death of the fungus.

PHARMACOKINETICS Nystatin is not absorbed from the skin or mucous membranes. It is therefore used for its local effect in the treatment of candidiasis (candidosis) on the skin or any part of the alimentary tract.

UNWANTED EFFECTS

These are exceedingly rare. The occasional patients feels nauseated after oral administration. There have been no reports of hypersensitivity reactions. The drug has a very unpleasant taste.

USES

Nystatin is used primarily to treat infections caused by *C. albicans*, such as thrush, denture stomatitis, antibiotic stomatitis, and some forms of mucocutaneous candidiasis.

Topical nystatin has been used for many years to treat oral lesions due to candidal infections. Usually, one pastille of nystatin (100 000 units) is allowed to dissolve in the mouth, four times daily, for a period that depends on the response to treatment. In treating candidal leukoplakia the regimen may have to be maintained for many months. An alternative is to use nystatin oral suspension (100 000 units per mL) when 1 mL is placed in the mouth after food, four times daily. The suspension is retained as long as possible near the lesions. The advantage of the pastilles is that they are pleasantly flavoured.

Although the precise cause of denture stomatitis is uncertain, candidal infection is one associated factor. Patients who have denture stomatitis should be advised to leave out their dentures as much as possible, and certainly overnight, and to keep them in a cleansing agent such as sodium hypochlorite solution. The treatment regimen is as indicated above. Many patients are understandably reluctant to leave out their dentures for any length of time, so a compromise is to smear the fitting surfaces with an antifungal ointment such as miconazole oral gel (see below) before insertion.

Mucocutaneous lesions and the lesions associated with AIDS are generally not susceptible to nystatin.

Candidal vaginitis is a common sexually transmitted disease and generally responds well to local applications of nystatin.

Amphotericin B

This is effective against a number of fungi, including *Candida* species. Its mode of action is thought to be like that of nystatin, and it has no effect on bacteria.

The treatment of fungal infections by either nystatin or amphotericin B is not always completely effective. Once the symptoms and signs have disappeared it may be necessary to continue medication for some time (perhaps as long again) to ensure that the infection has been totally eradicated.

PHARMACOKINETICS Amphotericin is poorly absorbed from the gastrointestinal tract and probably not at all from unbroken skin. It is used locally to treat conditions for which nystatin could be used. Amphotericin B is available for intravenous injection, when it can be used for the treatment of systemic fungal infections such as candidal septicaemia and histoplasmosis. The drug is excreted in an inactive form in the urine, and there is also biliary excretion.

UNWANTED EFFECTS

The parenteral use of amphotericin B is associated with a host of unwanted effects, including fever, nausea, and vomiting. Some undesirable effects on the kidney are almost inevitable; a rise in blood urea may occur.

USES

Amphotericin B is one of the relatively few antimicrobials effective against systemic fungal infections and is, therefore, a valuable weapon in the medical armamentarium, particularly as nystatin is too toxic to be used systemically. In dentistry, amphotericin B (10 mg) lozenges may be used locally in the mouth as an alternative to nystatin. In severe infections the dose may be doubled. Amphotericin oral suspension can be substituted for nystatin suspension.

Azole agents

The azole agents are divided into two broad classes: the imidazoles and the triazoles. They have a broad spectrum of activity. The imidazoles include miconazole, ketoconazole, and clotrimazole. The imidazole used most often in dentistry is miconazole. Among the triazoles are fluconazole and itraconazole.

The triazoles are more slowly metabolized than the imidazoles and also have less of an effect on host steroid synthesis.

MECHANISM OF ACTION The azoles suppress the synthesis of ergosterol. Lack of ergosterol interferes with fungal membrane function. This inhibits both fungal replication and transformation of *Candidal* cells into the pathogenic hyphal form.

PHARMACOKINETICS Miconazole is available for oral and parenteral administration. It has many unwanted effects when given intravenously and is not the antifungal drug of choice for systemic use.

Ketoconazole is available for oral administration, and peak plasma concentrations appear about 2 hours after a dose of 400 mg. The drug is metabolized in the liver, and most is excreted as metabolites in the urine.

Fluconazole may be administered orally or by intravenous injection. Fungicidal concentrations of the drug may be obtained in saliva. It is excreted unchanged in urine.

Itraconazole is administered orally. However, absorption is variable and the drug is extensively metabolized in the liver.

UNWANTED EFFECTS

Although the most commonly encountered unwanted effects with parenteral ketoconazole are nausea and vomiting, other untoward effects have occurred, including headache, photophobia, rash, and thrombocytopenia. Hepatic toxicity occasionally produces hepatic dysfunction. Unwanted effects when miconazole is used intravenously are frequent, and include anaemia, anaphylactoid reactions, and central nervous system involvement (hallucinations, blurred vision).

A number of drug interactions occur between the azoles and other drugs dental patients may be receiving. Like the antibacterial erythromycin, the antifungals ketoconazole, itraconazole, and other imidazoles should not be prescribed to patients receiving the newer antihistamines astemizole and terfenadine as cardiac dysrhythmias may occur.

The azoles enhance the anticoagulant effect of warfarin. It is important to appreciate that this interaction can occur even after topical antifungal use. The plasma concentration of midazolam is increased by the azoles. Miconazole increases the antiepileptic effects of phenytoin and increases the plasma concentrations of the sulfonylurea oral hypoglycaemics.

USES

Ketoconazole finds a use in the treatment of systemic fungal infections and candidiasis. It is also useful as a prophylaxis in patients who are on immunosuppressive therapy and in the treatment of such patients who have chronic candidal leukoplakia. A once-daily dose of ketoconazole (200 mg tablet) is taken with food, and the treatment is continued for 1–2 weeks after symptoms have disappeared and cultures are negative.

Miconazole has found a place in dentistry, and its primary use is topical. One miconazole tablet (250 mg) is taken 6-hourly. Topical treatment is achieved by allowing the tablets to dissolve in the mouth. Treatment should be continued for some time after symptoms and signs have resolved.

The drug is also presented as a sugar-free oral gel (25 mg mL^{-1}). The dosage is 5–10 mL in the mouth after food, taken four times daily, and being retained near to the lesions if possible before swallowing. This oral gel can be smeared onto the denture surface when treating patients with denture stomatitis. The gel is also thought to be useful in the treatment of candidal leukoplakia or chronic mucocutaneous candidiasis.

Angular cheilitis is an infection of the skin at the angle of the mouth, which is usually a mixed infection, possibly candidal and staphylococcal. Miconazole cream is applied to the lesions twice daily. It is not only effective against the candida, but also against Gram-positive organisms such as *Staphylococcus* and *Streptococcus* species. After resolution of the lesions, treatment should be continued for up to 10 days. There may be an underlying factor behind angular cheilitis, such as iron deficiency anaemia, and clearly this must be investigated and treated appropriately.

Miconazole is usually effective against all oral candidal infections.

Fluconazole capsules or suspension may be used to treat oral fungal infections that do not respond to topical applications. A dose of 50 mg daily (up to a maximum of 14 days) is used for adults.

Key facts
Antifungal drugs

- Antifungal drugs affect the permeability of mycelial cell membranes, interfere with membrane transport, and inhibit membrane-bound enzymes.
- In dentistry, antifungal drugs are used topically to treat oral mucosal infections.
- The azole group of antifungals enhance the effects of warfarin even after topical application.

Antiviral agents

The action of viruses can be arrested by a number of mechanism including:

(1) immunostimulation of the host;

(2) inhibition of viral nucleic acid synthesis;

(3) inhibition of viral proteins.

The recognition of HIV has led to an increase in research into antiviral therapy and there can be little doubt that advances will occur rapidly in this field. The advent of new therapies based on immunostimulation for serious viral infection is one area of potential growth.

Immunostimulation can be achieved by the:

(1) administration of human immune globulin;

(2) administration of immunostimulant drugs.

Cytokines (see Chapter 4) can be used to activate host cells such as lymphocytes, and such drugs may prove useful in treating serious viral diseases as well as playing a role in anticancer therapy.

The classic antiviral drugs used in dental practice are nucleoside analogues, which interfere with the replication of viral nucleic acid. These agents plus those used in the treatment of AIDS will be described below.

Viral infections differ from other types of infection because viruses are obligate intracellular parasites that require for their survival the active participation of the metabolic processes of the invaded cell. Thus, agents used to destroy viruses may also dam-

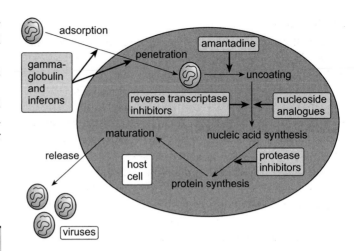

Fig. 11.7 The sites at which the different antiviral agents have their effects.

age the invaded cell. The sites at which the various antiviral drugs exert their effects are show in Fig. 11.7.

Antiherpetic agents

Most of these agents are nucleoside analogues.

Acyclovir (Aciclovir)

Developed in the early 1980s, this is an analogue of the purine nucleoside guanosine, and its antiviral activity is essentially confined to the herpesvirus. The drug can be given orally (200 mg), intravenously, and topically (5% cream).

MECHANISM OF ACTION Acyclovir is one of a group of antiviral agents, which are transformed by phosphorylation into their active state by viral enzymes. Acyclovir has much more affinity for viral than host enzymes and this selectivity makes it less toxic than other antiviral agents such as idoxuridine (see below). Viral enzymes phosphorylate acyclovir to form the compound acyclovir–GMP, which is then further catalysed by host cellular enzymes to acyclovir–GTP. Acyclovir–GTP is a potent inhibitor of viral DNA synthesis. It competes with viral nucleotides for incorporation into viral DNA. Once incorporated it terminates the DNA chain producing non-functional DNA strands, thus inhibiting replication of the virus (Fig. 11.8).

PHARMACOKINETICS When given orally, acyclovir has a half-life of 2.5 hours and is poorly bound to plasma protein (15%). The drug crosses the blood–brain barrier and is eliminated by the kidneys.

Resistance to acyclovir is rare, although it can occur in certain mucocutaneous herpetic infections.

UNWANTED EFFECTS

Unwanted effects arising from oral administration are few, and include nausea and headache. Topical application of acyclovir to mucous membrane can cause a transient burning sensation but this may be due to the polyethylene base.

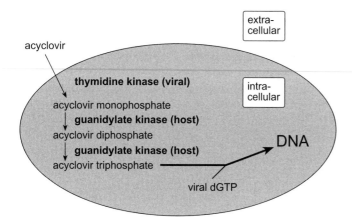

Fig. 11.8 The mechanism of action of acyclovir. The aberrant DNA produced by incorporation of acyclovir triphosphate is non-functional.

USES

Acyclovir is used to treat the following viral infections:

1. **HERPES SIMPLEX TYPE I VIRUS:** Acyclovir reduces the symptoms of the mucocutaneous lesions of the face and oropharynx associated with this infection. Immunocompromised patients (i.e. organ transplant patients, and those with AIDS) are particularly susceptible to herpes simplex type I, and systemic acyclovir may prevent the recurrence of this infection in these patients.

2. **HERPES SIMPLEX TYPE II VIRUS:** This virus causes genital herpes and may also be responsible for meningitis. Primary genital herpes responds to acyclovir, but does not prevent recurrence.

3. **VARICELLA–ZOSTER VIRUS:** Shingles is the principal disease caused by this virus and, in some patients, this is followed by postherpetic neuralgia. Acyclovir has been shown to reduce the symptoms of the initial attack of shingles, but is of little value in the treatment of the neuralgia.

The topical preparation is a 5% cream and it is applied five times daily. This formulation is available as an over-the-counter medicine for the treatment of herpes labialis ('cold sores'). When administered orally, acyclovir is given as a 200 mg tablet five times a day for 5 days. When given intravenously for severe infections, it is administered as an infusion over 1 hour at a dose of 5 mg kg^{-1}. This is given every 8 hours.

Valacyclovir

Valacyclovir is an ester of acyclovir used in the treatment of genital herpes and herpes zoster infection. It has an identical method of action to acyclovir but has the advantage of less frequent dosing (1 g every 8 hours for zoster infection).

Famciclovir

This is the pro-drug, the active agent being penciclovir. This latter agent is similar in many ways to acyclovir but has a lower affinity for DNA polymerase. It is active against herpes simplex I and II and also hepatitis B virus.

Gancyclovir

Gancyclovir is a guanosine analogue and, like acyclovir, is phosphorylated by viral enzymes. Unlike acyclovir it does not cause DNA chain termination; however, DNA replication is inhibited after incorporation of the triphosphate.

Gancyclovir is used to treat life-threatening cytomegalovirus infection in immunocompromised patients. It is much more active than acyclovir against cytomegalovirus. Gancyclovir has serious unwanted effects including bone-marrow suppression.

Idoxuridine

Idoxuridine is a thymidine analogue. It is phosphorylated within cells and the triphosphate so formed is incorporated into both cellular and viral DNA. Unlike acyclovir, idoxuridine does not block DNA synthesis but is incorporated into viral DNA. The resultant DNA is more susceptible to breakage, and altered viral proteins may result from faulty transcription. Hence, idoxuridine is mainly used against DNA viruses (herpes simplex type I, vaccinia, varicella, and cytomegalovirus). Due to its effects on cellular DNA, idoxuridine is too toxic for systemic administration and is therefore only used topically.

In the past, topical idoxuridine was used in the management of acute herpetic gingivostomatitis and herpes labialis; however, it has now largely been superseded. Acyclovir is the treatment of choice.

Vidarabine

This is an adenosine analogue, which, when phophorylated, suppresses DNA synthesis by inhibiting DNA polymerase. It is used systemically to treat life-threatening herpes zoster infection in immunocompromised patients. A topical application may be used to treat herpes simplex infections of the eye.

Foscarnet

This differs from the other antiviral agents discussed so far in that it is not a nucleotide derivative. It is a pyrophosphate analogue that suppresses DNA polymerase and RNA polymerase activity by binding at the pyrophosphate binding site. It is used in the management of acyclovir-resistant herpetic infection and in the treatment of retinitis due to cytomegalovirus.

Reverse transcriptase inhibitors

Most reverse transcriptase (RNA-dependent DNA polymerase) inhibitors are nucleoside analogues, although newer drugs such as nevirapine and delavirdine are non-nucleosides.

Nucleoside analogues

ZIDOVUDINE (AZT)

Zidovudine is a thymidine analogue and was first developed as an anticancer drug. Interest in it was reawakened when it was demonstrated to be cytopathic against the human immunodeficiency virus type I (HIV-1), the causative agent of AIDS.

The drug inhibits viral RNA-dependent DNA polymerase. In addition, it causes chain termination during DNA synthesis; this prevents further nucleotides from being incorporated into the growing strand of DNA. The antiviral action of zidovudine can be enhanced by acyclovir and interferon.

Zidovudine can be given orally (250 mg) or by continuous intravenous infusion. After oral dosage, it is rapidly absorbed from the gastrointestinal tract and peak plasma concentrations are achieved after 30–90 minutes. AZT has a short half-life (approximately 1 hour), is metabolized in the liver, and excreted via the kidney.

Granulocytopenia and anaemia are the main unwanted effects associated with zidovudine therapy. The haematological disturbances usually occur 6–8 weeks after commencement of therapy. Regular (two-weekly) blood counts should be carried out throughout. Aspirin, NSAIDs, and paracetamol increase the risk of zidovudine-induced haematological disturbances. Other unwanted effects of the drug include severe headache, nausea, insomnia, and muscle pains. Resistance to the drug occurs.

The main use of AZT is in the treatment of symptomatic HIV-positive and AIDS patients. The antiviral agent does not appear to delay the development of signs and symptoms of AIDS in those patients who are asymptomatic, but who are HIV positive.

DIDANOSINE

This drug is used in the treatment of AIDS. It is a nucleic-acid chain terminator and inhibits viral reverse transcriptase. Resistance to the effects of the drug occur but to a lesser extent than is the case with zidovudine.

ZALCITABINE

This is a reverse transcriptase inhibitor used in combination with zidovudine in the treatment of AIDS.

STAVUDINE

This is a new agent and is used in combination with other reverse transcriptase inhibitors in the management of AIDS.

LAMIVUDINE

This is again a new drug, which is used in combination with zidovudine to reverse viral resistance to the latter agent.

Non-nucleoside analogues

These are new drugs used in the treatment of AIDS and include nevirapine and delavirdine. Nevirapine was the first non-nucleoside, reverse transcriptase inhibitor synthesized, but due to resistance being readily developed it is only used in combined therapy. Nevirapine is an enzyme inducer and reduces the plasma concentration of carbamazepine and corticosteroids. Delavirdine, on the other hand, is an enzyme inhibitor and has similar drug interactions to the protease inhibitors described below.

Viral protein inhibitors

Unlike most of the agents described above these are not synthetic nucleosides.

Protease inhibitors

HIV-1 protease is an enzyme essential for the production of mature viral structural proteins and enzymes. Protease inhibitors are available for the treatment of HIV infection and include the agents indinavir, ritonavir, and saquinavir. They are used in combination with reverse transcriptase inhibitors.

Protease inhibitors counter the activity of drug metabolizing enzymes and this can affect concurrent drug therapy. Among the drugs used in dentistry whose plasma levels are increased by the protease inhibitors are lidocaine (lignocaine), midazolam, carbamazepine, and metronidazole. Care should therefore be exercised when prescribing these drugs in patients taking protease inhibitors.

Amantadine

Amantadine is a tricyclic amine. This drug is used in the prophylaxis of influenza A virus. Amantadine inhibits viral uncoating by blocking a viral membrane ion channel produced by the viral protein M2. This leads to a failure in viral replication.

Other antiviral agents

Interferons

Interferons are a group of cytokines (see Chapter 4). There are three types: interferon-α, interferon-β, and interferon-γ. All have antiviral actions. They are glycoproteins produced by the body in response to a viral infection. Their properties include the induction of resistance to viral infections and the regulation of other cell functions such as enhancing the cytotoxic ability of T lymphocytes.

Key facts
Antiviral drugs

- Most antiviral agents inhibit viral nucleic acid production.
- Most antiviral agents are nucleoside analogues.
- Some antiherpetic agents such as acyclovir block viral DNA synthesis, others such as idoxuridine are incorporated into DNA so forming unstable chains.
- Reverse transcriptase inhibitors may be nucleoside analogues such as zidovudine or they may be non-nucleoside analogues such as nevirapine.
- Protease inhibitors interfere with the production of mature viral proteins.
- Some antiviral agents such as interferons produce host immunostimulation.
- Antiviral agents are used topically and systemically to treat oral viral infections.

Infections due to prions

One of the most important recent advances in the molecular biology of infectious disease has been the recognition of those infective agents named prions.

Prions are unique as infective agents because they are pure proteins, they contain no genetic material. Prions differ from natural host proteins only in their conformation, and they can produce configurational changes in host protein by a prion–protein physical interaction. The therapeutic control of this interplay is an important challenge in modern pharmacology.

Diseases known at present to be produced by prions include bovine spongiform encephalitis (BSE) in cattle and Creutzfeldt–Jakob disease in humans. Our present knowledge of prions is in its infancy and their importance in oral and dental disease is unknown.

Further reading

Hardman, J. G. and Limbird, L. E. (ed.) (1996). Chemotherapy of microbial disease. In *Goodman and Gilman's the pharmacological basis of therapeutics*, Section IX. McGraw-Hill, New York.

Greenwood, I., Heylen, R., and Zakrzewska, J. M. (1998). Antiretroviral drugs—implications for dental prescribing. *British Dental Journal*, 184, 478–82.

Longman, L. P. and Martin, M. V. (1999). A practical guide to antibiotic prophylaxis in restorative dentistry. *Dental Update*, 26, 7–14.

Peterson, L. J. (1990). Antibiotic prophylaxis against wound infections in oral and maxillofacial surgery. *Journal of Oral Maxillofacial Surgery*, 48, 617.

12

Pharmacological control of dental caries and periodontal disease

- Dental caries
- Periodontal disease
- Dentine sensitivity
- References

Pharmacological control of dental caries and periodontal disease

Dental caries and periodontal disease are the two principal diseases that affect the morbidity of the dentition. Microbial plaque is the main aetiological factor in both diseases, although diet and the host response play vital roles. The incidence of dental caries can be considerably reduced by fluoride. Mechanical removal of plaque is the basis for controlling periodontal diseases, but this is often impracticable because of the high degree of motivation and dexterity required to make a mouth plaque-free. Research has been concentrated on the development of chemical methods for inhibiting plaque formation. This chapter discusses the various pharmacological methods for controlling dental caries and periodontal diseases.

Dental caries

This is caused by a biological interaction between bacteria, diet, and the tooth surface. There is now overwhelming evidence that refined carbohydrates are broken down by acid-producing bacteria, in turn these substances produce further acid causing demineralization of the enamel surface. *Streptococci mutans* are the main bacteria implicated in dental caries, which produce lactic acid from dietary carbohydrates.

The relationship between fluoride and dental caries was first realized in the early part of this century. Since then many epidemiological studies have demonstrated unequivocally the role of fluoride in preventing dental caries.

Mode of action of fluoride in reducing dental decay

The precise mode of action of fluoride is uncertain, but it probably acts via several mechanisms including an effect on enamel structure, an alteration in tooth morphology, and an action on bacterial plaque.

Fluoride and enamel structure

Enamel is mainly composed of crystals of hydroxyapatite, which readily loses its hydroxyl group in the presence of fluoride to form fluorapatite. Hydroxyapatite crystals dissolve more easily than fluorapatite in acid due to the presence of voids caused by the disordered arrangement of the hydroxyl group. Fluoride thus makes apatite crystals less soluble in acid by two mechanisms. First, crystals of fluorapatite have less voids than crystals of hydroxyapatite, thus reducing solubility. Second, fluoride displaces carbon and magnesium ions from apatite crystals: such displacement improves the crystalline structure. There is a greater concentration of fluorapatite on the surface of enamel, which further reduces enamel solubility.

Fluoride also has an effect on the remineralization of enamel after acid attack. Three possible mechanisms are suggested:

1. Fluoride reduces the more soluble carbonate of enamel, so reducing its solubility.

2. Acid attack causes the release of fluoride ions from the enamel surface. The released fluoride, together with fluoride ions contained in plaque and saliva, favours remineralization.

3. Fluoride accumulates in early carious lesions at concentrations that are sufficiently high to reduce enamel solubility.

The effects on remineralization are now considered to be the most important mechanisms of the anticaries action of fluoride. The earlier belief that the formation of fluorapatite exerted the greatest cariostatic effect has now been replaced by the view that it is a constant supply of soluble, ionic fluoride that is most effective.

Fluoride and tooth morphology

Fluoride ingested during dental development slightly alters the shape of teeth, resulting in wider fissures and more rounded cusps. Enamel and dentine are also thinner due to altered matrix formation caused by impaired protein synthesis. However, it is unlikely that these actions of fluoride are of any great clinical significance and may only have a slight effect on the incidence of pit and fissure caries.

Fluoride and plaque

Fluoride is an enzyme inhibitor and can have a significant effect on plaque metabolism. Furthermore, it is concentrated in bacterial plaque (over 100-fold when compared to saliva) and this facilitates enzyme inhibition in the plaque matrix. These high concentrations of fluoride are only possible because it binds to the plaque bacteria, the protein and polysaccharide matrix of plaque, and the tooth surface.

The Embden–Meyerhof pathway is the main mechanism of

acid production in plaque. This pathway involves the enzyme enolase, which converts phosphoglyceric acid to phospho-enolpyruvic acid. Fluoride ions inhibit enolase, so phospho-glyceric acid accumulates within plaque and later products such as phosphoenolpyruvic acid and lactic acid—implicated in the demineralization of enamel—are not formed.

Pharmacokinetics of fluoride

Fluoride is passively absorbed from the stomach, stored in skeletal tissue, and the excess is excreted via the kidney, sweat, and faeces. The placenta acts as a partial barrier to fluoride, which depends upon the maternal concentration of fluoride. The efficacy of therapeutic fluoride given to the pregnant mother to enhance the baby's teeth is uncertain. Most countries permit, but do not encourage, prenatal fluoride supplementation.

Fluoride administration

Fluoride can be administered systemically via the water supply, tablets, drops, milk, and salt, or topically in the form of solution, gels, varnishes, and toothpastes, or incorporated into restorative materials.

Systemic administration

WATER FLUORIDATION

Early epidemiological studies in areas with natural fluoride in the water supply clearly demonstrated its anticaries effect. In areas with no natural fluoride in the water supply, the addition of fluoride up to 1 part per million (p.p.m.) causes a significant reduction in the incidence of caries. This has the additional benefit of serving a large population at minimal cost.

When water fluoridation schemes are withdrawn, as occurred in Scotland in 1983, the dental health of children deteriorated.

FLUORIDE TABLETS AND DROPS

These are either the sodium or calcium salt, or the acidulated phosphate salt of fluoride. Current daily recommended dosage in the UK is as follows: 0.25 mg for those aged 6 months to 2 years, 0.5 mg for those aged 2–4, and 1.0 mg for those over 4 years. The dose of fluoride tablets or drops will need to be modified according to the concentration of fluoride in the drinking water. If the local water concentration is greater than 0.7 p.p.m., then no additional fluoride supplements should be given to the child since this will increase the risk of fluorosis. The effectiveness of fluoride tablets depends upon the age at which the child commences treatment; the earlier, the greater the percentage reduction in caries. Overall results from several studies indicate that this form of fluoride therapy produces a 40–80% reduction in the incidence of dental caries. Compliance with home-administered fluoride is poor, but school-based programmes might overcome this problem.

FLUORIDIZED MILK

Milk drinks are popular with young children, and would thus seem to be a good vehicle for delivering fluoride. Furthermore,

absorption of fluoride is not affected by the Ca^{2+} present in milk. There have been few studies to support the effectiveness of fluoridized milk in controlling dental caries, and other methods of fluoride delivery may be more acceptable. The amount of fluoride added to milk, in the form of sodium fluoride, is the equivalent of receiving 1 mg per day.

In warm climates, fluoridated fruit juices may be a practical alternative to fluoridated milk.

FLUORIDATED TABLE SALT

Salt is another excellent vehicle for dispensing fluoride. Concentrations of fluoride in salt vary between 200 and $350 \, mg \, kg^{-1}$ salt. Although widely used in the rest of Europe, there have been few studies into the efficacy of this fluoride delivery method for controlling dental caries. However, what findings there are suggest that it is effective, but not as good as fluoride in the water supply.

Topical administration

FLUORIDE SOLUTIONS

These can be classified into two types: an aqueous solution of sodium or stannous fluoride; and the acidulated phosphate fluoride system.

SODIUM AND STANNOUS FLUORIDE Sodium fluoride was the first topically applied fluoride solution. In clinical use, a freshly prepared 2% solution is applied to dried teeth for 3 minutes, usually three to four times per year. The long-term efficacy (over 4 years or more) of this fluoride application method is uncertain, but short-term results indicate a caries reduction of between 30 and 50%.

Stannous fluoride is more effective than sodium fluoride at reducing enamel dissolution by acid. In clinical practice, an 8–10% stannous fluoride solution is used, but it is unstable and each new application requires a fresh solution. A further disadvantage of stannous fluoride is the staining of teeth, especially at the margins of restorations.

ACIDULATED PHOSPHATE FLUORIDE This system was developed after studies had shown that the uptake of fluoride by enamel was enhanced by reducing the pH of the solution. Clinical trials have demonstrated that a 1.23% acidulated phosphofluoride solution brings about a 20–40% reduction in caries activity. The solution has to be applied to dried teeth for 4 minutes, usually twice a year. Application can present a problem with young children who have a copious salivary flow. Acidulated fluoride solutions cause nausea and sometimes vomiting if swallowed. This problem can be overcome by applying the solution in the form of a gel or by using a tray that fits closely to the teeth.

FLUORIDE VARNISHES

Fluoride applied in the form of a varnish allows a longer contact between the enamel surface and fluoride ions. Proprietary fluoride varnishes include Duraphat, Elmex, Protector, and Epoxylite 9070, and are usually applied twice a year. The effectiveness of this mode of applying fluoride is uncertain, and claims of caries reduction show marked variation between studies. Evidence suggests that this method of applying fluoride is the least effective.

FLUORIDE TOOTHPASTES

Fluoride in toothpaste is the commonest and easiest method of applying topical fluoride. Nearly all brands of toothpaste sold in the UK contain fluoride, usually as sodium monofluorophosphate. Regular use of a fluoride toothpaste causes a 30% reduction in the incidence of dental caries.

Research into the effectiveness of fluoride toothpaste has been directed along the following lines:

(1) changing the fluoride concentration from a yield of 1000 p.p.m. to 2500 p.p.m.;

(2) combining more than one fluoride agent, i.e. sodium fluoride and sodium monofluorophosphate; and

(3) adding other active agents such as calcium glycerophosphate, soluble pyrophosphate, and the co-polymer polyvinylmethylether maleic acid (PVM/MA).

PVM/MA is reported to enhance the retention of sodium fluoride.

MOUTH RINSES

A sodium fluoride solution at a concentration of 100–200 p.p.m. is widely used as a mouth rinse. The efficacy of this method of applying fluoride depends upon the frequency of rinsing, usually recommended once a week. Supervision at schools offers an ideal opportunity to carry out such a programme.

Unwanted effects of fluoride therapy

These can be classified as effects on skeletal tissue and effects on the teeth.

Effects on skeletal tissue

A high regular intake of fluoride (greater than 8 p.p.m.) can lead to skeletal fluorosis—characterized by an increase in bone density, especially in the lumbar spine and pelvis, and an increase in the thickness of long bones. In severe cases, calcification of the ligaments occurs. Histologically, skeletal fluorosis resembles osteomalacia, but biochemically the plasma calcium and phosphate levels are normal. The strength of fluorotic bone is poor, and spontaneous fractures are common.

There have been three possible mechanisms suggested to account for the action of fluoride on skeletal tissues:

(1) an increase in the number of osteoblasts and their activity;

(2) a fluoride-induced delay in bone demineralization; and

(3) an increase in the resorption of endosteal surfaces.

Effect on teeth

Excessive fluoride intake will cause dental fluorosis. The clinical appearance can range from white patches in the enamel to severe hypoplasia of the whole tooth. Dental fluorosis can develop if the daily fluoride intake exceeds 2 p.p.m.

Fluorosed enamel contains a higher protein content than normal enamel. This may arise as a result of the following actions:

(1) excessive secretion of proteins or differences in their amino acid composition;

(2) inhibition of the proteolysis of enamel proteins (amelogenins);

(3) reduction in the removal of amelogenins, which in turn would prevent normal mineralization.

Fluoride and cancer

There have been some data from the USA suggesting that water fluoridation was associated with an increased prevalence of cancer deaths. This has been contested, and further analysis of the American data has shown that the link between water fluoridation and cancer was not justified.

Fluoride overdose

The various fluoride preparations are readily available to the public and overdose can arise, especially in young children consuming excess tablets or drops. The lethal dose of sodium fluoride is 5 mg kg^{-1} body weight.

Signs and symptoms of acute fluoride poisoning are nausea, vomiting, and gastrointestinal pain. These are followed by muscle weakness, spasms, and tetany, since fluoride combines with blood calcium ions. An important site of toxic reaction is the stomach where fluoride reacts with the hydrochloric acid to form the highly irritant compound hydrofluoric acid, which can cause erosion of the gastric mucosa.

Treatment of fluoride overdose is by gastric lavage. In severe cases, the patient also requires the intravenous infusion of a 10% calcium gluconate solution to precipitate the excess fluoride and restore blood calcium levels.

Sugar-based medicines and dental caries

There has been considerable interest over the past few years in the relationship between dental caries in children and the chronic consumption of liquid formulations of drugs with a high sugar content. Sugar has been a constituent of paediatric medicines for many years, since it is cheap, makes the medicine more palatable, and acts as a preservative bulking agent.

Several studies have shown a link between the long-term administration of sugar-based medicines and dental caries. People with physical or learning disabilities or cardiac, respiratory, or kidney disease are at particular risk.

Sugar substitutes such as mannitol, sorbitol, and xylitol are virtually non-cariogenic, but the pharmaceutical industry has been reluctant to omit sugar from medicines for children. This situation is slowly improving and more and more sugar-free alternatives are becoming available. It is important that both dental and medical practitioners are aware of the problems associated with sugar-based medicines in chronically sick children. Where possible, alternatives should be prescribed.

Periodontal disease

The periodontal diseases are caused by bacterial plaque, although systemic disorders can modify the response of the periodontal tissues to bacterial toxins and enzymes. In essence, the diseases are a result of an interaction between the bacterial products and the host's immune and inflammatory responses. Periodontal disease is broadly classified as: gingivitis, where inflammatory changes are confined to the gingival connective tissue; and periodontitis, which involves loss of connective-tissue attachment to the root surface, apical migration of the junctional epithelium, pocket formation, and/or gingival recession and bone loss. The common form of periodontitis is the chronic adult type. Rarer types include prepubertal, juvenile, and rapidly progressive periodontitis. These conditions are now collectively referred to as early-onset periodontitis. A further form of periodontitis is now recognized and known as refractory periodontitis. As the name suggests, this type of periodontal disease does not respond to conventional treatment and appears to be associated with a specific microflora. Refractory periodontitis can only be diagnosed retrospectively and frequently requires systemic antimicrobial therapy to resolve the condition.

Pathogenesis of periodontal disease

There is overwhelming evidence that periodontal diseases are caused by bacterial plaque. However, several additional mechanisms may contribute towards the degradation of the gingival and periodontal connective tissues.

Activation of the host's immune cells (macrophages as well as T and B lymphocytes) by plaque toxins and enzymes can cause the release of a variety of cellular and biochemical mediators. Some of these mediators have the potential to cause degradation of gingival and periodontal connective tissue and alveolar bone resorption. The exact mechanism of plaque-induced periodontal destruction is uncertain. Interleukin-1, prostaglandins of the E series, and tumour necrosis factor released from macrophages and polymorphonuclear leucocytes can all modulate tissue destruction. In turn, these mediators activate metalloproteinases (i.e. collagenases) that degrade the connective tissue matrix.

Longitudinal studies in adults have shown that periodontal destruction is episodic and is characterized by bursts of activity, followed by periods of quiescence. Such bursts may be synchronous or occur at random times. There is uncertainty over the site specificity of such bursts and the initiating factors. Certain bacterial species, the so-called periodontopathogens (see later), are associated with active disease. *In-vitro* studies confirm the pathogenicity of these bacteria and the ability of their enzymes and toxins to destroy the periodontal tissues. However, it remains to be confirmed whether these bacteria are the initiators or the consequence of the burst of activity. It could also be argued that bursts are related to a localized failure of the host's response. An obvious cause for such a failure is a change in antigenic challenge arising from the subgingival microflora.

The pathogenesis of periodontal disease remains an area of intensive research. Perhaps the only fact that can be stated with confidence is that the disease is caused by the accumulation of bacterial plaque. The subsequent interaction between bacteria and their products with the host's immune and inflammatory responses probably leads to tissue breakdown and the progression of the disease. A thorough understanding of the disease process is mandatory since this will lead to more appropriate methods of control.

Dental plaque

Dental plaque is a bacterial aggregation on the teeth or other solid structures in the mouth. It is an uncalcified, soft material which is so tenaciously adherent to the tooth surface that it resists removal by salivary flow or a gentle spray of water across its surface. The dense bacterial masses are enveloped in a matrix that originates either from the host (salivary glycoproteins), or from the bacteria themselves (extracellular polysaccharides).

Composition of plaque

Approximately 70% of the volume of plaque is bacterial cells. The rest is made up of extracellular polysaccharides that act as a matrix for the cellular component. The carbohydrates include dextran, which is a predominantly α1–6-linked variety of glucan (a polymer of glucose), and mutan, which is a predominantly α1–3-linked glucan. These glucans are produced primarily by *Streptococcus mutans* and *Actinomyces* species during initial plaque formation.

In addition to the bacteria and matrix, plaque contains small numbers of epithelial cells and white blood cells probably derived from crevicular fluid.

The development of plaque

If a tooth surface is vigorously cleaned of all soft deposits, then a structure, distinct from dental plaque, begins to form within only a few minutes. This so-called pellicle is an amorphous layer, 0.1–1 μm thick, composed of salivary glycoproteins that have become selectively adsorbed on to the tooth surface. The adsorbed molecules of glycoprotein may penetrate the enamel surface and this can lead to difficulty in completely removing the pellicle (and subsequently plaque) from the tooth by normal brushing. The molecules of glycoprotein eventually undergo a biochemical transformation to produce a highly insoluble surface coating that is the base on which supragingival plaque formation occurs.

The first bacteria to colonize the pellicle are *Streptococcus sanguis* and *Streptococcus mitis*, followed by *Actinomyces* species. As the growth of plaque continues, the number of bacteria increases rapidly by further adsorption from saliva and by multiplication of the bacteria which have already colonized the teeth. There are concurrent qualitative changes in its bacterial composition. The proportions of Gram-negative cocci and Gram-positive and Gram-negative rods increase gradually and the percentage of Gram-positive cocci is reduced.

Filamentous and fusiform bacteria are seen in 2–4-day-old plaque and they eventually grow in to replace the coccal forms. Maturation of the plaque matrix increases the proportion of Gram-negative organisms to Gram-positive organisms, and the respiratory characteristics of the bacteria become predominantly anaerobic. These changes in metabolism usually coincide with the clinical features of gingivitis.

When inflammation develops in the marginal gingival tissues, they become oedematous and swollen. The primary source of nutrients of the microbial flora changes as the increased flow of crevicular fluid continuously bathes the subgingival bacteria. The most apical portion of the previously supragingival plaque becomes protected in the clinically deepened gingival sulcus, and may now be regarded as a subgingival deposit. The growth of subgingival plaque is enhanced by the downgrowth of bacteria into pockets from the supragingival location. This occurs partly by the movement of discrete colonies of pioneer bacteria by chemotaxis of motile forms, and predominantly by the migration of a continuous layer of plaque. The environment changes to further enhance the colonization and growth of Gram-negative anaerobic bacteria. The subgingival plaque is protected from the natural cleansing mechanisms of the oral cavity. A more loosely adherent bacterial layer can exist on the surface of the plaque mass.

The contents of a periodontal pocket are now rightly referred to as a biofilm—a biologically derived fluid that contains a suspension of either cells or bacteria. The major constituents of this biofilm are the Gram-negative bacteria of the subgingival plaque. The fluid mass of the biofilm is derived from gingival crevicular fluid. Other constituents include immunoglobulins, PMNs and other white blood cells, epithelial squames, and various proteolytic enzymes. The subgingival biofilm has a dynamic composition and its physicochemical properties have an important influence on local drug delivery that is sometimes used in the treatment of periodontal diseases.

Mechanisms of bacterial adherence to tooth surfaces

The bacteria that initially colonize the pellicle or tooth surface must possess a specific mechanism by which they adhere either to glycoprotein or to the hydroxyapatite. Many oral bacteria have ultrastructural appendages or fimbrae radiating from their surface. It is likely that such structures are important in the process of early bacterial attachment. The fimbrae have distinct lectin-like properties, which may be able to recognize specific sites within the pellicle or hydroxyapatite. One example is the ability of *Streptococcus mutans* to recognize β-galactoside residues of salivary glycoproteins in the pellicle. Similarly, bacterial co-aggregation can occur involving surface lectins on one micro-organism and carbohydrate-containing receptors on another cell. Such mechanisms would be responsible for the observation that several different types of bacteria are seen on a tooth surface after only a few days of abstaining from tooth cleaning.

Another mechanism of bacterial adherence involves the enzyme glycosyl transferase (GTF), which converts dietary sucrose to glucan polymers. GTF binds strongly to saliva-coated hydroxyapatite and may be able to bind bacteria directly to the surface. Alternatively, indirect mechanisms may involve GTF interactions with α1–3 glucose chains produced by the adsorbed enzyme on cell surfaces. This would explain why bacterial adherence to tooth surfaces is not improved by premade or commercially available glucans, as the active GTF enzyme is only available during bacterial production of glucan molecules.

Other factors such as electrostatic or electrodynamic forces can influence bacterial–tooth and bacterial–bacterial adherence, but evidence suggests it is the lectin–carbohydrate interaction that is of primary importance for bacterial adhesion to the tooth surface and the subsequent development of plaque.

The management of periodontal diseases

Periodontal diseases can be prevented by either inhibiting the formation of plaque on the tooth surface, or by completely removing plaque before inflammatory changes occur in the periodontal tissues. Complete plaque removal by mechanical means may be possible in well-motivated individuals, but most people leave plaque on some part of the tooth surface after brushing. It can be argued, of course, that a completely plaque-free dentition and absolute periodontal health are not just unattainable, but are unnecessary for many of the population. However, in certain types of particularly destructive forms of periodontal disease (for example in the early-onset periodontal conditions), even very thin, undetectable films of plaque may predispose to excessive periodontal destruction in a short period. In such cases, high standards of plaque control are essential if tooth loss in later life is to be avoided. Furthermore, certain physically or mentally handicapped patients are unable either to clean their teeth effectively or to attend a dentist regularly. These patients may also suffer from extensive periodontal disease.

A need exists for means of plaque control as adjuncts or alternatives to the time-honoured mechanical methods (Tables 12.1 and 12.2). There has been considerable research into developing plaque inhibitory agents and anticalculus agents that can be used in the management of periodontal disease. In addition, the role of bacterial plaque in the pathogenesis of periodontal disease is well established, and there is increasing evidence that specific bacteria may be more directly involved in the aetiology of the early-onset periodontal conditions (Table 12.3). Thus the development of specific antimicrobial agents directed towards such bacteria is an important advance in the management of this type of periodontal disease.

Prostaglandins of the E series are important mediators of the tissue destruction and bone loss seen in periodontal disease. Various studies have shown that non-steroidal anti-inflammatory

drugs (NSAIDs) may help stop bone loss and connective tissue breakdown (see later).

Properties and aims of antiplaque agents

The principles of chemical plaque control are based on certain criteria. Chemical agents should inhibit the microbial colonization of tooth surfaces and prevent the subsequent development of plaque. They should also eliminate or reduce the pathogenicity of already existing plaques, and prevent calculus formation.

A large number of compounds, including enzyme preparations, antibiotics, antiseptics, and surface-active substances, have been evaluated as antiplaque agents (see Table 12.1). The ideal properties of an antiplaque agent are listed in Table 12.2 above. No substance currently fulfils all these criteria.

First- and second generation agents

Antiplaque compounds have been categorized primarily according to their antimicrobial efficacy and relative substantivity. The term substantivity refers to the ability of a compound to be adsorbed on to a surface (or binding site) and then subsequently released from that surface over a period of time. When the compound is bound, it is in an inactive form.

First-generation compounds include antibiotics, phenols, quaternary ammonium compounds, and sanguinarine. They can reduce plaque scores by about 20–50%, and their efficacy is limited by their poor retention in the oral cavity.

Second-generation agents are more effectively retained by oral tissues and their slow-release properties reduce plaque scores by 70–90%. The bisbiguanides are examples. Using first-generation agents 4–6 times daily produces a similar effect to using the second-generation compounds once or twice a day.

Enzymes

Various enzymes have been used as antiplaque agents (see Table 12.1), on the basis of the theory that they would break down the matrix of already formed plaque and calculus. Furthermore, it was supposed that certain proteolytic enzymes would be bactericidal

---

Table 12.1 Classification of antiplaque agents

Cationic surfactants
Bisbiguanides, e.g. chlorhexidine digluconate, alexidine
Quaternary ammonium compounds, e.g. cetylpyridinium chloride,
    benzathonium chloride, benzalkonium chloride, domiphen bromide
Pyrimidine derivatives, e.g. hexetidine
Bispyridine derivatives, e.g. octenidine hydrochloride

Phenolic compounds
Listerine (thymol 0.06%, eucalyptol 0.09%, methyl salicylate 0.06%,
    methanol 0.04%)
Triclosan

Herbal extracts
Sanguinarine

Heavy metal salts
Zinc chloride and citrate
Stannous fluoride
Copper sulfate

Enzymes
Mucinase
Mutanase
Dextranase
Amyloglucosidase/glucose oxidase

Anionic surfactants
Aminoalcohols, e.g. octapinol, decapinol
Plax
Sodium dodecyl sulfate
Sodium lauryl sulfate

Table 12.2 Ideal properties of antiplaque agents

1.	Eliminate pathogenic bacteria only
2.	Prevent the development of resistant bacteria
3.	Exhibit substantivity
4.	Be safe to the oral tissues at the concentrations and dosages recommended
5.	Significantly reduce plaque and gingivitis
6.	Inhibit the calcification of plaque to calculus
7.	Not stain teeth or alter taste
8.	Have no adverse effects on the teeth or dental materials
9.	Be easy to use
10.	Be inexpensive

Based on Bral and Brownstein 1988.

Table 12.3 Pathogens which have been associated with different forms of periodontal disease

Disease	Associated micro-organisms
Localized juvenile periodontitis	*Actinobacillus actinomycetemcomitans*, *Prevotella intermedia*, *Capnocytophaga* spp., *Eikenella corrodens*, *Fusobacterium* spp., *Peptostreptococcus micros*, *Selenomonas* spp. Spirochaetes (*Treponema* spp.)
Rapidly progressive periodontitis	*Actinobacillus actinomycetemcomitans*, *Prevotella intermedia*,
(Early-onset/ generalized juvenile periodontitis)	*Eubacterium* spp., *Fusobacterium* spp., *Peptostreptococcus micros*, *Selenomonas*, Spirochaetes (*Treponema* spp.), *Wolinella recta*
Adult periodontitis	*Actinobacillus actinomycetemcomitans*, *Bacteroides*, *forsythus*, *Eikenella corrodens*, *Fusobacterium* spp., *Peptostreptococcus micros.*, *Selenomonas*, Spirochaetes (*Treponema* spp.), *Wolinella recta* *Prevotella intermedia*
Refractory periodontitis	*Actinobacillus actinomysetemcomitans*, *Porphyromonas gingivalis*, *intermedius*, and *forsythus*, *Eikenella corrodens*, *Fusobacterium* spp., *Peptostreptococcus micros*, Spirochaetes (*Trepenoma* spp.), *Wolinella recta*, *Candida* spp.
Periodontal abscess	*Porphyromonas gingivalis* and *Prevotella intermedia*, *Peptostreptococcus micros*, *Staphylococcus* spp., *Candida* spp.
Acute necrotizing ulcerative gingivitis (ANUG)	*Porphyromonas gingivalis* and *Prevotella intermedia*, Spirochaetes (*Treponema* spp.)

After Slots and Rams 1991

to plaque organisms and so act as 'disinfectants' when applied topically in the oral cavity.

Enzymes that have been used to destroy plaque include mucinases, extracts from dried pancreas (containing trypsin, chymotrypsin, carboxypeptidase, amylase, lipase, and nuclease), dextranase, and mutanase. These have been incorporated into chewing gum and toothpastes. However, although *in-vitro* findings showed promise, clinical trials produced indifferent results and a high incidence of unwanted effects. These enzymes are thus of little value in the control of periodontal disease.

A more effective enzymatic system for reducing plaque growth is based upon the production of an intrinsic salivary inhibitor by a series of humoral factors and biochemical pathways. This system is known as the lactoperoxidase–hypothiocyanite system, and is the basis for the pharmacodynamics of the commercially available dentifrice Zendium (Oral-B Laboratories).

Certain oral bacteria are known to produce hydrogen peroxide by the oxidation of the glycolytic enzyme $NADH_2$ oxidase. Normally, hydrogen peroxide is used to oxidize another $NADH_2$ molecule, or is inactivated by the enzyme catalase. However, when the level of hydrogen peroxide is increased it assists lactoperoxidase in the oxidation of thiocyanate to produce the hypothiocyanite ion ($OSCN^-$), which is the hypothalite of thiocyanogen. Hypothiocyanite ions interfere with cellular oxidation–reduction mechanisms, by upsetting the $NADH_2$–$NADPH_2$ balance. Lactoperoxidase and thiocyanate are essential to this reaction, and are both normal constituents of saliva.

The optimal level of hydrogen peroxide required for hypothiocyanite production is achieved by a further enzyme system involving amyloglucosidase and glucose oxidase. Both are constituents of Zendium toothpaste (Fig. 12.1).

In clinical trials, this toothpaste has been shown to inhibit plaque formation when compared with either placebo pastes containing no enzymes or other commercially available pastes.

Antibiotics as antiplaque agents

The bacterial nature of dental plaque and its primary role in the aetiology of periodontal disease has stimulated a considerable amount of research into the use of antibiotics to try to control the disease. Agents that have been evaluated include penicillin, vancomycin, erythromycin, and kanamycin. In all instances the drugs are used topically. However, since the mid-1970s, interest in this approach has waned. The potential problems of bacterial resistance, disturbances in the gut and oral flora, and the increased risks of hypersensitivity reactions are of more clinical significance than the antiplaque effects of these drugs. Furthermore, there are now many alternative antiplaque agents available for use instead of antibiotics.

Although the topical use of antibiotics has now ceased, the systemic use of these drugs is of benefit in the management of certain types of periodontal disease. This application is discussed later.

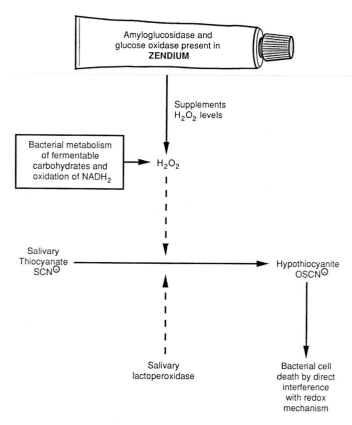

Fig. 12.1 Mechanism of Zendium in the lactoperoxidase–hypothiocyanite system.

Phenols

The phenols are a group of antiseptic compounds that have been used in medicine for over 100 years. Preparations of phenols and their derivatives have had widespread application as disinfectants and antiseptics (see Chapter 10). Most phenols exert a non-specific antibacterial action, which is dependent on the ability of the non-ionized form of the drug to penetrate the lipid component of the cell walls of Gram-negative organisms. The resulting structural damage affects the permeability control of the organisms. In addition, several metabolic processes that depend on enzymes in the cell membrane are also disrupted. Phenolic compounds also exhibit anti-inflammatory properties. This may result from their ability to inhibit neutrophil chemotaxis, neutrophil superoxide ion generation, and prostaglandin synthetase production.

Phenols have been incorporated into mouthrinses for topical use as antimicrobial/antiseptic agents to inhibit plaque formation. Listerine is an over-the-counter phenol preparation that contains thymol (0.06%), eucalyptol (0.09%), methyl salicylate (0.06%), and methanol (0.04%), i.e. in a hydroalcoholic vehicle.

The antiplaque activities of Listerine are well established. When compared to the vehicle or to water alone, Listerine was found to reduce both the wet and dry weights of plaque by more than 50% after 9 months' use. It also reduced the protein content

of plaque by about 60% and its toxicity by 75%. This suggests that the active agents in Listerine affect the pathogenicity of plaque by reducing its overall endotoxin activity.

TRICLOSAN

This compound is a non-ionic bisphenol with a broad spectrum of activity against both Gram-positive and Gram-negative bacteria as well as fungi. The compound exhibits poor substantivity and can be formulated into a mouthrinse or a toothpaste. The mechanism of Triclosan's antibacterial effect is uncertain. Due to its hydrophobic and lipophilic nature, it adsorbs on to the lipid portion of the bacterial cell membrane. At low concentrations, Triclosan interferes with vital transport mechanisms within the bacteria. When used alone, Triclosan possesses a moderate plaque-inhibitory effect. This activity is enhanced when the compound is combined with zinc citrate or incorporated into a co-polymer of methoxyethylene and maleic acid. These combinations are used extensively in proprietary toothpastes. The co-polymer increases the substantivity of Triclosan and acts as a reservoir. The combination of Triclosan and zinc citrate does not appear to be associated with the development of resistant strains, and long-term use has no adverse effects on the oral flora. No other unwanted effects have been have been reported with the long-term use of these combinations.

The clinical benefits of Triclosan and zinc citrate are small, but measurable. The impact of these compounds on the periodontal health of the population remains to be determined.

Key facts
Phenols

- Phenols exert their antibacterial actions by penetrating the lipid component of bacterial cell walls.

- In addition to their antibacterial actions, phenols also exhibit anti-inflammatory properties by inhibiting neutrophil chemotaxis, superoxide ion generation, and prostaglandin synthesis.

- Phenols are more effective against Gram-negative bacteria, and hence seem to be more efficacious in long-standing periodontal disease.

- Commercial preparations of phenols include Listerine and Triclosan.

- The plaque inhibitory actions of Triclosan are enhanced by combining the product with either a co-polymer or zinc citrate.

Quaternary ammonium compounds

Quaternary ammonium compounds are cationic antiseptics and surface-acting agents. The basic chemical structure is a central nitrogen atom linked to four alkyl groups by covalent bonds. An electrovalent bond connects the anion to the nitrogen atom (Fig. 12.2). The molecules have a net positive charge and react with the negatively charged, cell-membrane phosphates, disrupting its structure and so increasing permeability. Quaternary ammonium compounds tend to be more effective against Gram-positive than Gram-negative micro-organisms. This may suggest that these agents would be more beneficial as antiplaque agents when used against early developing plaque, which contains predominantly Gram-positive bacteria. Indeed, these compounds are used extensively as prebrushing rinses, that is they are rinsed around the mouth before toothbrushing. Prebrushing rinses are thought to disrupt plaque and thus facilitate its removal by mechanical means. Quaternary ammonium compounds used as antiplaque agents include benzethonium chloride, benzalkonium chloride, and cetylpyridinium chloride.

Many clinical trials support the effectiveness of quaternary ammonium compounds as antiplaque agents. However, comparison with chlorhexidine preparations (see later), suggests their clinical usefulness is somewhat limited. The oral retention of quaternary ammonium compounds is about twice that of chlorhexidine,

when assessed by their release into water rinses. However, the absorption of quaternary ammonium compounds into saliva is much more rapid. Factors in saliva could influence the relative absorption of these compounds. *In vitro*, calcium ions displace cetylpyridinium chloride from carboxyl groups at lower concentrations than those needed to displace chlorhexidine. Furthermore, the doubly charged chlorhexidine may bond more effectively to oral sites than the monovalent quaternary ammonium compounds. Such differences in physicochemical properties may account for the poorer efficacy of these compounds.

Quaternary ammonium compounds are not without unwanted effects and these include a burning sensation of the oral mucosa, brownish discoloration of the teeth and tongue, and a recurrent aphthous-type ulceration.

Key facts
Quaternary ammonium compounds (QACs)

- QACs are cationic antiseptics that are more effective against Gram +ve than Gram −ve bacteria.
- Examples include chloride salts of benzethonium, benzalkonium, and cetylpyridinium.
- Unwanted effects include a burning sensation of the oral mucosa, discoloration, and an increased susceptibility to aphthous-type ulceration.

Bisbiguanides

The bisbiguanide compounds, which include chlorhexidine gluconate and alexidine, are the most effective antiplaque agents currently in use. Bisbiguanides are the primary second-generation antiplaque agents and exhibit considerable substantivity, and they also have very broad antibacterial properties.

CHLORHEXIDINE DIGLUCONATE
Chlorhexidine is a cationic chlorophenyl bisbiguanide (Fig. 12.2) with outstanding bacteriostatic properties. It was synthesized by ICI in 1954 after extensive investigations of the biological properties of polydiguanide compounds.

Chlorhexidine is a well-tolerated and long-lasting antiseptic which is not neutralized by soaps, body fluids, or other organic compounds. Other medical uses of chlorhexidine are discussed in Chapter 10. Its application as an antiplaque agent was first proposed in 1969, and it is now available as a 0.2% or 0.12% aqueous solution, as a toothpaste gel (0.5–1%), and a local delivery device (a gelatin chip—the Periochip) for placement into periodontal pockets after root surface debridement.

PHARMACOKINETICS OF CHLORHEXIDINE When chlorhexidine is used as an antiplaque mouthrinse, its mode of action is purely topical. The drug does not penetrate through oral epithelium, and if some solution is inadvertently swallowed, the drug binds to the

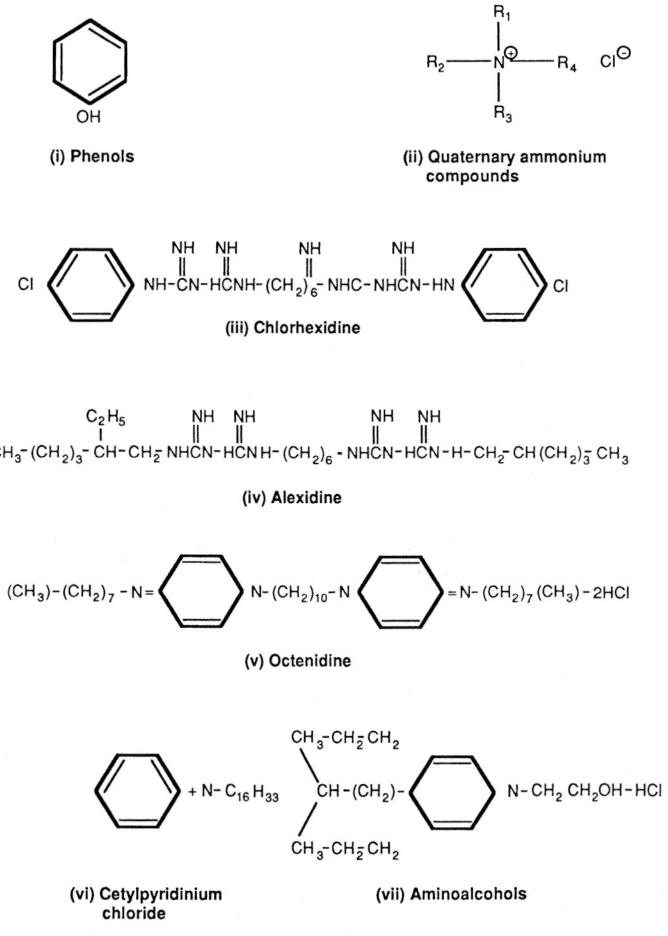

Fig. 12.2 Structures of antiplaque agents.

mucosal surfaces of the alimentary tract. These cells are desquamated and together with any unbound chlorhexidine are excreted in the faeces. The small amount of chlorhexidine that may be absorbed is metabolized in the liver.

BACTERICIDAL ACTION OF CHLORHEXIDINE The action of chlorhexidine in killing bacterial cells depends initially on the drug having access to the cell walls. This is facilitated by electrostatic forces between the negatively charged cells and the net positively charged, chlorhexidine molecules. Having gained access to the cell membrane, chlorhexidine disorientates its lipoprotein structure, destroying the osmotic barrier of the bacteria. Cell permeability increases and intracellular components such as potassium ions leak through the damaged membrane.

A secondary action of chlorhexidine is to cause intracellular coagulation, which effectively slows down the rate of cell-content leakage. This cytoplasmic coagulation is responsible for the bactericidal effect of chlorhexidine and is directly dependent on the concentration of the drug.

EFFECT OF CHLORHEXIDINE ON ORAL BACTERIA The short-term use of chlorhexidine causes a striking reduction in the number of oral micro-organisms. In the absence of other oral hygiene measures, chlorhexidine has been shown to reduce the number of bacteria in saliva by 85% after only 24 hours. A maximum reduction of 95% occurred after around 5 days. After this the numbers of bacteria gradually increased, but an overall reduction of 70–80% was maintained at 40 days. Cessation of chlorhexidine mouth rinses results in a rapid return of normal salivary bacterial counts.

Some bacteria are more susceptible to chlorhexidine than others. *Staphylococci* spp., *Strep. mutans*, *Strep. salivaris*, and *E. coli* are susceptible to chlorhexidine at a low minimum inhibitory concentration (MIC), whereas certain Gram-negative cocci resembling *Veillonella* spp. are the least susceptible.

The long-term use of any antimicrobial agent can be associated with increased microbial resistance and reduced sensitivity. Long-term studies of chlorhexidine are inconclusive in this respect. It has been suggested that the prolonged use of chlorhexidine tends to be more bactericidal towards strains of the more resistant bacteria in the oral flora. In effect, therefore, there is no change from susceptible organisms to resistant ones, so the effect on long-term plaque inhibition is negligible.

RETENTION OF CHLORHEXIDINE IN THE ORAL CAVITY Chlorhexidine is the most effective antiplaque agent. This is primarily due, not to its ability to destroy micro-organisms, but rather to the specific pharmacodynamics associated with the retention of the drug in the oral cavity.

After rinsing with 10 mL of a 0.2% aqueous solution of chlorhexidine for 1 minute, approximately 30% of the drug is retained in the mouth. The drug is believed to bind electrostatically to acidic protein groups such as phosphates, sulfates, and carboxyl ions which exist extensively on the oral tissues. Calcium ions in saliva are able to displace chlorhexidine from the carboxyl

binding sites. This displacement is comparatively slow and may help to explain the prolonged bacteriostatic effect of the drug in the mouth. Further, chlorhexidine can displace calcium ions that are bound to the sulfated glycoproteins of bacterial plaque. These findings suggest three possible mechanisms for the inhibition of plaque by chlorhexidine:

1. The blocking of acidic groups of salivary glycoproteins will reduce their adsorption to hydroxyapatite and the formation of the acquired pellicle.

2. The ability of bacteria to bind to tooth surfaces may be reduced by the adsorption of chlorhexidine to the extracellular polysaccharides of bacterial capsules or glycocalyces.

3. Chlorhexidine may compete with calcium ions for acidic agglutination factors in plaque.

Laboratory studies have also shown that chlorhexidine can bind to hydroxyapatite. However, the conditions under which this occurs are not usually comparable to those *in vivo*. Thus, it is now considered that the affinity of chlorhexidine for the acidic proteins in pellicle, plaque, and calculus and on the surfaces of bacteria and oral mucosa is of greater clinical significance than its affinity for hydroxyapatite.

FACTORS AFFECTING THE RETENTION OF CHLORHEXIDINE A number of factors have been demonstrated to affect the binding capacity and plaque-inhibitory effect of chlorhexidine *in vivo*. After an oral rinse, the concentration of the drug in saliva falls rapidly and logarithmically during the first 4–8 hours, although the drug may still be detected after 24 hours. The proportion of chlorhexidine retained depends directly on both the concentration and the volume of the rinse solution. Approximately half of the chlorhexidine retained during a 60-second rinse will have bonded to receptor molecules in the first 15 seconds.

The pH in the oral cavity significantly affects both the binding and the release of chlorhexidine. Reducing the pH of the rinsing solution from 6.4 to 3 greatly reduces drug retention. The mechanism probably involves a reduction in the available negatively charged receptor sites for chlorhexidine when the environment becomes more acidic. Increasing the pH, however, does not appear to affect retention. Reducing the pH of the oral cavity by using acidic after-rinses also reduces retention of the drug and the subsequent plaque-inhibition. Free calcium ions also reduce the oral binding of chlorhexidine and increase its release from protein binding sites. The mechanism is likely to involve direct competition between the ions and the drug for available carboxyl groups on oral tissues. This finding has an important implication with respect to the use of chlorhexidine mouthrinses and the use of toothpastes. Most proprietary toothpastes contain calcium salts as filler agents. Thus if chlorhexidine is used soon after toothbrushing, there will be a high concentration of calcium ions present in the mouth. This will affect the binding of chlorhexidine and reduce its substantivity. Patients should be advised to use chlorhexidine at least 30 minutes after toothbrushing to avoid an interaction between the calcium ions in toothpaste and the mouthwash.

UNWANTED EFFECTS OF CHLORHEXIDINE Chlorhexidine has been used for 30 years and its unwanted effects are of a local nature. Many patients find its initial taste unpleasant and repeated use often produces a disturbance in taste, which may last for several hours. Occasional cases of desquamative lesions of the oral mucosa and parotid swelling have been reported, but the incidence is low. The main unwanted effect of chlorhexidine mouthwash or gel is a brown staining of the teeth. Three possible mechanisms may all contribute to this problem:

1. *Non-enzymatic browning reactions (Maillard reactions)*: Carbohydrates and amino acids can act as substrates for the Maillard reaction. These food substances undergo a series of condensation and polymerization reactions leading to the formation of brown-pigmented substances known as melanoids. Melanoid production is catalysed by a high pH and chlorhexidine. The glycoprotein of the acquired pellicle covering the tooth surface may serve as a substrate for the Maillard reaction.

2. *Formation of pigmented metal sulfides*: The glycoprotein molecules of the tooth pellicle contain many disulfide bridges. When the glycoprotein is denatured, the disulfide bridges split yielding free sulfydryl groups, which react with ferric or stannous ions in the diet to form brown or yellow metallic sulfides. Chlorhexidine causes denaturation of the pellicle glycoprotein, and this may contribute towards the staining potential.

3. *Reaction between chlorhexidine and factors in the diet*: Many factors may be involved in the reaction between chlorhexidine and constituents of the diet to produce staining. It has been shown that aldehydes and ketones react with chlorhexidine to form coloured products and that these products would attach to a tooth surface. Staining from chlorhexidine is accentuated if there is a heavy consumption of tea, coffee, and red wine, these all contain tannin, which denatures the pellicle glycoprotein. Red wine also contains a high amount of iron.

Regular use of chlorhexidine causes thickening of the pellicle, so providing a larger than usual surface area for stain absorption. The thickened pellicle also predisposes towards supragingival calculus formation and this may counteract the benefit of chlorhexidine.

The efficacy of chlorhexidine appears to be less in the presence of blood. The compound binds to various proteins found in blood and the bound substance is inactive. There are obvious implications with the use of chlorhexidine in the subgingival environment where the tissues are inflamed and blood may be present. The use of chlorhexidine in these circumstances will be more beneficial once the inflammation is brought under control.

In-vitro studies have also shown that chlorhexidine is cytotoxic to gingival fibroblasts and inhibits their ability to bind to surfaces such as dentine. This finding could have an impact upon the healing of periodontal defects after regenerative procedures.

ALEXIDINE AND OTHER BISBIGUANIDES

Alexidine (2-ethylhexylbisbiguanide dihydrochloride) is structurally related to chlorhexidine and has very similar properties. In alexidine, the *p*-chlorophenyl groups of chlorhexidine are replaced by alkyl terminal groups (Fig. 12.2). The antiplaque activity of alexidine has been demonstrated following the use of 0.035% and 0.05% mouthwashes.

A number of other alkyl bisbiguanides, including hexocitidine, heptihexidine, hexidecidine, and hexhexidine, also have activity against oral micro-organisms comparable to that of chlorhexidine. The activity appears to be related to the structure of the molecules. For example, agents with branched terminal alkyl groups are more active against *Actinomyces* spp. than those with unbranched groups. Similarly, increasing the length of the methylene bridge increases the activity against species of *Bacteroides* and *Fusobacterium*.

From a clinical viewpoint, the structure modification of antiplaque agents to optimize their activity against specific bacterial species may prove a valuable field for future research. Such agents will become particularly useful if the precise roles of the peridontopathogens are clearly identified.

Key facts
Bisbiguanides

- Chlorhexidine is the most widely used bisbiguanide antiplaque agent.

- Electrostatic forces attract positively charged chlorhexidine to the negatively charged bacterial cell wall. On contact, chlorhexidine disorientates the lipoprotein structure.

- In addition to chlorhexidine's antibacterial properties, it also inhibits plaque formation by affecting the pellicle, inhibits further bacterial incorporation into the plaque mass, and reduces salivary agglutination factors, which in turn reduce plaque's adherence to tooth surfaces.

- Chlorhexidine is available in a variety of preparations including a mouthwash (0.2% or 0.12% (w/v)), a toothpaste gel (0.5–1%), and a controlled delivery system (Periochip).

- Unwanted effects of chlorhexidine include staining (enhanced by certain food substances), taste disturbances, and occasional parotid swelling.

Bispyridines

Octenidine hydrochloride is the main bispyridine used as an antiplaque agent. Twice-daily rinsing with a 0.1% solution in a glycerol base almost completely inhibits plaque formation. As with chlorhexidine, staining of the teeth and occasional epithelial desquamation are the main unwanted effects associated with octenidine.

Metallic salts

The salts of certain heavy metals can inhibit the growth of dental plaque and calculus formation. Salts of zinc and tin have received most attention and a number of commercial toothpastes now include these compounds in their formulation.

ZINC SALTS

Zinc citrate is the main zinc salt used for its antiplaque and anti-calculus activity. Toothpastes containing up to 4% zinc citrate significantly inhibit plaque growth. The antiplaque activity of zinc salts appears to be a direct inhibitory action against streptococci. These micro-organisms are the first to colonize the tooth surface and are thus important in plaque formation.

TIN SALTS

The ability of tin ions to inhibit plaque formation has been studied, primarily using stannous fluoride mouthrinses. Daily rinsing with a 0.1% stannous fluoride solution significantly reduces bacterial accumulation on the teeth.

The action of stannous ions is mediated through their ability to bind to lipoteichoic acid on the surface of Gram-positive bacteria. The surface net charge of the organism is therefore reversed and the adsorption of the cells on to teeth is consequently reduced. Furthermore, the effectiveness of a stannous fluoride solution in reducing bacterial adhesion is related to the stability of the stannous ions in aqueous solution and the rate at which they are taken up and retained by specific bacteria. The accumulation of tin in bacteria may alter their metabolism and other physicochemical characteristics.

Key facts
Metallic salts

- Salts of zinc (citrate) and tin (fluoride) have been shown to have an inhibitory effect on plaque formation.

- Zinc citrate has a direct inhibitory action against streptococci.

- Stannous fluoride binds to lipoteichoic acid on the bacterial cell wall, which then reduces adsorption on to tooth surfaces.

Herbal extracts

Sanguinarine is the main herbal extract used for its antiplaque activity. It is a benzophenathridine alkaloid derived from the plant *Sanguinaria canadensis*. It is structurally related to the alkaloids found in the plant *Fagara zanthoxyloides*—in Third World countries this plant is chewed as a method for cleaning teeth. Sanguinarine, in its quaternary iminium form, has antimicrobial properties that have led to its introduction as an antiplaque agent. *In-vitro* analysis of minimum inhibitory concentration (MIC) values of sanguinarine has determined that, in the range of 1 to $16\,\mu g\,mL^{-1}$, the drug can inhibit the growth of a wide range of oral bacteria.

In addition to its antimicrobial properties, a further important feature of sanguinarine is its retention in dental plaque when used as a mouthrinse. The levels in plaque can exceed the MIC values for up to 2 hours after rinsing.

Sanguinarine has been incorporated into mouthrinses and toothpastes and 0.03% is the most frequently tested concentration. Few unwanted effects are associated, but many patients find the taste unacceptable.

Surfactants

Surfactants or 'wetting agents' were introduced as an alternative method of plaque inhibition. Agents with low surface tension and lipophilic–hydrophilic properties can interfere with plaque growth by preventing bacterial adhesion to both the pellicle and within the plaque mass. Thus a plaque inhibitory effect occurs without affecting the ecological balance of the oral flora. A number of antimicrobial agents, including chlorhexidine, possess surfactant properties. This section, however, is concerned primarily with products whose effects are mediated mainly through their wetting abilities. Examples include the aminoalcohols and the proprietary mouthwash Plax.

AMINOALCOHOLS

The substituted aminoalcohols have comparatively low antibacterial properties. They also have a lower surface tension than the tooth surface and so the low antimicrobial effect may be compensated by a high local concentration on the enamel surface. Early studies have shown that a 1% octapinol solution causes complete plaque inhibition for between 3 and 12 days. Octapinol also prevented further plaque growth and was able to partly dissolve the plaque that had already formed on teeth. Similar efficacy has also been demonstrated with 1% decapinol.

The unwanted effects of aminoalcohols include a slight local anaesthetic effect on soft tissues, a slightly bitter taste, and light brown staining of the teeth, fortunately this is easily removed with a toothbrush.

PLAX

Plax is a commercial mouthrinse with surfactant properties. The rinse comprises a combination of anionic and ionic surfactants, including sodium lauryl sulfate, polysorbate 20, triclosan 0.3%, and a co-polymer of methoxyethylene and maleic acid. These ingredients act on already formed plaque to loosen and remove the deposits. The manufacturers recommend it is used before daily toothbrushing. It must be emphasized that, although Plax may be a useful adjunct to toothbrushing, it is not a substitute for daily mechanical plaque removal.

Application of antiplaque agents

The efficacy of any antiplaque agent depends not only on its activity but also on the length of contact time between tooth surface and agent. Furthermore, it is essential that the agent gains access to the specific sites on the teeth where the maximum antiplaque effects will be achieved. In health, these sites are primarily interproximally and at the gingival margins. Where there is periodontal disease, subgingival application is required.

The most frequently used modes of application for antiplaque agents are mouthrinses and toothpastes. The main problem with both these methods is the relative short contact time between the active agents and the teeth. Consequently, the well-proven success of chlorhexidine as a plaque inhibitor is related to its substantivity rather than to any unique action upon the oral flora.

Mouthrinses are unable to penetrate subgingivally and so where periodontal pockets exist, direct subgingival irrigation is required. Toothpastes may, to some extent, be applied directly into pockets using a crevicular brushing technique. However, it is doubtful that such methods can satisfactorily introduce antiplaque agents to the bases of deep periodontal pockets.

Some of the plaque inhibitory agents listed in this section are used as prebrushing rinses, that is they are used just before toothbrushing or other mechanical methods of plaque control. The manufacturers of these prebrushing mouthrinses advocate that such an application will 'loosen' plaque and perhaps facilitate its removal. At the same time, the antibacterial actions of the mouthrinses may help to reduce the pathogenicity of the bacterial plaque. Whilst some patients may find a cosmetic benefit from using prebrushing rinses, there is little evidence to support their efficacy in the application suggested. Furthermore, there is the very real risk that patients may rely solely on such mouthrinses as their only means of plaque control. This will certainly be detrimental to their dental and periodontal health.

Interproximal applications of chlorhexidine can be made by using the gel preparation together with floss, woodsticks, or interproximal brushes. In attempts to increase their contact time with the tooth surface, drugs have been incorporated into chewing gum, lozenges, and periodontal dressings. Further, a number of so-called slow-release devices have been used to increase the length of time the drugs spend in the gingival crevice or periodontal pocket. Antiplaque agents have been incorporated into pieces of dialysis tubing, hollow cellulose acetate fibres, acrylic strips, and ethyl cellulose films to prolong delivery time. Clinically and microbiologically, the effects of such systems have been promising.

Anticalculus agents

Dental calculus is an ectopic mineralized structure that arises as a result of the calcification of bacterial plaque. Many toothpastes contain active ingredients that attempt to reduce calculus formation. These are referred to commercially as tartar-control toothpastes. The active ingredients of such preparations are:

- soluble pyrophosphates;
- zinc salts (chloride and citrate);
- diphosphonates;
- Triclosan with either a polymer system or zinc citrate.

The active ingredients have several mechanisms of action that can lead to a reduction in calculus formation. These include active retention within saliva and plaque, an inhibition of the phase transformations within developing calculus, and an inhibitory effect on the accumulative factors affecting the rate of supragingival plaque mineralization.

The efficacy of commercially available antitartar toothpastes in reducing supragingival calculus formation has been demonstrated in both short- and long-term studies. Whether this reduction in calculus formation has any clinical significance with respect to periodontal health remains to be determined.

Antimicrobials in the management of periodontal diseases

Antimicrobials are typically used in medicine to eliminate infections caused by foreign pathogenic micro-organisms (see Chapter 11). The microbial aetiology of inflammatory periodontal diseases has provided the basis for the introduction of antimicrobials in the management of these diseases. This section will assess the ability of specific antimicrobial agents to reduce the pathogenicity of the subgingival microflora, and affect the clinical signs of disease.

Rationale for the use of antimicrobials in periodontal diseases

There is little doubt that specific micro-organisms are closely associated with some forms of periodontal disease (see Table 12.3). Between 6 and 12 microbial species may be responsible for most cases of periodontitis, or be causative in active episodes of the disease process. Unlike the majority of general infections, all the suspected periodontal pathogens are indigenous to the oral flora. Consequently, long-term and total elimination with antimicrobials will be very difficult to achieve. On cessation of the drug, repopulation of the indigenous bacteria will occur. Antimicrobial agents should only be considered as an adjunct to conventional periodontal therapy.

Nevertheless, in certain forms of periodontitis, the loss of connective tissue attachment is rapid. Extremely virulent Gram-negative organisms populate the deep pockets and can actually invade the gingival connective tissue. Under these circumstances, antimicrobials provide a useful adjunct to root planing; this, by itself, may not remove all subgingival deposits and certainly would not affect any invading organisms which had already penetrated the soft tissues. The micro-organisms listed in Table 12.3 are sensitive to a number of antimicrobials, especially the tetracyclines and metronidazole, hence these drugs are extensively used in the management of periodontal disease.

Routes of administration

The aim of using an antimicrobial is to achieve a concentration of the drug in the periodontal environment sufficient either to kill or arrest the growth of pathogenic micro-organisms. The most effective and reliable method is systemic administration, which enables the drug to bathe the subgingival flora by passing into the crevicular fluid. Indeed, certain drugs such as tetracycline have been found to concentrate in crevicular fluid at higher levels than those found in serum following oral administration. The drug can then bind to the tooth surfaces, from where it is released in active form.

In an attempt to minimize the risks of adverse reactions, antimicrobials have been applied topically to periodontal pockets by techniques such as subgingival irrigation, acrylic strips, gels, and fibres filled with drug. Such methods permit lower doses of antimicrobials to be administered than for oral dosing, although the extent to which the drugs penetrate the pockets is less predictable. Furthermore, the insertion and removal of multiple acrylic strips and fibres is time-consuming and this may preclude their widespread clinical use. It is now accepted that the use of local antimicrobial delivery into a periodontal pocket is an adjunct to root surface debridement and not an alternative to such treatment. Moreover, debridement will also serve to disrupt the subgingival biofilm and permit better contact between the antimicrobial agent and the subgingival flora. With some of the subgingival antimicrobials, it is recommended that they be administered up to a week after root planing. This allows for resolution of the inflammatory response and a concomitant reduction in the flow of gingival crevicular fluid. Both changes will reduce drug clearance from the pocket and prevent the delivery device from blocking the natural drainage from the periodontal defect.

Tetracyclines

The tetracyclines comprise a group of closely related bacteriostatic antibiotics that provide a broad spectrum of activity against both Gram-positive and Gram-negative micro-organisms. Tetracyclines are effective against many anaerobic and facultative anaerobic bacteria, which is a particularly important consideration when they are used in the management of periodontal diseases. Tetracyclines are also active against most spirochaetes. The general pharmacology of these drugs is discussed in Chapter 11.

TETRACYCLINES AND PERIODONTAL DISEASES

Cases of moderately severe and advanced periodontal disease are usually treated with oral hygiene instruction, scaling, and root surface debridement. This usually results in a reduction in plaque scores and gingival inflammation, a decrease in periodontal pockets, and the establishment of a periodontal microbial flora compatible with the maintenance of periodontal health. In such cases, the adjunctive use of tetracycline therapy is not indicated because it is unlikely to achieve any short-term or long-lasting clinical effects not provided by mechanical debridement alone. Occasionally, a case of chronic adult periodontitis will show no clinical improvement after routine therapy and the periodontal flora will continue to be a mixture of spirochaetes and Gram-negative anaerobic rods. These refractory cases of periodontitis can benefit from a 2-week course of systemic tetracycline therapy of 1 g daily.

The effects of tetracycline therapy on the subgingival flora associated with periodontitis have been well documented. A 2-week course of 1 g tetracycline daily produces a shift from an essentially complex Gram-negative flora to one which is essentially Gram-positive and associated with healthy tissues. Bacterial resistance amongst the indigenous flora is not uncommon, both before and following tetracycline therapy. Species of *Streptococcus* and *Actinomyces* have been found to be resistant. However, the association between these bacteria and gingival health may negate the importance of this resistance. In refractory cases of periodontitis, a short course of systemic tetracycline will reduce spirochaetes and Gram-negative rods to low or undetectable levels.

Tetracycline is of considerable value in the treatment of the early-onset periodontal conditions. The prime pathogen in this unusual destructive form of periodontal disease is *Actinobacillus actinomycetemcomitans* (*A.a*). This is very susceptible to tetracycline. *A.a.* is difficult to eliminate by mechanical debridement alone, presumably because of its ability to invade the gingival connective tissue. Systemic administration of tetracycline 1 g daily for 3–6 weeks in conjunction with supragingival plaque control can halt the progression of juvenile periodontitis. However, it is more usual to give a 2-week course of tetracycline as an adjunct to surgical management.

In addition to the antimicrobial effects of tetracyclines, a further mechanism has been proposed to explain their efficacy in the management of periodontal diseases. In laboratory experiments and clinical trials on patients with diabetes, it has been shown that tetracycline, doxycycline, and minocycline can all suppress the activity of collagenases, especially those derived from PMNs (also referred to as MMP-8). Collagenases are also produced by fibroblasts which maintain collagen and gingival connective tissue homeostasis. Mammalian collagenases are calcium-dependent enzymes and, as tetracyclines bind to calcium ions, this may be the mechanism of inhibition. The conversion of tetracycline to a non-antimicrobial analogue, de-dimethylaminotetracycline, does not reduce the anticollagenolytic action of the drug. This suggests that this action is independent of antimicrobial activity. A further mechanism may be associated with the ability of the tetracyclines to scavenge oxygen radicals (e.g. hydroxyl groups or hypochlorous acid) produced by PMNs. These oxygen radicals activate latent collagenases, and their inhibition may result in further antiproteolytic effects such as inactivation of α-1 proteinase inhibitor and neutrophil elastase. These antiproteolytic properties of the tetracyclines may contribute to the general anti-inflammatory effects attributed to these drugs, and also their ability to inhibit bone resorption.

A further important property of the tetracyclines in the

management of periodontal diseases is their ability to enhance fibroblast attachment to root surfaces. This will facilitate regenerative procedures that attempt to create new periodontal attachment.

LOCAL DELIVERY

A number of slow-release devices have been used to facilitate the local delivery of tetracyclines (and other antimicrobials) into periodontal sites. Monolithic, ethylene vinyl acetate fibres have been found to be the most efficacious in achieving prolonged delivery of the drug from the entire length of the fibres. Furthermore, the concentrations of tetracyclines achieved in crevicular fluid by controlled local delivery are up to 100 times those obtained following systemic dosing ($1500\,\mu g\,mL^{-1}$ vs. 15 $\mu g\,mL^{-1}$). Thus, the chances of complete suppression of bacterial growth (and/or collagenase activity) are increased. Local application of fibres impregnated with tetracycline (Actisite) has been shown to be as effective as root surface debridement in reducing bleeding on probing and probing pocket depth. However, the fibre may be difficult to apply and be retained within the pocket.

Minocycline has also been incorporated into a local delivery system (Dentomycin gel). This gel is used as an adjunct to root surface debridement and is applied three to four times over an 8-week period. The gel is easy to apply and appears to be more effective in the treatment of deep periodontal pockets.

Key facts
Tetracyclines in periodontal disease

- Tetracyclines are bacteriostatic antibiotics and are effective against many periodontopathogens.

- In addition to their antibacterial properties, tetracyclines inhibit PMN-derived collagenases (MMP-8), scavenge free oxygen radicals, inhibit bone resorption, and condition the root surface to facilitate fibroblast attachment.

- Systemic tetracyclines are used as adjuncts in the management of early-onset periodontal conditions and refractory periodontitis.

- Normal course of treatment of tetracycline is 1 g daily in divided doses for 3–6 weeks.

- Tetracyclines can be incorporated into local delivery systems (fibres and gels) for direct placement into periodontal pockets.

Metronidazole

Metronidazole is a nitroimidazole that has a broad spectrum of activity against protozoa and anaerobic bacteria. The antimicrobial activity of this drug against anaerobic cocci, and anaerobic Gram-negative and Gram-positive bacilli has led to its extensive use in the management of periodontal diseases. Its general pharmacology is discussed in Chapter 11.

METRONIDAZOLE AND PERIODONTAL DISEASES

The rationale for the use of metronidazole in the treatment of periodontal diseases and other oral infections has revolved around the drug's specificity for anaerobes and the apparent inability of susceptible organisms to develop resistance. However, the plasma (or crevicular fluid) levels of metronidazole required for the drug to be effective against the majority of anaerobes have not been clearly established. Plasma levels of $6\,\mu g\,mL^{-1}$ are adequate to deal with most anaerobic infections, and these levels can be achieved by a regimen of 200 mg three times a day. However, another study showed that a concentration of $8\,\mu g\,mL^{-1}$ was inhibitory to more than 90% of bacteria in subgingival plaque. Crevicular fluid levels of $15\,\mu g\,mL^{-1}$ would be necessary for maximal inhibition. Such levels may be achieved following the administration of metronidazole 400 mg twice a day.

Many studies have shown that metronidazole has a clinical, histopathological, and microbiological benefit to the periodontal tissues. This benefit is enhanced when drug therapy is combined with conventional treatment. Metronidazole has been shown to be particularly useful in the management of advanced cases of periodontal destruction, and in the management of the early-onset periodontal conditions.

LOCAL DELIVERY OF METRONIDAZOLE

A commercially available local metronidazole preparation (Elyzol) is now available for direct application into a periodontal pocket. The product contains 25% metronidazole in a delivery vehicle containing glyceryl mono-oleate and sesame oil. Efficacy studies suggest that two applications of the gel (1 week apart) are as effective as conventional non-surgical management in reducing probing depths and bleeding on probing. Furthermore, the clinical benefit of such local drug delivery was evident up to 18 months after treatment. In this instance, the local application of metronidazole is being used as an alternative to conventional therapy, not as an adjunct.

METRONIDAZOLE AND ACUTE ULCERATIVE NECROTIZING GINGIVITIS (ANUG)

Metronidazole is the treatment of choice for ANUG. Gingival ulceration, bleeding, pain, and halitosis usually resolve rapidly within about 48–72 hours of starting metronidazole treatment (200 mg, three times a day). These clinical changes are accompanied by the rapid disappearance of the spirochaete–fusobacteria complex, which is a feature of this acute disease. However, it is essential that once the acute phase of the disease has been controlled, mechanical debridement should be carried out immediately. Failure to do so will result in the recurrence of infection.

Key facts
Metronidazole in periodontal disease

- Metronidazole is effective against the anaerobic Gram –ve bacteria associated with destructive forms of periodontitis.

(cont.)

- Bacterial resistance to metronidazole rarely occurs and is not a problem with the periodontopathogens.

- The drug is particularly useful in the management of ANUG, where normal dosing is 200 mg, three times a day for 5 days.

- A local delivery preparation of metronidazole is available (Elyzol) for direct placement into periodontal pockets after debridement.

Combination antimicrobial therapy

There is increasing evidence that a combination of 375 mg amoxicillin (amoxycillin) and 250 mg metronidazole, three times a day for a week, is of value in the management of refractory and other rapidly progressive forms of periodontitis. This combination therapy has also been shown to be effective in treating refractory cases of localized juvenile periodontitis where patients still harboured *Actinomyces actinomycetemcomitans* after treatment with a systemic tetracycline. Before such a combination of antimicrobials is prescribed, it is essential that the periodontal diagnosis is correct, and that some attempt has been made to identify the microorganisms and their sensitivity.

NSAIDs in the management of periodontal diseases

NSAIDs are a heterogeneous group of compounds whose analgesic, anti-inflammatory, and antipyretic properties are due to the inhibition of eicosanoid synthesis (see Chapters 4 and 6). The eicosanoids are important mediators of inflammation in periodontal disease, and prostaglandins of the E series are potent stimulators of osteoclasts. This latter activity is one of the factors contributing towards bone loss, a major feature of periodontal disease. Further evidence that prostaglandins may be important in the pathogenesis of periodontal disease came from cross-sectional studies on patients on long-term NSAID therapy. These patients had less alveolar bone loss and gingival inflammation than age-matched, otherwise healthy controls.

Others studies have shown that topical and systemic flurbiprofen have a marked inhibitory effect on the development of gingival inflammation in the experimental gingivitis model. Systemic flurbiprofen (50 mg twice daily for 2 months) has been evaluated on patients with refractory periodontitis. The rate of bone loss was considerably reduced and some sites actually gained bone. Long-term systemic flurbiprofen (3 years) reduced bone loss for 12–18 months of treatment. This benefit does not extend beyond 2 years, although this may be due to lack of compliance by patients taking the flurbiprofen therapy, or to a true loss of the effect of flurbiprofen such that other pathways of bone resorption became active.

The precise mechanism of the action of NSAIDs in preventing periodontal bone loss needs to be established. Subsequently, the dose, frequency of dosing, and the most suitable method of administration of the drug can be determined. It would be unrealistic to expect patients with periodontal disease to undertake regular and prolonged systemic NSAID therapy, especially as periodontal disease is not outwardly disabling. However, if relatively small, but active, amounts of an NSAID such as flurbiprofen could be incorporated into a gel or toothpaste for topical application, then compliance would be better.

Studies of NSAIDs and periodontitis over the next few years should provide new methods for preventing and controlling the onset and progression of a disease which is currently the major cause of tooth loss in adults.

Key facts
NSAIDs in periodontal diseases

- NSAIDs inhibit prostaglandin synthesis, which stimulates osteoclasts and hence causes bone resorption.

- Flurbiprofen, applied both topically and systemically, has a marked inhibitory effect on the development of gingival inflammation.

- Widespread use of NSAIDs in the management of periodontal diseases is unlikely since these drugs are associated with significant unwanted effects.

Oxygen-releasing agents

Hydrogen peroxide and sodium peroxyborate (Bocasan) are the main oxygen-releasing agents used in the treatment of periodontal disease. Both are restricted to the treatment of acute necrotizing ulcerative gingivitis, which is thought to be caused by anaerobic bacteria. It is doubtful if the oxygen released has a significant action on the metabolism of anaerobic organisms during the short period of exposure. This painful gingival condition is more appropriately treated with metronidazole.

Conclusion

There is little doubt that antiplaque agents and antimicrobials are of significant value in the management of periodontal diseases. The antiplaque agent of choice is chlorhexidine. This agent can be applied in a variety of ways. Subgingival irrigation or other means of direct placement of the drug into the periodontal pocket is a useful adjunct to conventional periodontal treatment. Rinsing the mouth with a 0.2% solution is of value after periodontal surgery and in the management of oral mucosal lesions such as aphthous ulceration and stomatitis secondary to radiotherapy and chemotherapy.

Tetracycline is of proven benefit as an adjunct to surgery in the treatment of juvenile periodontitis. It is also useful in cases of refractory and rapidly progressive periodontitis. A 2–4-week course is usually advocated. Tetracycline concentrates in the crevicular fluid and inhibits collagenase. These two properties make it of particular value in the management of periodontal disease.

Dentine sensitivity

Painful symptoms arising from exposed dentine are a common finding in the adult population, with an incidence of 1/7. Exposure of dentine can arise from either the removal of enamel or denudation of the root surface. Loss of enamel occurs in attrition, erosion, toothbrush abrasion, or caries. Several factors can cause denudation of the root surface including gingival recession with increasing age, chronic periodontal disease, periodontal surgery, incorrect toothbrushing, and trauma.

Dentine sensitivity (erroneously termed hypersensitivity) is characterized by pain, elicited by various stimuli, that disappears when the stimulus is removed. Some people are sensitive to cold alone; others to touch, sweet, or sour foods; and some to a combination of any of these stimuli. The pain may be so severe that they find eating difficult.

Theories of dentine sensitivity

Precisely how external stimuli are transmitted through dentine to pulp is not established and, although evidence suggests that dentine is innervated, the extent of this innervation is uncertain. There are three theories of dentine sensitivity:

(1) the dentinal receptor mechanism;

(2) the hydrodynamic mechanism; and

(3) the modulation of nerve impulses by polypeptides.

Dentinal receptor mechanism

This theory suggests that the odontoblast has a sensory function, perhaps serving as a transducer between external stimuli and the nearby pulpal nerve plexus. Certainly, when there is disruption of odontoblasts, the dentine becomes very sensitive. However, pain-inducing substances, such as potassium chloride, 5-hydroxytryptamine, and histamine, have failed to evoke pain when applied to exposed dentine. This finding would question the nociceptive role of the odontoblast.

Hydrodynamic mechanism

This is the most widely accepted theory. Dentinal tubules contain fluid, so a blast of air, or hot and cold stimuli will cause a rapid movement of this fluid within the tubules. This movement will cause deformation of both the odontoblastic process and adjacent nerve fibres. Nerve deformation causes pain.

Modulation of nerve impulses by polypeptides

Pulpal tissue contains a number of polypeptides that can act as regulators of neural transmission. These include substance P and bradykinin, which may alter the permeability of the odontoblast cell membrane (depolarization). Such depolarization could make the pulp more sensitive to various external stimuli. Thus, substance P and bradykinin may act as modulators of nerve impulses in the pulp.

Desensitizing agents

Ideally, a desensitizing agent should:

- be non-irritant to the pulp;
- be relatively painless on application;
- be easily applied;
- have a rapid onset of action;
- be permanently effective;
- not stain the teeth;
- be consistently effective.

Many agents have been used to treat dentine sensitivity, and some are discussed below.

Sodium fluoride

This is conveniently applied as a paste, for example Lukomsky's paste, which contains equal parts by weight of sodium fluoride, kaolin, and glycerin. The paste is burnished into the previously dried sensitive area, and left on for about 3 minutes before the patient is allowed to rinse. Occasionally, application may cause a marked but transitory pain. Fluoride from the sodium salt will be taken up by the dentine thus making it more resistant to acid decalcification. The fluoride may also lead to an increase in secondary dentine formation, thus blocking dentinal tubules. Sodium fluoride either in pastes, gels, or mouthwashes has to be applied frequently for maximum effectiveness.

Stannous fluoride

This also reduces dentine sensitivity. In solution it undergoes spontaneous hydrolysis and oxidation, so it is applied in the form of a gel mixed with carboxymethylcellulose or glycerine. Stannous fluoride acts as an enzyme poison and may inactivate enzymatic activity in the odontoblastic process. Like sodium fluoride, stannous fluoride induces mineralization within the dentinal tubules, thus creating a calcific barrier on the dentine surface.

Sodium monofluorophosphate

This fluoride salt is widely used in toothpastes, but is of uncertain efficacy as a desensitizing agent. It is suggested that monofluorophosphate is hydrolysed by hydroxyapatite on the surface of enamel and dentine. The hydrolysis releases fluoride ions, which are then incorporated into the lattice work of the apatite crystal.

Calcium hydroxide

Although this compound occludes dentinal tubules, its use as a desensitizing agent is uncertain, probably because of its poor adhesion to exposed dentine.

Strontium chloride

Strontium ions have a strong affinity for calcified tissues, and also accelerate the rate of calcification. Thus, strontium salts will obliterate the dentinal tubules. Sensodyne toothpaste contains 10% strontium chloride, but the efficacy of this compound in controlling dentine sensitivity is uncertain.

Formaldehyde

Toothpastes containing 1.3–1.4% formalin (for example Emoform) are used as desensitizing agents, but their unpleasant taste may limit their use. Formalin is thought to precipitate proteins in the dentinal tubules and hence reduce sensitivity.

Resins and adhesives

Various resins and adhesives can be applied to exposed dentine, sealing off the tubules and hence acting as a mechanical barrier to external stimuli. Tooth preparation, such as acid-etching, is required before some of these materials can be applied, so their use should be restricted to the more persistent cases of dentine sensitivity.

Key facts
Dentine sensitivity

- Exposure of dentine can arise as a result of toothbrush trauma or periodontal disease.

- Agents used in the treatment of dentine hypersensitivity include sodium and stannous fluoride, sodium monofluorophosphate, calcium hydroxide, strontium chloride, formaldehyde, and various resins and adhesives.

References

Bral, M. and Brownstein, C. N. (1988). Antimicrobial agents in the prevention and treatment of periodontal diseases. *Dental Clinics of North America*, **32**, 217–41.

Slots, J. and Rams, T. E. (1991). Antibiotics in periodontal therapy: advantages and disadvantages. *Journal of Clinical Periodontology*, **17**, 479–93.

13

Haemostasis and haemostatic agents

- Haemostasis
- Anticoagulants
- Antiplatelet drugs
- Fibrinolytic and antifibrinolytic agents
- Dental management of patients with haemostatic problems
- The management of postextraction haemorrhage
- Further reading

Haemostasis and haemostatic agents

Haemostasis

Several factors play an integrated role in the arrest of haemorrhage after a tooth extraction or dental surgical procedure. These include the ability of vessel walls to contract, the adhesion and aggregation of platelets, the ability of blood to coagulate, and the breakdown of blood clots (fibrinolysis). A variety both of diseases and drugs can affect these factors. However, in this chapter only the effect of drugs will be discussed.

Vessel wall contraction

In the early stages of injury, contraction of the smooth muscles in vessel walls is an important factor in the control of haemorrhage. This vasoconstriction is only of short duration (usually 5–20 minutes) but can be prolonged by topical or local infiltration of epinephrine (adrenaline).

Platelets

These are non-nuclear cells with a cytoplasm rich in granules. They are formed by the fragmentation and detachment of delicate processes from megakaryocytes. The normal platelet count in humans is in the range 150 000 to 400 000 cells per mL, and their half-life is 7–10 days. Platelets play an essential role in haemostasis: when a blood vessel is cut or damaged, they rapidly adhere to the exposed subendothelial tissues, especially collagen. Adhesion involves the linking of subendothelial components to glycoprotein IIb-receptors on the platelet membrane by the von Willebrand factor. This factor is a large glycoprotein synthesized by endothelial cells, and is missing in the hereditary haemorrhagic disease of the same name. Platelet adhesion is followed by the release from the platelet granules of adenosine diphosphate (ADP), fibrinogen, 5-HT, platelet-aggregating factor (PAF), and the powerful pro-aggregating substance, thromboxane A_2 (TXA_2). Both ADP and thromboxane induce platelets to stick to each other (platelet aggregation) to form a platelet plug. The plug will arrest haemorrhage, but it must be further stabilized by fibrin. Fibrin formation is stimulated by the exposed cut collagen, platelet membranes, and chemicals released by the platelets themselves, such as 5-HT and PAF.

Platelets also release factors that increase vascular permeability, and that are chemotactic to WBCs. They also produce platelet-derived growth factor (PDGF), which is important in the repair process.

Blood coagulation

This is a complex process involving the initiation and interaction of several factors in blood and damaged tissues (Fig. 13.1). The final event in the blood coagulation cascade is the conversion of prothrombin (factor II) to thrombin, which in turn converts fibrinogen (factor I) to fibrin. Fibrin is further polymerized by factor XIII.

There are two pathways to blood coagulation: an intrinsic pathway (all components present in blood), and an extrinsic pathway (some components derived from outside the blood). Activation of the intrinsic system occurs when blood contacts an abnormal surface. This leads to the sequential activation of factors XII, XI, IX, VIII, and X. Activated factor (Xa) together with factor V and phospholipids derived from activated platelets, result in the conversion of prothrombin to thrombin (Fig. 13.1). The extrinsic system is activated by tissue damage, resulting in the release of a 'tissue factor', which is a membrane protein. The tissue factor, together with factor VII and platelet phospholipids, activates factor X. The sequence of events is then the same as in the intrinsic system. The two pathways are described separately. However, various feedback loops exist that enhance the rates of reaction—activation of one factor catalyses the formation of larger amounts of the next factor and so on. This amplification results in the rapid formation of fibrin. In addition, calcium ions (factor IV) are essential for many of the stages of blood coagulation.

Once the blood coagulation cascade has been initiated, there is an acceleration in the reactions that could, if not controlled, result in clotting of all the blood in the body. This catastrophe is prevented by several mechanisms, including:

- the generation by intact endothelium of several antithrombotic substances, including thrombomodulin (which binds to thrombin) and protein C (which inhibits factors Va and VIIa and stimulates fibrinolysis);

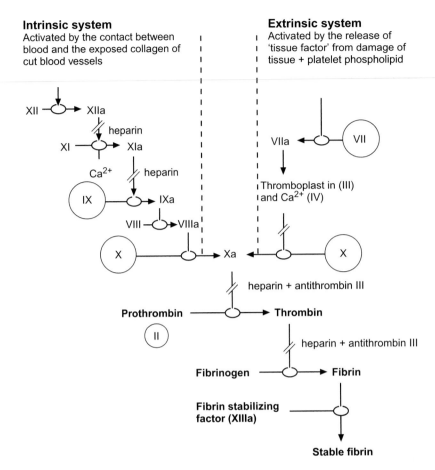

Fig. 13.1 Schematic representation of the blood clotting cascade (factors in circles are dependent on vitamin K for their synthesis, and are affected by warfarin).

- the synthesis of α_2-globulin (also known as antithrombin III), which neutralizes thrombin and activated factors Xa, IXa, XIa, and XIIa;

- the release from vessel endothelium of heparan sulfate and heparin, which are both co-factors for antithrombin III (see below).

Vitamin K

Vitamin K is a fat-soluble vitamin that is essential for the normal hepatic biosynthesis of several factors required for blood clotting (II, VII, IX, X). Its pharmacology is dealt with in more detail in Chapter 21.

The main use of vitamin K is in the correction of hypoprothrombinaemia—either congenital, or induced by the coumarin group of anticoagulants (see later). Excessive bleeding in patients on these drugs can be corrected by the administration of vitamin K. Natural vitamin K (phytomenadione) may be given orally or by intramuscular or intravenous injection. However, it requires bile salts for absorption if given by mouth. A synthetic preparation, menadiol sodium phosphate, is also available. This compound is water-soluble, but takes longer to act. Careful moni-toring of the patient's INR (see later) and anticoagulant levels are necessary following this procedure. Vitamin K is also used to treat hypoprothrombinaemia of the newborn.

Fibrinolysis

The final stage of haemostasis—the breakdown of a blood clot by proteolytic enzymes—is known as fibrinolysis. Extravascularly, as in the case of a haematoma, enzymes are produced by white blood cells. Intravascularly, blood clots are broken down by plasmin, which is derived from the plasma protein plasminogen. The conversion of plasminogen to plasmin may be caused by either tissue or blood activators (Fig. 13.2). The tissue factor has not been identified, but may be released as a result of tissue damage. The blood activator is formed by the action of kinases on a blood pro-activator. The kinases are liberated from blood tissues, and certain bacteria, for example streptococci produce streptokinase (see later).

Fibrinolysis can be influenced by a whole range of factors; for example age, sex, diet, smoking, altitude, and exercise. It can be inhibited by the inactivation of plasmin by the protein α_2-antiplasmin.

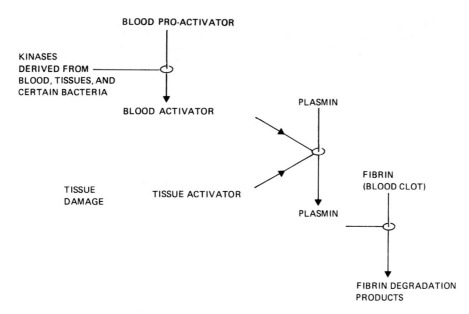

Fig. 13.2 Schematic representation of the stages involved in fibrinolysis.

Key facts
Haemostasis

- Haemostasis is the arrest of blood loss from damaged vessels and the formation of a fibrin-reinforced blood clot.

- Four distinct stages can be identified: vessel wall contraction; platelet aggregation; blood coagulation; and fibrinolysis.

- Vessel wall contraction is of short duration (5–20 min), but can be prolonged by epinephrine (adrenaline).

- Platelets adhere to the exposed collagen of cut blood vessels and release ADP and thromboxane A_2.

- Thromboxane A_2 is a powerful inducer of platelet aggregation, which facilitates the formation of the platelet plug.

- The platelet plug is reinforced with fibrin, which is formed during the clotting cascade.

- Vitamin K is essential for the formation of the clotting factors II, VII, IX, and X.

- Fibrinolysis is the final stage of haemostasis and involves the breakdown of the clot by plasmin.

Anticoagulants

These either directly or indirectly interfere with the normal clotting mechanisms of blood, and thus reduce the incidence of thromboembolic disorders. Patients likely to be receiving anticoagulant therapy include those with a history of myocardial infarction, cerebrovascular thrombosis, venous thrombosis, pulmonary embolism, and patients with prosthetic heart valves. Those on renal dialysis also receive anticoagulant therapy before and during dialysis.

Heparin

Heparin is not a single substance, but a family of sulfated glycosaminoglycans. Heparin occurs in minute accounts in mast cells, but its physiological function is unclear. The drug was 'accidentally' discovered in 1916, although it was not widely used as an anticoagulant until the early 1940s. Fragments of heparin with slightly different anticoagulant activity from the parent molecule are now available. They have lower molecular weights and are hence referred to as low molecular weight heparins (LMWHs). The synthetic drug is the only effective, direct-acting anticoagulant immediately effective on fresh blood.

Pharmacodynamics

Heparin interferes with blood coagulation at several stages of the cascade reaction (see Fig. 13.1). These actions are due to the drug enhancing the activity of antithrombin III, which is a glycosated polypeptide synthesized in the liver. Antithrombin III neutralizes several of the activated clotting factors, namely factors IXa, Xa, XIa, and XIIa. It also inactivates prothrombin (II) by forming an irreversible complex with this clotting protein. Heparin facilitates the inhibitory action of antithrombin III by at least 1000-fold, thus acting as a catalytic template. The long-term use of heparin therapy is associated with a depletion of antithrombin III; this decreases the effect of subsequent heparin therapy.

Pharmacological properties

Because it is highly ionized and is very poorly absorbed from the gut, heparin must be administered parenterally. It is metabolized in the liver by the enzyme heparinase, and the metabolites excreted via the kidney. After intravenous administration, heparin has an immediate onset of action, and a half-life of between 1–5 hours. The higher the dose, the longer the half-life, since metabolism is readily saturated. Heparin is bound to a number of plasma proteins thereby decreasing its bioavailability. The drug appears to be metabolized by the reticuloendothelial system.

Low doses of heparin can be given subcutaneously, but high doses should be given via a slow intravenous infusion. Intramuscular injections of heparin should be avoided because large haematomas can form at the site of injection.

Low molecular weight heparins (LMWHs)

The action of antithrombin III on factor Xa is increased with these newer heparins. They also show less protein binding and thus greater bioavailability following subcutaneous injection than standard heparin. Recent clinical trials suggest that LMWHs are more effective than standard heparin preparations in the prevention of various thromboembolic disorders.

Unwanted effects

Haemorrhage is the principal unwanted effect associated with heparin, usually occuring from the gastrointestinal or genitourinary tract. Hence, heparin should not be given to any patient with a bleeding disorder or ulceration of the gastrointestinal tract. The anticoagulant effects of heparin are monitored by testing the kaolin–cephalin clotting time (KCCT) which should be increased by a factor of 1.5 to 2.5 mins. The KCCT assesses the plasma concentration of factors VIII, IX, XI, XII, and also pre-kallikrein and high molecular weight kininogen.

A mild transient thrombocytopenia is reported in about 25% of patients receiving heparin. However, in a few, thrombocytopenia can be severe and deaths have occurred. Platelet counts should be carried out at regular intervals for all those on heparin therapy.

Commercial preparations of heparin are obtained from animal tissues, and care should be exercised in their use on patients with any history of allergy. Long-term heparin therapy can cause osteoporosis, alopecia, and abnormalities of hepatic function.

The anticoagulant effects of heparin can be reversed by the specific antagonist protamine sulfate, at the dose regimen of 1 mg of protamine for every 100 units of heparin. Protamine combines with heparin to form a stable complex with no anticoagulant properties. This complex is formed because heparin is electronegative and protamine electropositive. However, protamine sulfate, by interacting with platelet function and fibrinogen, has an anticoagulant effect of its own. Thus, the minimum amount of protamine sulfate should be given to reverse the anticoagulant effect of heparin.

Coumarin anticoagulants

This group, also known as the oral anticoagulants, includes warfarin sodium and phenindione. Coumarin anticoagulants are derived from a substance found in the spoiled, sweet-clover plant.

Pharmacodynamics

Coumarin anticoagulants are antagonists to vitamin K. Hence, they will reduce the synthesis of the vitamin K-dependent clotting factors (II, VII, IX, and X). Synthesis of these factors requires a reduced form of vitamin K, but coumarin anticoagulants block the regeneration of reduced vitamin K thus inducing a state of deficiency.

Because of the varying rate of synthesis of these factors, there is a delay of 8–12 hours before a therapeutic response can be obtained following the administration of a coumarin anticoagulant. Many factors can affect the activity of these anticoagulants, including diet, small-bowel disease, pyrexia, age, pregnancy, concurrent drug therapy, and liver disease.

The effect of coumarin anticoagulants on haemostasis is evaluated by the International Normalized Ratio (INR). This is essentially a measure of prothrombin activity with the therapeutic range for patients on coumarin anticoagulants being between 2 and 4.

Pharmacological properties

Warfarin sodium, which is the archetypal coumarin anticoagulant, is rapidly absorbed and extensively (98%) bound to plasma protein. Its plasma half-life is 35–37 hours. The drug is metabolized in the liver, and the metabolites are excreted in the urine and faeces. Coumarin anticoagulants differ from heparin in that they are effective when given by mouth and have a much longer duration of action (2–5 days).

Unwanted effects

Haemorrhage is the most common unwanted effect, and regular monitoring of the prothrombin time, to assess the efficacy of the anticoagulant, is essential for patients on these drugs. Haemorrhagic problems include haematuria, ecchymosis, epistaxis, and gingival bleeding. Such problems are treated by withdrawal of the drug, followed by the oral or intravenous administration of vitamin K (10–20 mg) depending on the severity of the haemorrhage. For less severe haemorrhages, fresh frozen plasma can be given intravenously. Withdrawal of anticoagulant therapy must be done in consultation with the patient's physician.

DRUG INTERACTIONS

Coumarin anticoagulants are frequently implicated in drug interactions that can either increase or decrease the anticoagulant response. Drugs that increase this response include aspirin, metronidazole, and co-trimoxazole.

Aspirin should not be given to patients on coumarin anticoagulant therapy: as few as one or two aspirin tablets can impair platelet function by blocking the release of ADP and the powerful aggregatory substance thromboxane A$_2$ (see earlier). As a consequence, there is a weak and poorly formed platelet plug: the impairment of platelet function, together with the impairment in blood coagulation, can lead to a fatal haemorrhage. Other aspirin-like drugs, such as non-steroidal anti-inflammatory agents (see

Chapter 6), may also affect platelet aggregation, and should also be avoided in patients on coumarin anticoagulants.

Aspirin and other NSAIDs displace warfarin from plasma-protein binding sites, so increasing the amount of unbound (pharmacologically active) warfarin. In theory, such a displacement could lead to a more pronounced anticoagulant effect. However, the increase in unbound warfarin initiates further hepatic metabolism of the drugs, thus cancelling out the enhanced anticoagulant effect.

Metronidazole and co-trimoxazole inhibit hepatic microsomal enzymes that metabolize warfarin, resulting in an increase in the drug's half-life. Hence concomitant administration of these antimicrobials with warfarin will enhance the anticoagulant effect.

Carbamazepine decreases the anticoagulant response of warfarin by inducing hepatic microsomal enzymes. This action increases the metabolism of the anticoagulant, and causes a decrease in hypoprothrombinaemia.

Cephalosporins inhibit the reduction of vitamin K and thus reduce the anticoagulant properties of warfarin.

Vitamin C in massive doses can reduce the hypoprothrombinaemic effect of coumarin anticoagulants in some patients. The mechanism of this interaction is unclear, but vitamin C may reduce the absorption of these drugs.

Other anticoagulant agents

New anticoagulation agents include dermatan sulfate—a heparinoid drug that only inhibits thrombin. Other new antithrombin III-independent inhibitors are based upon the substance hirudin, obtained from the medicinal leech. Examples include Hirugen, argatroban, and PPACK.

Key facts
Anticoagulants

- Heparin and warfarin are the main anticoagulants used in clinical practice.

- Heparin can only be given parenterally and acts by increasing the activity of antithrombin III.

- The onset of heparin-induced anticoagulation is rapid, and the effects are reversed by protamine sulfate.

- Low molecular weight heparins (LMWHs) have less effect on thrombin than standard heparin, and are associated with fewer unwanted effects.

- Warfarin is the main oral anticoagulant that inhibits the vitamin K-dependent clotting factors (II, VII, IX, and X).

- Warfarin has a long half-life (37–38 hours) and is extensively protein-bound.

- Onset of anticoagulation with warfarin can take up to 16 hours due to the variable rate of synthesis of the clotting proteins.

- Anticoagulant effects of warfarin are assessed by the INR, which should be in the range of 2 to 4.

- The anticoagulant effects of warfarin are reversed by vitamin K, and excessive bleeding may also require the use of fresh frozen plasma.

- Warfarin is often implicated in drug interactions; especially those that involve displacement from the plasma-protein binding site, or that inhibit the hepatic metabolism of the drug.

Antiplatelet drugs

Antiplatelet, or antithrombotic, drugs decrease thrombin formation. Aspirin has been widely investigated for this purpose; other antithrombotic drugs are dipyridamole and abciximab.

Aspirin and platelet aggregation

Aspirin causes an increase in bleeding time by reducing platelet aggregation. The haemostatic response to aspirin shows marked interindividual variation. Aspirin inhibits the release of ADP from platelets and prevents their aggregation by irreversibly blocking (acetylating) the platelet cyclo-oxygenase (COX-1) enzyme system. This prevents the formation of the powerful platelet aggregating substance, thromboxane A_2. The antiaggregatory effect of aspirin lasts for the life-span of the platelet (7–10 days), and a single dose of 600 mg may produce detectable effects on platelet aggregation and bleeding time for several days. Normal platelet aggregation is only restored when new platelets are released into the circulation.

In addition to the action on platelet cyclo-oxygenase, aspirin also inhibits the synthesis of vessel-wall prostacyclin. It is thought that prostacyclin inhibition occurs with higher doses of aspirin (over 1 g per day). Furthermore, vascular endothelial cells are less sensitive to aspirin than are platelets, so the cyclo-oxygenase activity in vessel walls can be quickly restored. Also, endothelial cells can synthesize fresh cyclo-oxygenase whilst platelets, with no nucleus, are unable to do this.

Other NSAIDs also affect platelet cyclo-oxygenase, but, unlike aspirin, the action of these drugs on this enzyme is reversible and the effect only lasts for 8–10 hours.

Use of aspirin in the prevention of thromboembolic disorders

There has been much interest in the use of aspirin for the prevention of thromboembolic disorders such as transient ischaemic attacks (TIAs), myocardial infarction, cerebrovascular disease, and venous thromboembolism. However, there remains much controversy as to the most suitable dose of aspirin for such conditions. The confusion has arisen from reports claiming that large doses of aspirin inhibit both thromboxane and prostacyclin biosynthesis, whereas low doses of aspirin selectively inhibit platelet thromboxane synthesis.

Aspirin (600 mg per day) has been shown to be effective in reducing the incidence of TIAs. It has also been extensively evaluated in the prevention of primary myocardial infarction and of secondary reinfarction. A placebo-controlled study showed that 325 mg aspirin per day produced a 45% reduction in the incidence of myocardial infarction and a 72% reduction in the incidence of fatal myocardial infarction. In the prevention of secondary myocardial infarction, low doses of aspirin (150–300 mg per day) produced a 30% reduction in vascular mortality. The current consensus is that daily, low-dose aspirin (150–300 mg) is effective in the prevention of myocardial infarction in 'at-risk' patients. The drug appears to be of little benefit in healthy people.

Dipyridamole

Dipyridamole is a phosphodiesterase inhibitor with an anti-thrombotic action based upon its ability to modify various aspects of platelet function such as aggregation, adhesion, and survival. In addition, the drug is a potent vasodilator and should be used with caution in patients with rapidly worsening angina or haemodynamic instability following a recent myocardial infarction. It should obviously be avoided in patients with an inherited or disease-induced coagulation disorder. The main use of dipyridamole is as an adjunct to oral anticoagulation for the prophylaxis of thromboembolism associated with prosthetic heart valves.

Abciximab

This compound is a monoclonal antibody that inhibits platelet aggregation and thrombus formation. Its use is restricted to hospital practice where it is used as an adjunct to heparin and aspirin therapy. The antibody should only be used once, and the indications are for high-risk patients undergoing coronary bypass surgery.

Fibrinolytic and antifibrinolytic agents

Fibrinolytic drugs

This group of drugs promotes the breakdown of thrombi by activating plasminogen to form plasmin. Examples include streptokinase, urokinase, and tissue-plasminogen activator. Fibrinolytic drugs have a prolonged effect on haemostasis and can cause extensive problems if not used carefully.

Streptokinase

This is a protein derived from β-haemolytic streptococci, which interacts with the proactivator of plasminogen to catalyse the conversion of plasminogen to plasmin. Bleeding from the site of injection is a common problem associated with streptokinase administration and allergic reactions to the drug have been reported. Streptokinase is used to treat acute pulmonary embolism and deep vein thrombosis. It is also used to reduce mortality after a myocardial infarction. The drug is extremely expensive, and this imposes restrictions on its routine use.

Urokinase

This is a proteolytic enzyme that activates the conversion of plasminogen to plasmin. It is as active as streptokinase and is used in patients who are allergic to streptokinase.

Tissue plasminogen activator (alteplase)

Tissue plasminogen activator (t-PA) is a protease which activates bound plasminogen. It is mainly used in the management of acute myocardial infarction, where it is administered as a 10 mg IV bolus, followed by slow IV infusion. Like all fibrinolytic drugs, the main unwanted effect is haemorrhage.

Anistreplase

This is a complex of human plasminogen and streptokinase, and is thus essentially a pro-drug for streptokinase. It is given as a single intravenous infusion over 4–5 minutes, and fibrinolytic activity is maintained for up to 6 hours.

Antifibrinolytic drugs

These encourage the stabilization of fibrin by inhibiting plasminogen activation. Examples include epsilon-aminocaproic acid or the more potent tranexamic acid.

Antifibrinolytic agents may be useful in controlling persistent haemorrhage after tooth extraction, in conjunction with local measures. However, their main use is in haemophiliac patients as an adjunct to factor VIII therapy. Unwanted effects associated with antifibrinolytic drugs include nausea, diarrhoea, and hypotension.

Key facts
Fibrinolytic and antifibrinolytic agents

- As their name suggests, these drugs either promote or inhibit fibrinolysis.
- Fibrinolytic agents include streptokinase, urokinase, and t-PA; they all enhance the conversion of plasminogen to plasmin.
- Fibrinolytic drugs are used in the management of acute thromboembolic disorders such as myocardial infarction.
- Antifibrinolytic agents include epsilon-aminocaproic acid and tranexamic acid.
- These drugs encourage stabilization of thrombin, and are useful in the management of postextraction haemorrhage.

Dental management of patients with haemostatic problems

Haemostatic problems that the dental surgeon is likely to encounter can be broadly classified into three groups:

(1) impaired platelet function;

(2) vascular defects;

(3) impaired coagulation.

In all patients with haemostatic problems, careful treatment planning and consultation with their physician are essential. When surgery is required, such patients are best treated in a dental hospital or oral surgery department. Every attempt should be made to obtain adequate haemostasis during the operative procedure (i.e. by suturing and packing sockets).

Impaired platelet function

This may be due to a reduction in platelet count (thrombocytopenia), or impaired aggregation resulting from drug therapy.

Thrombocytopenia occurs when the platelet count (normal range 150 000–400 000 cells mL blood^{-1}) falls below 100 000 cells mL^{-1}. It can be caused by a variety of factors such as radiotherapy, connective tissue disease, or leukaemia. In patients with a low platelet count (less than 50 000 cells mL^{-1}), a platelet transfusion may be necessary just before a dental surgical procedure (i.e. tooth extraction or periodontal surgery). If the thrombocytopenia is due to the immune destruction of platelets, as occurs in idiopathic thrombocytopenic purpura, corticosteroids need to be administered, either instead of or as well as the platelet infusion.

Drugs that impair platelet aggregation and increase bleeding time include aspirin and non-steroidal anti-inflammatory drugs (see above), sodium valproate, and phenytoin. When tooth extractions are carried out on patients taking these drugs it is a wise precaution to suture and pack the socket to minimize the risk of postextraction haemorrhage.

Vascular defects

Defects that can cause impairment of haemostasis are associated with vitamin C deficiency (ascorbutic) and long-term corticosteroid therapy. Vitamin C is essential for collagen synthesis and a deficiency causes scurvy. Ascorbutic patients have increased capillary fragility, which can cause bleeding problems after surgery. Long-term corticosteroid therapy can cause both a thrombocytopenia and an inadequate constriction of the small vessels after surgery, and these can lead to haemorrhagic problems. Patients with such vascular defects undergoing dental surgery can present with these haemorrhagic problems, but usually they can be controlled by pressure, suturing, and packing.

Impaired coagulation

This can be due to either an inherited coagulation defect, or to anticoagulant therapy.

Coagulation defects

HAEMOPHILIA

This is a sex-linked, inherited coagulation disorder that usually only affects males. Patients have a reduced factor VIII activity, although this can be corrected by replacement therapy of freeze-dried factor VIII (cryoprecipitate). Any dental procedures involving haemorrhage, such as extractions or scaling, will put the haemophiliac patient at risk. All dental procedures should be carefully planned and carried out with factor VIII cover. The dose is dependent upon the severity of the haemophilia. Factor VIII cover may need to be repeated as it is only effective for 12 hours. Other drugs used in conjunction with factor VIII include the antifibrinolytic agent, epsilon aminocaproic acid, which reduces the factor VIII requirements. This drug should be started preoperatively and continued until all risk of haemorrhage has ceased.

CHRISTMAS DISEASE

This is associated with a deficiency of Factor IX and, clinically, the disease is identical to haemophilia. Factor IX is derived from plasma, but is absent in cryoprecipitates. The half-life of Factor IX is greater than that of Factor VIII, so replacement therapy is given at longer intervals. The dental management of patients with Christmas disease is the same as for haemophiliacs.

VON WILLEBRAND'S DISEASE

This is an inherited disorder associated with a prolonged bleeding time together with a deficiency of both von Willebrand's factor and Factor VIII, although the latter shows marked individual variation. When Factor VIII levels are low, replacement therapy is necessary if surgery is to be carried out on these patients.

Anticoagulant therapy

HEPARIN

Heparinized patients are usually confined to hospital; this group will include those with recent thromboembolic disorders and those undergoing renal dialysis. The anticoagulant effects of heparin last for 4–6 hours after a single dose. If an emergency extraction is needed on a heparinized patient it should be carried out when the anticoagulant effect is minimal. Patients on continuous heparin therapy should be given intravenous protamine sulfate at a dosage of 1 mg per 100 units of heparin. Monitoring the patient's kaolin–cephalin clotting time (KCCT) is essential.

COUMARIN ANTICOAGULANTS

Consultation with the patient's physician is essential if elective surgery, such as the removal of an impacted lower third molar, is required for patients taking coumarin anticoagulants so that dose regimes can be altered. In most instances, the patient will be required to stop their warfarin for 48 hours prior to the planned procedure. This long time period is required since the drug has a long half-life (37–38 hours) and because of the variable rate of hepatic synthesis of the clotting proteins. Prior to surgery, the patient's INR should be reassessed.

Emergency single extractions can be carried out on patients

taking coumarin anticoagulants, provided their prothrombin time does not exceed 2–2.5 times the normal value. Sockets should be packed and sutured. If haemorrhage does occur, the anticoagulant effect can be reversed by the intravenous administration of fresh-frozen plasma. In very severe cases, vitamin K (phytomenadione, 10–20 mg) should be given via an intravenous drip. Intravenous vitamin K and fresh-frozen plasma are also used to treat a warfarin-induced bleed (e.g. a bleeding tooth socket, or a surgical wound) that does not respond to local measures.

In some situations, a physician may be reluctant to stop a patient's anticoagulant therapy, since warfarin cessation may be potentially life threatening to the patient. In such instances, the patient is admitted to hospital and their anticoagulant control switched to heparin. It may take several days to achieve the appropriate haematological profile, however the short half-life of heparin (1–2 hours) allows for greater flexibility in controlling the patient's INR.

The management of postextraction haemorrhage

A careful and detailed history should be taken from all patients presenting with a postextraction haemorrhage. This is essential to ensure that there is no underlying systemic disease or drug therapy (for example aspirin or anticoagulant therapy) contributing to the haemorrhage. If the patient has a predisposing prob-lem, then the appropriate treatment should be carried out as pre-viously outlined.

Most cases of postextraction haemorrhage are due to tears in the mucoperiosteum around the tooth socket. Generally, a suture will effectively control the haemorrhage. Further aids to haemostasis can be obtained by placing an absorbable material in the socket. These materials are made of either cellulose, alginate, gelatin, or fibrin, and provide a network that activates the clot-ting mechanisms. Surgicel (oxidized regenerated cellulose) is the most widely and easily applied resorbable material. It is available in strips and can be cut and placed in the tooth socket. Surgicel resorbs within 7–10 days, and foreign-body reactions are rare.

Further reading

Hamberg, M., Svenson, J., and Samuelsson, B. (1975). Thromboxanes: a new group of biologically active compounds derived from prostaglandin endoperoxides. *Proceedings of the National Academy of Sciences USA*, 72, 2994–8.

O'Reilly, R. A. (1976). Vitamin K and the oral anticoagulant drugs. *Annual Review of Medicine*, 27, 245–61.

Roth, G. J. and Majerus, P. W. (1975). The mechanism of the effects of aspirin on human platelets I: acetylation of a particular fraction protein. *Journal of Clinical Investigation*, 56, 624–32.

Vane, J. R. (1978). Inhibitors of prostaglandin, prostacyclin and thromboxane synthesis, *Advances in Prostaglandin and Thromboxane Research*, 4, 27–44.

14

Drugs and the autonomic nervous system

- Organization
- Parasympathetic and sympathetic nervous systems
- Cholinergic transmission
- Noradrenergic transmission
- Further reading

Drugs and the autonomic nervous system

Organization

The autonomic nervous system is responsible for those vital bodily functions requiring constant monitoring and adjustment. It is part of the nervous system that is largely outside the influence of voluntary control. The organization of the autonomic nervous system involves three basic elements (Fig. 14.1):

1. An afferent limb that arises from, for example, visceral afferent, vagal afferent, and nociceptive fibres.

2. A central control element within the hypothalamus that integrates information from afferent fibres and from other parts of the brain such as the limbic system. In addition, the hypothalamus receives and integrates information about the 'internal milieu' from temperature-sensitive receptors, and from plasma osmolarity and hormone concentrations.

3. An efferent limb principally consisting of the parasympathetic and sympathetic nervous systems that deliver appropriate signals from the central nervous system (CNS) to the effector organs.

This chapter is concerned with the processes of neurotransmission in the parasympathetic and sympathetic nervous systems and drugs which affect these processes.

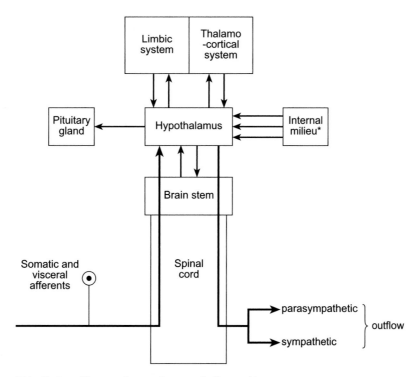

* Monitoring of temperature, salt concentration and hormone concentration within the hypothalamus itself

Fig. 14.1 The organization of the autonomic nervous system, which consists of an afferent limb, a central control element within the hypothalamus, and an efferent limb comprising parasympathetic and sympathetic outflows.

Parasympathetic and sympathetic nervous systems

The pathways for both the parasympathetic and sympathetic nervous systems consist of two neurones (preganglionic and postganglionic) connected by synapsing in a ganglion that lies outside the central nervous system (Fig. 14.2).

The sympathetic preganglionic neurones have cell bodies in the grey matter of the lateral horns of the first thoracic to the third lumbar segments of the spinal cord. The preganglionic fibres pass out of the spinal cord in the spinal nerves and enter the paravertebral chain of sympathetic ganglia lying on either side of the spinal cord. The preganglionic fibres may run up or down the sympathetic chain before synapsing in one of the ganglia with a postganglionic fibre that innervates the target organ. There are some exceptions to this arrangement: (1) the adrenal medulla is innervated by sympathetic nerves that do not relay in sympathetic ganglia; and (2) those sympathetic preganglionic nerves innervating viscera in the abdomen and pelvis do not relay in paravertebral ganglia but synapse in unpaired prevertebral ganglia in the abdomen. The cells of the adrenal medulla can be viewed as a modified sympathetic ganglion, secreting epinephrine (adrenaline) in response to an increase in activity of the nerves supplying it that are the equivalent of preganglionic fibres.

In contrast to the thoracolumbar outflow of the sympathetic nervous system, the parasympathetic has a craniosacral outflow. Preganglionic parasympathetic nerves emerge from the CNS in certain cranial nerves:

- the oculomotor nerve supplying parasympathetic fibres to the eye;
- the facial and glossopharyngeal nerves delivering fibres to

the salivary glands as well as the mucous glands of the nose and pharynx; and

- the vagus nerve carrying fibres to the heart, pulmonary tree, and abdominal viscera.

These parasympathetic preganglionic fibres synapse in ganglia which, in contrast to sympathetic ganglia, lie within or close to the innervated organ. Preganglionic parasympathetic nerves also emerge with pelvic nerves originating in the second, third, and fourth sacral segments of the spinal cord. Similar to parasympathetic nerves which have a cranial origin, the associated postganglionic fibres are short because the parasympathetic ganglia lie in close proximity to their target organs, for example the bladder, rectum, and genital organs.

Nerve impulses produce responses in postsynaptic neurones and effector organs such as heart, smooth muscle, and exocrine glands through the release of specific chemical mediators or transmitters, a process known as neurotransmission. The neurotransmitters released at synapses in the autonomic nervous system are acetylcholine and norepinephrine (noradrenaline). Transmission involving acetylcholine is termed cholinergic transmission; it occurs at autonomic ganglia, the adrenal medulla, and postganglionic parasympathetic nerve terminals, with released acetylcholine acting on postsynaptic receptors classified as either nicotinic or muscarinic (Fig. 14.2). In addition, those postganglionic sympathetic nerves innervating sweat glands release acetylcholine that acts on muscarinic receptors. However, all other postganglionic sympathetic fibres release norepinephrine which stimulates either α- or β-adrenoceptors. A fuller description of the classification of receptors in the autonomic nervous system is given in later sections. Neurotransmission involving norepinephrine is referred to as noradrenergic transmission, although sometimes less accurately as adrenergic transmission. Neurotransmission in the autonomic nervous system does not involve a single transmitter since other transmitters, known as co-transmitters, are also released when autonomic nerves are stimulated. For example, ATP is released along with norepinephrine, and vasoactive intestinal peptide (VIP) is released along with acetylcholine. Whilst the main function of neurotransmission is carried out by the primary transmitter (acetylcholine or norepinephrine), co-transmitters may modulate the response of the postsynaptic cell.

A number of organs and tissues receive innervation from both divisions of the autonomic nervous system. For example, the heart is innervated by sympathetic nerves, stimulation of which produces an increase in heart rate, whilst stimulation of parasympathetic nerves leads to a fall in heart rate. In this example, the sympathetic and parasympathetic systems produce opposing effects; however, the activity of some tissues is regulated by only one division of the autonomic nervous system. For example, the tone of blood vessels and secretion from sweat glands is controlled solely by the sympathetic system. Moreover, in some tissues, such as the salivary glands, the sympathetic and parasympathetic systems

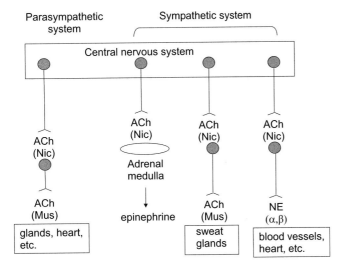

Fig. 14.2 The neurotransmitters and receptors in the parasympathetic and sympathetic nervous systems. ACh, acetylcholine; NE, norepinephrine; Nic, nicotinic receptors; Mus, muscarinic receptors; α,β, α- and β-adrenoceptors.

have similar effects. Sympathetic activity increases in stressful situations, 'fight-or-flight responses', whereas the parasympathetic system dominates at rest or during digestion of a meal. However, these situations apart, both systems contribute to the physiological control of the majority of organs and tissues during normal conditions. Some of the effects of the sympathetic and parasympathetic nervous systems, and the postsynaptic receptors at postganglionic nerve terminals mediating these effects are given in Table 14.1.

Key facts
The autonomic nervous system

- The autonomic nervous system controls smooth muscle activity, secretions, cardiac activity, and some metabolic processes such as glycogenolysis.

- Sympathetic and parasympathetic systems have opposing actions in some organs/tissues, e.g. control of heart rate. In some tissues, one system exerts sole control, e.g. sympathetic control of vascular smooth-muscle activity, whilst in other tissues, both systems produce similar effects (salivary glands).

- The principal neurotransmitters are acetylcholine (cholinergic transmission) and norepinephrine (noradrenergic transmission).

- Cholinergic transmission occurs at autonomic ganglia, the adrenal medulla, postganglionic parasympathetic nerves, and postganglionic sympathetic nerves which innervate sweat glands.

- Noradrenergic transmission occurs at postganglionic sympathetic nerves (except those to sweat glands).

Table 14.1 The main effects of the sympathetic and parasympathetic nervous systems and the postsynaptic receptors at postganglionic nerve terminals that mediate these effects

Organ/tissue	Sympathetic	Receptor	Parasympathetic	Receptor
Blood vessels	Constriction	α_1, α_2	No effect	
	*Dilatation	β_2	No effect	
Heart				
Sinoatrial node	↑Rate	β_1	↓Rate	M_2
Atrial muscle	↑Force	β_1	↓Force	M_2
Ventricular muscle	↑Force	β_1	No effect	
Viscera				
Bronchioles				
– smooth muscle	*Relaxation	β_2	Contraction	M_3
– glands	↓Secretion	β_2	↑Secretion	M_3
GI tract				
– smooth muscle	↓Motility	α_1, β_1	↑Motility	M_3
– sphincters	Constriction	α_1	Dilatation	M_3
– glands	No effect		Secretion	M_3
Eye				
Pupil	Dilation	α_1	Constriction	M_3
Ciliary muscle	Slight relaxation	β_2	Contraction	M_3
Salivary glands	K^+ secretion	α_1	Water and K^+ secretion	M_3
	Amylase secretion	β_1		
Skeletal muscle	*Tremor	β_2	No effect	
Liver	Glycogenolysis	α_1, β_2	No effect	
Fat	Lipolysis	β_3	No effect	

α and β indicate α and β adrenoceptors; M indicates muscarinic receptors. A description of the classification of muscarinic and adrenoceptors is given later in the text.

*Effect produced by circulating epinephrine (adrenaline) released from the adrenal medulla.

Cholinergic transmission

Cholinergic transmission, as all forms of neurotransmission, involves a number of processes, namely the:

- synthesis of transmitter;
- storage of transmitter in vesicles;
- influx of Ca^{2+} in response to depolarization produced by an action potential;
- release of neurotransmitter by exocytosis, a process where vesicles fuse temporarily with the cell membrane to discharge their contents;
- diffusion of transmitter to postsynaptic membrane;
- stimulation of postsynaptic receptors;
- stimulation of presynaptic receptors;
- inactivation of neurotransmitter;
- reuptake of neurotransmitter or breakdown products by a selective carrier protein.

Figure 14.3 illustrates this sequence of processes for cholinergic transmission. Acetylcholine is synthesized by the acetylation of choline (with acetyl-coenzyme A being the source of the acetyl groups), a reaction catalysed by the enzyme choline acetyltransferase. The synthesized acetylcholine is packaged into vesicles that release their contents in response to depolarization of the

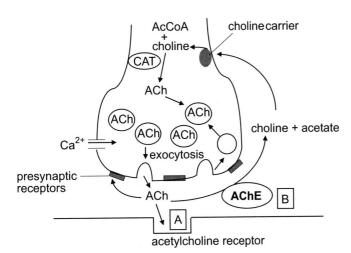

Fig. 14.3 A diagram of the various stages in cholinergic transmission showing: synthesis of acetylcholine (ACh) from choline and acetyl-coenzyme A (AcCoA), by the enzyme choline acetyltransferase (CAT); release of ACh which diffuses across the synapse to stimulate postsynaptic acetylcholine receptors; metabolism of acetylcholine by the enzyme acetylcholinesterase (AChE); and uptake of choline for reuse in the synthesis of acetylcholine. The sites of action of clinically useful drugs are: (A) agonists and antagonists at acetylcholine receptors; and (B) inhibitors of acetylcholinesterase.

nerve terminal. Upon release, acetylcholine stimulates the postsynaptic receptor which produces the tissue response. In addition, acetylcholine stimulates those presynaptic muscarinic receptors that have an inhibitory effect on acetylcholine release, which therefore acts as a negative feedback system. Receptors located on the presynaptic membrane stimulated by the transmitter released from the same nerve are referred to as presynaptic autoreceptors. The action of acetylcholine is terminated by the enzyme acetylcholinesterase; this breaks down acetylcholine to acetate and choline which is taken back up into the nerve terminal for reuse in the synthesis of acetylcholine. Therapeutically useful drugs either act as agonists or antagonists at the postsynaptic receptor (site A, Fig. 14.3), or inhibit acetylcholinesterase (site B).

In addition to the sites of cholinergic transmission outlined in Fig. 14.2, cholinergic transmission also occurs in the central nervous system and at the neuromuscular junction, i.e. the junction between somatic nerves and skeletal muscle. This latter site is of interest because drugs interacting with these receptors (neuromuscular blocking drugs) produce muscle paralysis, which is useful during general anaesthesia (see Chapter 9).

Classification of acetylcholine receptors (cholinoceptors)

Receptors for acetylcholine are divided into two principal categories: muscarinic and nicotinic, so-called because the two types of receptor are selectively stimulated by the naturally occurring compounds muscarine and nicotine, respectively. Nicotinic receptors are ligand-gated ion channels present in the adrenal medulla, autonomic ganglia, and the neuromuscular junction. There are differences in the amino acid composition of nicotinic receptor subunits present at autonomic ganglia and those at the neuromuscular junction. This explains why ganglion blocking drugs (described below) and neuromuscular blocking drugs, both of which interact with nicotinic receptors, are selective for their respective sites of action.

Muscarinic receptors are G-protein-coupled to a range of effectors, including potassium channels, phospholipase C, and adenylyl cyclase (inhibition). A number of subtypes of muscarinic receptor have been cloned, three types of which have been identified pharmacologically:

1. M_1, present in the CNS and autonomic ganglia;

2. M_2, found in the heart and on the presynaptic membrane of nerve terminals; and

3. M_3, present in glands and smooth muscle (see Table 14.1).

In contrast to nicotinic receptors, M_1 receptors present in ganglia generally play only a minor role in transmission. With the exception of pirenzepine (see below), those muscarinic agonists or antagonists currently used clinically do not discriminate between muscarinic receptor subtypes and therefore show similar activity at all subtypes.

Key facts
Cholinergic transmission

- Acetylcholine is synthesized from choline and acetyl groups provided by acetyl-coenzyme A, a reaction catalysed by choline acetyltransferase.

- Acetylcholine stimulates two principal types of receptor: muscarinic and nicotinic.

- Nicotinic receptors are ligand-gated ion channels present at the postsynaptic membrane of autonomic ganglia, the adrenal medulla, and the neuromuscular junction.

- Muscarinic receptors, of which three subdivisions have been characterized, are G-protein-coupled and are present at the postsynaptic membrane of postganglionic parasympathetic nerves, and postganglionic sympathetic nerves innervating sweat glands.

- The action of acetylcholine is terminated by acetylcholinesterase, which splits acetylcholine into acetate and choline.

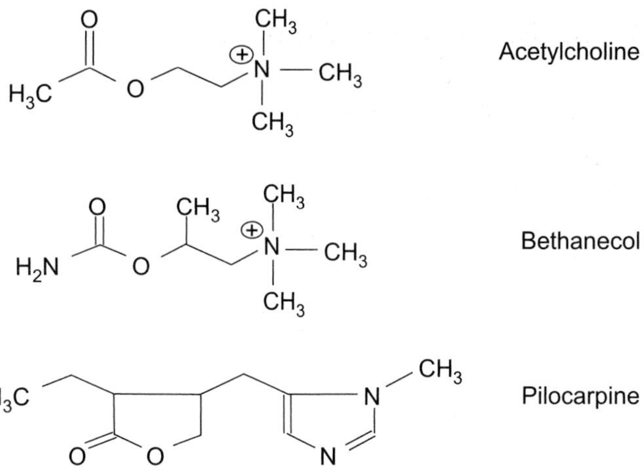

Muscarinic agonists

Since muscarinic receptors are present on the postsynaptic membrane of postganglionic parasympathetic nerve terminals, drugs that selectively stimulate muscarinic receptors, i.e. muscarinic agonists, will produce effects mimicking those of the parasympathetic nervous system. However, therapeutic uses for such drugs is limited. One muscarinic agonist with a clinical use is bethanecol, which can be used to overcome urinary retention and inadequate emptying of the bladder when there is no obstruction in the urinary tract. Such urinary retention may occur postoperatively or as a result of neurological disease. A further use for muscarinic agonists is in the treatment of glaucoma, an abnormally raised intraocular pressure which, if untreated, can cause blindness. In some cases of glaucoma, the drainage of aqueous humour is impaired when the pupil is dilated—because folding of the iris occludes drainage into a canal (canal of Schlemm) close to the margin of the iris. This obstruction to the drainage of aqueous humour results in the elevation of intraocular pressure. Stimulation of muscarinic receptors in the constrictor pupillae (circular muscles in the iris) produces constriction of the pupil (miosis), lowering an elevated intraocular pressure by improving drainage via the canal of Schlemm. Pilocarpine, administered as eye drops, is the most effective muscarinic agonist in the treatment of glaucoma since it is lipid-soluble and crosses the conjunctival membrane. Pilocarpine is lipid-soluble because it is a tertiary amine and carries no charge, unlike acetylcholine and most other muscarinic agonists which are quaternary ammonium compounds with a positive charge that results in poor lipid-solubility (Fig 14.4). A further use for pilocarpine is in the treatment of dry mouth which occurs following radiotherapy to the jaws

Fig. 14.4 The structures of acetylcholine, bethanecol, and pilocarpine.

where salivary function is compromised as a result of radiation damage. In this case, it stimulates salivation and is administered orally in tablet form. Both pilocarpine and bethanecol are resistant to hydrolysis by cholinesterases and therefore have a longer duration of action than acetylcholine.

Muscarinic antagonists

Muscarinic antagonists, which are reversible competitive antagonists, reduce or abolish the effects of the parasympathetic nervous system and, as a consequence, are sometimes referred to as parasympatholytic agents. The effects produced by muscarinic antagonists include: an increase in heart rate; inhibition of secretions; and relaxation of smooth muscle. These drugs will also inhibit sweating since sweat glands are innervated by sympathetic cholinergic nerve fibres (see Fig 14.2). Most muscarinic antagonists are sufficiently lipid-soluble to be absorbed from the gastrointestinal tract and to cross the blood–brain barrier. There are two naturally occurring muscarinic antagonists, atropine and hyoscine, which are alkaloids (basic substances derived from plants) found in solanaceous plants such as deadly nightshade (*Atropa belladonna*). A range of synthetic muscarinic antagonists is also available with particular therapeutic uses, as outlined below. All muscarinic antagonists produce similar peripheral effects, although some do exhibit a degree of selectivity for muscarinic receptors present in a particular tissue. These drugs also have effects on the CNS. For example, atropine overdose, which can occur in children who eat deadly nightshade berries, produces excitement, irritability, and a rise in body temperature that is enhanced by the loss of sweating.

There a number of situations when the blockade of muscarinic receptors in a particular tissue or organ produces useful clinical effects; although, when administered systemically, the adverse effects will be those produced by muscarinic receptor blockade in tissues other than the target organ. For example, when hyoscine is used as an antiemetic it can produce a dry mouth, blurred vision, and difficulty in micturition.

THE CLINICAL USES OF MUSCARINIC ANTAGONISTS

These are outlined below:

- *ophthalmic*—dilatation of the pupil to facilitate ophthalmic examination (tropicamide and cyclopentolate eyedrops—shorter acting than atropine);

- *antiemetic*—useful in motion sickness, a CNS effect (oral or transdermal hyoscine);

- *cardiovascular*—treatment of sinus bradycardia, which can occur during surgery or following myocardial infarction—also used as one component in the treatment of cardiac arrest (IV atropine);

- *anaesthesia*—sometimes useful during general anaesthesia to inhibit excessive salivation and bronchial secretions (IV hyoscine);

- *gastrointestinal*—relaxation of gastrointestinal smooth muscle to facilitate endoscopy (IV hyoscine) and in the treatment of irritable bowel syndrome (oral dicycloverine (dicyclomine))—inhibition of gastric acid secretion which is useful in the treatment of peptic ulcers (oral pirenzepine, a selective M_1 antagonist, although now superseded by histamine H_2-receptor antagonists) (see Chapter 18);

- *asthma*—bronchodilatation (inhaled ipratropium) (see Chapter 17);

- *Parkinson's disease*—control of tremor, a CNS effect (oral benzhexol) (see Chapter 15).

Nicotinic receptor, ganglion blocking drugs

Drugs that block nicotinic receptors at autonomic ganglia were the first drugs introduced to treat hypertension. Their antihypertensive effect resulted from the blockade of sympathetic ganglia, which reduced sympathetic tone to the heart and blood vessels resulting in vasodilatation and a reduction in cardiac output. However, these drugs produced a wide range of adverse effects (including constipation, urinary retention, blurred vision, and dry mouth) due to the blockade of transmission at parasympathetic ganglia. The only ganglion blocker still in clinical use is trimetaphan, which is administered by intravenous infusion in hypertensive emergency associated with a dissecting aortic aneurysm and for certain surgical procedures requiring controlled hypotension.

Anticholinesterase drugs

Inhibition of acetylcholinesterase results in the accumulation of acetylcholine and therefore enhancement of cholinergic transmission. Anticholinesterase agents can be divided into three groups:

(1) short-acting anticholinesterases, of which edrophonium is the only example;

(2) intermediate-duration anticholinesterases such as physostigmine, pyridostigmine, and neostigmine;

(3) irreversible anticholinesterases, which are organophosphorous compounds. These have no clinical uses but have been developed as chemical warfare agents, e.g. sarin, or as insecticides, e.g. parathion.

PHYSOSTIGMINE

This anticholinesterase agent is administered as eyedrops for the treatment of glaucoma. The accumulation of acetylcholine produces constriction of the pupil, thus lowering an elevated intraocular pressure.

NEOSTIGMINE, PYRIDOSTIGMINE, AND EDROPHONIUM

These drugs are used not for their effect on the autonomic nervous system but for their ability to improve cholinergic transmission at the neuromuscular junction. Myasthenia gravis is an autoimmune disease characterized by muscle weakness due to the presence of antibodies directed against nicotinic receptors at the neuromuscular junction. As a consequence of these antibodies, there is a reduction in the numbers of nicotinic receptors. Anticholinesterase drugs such as neostigmine and pyridostigmine, by inhibiting acetylcholine breakdown, increase the probability of any given acetylcholine molecule interacting with the remaining nicotinic receptors. The net result is an improvement in cholinergic transmission and an increase in muscle strength in patients with myasthenia gravis. Edrophonium is used in the diagnosis of myasthenia gravis, since an improvement in muscle strength on intravenous injection indicates that the patient is suffering from myasthenia gravis as opposed to other causes of muscle weakness. The adverse effects of anticholinesterase drugs used in the treatment of myasthenia gravis are those arising from increased concentration of acetylcholine at muscarinic receptors. This can produce bradycardia, increased salivation, abdominal cramps, and diarrhoea, but these effects can be controlled by the administration of a muscarinic antagonist such as atropine, although tolerance to the muscarinic effects of anticholinesterase drugs frequently develops.

Key facts
Drugs that interfere with cholinergic transmission

- The muscarinic agonist pilocarpine produces constriction of the pupil and is used in the treatment of glaucoma. It is also sometimes used to treat radiation-induced dry mouth.

- Muscarinic antagonists, such as atropine and hyoscine, have a range of clinical uses as a result of their ability to:
  – dilate the pupil;
  – inhibit secretions;
  – produce relaxation of smooth muscle; and
  – increase heart rate.

- Drugs that inhibit acetylcholinesterase are used in the treatment of glaucoma (a raised intraocular pressure) and myasthenia gravis (a muscle weakness disease).

Noradrenergic transmission

The precursor for the biosynthesis of the catecholamine norepinephrine is tyrosine, which is taken up into the neurone by a specific transport system. (A catecholamine is a compound with a catechol nucleus, i.e. a benzene ring with two adjacent hydroxyl groups, linked to a side chain containing an amine group.) The various enzymes and intermediate compounds in the synthesis of norepinephrine are shown in Fig. 14.5. The rate-limiting step in this synthetic pathway is the conversion of tyrosine to dihydroxyphenylalanine (DOPA). This stage and the conversion of DOPA to dopamine occur in the cytosol, dopamine is then taken up into the vesicles where it is hydroxylated to produce norepinephrine (Fig. 14.6). The synthesis of epinephrine, which only takes place in the adrenal medulla, occurs by the same pathway but with an additional methylation step to convert norepinephrine to epinephrine (Fig. 14.5). Some nerves, particularly in the CNS, utilize dopamine as a neurotransmitter (dopaminergic nerves) and, in these nerves, neurotransmitter synthesis is by the same pathway but terminates following the decarboxylation of DOPA.

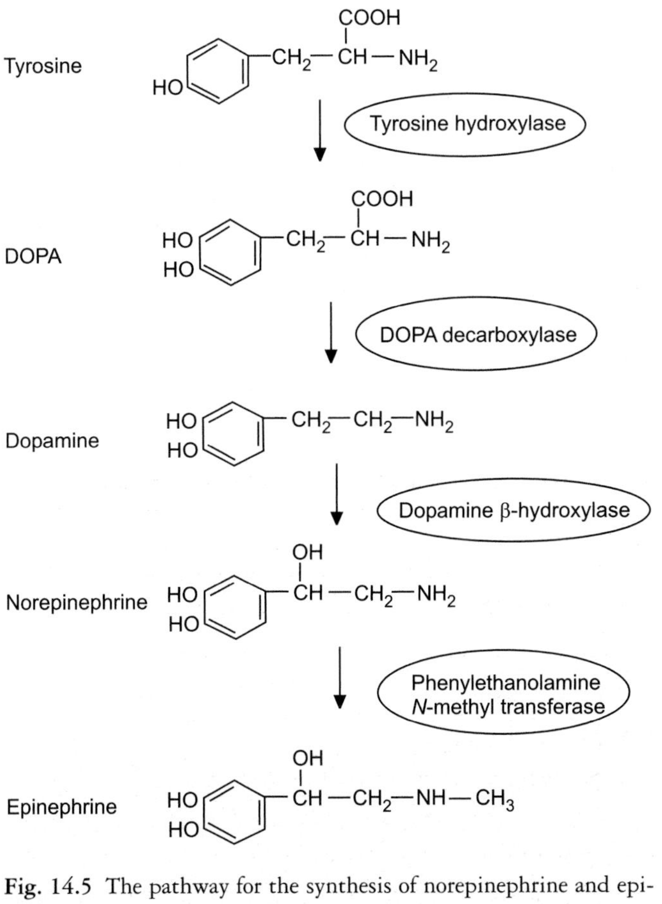

Following its release, norepinephrine stimulates postsynaptic adrenoceptors, which results in the tissue response, such as an increase in heart rate. Presynaptic α_2- adrenoceptors are also stimulated thereby inhibiting the further release of norepinephrine, a mechanism that depends on the inhibition of adenylyl cyclase (Fig. 14.6). Although not shown in Fig. 14.6, sympathetic nerve terminals also possess β-adrenoceptors, positively coupled to adenylyl cyclase, which cause an increase in norepinephrine release. Blockade of these receptors may be involved in the antihypertensive action of β-adrenoceptor antagonists (see Chapter 16). In contrast to cholinergic transmission, where the action of acetylcholine is terminated by an enzyme located in the synapse, the action of norepinephrine is terminated by its reuptake into the nerve terminal and uptake into postsynaptic tissue. Both uptake systems are saturable active-transport systems capable of operating against concentrations gradients. Neuronal uptake (uptake 1) is relatively selective for norepinephrine, whilst extraneuronal uptake (uptake 2) shows less selectivity, transporting epinephrine and other catecholamines, such as the β adrenoceptor agonist isoprenaline, in addition to norepinephrine. Uptake 1 is the most important mechanism for terminating the action of norepinephrine and can be blocked by tricyclic antidepressant drugs (see Chapter 15).

Following uptake into the nerve terminal, norepinephrine can either be transported back into vesicles for reuse or metabolized by monoamine oxidase (MAO) (Fig. 14.6). In addition to noradrenergic nerve terminals, MAO is also present in the liver and

Fig. 14.5 The pathway for the synthesis of norepinephrine and epinephrine. Note that the final stage, the methylation of norepinephrine to form epinephrine, only occurs in the adrenal medulla.

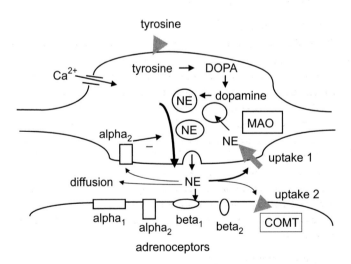

Fig. 14.6 A diagram of the various stages in noradrenergic transmission. Following its release and activation of postsynaptic and presynaptic receptors, the action of norepinephrine (NE) is primarily terminated by uptake in the nerve terminal (uptake 1) where it is either metabolized by monoamine oxidase (MAO) or transported back into vesicles. Some norepinephrine is taken up into extraneuronal tissue (uptake 2) where it is metabolized by catechol-o-methyl transferase (COMT).

intestinal epithelium. MAO converts norepinephrine to an aldehyde, which in turn is metabolized by aldehyde dehydrogenase to a carboxylic acid, dihydroxymandelic acid (DOMA). There are drugs available that inhibit MAO and these have a role in the treatment of depression (see Chapter 15). Norepinephrine is transported by the uptake 2 process and is metabolized by the enzyme catechol-*o*-methyl transferase (COMT), which has a widespread tissue distribution. COMT, as it name suggests, catalyses the *o*-methylation of norepinephrine to produce the metabolite normetanephrine. Norepinephrine or its metabolites are subject to the action of both MAO and COMT, the final product being 3-methoxy-4-hydroxymandelic acid (vanillylmandelic acid, VMA) which is excreted in the urine.

Classification of adrenoceptors

Adrenoceptors, which are G-protein-coupled, are divided into two basic subdivisions— α and β—on the basis of the rank orders of potency of norepinephrine, epinephrine, and isoprenaline (a synthetic catecholamine), i.e.:

α   norepinephrine > epinephrine > isoprenaline;

β   isoprenaline > epinephrine > norepinephrine.

Following this original classification, further subdivisions of both α- and β-receptors have been identified. The main subdivision of α-adrenoceptors is into α_1- and α_2-receptors, although molecular biology has revealed further divisions of both α-adrenoceptor subtypes. α_1-Adrenoceptors are coupled to phospholipase C and produce their effects by an elevation of intracellular calcium, whereas α_2-receptors are negatively coupled to adenylyl cyclase which results in a reduction in cyclic 3',5'-AMP (cAMP) production. There is a difference in the relative pre- and postsynaptic locations of α_1- and α_2-adrenoceptors: α_1-receptors are located exclusively postsynaptically, while α_2-receptors are present at both pre- and postsynaptic sites. α_2-Adrenoceptors produce an inhibitory effect on norepinephrine release, although some of the effects of released norepinephrine, for example on the smooth muscle of blood vessels, are also mediated by this α-receptor subtype (Table 14.1 and Fig. 14.6).

β-Adrenoceptors have also been divided into two principal subdivisions—β_1 and β_2—both of which are positively coupled to adenylyl cyclase therefore resulting in an elevation in levels of cAMP. The distinction between β_1- and β_2-receptors is of therapeutic interest since this has led to development of agonists and antagonists selective for a particular receptor subtype. Such selectivity allows drugs to target particular organs or tissues. For example, selective β_2-agonists such as salbutamol produce bronchodilatation—a property useful in the management of asthma (see Chapter 17)—but with little effect on the heart which contains β_1-receptors (see Table 14.1). A further subdivision of β-receptors has recently been identified known as β_3-receptors, these are present in fat cells and, when stimulated, produce lipolysis.

Adrenoceptor agonists (sympathomimetics)

The endogenous adrenoceptor agonists norepinephrine and epinephrine differ in their selectivity at the four main types of adrenoceptor; norepinephrine has similar potency at α_1-, α_2-, and β_1-receptors but is less potent at β_2-receptors, whilst epinephrine has similar potency at all four receptor types. By contrast to norepinephrine, epinephrine has a number of clinical uses, namely:

- *in the treatment of cardiac arrest*—IV administration (cardiac stimulation produced by β_1-adrenoceptor stimulation);

- *as a vasoconstrictor in local anaesthetic solutions*—SC and submucosal administration (an α_1-/α_2-adrenoceptor-mediated effect);

- *for the emergency treatment of asthma*—IM administration (bronchodilatation produced by β_2-adrenoceptor stimulation);

- *in the management of anaphylactic shock*—IM administration (increase in blood pressure as a result of α-adrenoceptor-mediated vasoconstriction and dilatation of bronchioles due to β_2-adrenoceptor stimulation).

Drugs that produce effects similar to those of norepinephrine and epinephrine are referred to as sympathomimetics. Some of these drugs act directly, i.e. they stimulate adrenoceptors and are termed directly acting sympathomimetics whilst others, indirectly acting sympathomimetics, are dependent upon the release of norepinephrine. Directly acting sympathomimetics produce some, but not all, of the effects of norepinephrine and epinephrine depending on their selectivity for the various types of adrenoceptor. Indirectly acting agents enter nerve terminals by the uptake-1 process and displace norepinephrine from the storage vesicles. The displaced norepinephrine diffuses across the presynaptic membrane to stimulate the postsynaptic receptors. However, indirectly acting sympathomimetics are not specific in their actions and act, in part, by directly stimulating the receptors, inhibiting uptake 1, or inhibiting MAO. In addition to actions in the periphery, indirectly acting sympathomimetics may also have actions in the CNS. For example, amfetamine (amphetamine) (see Chapter 25) has a stimulant action in the CNS as a result of the release, not only of norepinephrine, but also of dopamine and 5-hydroxytryptamine from nerve terminals. A summary of the properties and clinical uses of sympathomimetics is given in Table 14.2.

Key facts
Noradrenergic transmission

- The starting substance for the synthesis of norepinephrine is tyrosine.

- Norepinephrine and epinephrine stimulate two principal types of G-protein-coupled receptors; α-adrenoceptors which have been further subdivided into α_1 and α_2, and β-adrenoceptors divided into β_1, β_2, and β_3 subtypes.

Table 14.2 The pharmacological properties and clinical use of sympathomimetic agents

Sympathomimetic	Action	Clinical use/effect	Administration	Comments
Directly acting				
Epinephrine (adrenaline)	α/β agonist	Cardiac arrest, vasoconstrictor in local anaesthetic solutions, anaphylactic shock, asthma (emergency only)	IV/IM/SC	
Dobutamine	β_1 agonist	Cardiogenic shock	IV	
Salbutamol	β_2 agonist	Asthma	Inhalation, occasionally orally or IV infusion in severe acute asthma	4–6 h duration of action following inhalation
Salmeterol	β_2 agonist	Asthma	Inhalation	12 h duration of action
Oxymetazoline	α_2 agonist	Nasal decongestant (constriction of nasal muscosa)	Nasal drops or spray	
Phenylephrine	α_1 agonist	Nasal decongestant, mydriatic, acute hypotension in spinal anaesthesia	Nasal drops, eye drops, IV injection, or infusion	
Clonidine	α_2 agonist	Antihypertensive	Oral	Lowers blood pressure by a central action (see Chapter 16)
Indirectly acting				
Tyramine	Norepinephrine (noradrenaline) release	No clinical use Present in foods		Interaction with MAO inhibitors used as antidepressants (see Chapter 15)
Ephedrine or one of its isomers, pseudoephedrine	Norepinephrine (noradrenaline) release, β-agonist	Nasal decongestant Weak CNS stimulant	Oral or nasal drops	
Amfetamine (amphetamine)	Norepinephrine release, uptake 1 and MAO inhibitor	CNS stimulant, Drug of abuse, Treatment of narcolepsy and hyperkinetic children (paradoxical use)	Oral	

- Postsynaptic α_1- and α_2-adrenoceptors produce constriction of vascular smooth muscle.
- Presynaptic α_2-adrenoceptors mediate the inhibition of norepinephrine release.
- β_1-Adrenoceptors produce cardiac stimulation, whilst β_2-receptors produce relaxation of bronchial smooth muscle and vasodilatation.
- The action of norepinephrine is primarily terminated by uptake into the nerve terminal.

- Sympathomimetic agents produce stimulation of adrenoceptors by directly stimulating adrenoceptors or indirectly by causing the release of norepinephrine.
- Epinephrine is used as a vasoconstrictor in local anaesthetic solutions, and in the treatment of anaphylactic shock, cardiac arrest, and a life-threatening asthmatic attack.

Alpha-adrenoceptor antagonists

A range of compounds have been synthesized possessing α-adrenoceptor blocking activity; either non-selective, showing similar affinity for α_1- and α_2-adrenoceptors, or selective for a particular α-adrenoceptor subtype. However, only phenoxybenzamine and selective α_1-adrenoceptor antagonists such as prazosin have found clinical uses.

Phenoxybenzamine is a non-selective, irreversible, competitive α-adrenoceptor antagonist used solely in the management of phaeochromocytoma—a catecholamine-secreting tumour of chromaffin tissue of the adrenal glands which produces episodes of severe hypertension. It is administered prior to surgery to block α-adrenoceptor-mediated vasoconstriction produced by the release of epinephrine which can occur on handling the tumour. An irreversible antagonist is required since the quantities of epinephrine suddenly released from the tumour may overcome the blockade produced by a reversible antagonist. To ensure the effective control of blood pressure, a β-adrenoceptor antagonist such as atenolol is also administered to block the cardiostimulant effects of released epinephrine.

The selective, competitive, reversible α_1-adrenoceptor antagonist prazosin and the longer acting doxazosin and terazosin produce vasodilatation and are used in the treatment of hypertension. Non-selective α-adrenoceptor antagonists are not used to control hypertension since they produce tachycardia and cardiac dysrhythmias due to an increase in norepinephrine release from sympathetic nerve terminals in the heart. This increased norepinephrine release results from the blockade of presynaptic α_2-adrenoceptors which have an inhibitory effect on norepinephrine release. By contrast to non-selective α-adrenoceptor antagonists, prazosin does not produce significant cardiac stimulation. However, postural hypotension (a marked fall in blood pressure upon standing, resulting in dizziness and possibly fainting) can be a problem which is particularly pronounced on starting treatment, the so-called 'first-dose phenomenon'. The risk of this phenomenon is minimized by using a low initial dose and then gradually increasing the dose until satisfactory control of blood pressure is achieved. α_1-Adrenoceptors are present in the trigone muscle of the bladder and urethra and stimulation increases resistance to the outflow of urine. Selective α_1-adrenoceptor antagonists reduce this resistance and are used to provide relief of urinary retention in patients with benign prostatic hyperplasia.

β-Adrenoceptor antagonists (β-blockers)

This is an important class of adrenoceptor antagonist because they have a number of clinical uses, particularly in the treatment of cardiovascular disease. The first competitive reversible β-adrenoceptor antagonist to be introduced for clinical use was propranolol and this has been followed by the development of a range of compounds with β-blocking activity. β-adrenoceptor antagonists are categorized according to receptor selectivity, partial agonist activity, and pharmacokinetic properties.

SELECTIVITY

A number of β-adrenoceptor antagonists such as propranolol have similar affinity for β_1- and β_2-adrenoceptors and are termed non-selective antagonists. By contrast, other antagonists, for example atenolol, have a greater affinity for β_1- compared to β_2-adrenoceptors. These antagonists are referred to as selective β_1-antagonists or cardioselective antagonists since their principal site of action is the heart, which contains predominately β_1-adrenoceptors. Most β-adrenoceptor antagonists have no affinity for β_3-adrenoceptors and therefore do not influence lipolysis (see Table 14.1). A small number of β-adrenoceptor antagonists, such as labetalol, also have affinity for α_1-adrenoceptors and therefore possess both α- and β-adrenoceptor blocking activity.

PARTIAL AGONIST ACTIVITY

β-Adrenoceptor antagonists possessing this property, such as pindolol, produce a low level of stimulation of β-adrenoceptors whilst antagonizing the action of full agonists such as norepinephrine and epinephrine. Those β-adrenoceptor antagonists that are partial agonists have potential clinical advantages, such as a reduced likelihood of precipitating cardiac failure.

PHARMACOKINETICS

Most β-adrenoceptor antagonists are well absorbed after oral administration, with elimination half-lives ranging from 3 to 24 hours. One exception is esmolol, this has an elimination half-life of 10 min due to a structure with an ester linkage that is rapidly hydrolysed by esterase enzymes present in erythrocytes. This particular β-adrenoceptor antagonist is given by intravenous infusion and used when a short-duration β-blockade is required, such as the control of supraventricular dysrhythmias in acutely ill patients. The oral bioavailability of β-adrenoceptor antagonists varies between 20% for labetalol to as high as 90% for sotalol. The low bioavailability of some β-adrenoceptor antagonists is due either to incomplete absorption (atenolol) or extensive first-pass metabolism (propranolol), the latter contributing to large variations in plasma concentrations (see Chapter 1). β-Adrenoceptor antagonists vary in their lipid-solubility with some, such as propranolol, having high lipid-solubility whilst others, for example atenolol, having low lipid-solubility. The degree of lipid-solubility influences the extent to which these drugs pass the blood–brain barrier and therefore the potential to exert actions in the CNS. A number of β-antagonists, such as propranolol and metoprolol, are metabolized extensively in the liver with little unchanged drug appearing in the urine, whilst others, such as atenolol and nadolol, are excreted in the urine largely unchanged. A summary of the properties of several β-adrenoceptor antagonists is given in Table 14.3.

Actions of β-adrenoceptor antagonists

The pharmacological actions of β-adrenoceptor antagonists can be deduced from the location of β-adrenoceptors and the effects they mediate as outlined in Table 14.1. The main effects of β-adrenoceptor antagonists are on the cardiovascular and respiratory systems, with some metabolic effects in diabetic patients. Their effects will depend upon the degree of sympathetic nerve activity which is low in patients at rest. Non-selective β-adrenoceptor antagonists produce little change in heart rate, cardiac output, or

Table 14.3 Properties of several β-adrenoceptor antagonists

Type	Partial agonist activity	Lipid solubility	$t_{0.5}$	Oral bioavailability (%)	Comments on absorption/metabolism/excretion
Non-selective ($\beta_1 + \beta_2$)					
Propranolol	0	High	3–5 h	25	Extensive first-pass metabolism
Nadolol	0	Low	10–20 h	35	Incomplete absorption; excreted in urine unchanged
Sotalol	0	Low	12 h	90	Excreted mainly unchanged in the urine
Timolol	0	moderate	3–5 h	50	Undergoes moderate first-pass metabolism
Labetalol*	+	Moderate	4–6 h	20	Extensive first-pass metabolism
Pindolol	++	Moderate	3–5 h	75	50% metabolized in liver
Selective (β_1)					
Atenolol	0	Low	6–9 h	50	Incomplete absorption; excreted mainly unchanged in the urine
Esmolol	0	Low	10 min	—	Only given IV; hydrolysed in blood
Metoprolol	0	Moderate	3–4 h	40	Undergoes moderate first-pass metabolism
Acebutolol	+	Low	3–4 h	50	Undergoes moderate first-pass metabolism

*Labetalol is also a potent α_1 antagonist and has partial agonist activity at β_2 receptors only.

blood pressure in subjects at rest, although they will reduce the cardiovascular effects of exercise or emotional excitement when the sympathetic system is activated. β-Adrenoceptor antagonists with partial agonist activity will similarly reduce the cardiovascular response to activation of the sympathetic system, but, by contrast to β-adrenoceptor antagonists devoid of partial agonist activity, will increase the heart rate at rest.

β-Adrenoceptor antagonists have little effect on airway resistance in normal subjects, but non-selective antagonists, such as propranolol, can produce dangerous bronchoconstriction in asthmatic patients due to the blockade of β_2-adrenoceptors that mediate the relaxation of bronchial smooth muscle. The possibility of producing bronchoconstriction in asthmatic patients or patients with other forms of obstructive airway diseases is less with selective β_1-adrenoceptor antagonists. However, these antagonists are not so selective as to eliminate the risk, and therefore even selective β_1-antagonists should not be given to asthmatic patients.

The metabolic effects of β-adrenoceptor antagonists in normal subjects are minor, but non-selective antagonists increase the likelihood of exercise-induced hypoglycaemia in insulin-dependent diabetics. This occurs because, during exercise, epinephrine induces the release of glucose from the liver as a result of β_2-adrenoceptor stimulation of glycogenolysis. This effect is less likely to occur with selective β_1-antagonists. The use of β-antagonists in diabetic patients presents an additional hazard since sympathetically mediated muscle tremor, as well as increases in

cardiac rate and force of contraction are important warning signs of hypoglycaemia. Consequently, hypoglycaemia is likely to go unnoticed with no remedial action taken (usually a sugary drink) if diabetic patients are treated with a β-antagonist. Since β_1-receptors mediate the increase in heart rate, this effect will occur with either non-selective or β_1-selective antagonists.

CLINICAL USE

The main use of these drugs is in the treatment of cardiovascular diseases, namely *hypertension, angina*, and *cardiac dysrhythmias*. Their use in these diseases is discussed in detail in Chapter 16. β-Adrenoceptor antagonists have other clinical uses, namely:

- *Hypertrophic obstructive cardiomyopathy*: Propranolol reduces the angina, palpitations, and syncope in patients with this disorder. The beneficial effects result from slowing of ventricular ejection.

- *Migraine*: A number of β-antagonists such as propranolol and timolol are effective in the prophylaxis of migraine, although the mechanism of action is unclear.

- *Hyperthyroidism (thyrotoxicosis)*: Many of the symptoms of hyperthyroidism, such as tachycardia and tremor, are similar to excessive activity of the sympathetic nervous system although catecholamines levels are not increased. These effects are probably a result of up-regulation of β-adrenoceptors or an enhancement of receptor–effector coupling mechanisms. β-Adrenoceptor antagonists control many of the symptoms of hyperthyroidism and propranolol inhibits the conversion of levothyroxine (thyroxine) to triiodothyronine (see Chapter 19), although this effect may not be related to β-blockade.

- *Glaucoma*: β-Adrenoceptor antagonists decrease intraocular pressure by decreasing the rate of production of aqueous humour by the ciliary body (a β_1-receptor-mediated effect). Timolol administered as eye drops is the most popular treatment for glaucoma because of the convenience (once or twice daily dosing) and the lower incidence of unwanted effects compared to pilocarpine and physostigmine. However, timolol is systemically absorbed and can produce adverse cardiovascular and pulmonary effects.

- *Anxiety*: Acute anxiety attacks are characterized by tachycardia and muscle tremors resulting from increased sympathetic activity. Propranolol and other β-antagonists are useful in controlling the symptoms of these anxiety attacks. Propranolol may also be useful in the treatment of benign essential tremor.

ADVERSE EFFECTS

- *Cardiac failure*: Patients with heart disease may be dependent on sympathetic drive to the heart to maintain an adequate cardiac output. Removal of this sympathetic drive with a β-antagonist may precipitate some degree of heart failure. Drugs with partial agonist activity, e.g. pindolol, have the potential advantage of producing cardiac stimulation in patients at rest, and therefore should be less likely to produce cardiac failure. However, clinical studies have failed to produce clear evidence of any advantage.

- *Hypoglycaemia*: As discussed above, β-adrenoceptor antagonists may precipitate hypoglycaemia by reducing the release of glucose in response to epinephrine as well as blocking the warning signs of hypoglycaemia.

- *Fatigue*: This is experienced during exercise by patients taking β-adrenoceptor antagonists and is due to reduced cardiac output and reduced muscle blood flow, the latter as a result of vasodilator β_2-adrenoceptor blockade.

- *Bronchoconstriction*: Both non-selective and β_1-selective antagonists have the potential to produce life-threatening bronchoconstriction in asthmatic patients, as described above. As a result all β-antagonists are contraindicated in asthmatics and patients with other forms of obstructive airway disease such as chronic bronchitis and emphysema.

- *Cold extremities*: Some patients complain of cold extremities whilst taking β-adrenoceptor antagonists and symptoms of peripheral vascular disease may be aggravated. These effects result from the blockade of β_2-adrenoceptor-mediated vasodilatation in skin and skeletal muscle. β_1-Selective antagonists or drugs with partial agonist activity should be less likely to produce these effects, although it is not known whether this is the case in practice.

- *Central nervous system effects*: β-Adrenoceptor antagonists can produce sleep disturbances, including insomnia and nightmares, and depression as a result of their actions in the CNS. The incidence of these effects is believed to be lower with poorly lipid-soluble drugs such as atenolol than with highly lipid-soluble drugs such as propranolol (see Table 14.3), since the latter cross the blood–brain barrier more easily.

Key facts
α-, β-Adrenoceptor antagonists

- Phenoxybenzamine, a competitive, irreversible, non-selective α-antagonist, is used to control blood pressure during surgery in patients with a phaeochromocytoma.

- Selective α_1-antagonists such as prazosin produce vasodilatation and are used in the treatment of hypertension.

- A number of β-adrenoceptor antagonists, such as propranolol, have similar affinity for β_1- and β_2- receptors and are termed non-selective antagonists, whilst others, such as atenolol, have a greater affinity for β_1-receptors (β_1-selective).

- Labetalol is both a non-selective β-antagonist and an α_1-antagonist.

- β-Adrenoceptor antagonists are an important class of drugs with a range of clinical uses, including the treatment of: hypertension; angina; cardiac dysrhythmias; glaucoma; anxiety; and hyperthyroidism.

- Adverse effects of β-adrenoceptor antagonists include: bronchoconstriction in asthmatics; cardiac failure; hypoglycaemia in patients with diabetes mellitus; cold extremities; fatigue; depression; and sleep disturbances.

Further reading

Brown, J. H. and Taylor P. (1996). Muscarinic receptor agonists and antagonists. In: *Goodman and Gilman's the pharmacological basis of therapeutics* (9th edn) (ed. J. G. Hardman, L. E. Limbird, P. B. Molinoff, R. W. Ruddon, and A. G. Gilman), pp 141–60. McGraw Hill, New York.

Hoffman, B. B. (1998). Adrenoceptor antagonist drugs. In: *Basic and clinical pharmacology* (7th edn) (ed. B. G. Katzung), pp 136–51. Appleton and Lange, Stamford, Connecticut.

Parsons, S. M., Prior, C., and Marshall, I. G. (1993). Acetylcholine transport, storage and release. *International Review of Neurobiology*, 35, 279–390.

Ruffolo, R. R., Nichols, A. J., Stadel, J. M., and Hieble, J. P. (1991). Structure and function of α-adrenoceptors. *Pharmacological Reviews*, 43, 475–505.

Starke, K., Göthert, M., and Kilbinger, H. (1989). Modulation of transmitter release by presynaptic autoreceptors. *Physiological Reviews*, 69, 864–989.

15

Drugs and the central nervous system

- Psychoses and neuroleptic drugs
- Depression and antidepressants
- Parkinson's disease and its drug treatment
- Hypnotics and anxiolytics
- Epilepsy, facial neuralgias, and anticonvulsants
- Migraine
- Further reading

Drugs and the central nervous system

This chapter is concerned with disorders of the central nervous system (CNS) and their treatment. The following will be considered:

- psychoses and neuroleptic drugs;
- depression and antidepressants;
- Parkinson's disease and its drug treatment;
- hypnotics and anxiolytics;
- epilepsy, facial neuralgias, and anticonvulsants;
- migraine, and drugs used in the prophylaxis and treatment of migraine.

Other categories of drugs act on the CNS but are discussed elsewhere; these include opioid analgesics (see Chapter 7), general anaesthetic agents (see Chapter 9), and antiemetic drugs (see Chapter 18).

Psychoses and neuroleptic drugs

Psychoses

Psychosis is a mental state in which there is an impairment in behaviour associated with an inability to think coherently and to comprehend reality. Symptoms may include delusions, hallucinations, and thought alienation whereby patients believe that their thoughts are under the control of an external agency. The patient also has no insight into these abnormalities, that is to say the patient is unaware there is a problem. Psychosis is not a specific disorder but a series of characteristic symptoms that, in addition to psychotic illness such as schizophrenia and delusional disorders, may occur in some depressive illnesses. Psychosis may be a result of damage to the brain—arising, for example, from a head injury, an infection such as encephalitis, or alcoholism. These types of psychoses are referred to as organic psychoses. Many forms of psychosis have no obvious cause, although subtle changes in the levels of neurotransmitters or their receptors have been postulated to underlie the changes in behaviour.

Schizophrenia is the most common psychotic illness, having an incidence in the population of 0.2–1%, with a strong hereditary component. It features the positive symptoms described above in addition to negative symptoms, such as withdrawal from family and friends, flattening of emotions, attention impairment, and restriction of spontaneous speech. Positive symptoms are characteristic of the acute phase of the disorder, whilst negative symptoms predominate in chronic schizophrenia. Schizophrenia may completely resolve in some patients with no further recurrence. However, the illness recurs repeatedly in the majority of patients, of whom a proportion may have incomplete recovery with more severe symptoms present with each successive relapse. Hypotheses to explain the cause of schizophrenia have implicated changes in the levels of various central neurotransmitters including dopamine, 5-hydroxytryptamine (5-HT), glutamate, and γ-aminobutyric acid (GABA). The role of excess dopamine in schizophrenia has received the greatest attention, in part because many drugs used in the treatment of schizophrenia block dopamine receptors. However, postmortem studies of dopamine levels in the brains of schizophrenics have produced equivocal results.

Neuroleptic drugs (antipsychotic drugs)

The terms neuroleptic, antipsychotic, and antischizophrenic are used interchangeably and describe drugs used in the treatment of psychoses. A further term for these drugs is major tranquillizers, but this can give rise to confusion with the anxiolytic drugs, such as the benzodiazepines, and therefore should be avoided. Typical or classical neuroleptic drugs block dopamine D_1- and D_2-receptors, particularly in the mesocortical and mesolimbic regions of the brain. To date, five different types of dopamine receptor have been pharmacologically identified and cloned, D_1–D_5; stimulation of these G-protein-coupled receptors produces increases (D_1 and D_5) or decreases (D_2, D_3, and D_4) in cAMP levels, resulting in either presynaptic or postsynaptic inhibition. The more recently developed atypical neuroleptics have, in general, a lower affinity for D_2 receptors but with higher affinities for dopamine D_4 receptors in the limbic cortex and 5-HT$_2$ receptors in the frontal cortex. In addition, atypical neuroleptics have a lower incidence, compared to typical neuroleptics, of unwanted motor disturbances. Neuroleptic drugs can be divided into two main groups: the typical and atypical neuroleptics.

TYPICAL NEUROLEPTICS
Namely:

- phenothiazines, which are further classified into:
  - drugs with an aliphatic side chain, e.g. chlorpromazine,

– piperidine derivatives, such as thioridazine,
– piperazine derivatives, e.g. trifluoperazine;

- thioxanthenes, e.g. flupentixol (flupenthixol);

- butyrophenones (e.g. haloperidol and droperidol) and diphenylbutylpiperidines (e.g. pimozide, which is a selective D_2 antagonist).

ATYPICAL NEUROLEPTICS

These are the:

- benzamides, such as sulpiride;

- dibenzodiazepines, e.g. clozapine and loxapine;

- benzisoxazoles, e.g. risperidone.

Psychotic patients successfully treated with neuroleptic drugs, either typical or atypical, initially become less aggressive and withdrawn. Over the following days there is a marked reduction in psychotic symptoms of hallucinations, delusions, and disorganized thoughts. The negative symptoms of schizophrenia, such as flattening of emotions, may also improve, although some reports suggest that neuroleptics have less ability to relieve negative symptoms compared to positive symptoms. Patients may not respond to a particular drug or respond better to one than another, and selection of the best treatment may be a process of trial and error with each drug assessed over a period of 4–6 weeks. Some authorities recommend that initial treatment of psychotic illnesses is with the atypical neuroleptic risperidone since this drug has a reduced incidence of extrapyramidal symptoms (see below). Should this prove ineffective a typical neuroleptic such as a phenothiazine should be given. However, the selection of antipsychotic treatment is very much dependent on a psychiatrist's experience with a particular drug(s). Neuroleptic drugs can be administered orally or by intramuscular injection, the latter route is of use in acutely disturbed and agitated patients. A number of esters of typical neuroleptics are formulated as depot preparations. These are given as deep intramuscular injections, with dosing intervals of between 2 and 4 weeks, and are useful for maintenance treatment to ensure patient compliance, although they have a higher rate of extrapyramidal reactions. The use of depot preparations allows patients to be cared for and treated in the community rather than as hospital in-patients. As a result of the blockade of dopamine D_2 receptors, a number of neuroleptic drugs have useful antiemetic properties (see Chapter 18).

Adverse effects of neuroleptics

Neuroleptic drugs can produce a wide range of adverse effects:

- *Sedation*: Many neuroleptic drugs, particularly chlorpromazine, have a pronounced sedative effect, although tolerance to this effect usually develops. The sedative effect is probably due to antagonism of histamine H_1-receptors.

- *Neuroendocrine effects*: A dopaminergic pathway exerts an inhibitory effect on prolactin secretion from the anterior pituitary. Blockade of the relevant dopamine D_2 receptors by neuroleptic drugs results in an increased secretion of pro-

lactin, which produces amenorrhoea (absence of menstruation), and breast enlargement and lactation in men as well as women.

- *Autonomic effects*: Many neuroleptics have antagonistic actions at muscarinic receptors and these can result in decreased sweating, dry mouth, constipation, and blurred vision. Chlorpromazine, thioridazine, and to a lesser extent haloperidol and risperidone have α-adrenoceptor blocking actions that can result in postural hypotension.

- *Immunological hypersensitivity reactions*: Skin reactions are common, occurring in 5% of patients taking chlorpromazine, and include urticaria, dermatitis, and photosensitivity that resembles severe sunburn. Cholestatic jaundice is a rare hypersensitivity reaction to chlorpromazine, but the jaundice is mild and disappears quickly on withdrawal of the drug. Leucopenia and agranulocytosis, potentially fatal reactions, may occur but the incidence is low (1 in 10 000 patients) with most neuroleptic drugs. However, the incidence is much higher with clozapine (in 1% of patients within a few months of treatment) and its use requires regular monitoring of white cell numbers. As a consequence of this reaction, clozapine is only indicated for the treatment of schizophrenia if patients are unresponsive to, or intolerant of other neuroleptics.

- *Neurological effects*:
  - *Acute dystonic reactions* can occur within days of starting treatment and consist of muscle spasms of the tongue, face, neck, and back, which can cause severe distress. They are most common in young males and dramatically improve following the intramuscular or intravenous administration of muscarinic antagonists used in the treatment of Parkinson's disease, benzatropine (benztropine) and procyclidine.
  - *Akathisia* is subjective feelings of restlessness and discomfort with a need to be constantly moving, i.e. motor restlessness. Treatment is a reduction in neuroleptic drug dosage.
  - *Parkinsonism* (see below) results from a blockade of dopamine D_2 receptors in basal ganglia. The symptoms can appear days to weeks after starting neuroleptic treatment and are managed either by a reduction in dose; transfer to an atypical neuroleptic (for example risperidone, which is less likely to produce such effects), or use of muscarinic antagonists such as procyclidine.
  - *Neuroleptic malignant syndrome* is a rare but life-threatening disorder (mortality rate of 10–20%), which can occur within days or weeks following initiation of neuroleptic treatment. Symptoms are hyperthermia, muscle rigidity with possible muscle damage, labile blood pressure, and fluctuating consciousness. Management is immediate withdrawal from the neuroleptic drug and treatment with the muscle-relaxant drug dantrolene (also used in

the treatment of malignant hyperthermia—see Chapter 9) or the dopamine agonist bromocriptine to reverse dopamine receptor blockade.

- *Tardive dyskinesia* appears after months or years of neuroleptic treatment and is characterized by stereotyped repetitive involuntary tic-like (choreiform) movements of the face, eyelids, mouth (lip smacking), tongue, and limbs. There may also be twisting movements of the trunk and sustained postures. Symptoms can persist indefinitely after withdrawal of treatment, but they frequently diminish or disappear over the ensuing months. The mechanism for tardive dyskinesia is unclear but may involve the upregulation of dopamine receptors. There is no effective treatment and therefore early recognition is important. An increase in the dose of the neuroleptic drug may provide temporary relief, whilst the incidence of tardive dyskinesia is less with atypical neuroleptics.

Key facts
Psychoses and neuroleptic drugs

- Psychoses such as schizophrenia are characterized by thought disorder, hallucinations, and delusions (positive symptoms) as well as flattening of emotions, attention impairment, and withdrawal from social contacts (negative symptoms).

- Treatment is with neuroleptic drugs (antipsychotic drugs). These are categorized as typical neuroleptics (e.g. chlorpromazine, flupentixol (flupenthixol), and haloperidol) and atypical neuroleptics (e.g. risperidone). Typical neuroleptics are dopamine D_1- and D_2-receptor antagonists whilst atypical neuroleptics have, in general, low affinity for D_2 receptors but high affinity for either dopamine D_4 and/or $5-HT_2$ receptors. Atypical neuroleptics have a lower incidence, compared to typical neuroleptics, of the neurological adverse effects that produce motor disturbances.

- Neuroleptics produce a range of adverse effects, of which the most distressing to the patient are the motor disturbances, i.e.:
  - dystonias (muscle spasms);
  - akathisia (motor restlessness);
  - parkinsonism (tremor at rest, muscle rigidity, and difficulty in initiating movement—akinesia);
  - neuroleptic malignant syndrome (a rare but life-threatening disorder characterized by hyperthermia, muscle rigidity, labile blood pressure, and fluctuating consciousness);
  - tardive (late) dyskinesia, appearing after months or years of neuroleptic treatment with symptoms of stereotyped repetitive involuntary choreiform movements.

- Other adverse effects include: sedation; increased prolactin secretion (causing breast enlargement and lactation); dry mouth, etc. (due to muscarinic receptor blockade); postural hypotension (due to α-adrenoceptor blockade); skin rashes, jaundice (a reaction to chlorpromazine); and leucopenia and agranulocytosis (most common with clozapine).

Depression and antidepressants
Depression

Depression and mania are affective disorders, referring to changes in mood as opposed to the disturbances of thought characteristic of psychoses. Depression is one of the most common mental illnesses, with an estimated 10% of the population becoming depressed at some time during their lives. The symptoms of depression include feelings of apathy, pessimism, and misery; lack of self-esteem; loss of concentration; sleep disturbances characterized by difficulty getting to sleep and early morning waking; loss of appetite; and suicidal thoughts, which occur in 10–15% of depressed individuals. Depressive conditions can be broadly divided into unipolar and bipolar depression, i.e. when the patient is depressed or oscillates between episodes of depression and mania. Episodes of mania are characterized by excessive elation, hyperactivity, insomnia, excessive physical activity in combination with irritability and impatience. Unipolar depression may be precipitated by specific stimuli such as bereavement and serious illness (reactive depression), whilst depression may have no obvious cause (endogenous depression or major depression). The latter form of depression is normally associated with disturbances of sleep and appetite, and usually responds specifically to antidepressant treatment, whereas reactive depression may resolve spontaneously. Unipolar and bipolar depression are treated differently, unipolar with antidepressants and bipolar with mood-stabilizing drugs. Treatment, other than with drugs, is also available such as psychotherapy and electroconvulsive therapy (ECT), the latter can be used in patients unresponsive to antidepressant treatment. Both unipolar and bipolar depression may be associated with anxiety, or delusions and hallucinations (psychotic depression).

The main theory proposed to explain depression is the monoamine hypothesis, which states that depression is a result of a functional deficit in monoamine neurotransmitters (norepinephrine (noradrenaline), dopamine, or 5-HT) at key locations in the brain. The converse of this theory is that mania is the result of an functional excess of monoamines. The theory arose from pharmacological evidence that antidepressants potentiate the actions of monoamines, whereas reserpine—an obsolete antihypertensive drug, which lowers blood pressure by depleting monoamines—caused depression. The monoamine hypothesis was originally advanced in relation to norepinephrine, although more recent work has highlighted the importance of 5-HT (four main types of 5-HT receptor have been identified, $5-HT_{1-4}$, with further subdivisions of types 1 and 2; all receptors are G-protein-coupled to either adenylyl cyclase or phospholipase C with the exception of the 5-HT$_3$ receptor which is a ligand-gated ion channel).

Biochemical studies of monoamine levels in blood, cerebrospinal fluid, urine, and postmortem brain tissue from depressed patients have, in general, provided little support for the hypothesis. Furthermore, whilst the biochemical action of antidepressants occurs rapidly, the relief of depression can take weeks to develop. This delay in clinical response has been attributed to receptor downregulation in response to elevation in monoamine levels. Downregulation (a reduction in density) of 5-HT$_{1A/2}$ receptors, and α_2- and β-adrenoceptors has been demonstrated following chronic antidepressant treatment (see Fig. 15.1), although the relationship between these changes and an antidepressant action is unclear. In summary, whilst the majority of antidepressant drugs enhance the actions of monoamines, the monoamine theory of depression still remains to be accepted.

Tricyclic antidepressants

Tricyclic antidepressants (TCA), so named because of a characteristic 3-ring structure, include amitriptyline, imipramine, nortriptyline, doxepin, and clomipramine. These drugs block the reuptake of neurotransmitter monoamines into the nerve terminal by competing with the monoamines for the transporter protein (Fig 15.1). They block the uptake of both norepinephrine and 5-HT with less effect on the uptake of dopamine, although their antidepressant effect is probably a result of their ability to augment 5-HT neurotransmission rather than noradrenergic transmission. Their antidepressant effect can take up to 2 weeks to occur and treatment is ineffective in 30–40% of depressed patients. The delay to onset of an antidepressant effect may produce problems of patient compliance; patients may stop taking the drugs in the belief that they are ineffective or in response to minor adverse effects. In addition to binding to the monoamine

carrier, tricyclic antidepressants also have affinity for histamine H$_1$-receptors and muscarinic receptors therefore accounting for some of their adverse effects:

- sedation (due to histamine H$_1$ receptor blockade), although this may be an advantage in patients with sleep disturbances;

- dry mouth, blurred vision, constipation, urinary retention (due to muscarinic receptor antagonism);

- postural hypotension;

- weight gain.

These drugs are frequently used in suicide attempts, resulting in life-threatening toxic effects on the heart and CNS. Cardiac dysrhythmias are common and the initial CNS effects are excitement, delirium, and sometimes convulsions followed by coma and respiratory depression which may persist for days.

Tricyclic antidepressants are well absorbed following oral administration and metabolism in the liver can generate pharmacological active metabolites. For example, imipramine and amitriptyline undergo N-demethylation resulting in the production of desmethylimipramine and nortriptyline, respectively, both of which have antidepressant actions.

In addition to the treatment of depression, tricyclics are used in the treatment of:

- Obsessive–compulsive disorders (clomipramine).

- Chronic pain: A number of chronic pain states with no obvious causes respond to treatment with tricyclics. It is unclear whether these drugs interfere with pain pathways or that the pain is an expression of underlying depression.

- Enuresis (urinary incontinence): Drug treatment is not the preferred approach to this condition but tricyclics, such as amitriptyline and imipramine, may be effective in controlling the problem.

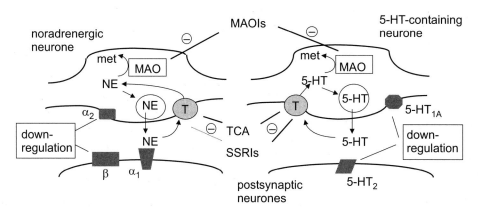

Fig 15.1 Sites of action of antidepressant drugs. Tricyclic antidepressants (TCA) inhibit the reuptake of norepinephrine (NE) and 5-HT into noradrenergic and 5-HT-containing neurones by binding to the respective transporters (T), whilst selective serotonin (5-HT) reuptake inhibitors (SSRIs) block the reuptake of 5-HT with only a minor effect on norepinephrine uptake. Monoamine oxidase inhibitors (MAOIs) inhibit the deamination of norepinephrine and 5-HT, thus elevating the cytoplasmic pool of these monoamines. A secondary response to antidepressants is down-regulation of α_2-adrenoceptors (α_2), β-adrenoceptors (β), and 5-HT$_{1A/2}$ receptors. met, metabolites.

Selective serotonin reuptake inhibitors (SSRIs)

These drugs, which include fluoxetine, fluvoxamine, paroxetine, and sertraline, are as effective as tricyclics in treating depression with fluoxetine (Prozac)—currently the most prescribed antidepressant. In contrast to tricyclics, they selectively block the reuptake of 5-HT (serotonin) and therefore enhance 5-HT-mediated transmission with only a minor effect on norepinephrine reuptake (Fig 15.1). Compared to tricyclics, they have little affinity for histamine H_1 and muscarinic receptors but show a similar delay of 2–4 weeks before an antidepressant effect is evident. SSRIs are less sedative with lower cardiotoxicity than the tricyclics. However, they have their own adverse-effect profile:

- gastrointestinal effects: nausea, vomiting, and diarrhoea;
- headache;
- anxiety and restlessness that resembles akathisia;
- insomnia;
- sexual dysfunction, including inhibition of ejaculation.

SSRIs are well absorbed after oral administration. Fluoxetine undergoes demethylation to an active metabolite norfluoxetine, which has a plasma half-life of 7–9 days, i.e. slightly longer than the half-life of the parent drug.

Other therapeutic uses of SSRIs include the treatment of eating disorders (bulimia) and obsessive–compulsive disorders.

Monoamine oxidase (MAO) inhibitors

Inhibitors of MAO were the first drugs to be introduced for the treatment of depression but, due to their adverse effects and interactions with certain foods, they have been largely superseded by tricyclic antidepressants and SSRIs. MAO is found in one of two forms in nearly all tissues; MAO-A which has a substrate preference for 5-HT and MAO-B with preference for phenylethylamines. Both forms of the enzyme will metabolize dopamine and norepinephrine. MAO-A has wide tissue distribution, whilst MAO-B predominates at sites of dopaminergic transmission in the CNS.

Most of the available MAO inhibitors—such as phenelzine, isocarboxazid, and tranylcypromine—irreversibly inhibit both forms of the enzyme, although the antidepressant action and adverse effects have been attributed to inhibition of MAO-A. However, moclobemide, a more recent MAO inhibitor, acts reversibly and is selective for MAO-A. MAO is contained within the cytosol of noradrenergic, dopaminergic, and 5-HT-containing neurones and metabolizes monoamines in the cytosol that are not contained within storage vesicles (Fig. 15.1 and see Chapter 14). Inhibition of MAO increases the levels of norepinephrine, dopamine, and 5-HT within neurones in the brain and peripheral tissues, with levels of 5-HT most affected. This results in an increased rate of spontaneous leak of monoamines from the cytoplasm, whilst the response to nerve stimulation is little affected since MAO inhibition does not have a great effect on vesicular stores of monoamines. This lack of effect on neurotransmission contrasts with tricyclics and SSRIs which enhance transmission although, similar to these antidepressant drugs, monoamine oxidase inhibitors produce receptor downregulation (Fig. 15.1)

One of the most serious problems with MAO inhibitors is an interaction with foods containing tyramine, 'the cheese reaction'. Tyramine is an indirect sympathomimetic which displaces norepinephrine from vesicles into the cytosol, from where it is either metabolized by MAO or leaks out to produce a response via interaction with postsynaptic receptors. When foods containing tyramine are ingested, the amine is normally metabolized by MAO in the gut wall and little tyramine is absorbed. However, in the presence of MAO inhibition, this does not occur and tyramine reaches the systemic circulation. When taken up by noradrenergic nerve terminals, the response to tyramine is enhanced, since MAO present in the nerve terminals is also inhibited and is unable to metabolize the displaced norepinephrine. The result of tyramine ingestion in patients taking MAO inhibitors is a sudden rise in blood pressure producing a throbbing headache with the possibility of intracranial haemorrhage. To avoid this interaction, patients taking MAO inhibitors are given a list of foods containing tyramine that must avoided, examples of which are mature cheeses and yeast products. Drugs such as ephedrine, an indirect sympathomimetic used as a nasal decongestant, should also be avoided. The risk of these interactions is less with the reversible inhibitor moclobemide. Other adverse effects of MAO inhibitors include:

- antimuscarinic effects such as dry mouth, blurred vision etc.;
- tremors, excitement, insomnia, with convulsions in overdose;
- weight gain due to increased appetite;
- hypotension (paradoxical);
- hepatotoxicity with phenelzine although this is rare.

MAO inhibitors are used to treat depression in patients who are refractory to tricyclics and SSRIs and, similar to other antidepressants, a therapeutic effect can take 3 weeks to develop with an additional 1–2 weeks before the response is maximal. Depressed patients with severe anxiety and hypochondrial symptoms respond well to MAO inhibitors and these drugs are also effective in the treatment of phobias and panic disorder.

Atypical antidepressants (heterocyclics)

These are a group of compounds, including maprotiline, mianserin, and trazodone, that have efficacy as antidepressants but do not neatly fall into the previous categories of antidepressant drugs. They have advantages over tricyclics in that they have a lower incidence of sedation and antimuscarinic effects and reduced toxicity in overdose, although they show a similar delay in onset of action. Atypical antidepressant are no more effective than tricyclics but they are of use in patients who are intolerant of their adverse effects. The proposed modes of action of atypical antidepressants include blockade of monoamine uptake, although with little activity against 5-HT (maprotiline), and blockade of presynaptic α_2-adrenoceptors on noradrenergic nerve terminals which, by reducing inhibitory feedback, enhances norepinephrine release (mianserin). The adverse effects of atypical antidepressants include rashes and an increased risk of convulsions (maprotiline), and leucopenia and influenza-like syndrome (mianserin).

Mood stabilizing drugs

LITHIUM

Lithium, administered orally in the form of lithium carbonate or citrate, prevents mood swings in patients with bipolar depression as well as being effective in particular cases of unipolar depression. Specific uses are:

- prophylaxis of both depressive and manic phases of bipolar depression;
- treatment of acute mania, although neuroleptics are as effective and act more quickly;
- prophylaxis of recurrent unipolar depression;
- as an adjunct to tricyclics or SSRIs when these antidepressants fail to fully relieve depression.

The precise mode of action of lithium is unclear but it appears to result from an inhibitory effect on receptor–effector transduction mechanisms. Lithium inhibits the recycling of inositol phosphates, which reduces the release of the second messengers IP_3 and DAG produced by phospholipase C (see Chapter 2). This action will have a depressant effect on neurotransmission involving the phospholipase-C transduction pathway, such as transmission mediated via α_1-adrenoceptors, and could explain lithium's suppression of mania. In addition, lithium also inhibits agonist-induced stimulation of adenylyl cyclase, possibly by modifying the function or abundance of G-proteins. This action might contribute to both its antimania and antidepressant actions.

Lithium is cleared by the kidneys: about 50% of an oral dose is excreted over the following 6–12 hours whilst the remainder is slowly excreted over the next 10–14 days. As a result, lithium accumulates during initial treatment, with a steady-state plasma concentration reached after 14 days. Lithium has a narrow therapeutic range, which necessitates regularly monitoring of plasma concentrations to avoid toxicity. A concentration of 0.75–1.25 mM is considered to be effective and reasonably safe. The toxic effects of lithium are:

- nausea, vomiting, and diarrhoea;
- tremor;
- polyuria and associated polydipsia, due to inhibition of the action of antidiuretic hormone on the collecting ducts of the kidney;

- inhibition of thyroid function, with thyroid enlargement noted in some patients;
- weight gain due, in part, to oedema produced by sodium retention.

Acute lithium toxicity (plasma concentrations, 3–5 mM) produces neurological effects, which range from confusion to coma, convulsions, and death.

CARBAMAZEPINE AND SODIUM VALPROATE

These anticonvulsant drugs, which are used in the treatment of epilepsy, are also of benefit in the prophylaxis of bipolar depression. They are given either alone or in combination with lithium to patients who are unresponsive to monotherapy with lithium. The details of the mechanisms of action and adverse effects of carbamazepine and sodium valproate are described later.

Key facts
Depression and antidepressant drugs

- Depression and mania are affective disorders characterized by changes in mood. Depressive conditions can be divided into unipolar depression (depression only) and bipolar depression (episodes of depression alternating with mania).

- Unipolar depression can be treated with tricyclic antidepressants, selective serotonin reuptake inhibitors (SSRIs), monoamine oxidase inhibitors, and atypical antidepressants.

- Tricyclics, such as amitriptyline and imipramine, inhibit the neuronal uptake of the neurotransmitters norepinephrine (noradrenaline) and serotonin (5-HT), whilst SSRIs, e.g. fluoxetine, block the reuptake of 5-HT with little effect on norepinephrine uptake. Inhibition of monoamine uptake enhances neurotransmission.

- Monoamine oxidase (MAO) inhibitors prevent the deamination of norepinephrine, dopamine, and 5-HT, thus elevating cytoplasmic levels of these transmitters in nerve terminals. Antidepressant activity results from inhibition of MAO type A. Most MAO inhibitors, e.g. phenelzine and tranylcypromine, are irreversible inhibitors of type A and type B MAO, whilst moclobemide is a selective reversible inhibitor of MAO-A. Moclobemide is less likely, compared to irreversible inhibitors, to produce hypertension following ingestion of foods containing tyramine. MAO inhibitors are used to treat depression in patients who are refractory to tricyclics and SSRIs.

- Atypical antidepressants, such as mianserin, have a variety of ill-defined mechanisms of action. There are useful in individual patients who find the adverse effects of tricyclics and SSRIs unacceptable.

- Although their biochemical effects develop quickly, all antidepressants take 2–3 weeks before producing a beneficial effect. This indicates that secondary effects underlie their antidepressant action. Such secondary effects include the downregulation of 5-HT$_{1A}/_2$ receptors, and α_2- and β-adrenoceptors, although the relationship between these changes in receptor density and antidepressant action is unclear.

- Lithium, as lithium carbonate or citrate, is used principally in the prophylaxis of both depressive and manic phases of bipolar depression. It has an inhibitory effect on receptor–effector transduction mechanisms. Lithium has a narrow 'therapeutic window' and therefore monitoring of plasma concentrations is essential to avoid toxic effects.

Parkinson's disease and its drug treatment

Parkinson's disease

This is a progressive neurological disease that results in impaired voluntary movement. There are two systems involved in the control of movement: (1) neuronal pathways of the corticospinal system travelling in pyramidal tracts to directly affect lower motor neurones in the spinal cord; and (2) additional descending pathways (extrapyramidal tracts) that indirectly affect lower motor neurones. The corticospinal and additional descending systems are interconnected and co-operate to control complex voluntary movement. A major influence on the additional descending pathways are the basal ganglia (caudate nucleus, globus pallidum, thalamus, and substantia nigra). Parkinson's disease, currently of unknown cause, is a condition in which dopaminergic neurones in the basal ganglia, particularly the substantia nigra, deteriorate and eventually die. This neurodegenerative disease was first described by James Parkinson in 1817 in a publication entitled 'An essay on the shaking palsy'. The connections between the basal ganglia involved in Parkinson's disease are shown in Fig 15.2.

The result of degeneration of the dopaminergic pathway from the substantia nigra to the corpus striatum is a loss of an inhibitory influence on cholinergic neurones, resulting in their overactivity thus producing the characteristic symptoms of Parkinson's disease:

- muscle rigidity;

- resting tremor with the hands involved in 'pill-rolling movements';

- akinesia/hypokinesia (lack of movement) and bradykinesia (slowness of movement);

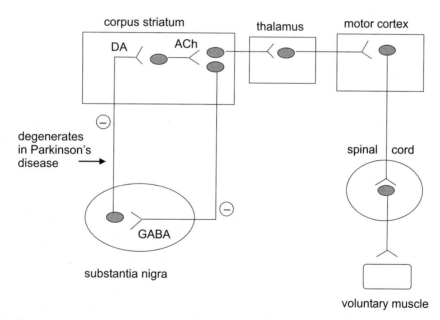

Fig. 15.2 Organization of basal ganglia involved in Parkinson's disease. Degeneration of dopaminergic nerves running from the substantia nigra to the corpus striatum produces loss of an inhibitory influence on cholinergic neurones. The resulting overactivity of cholinergic neurones produces the characteristic motor symptoms of Parkinson's disease. Control of symptoms is achieved by augmenting the influence of dopamine and/or decreasing the influence of acetylcholine. Acetylcholine released from cholinergic neurones also stimulates GABA-containing neurones, which in turn inhibit dopaminergic neurones. Theoretically, blocking the action of GABA would help to restore the balance between dopamine and acetylcholine. However, GABA has an inhibitory action at a number of sites in the brain, and blocking its action would have a range of adverse effects including convulsions. DA, dopamine; ACh = acetylcholine; GABA, gamma-aminobutyric acid.

- abnormal posture;

- akathisia (see above);

- excessive salivation.

There is currently no cure for Parkinson's disease, although transplantation of fetal tissue is under investigation. The objective of treatment is to control the symptoms. Treatment is directed at re-establishing the normal balance of dopamine and acetylcholine by increasing the influence of dopamine and decreasing the influence of acetylcholine.

Treatment of Parkinson's disease

L-dopa/levodopa

Dopamine does not cross the blood–brain barrier and therefore its precursor L-dopa (see Chapter 14) is used to increase dopamine levels in the corpus striatum. L-dopa crosses the blood–brain barrier by an aromatic amino-acid transport pathway and is subsequently decarboxylated to dopamine. L-dopa is rapidly absorbed from the gastrointestinal tract but—due to metabolism in the gut wall, blood, and peripheral tissues by either dopa decarboxylase, MAO, or catechol-O-methyl transferase (COMT)—only about 1% of an oral dose enters the brain (Fig 15.3). To increase the proportion of a dose of L-dopa entering the brain, it is normally given in combination with a dopa-decarboxylase inhibitor such as carbidopa and benserazide. These inhibitors prevent the decarboxylation of L-dopa in the periphery but, since they do not cross the blood–brain barrier, there is no inhibition of their conversion to dopamine in the brain. The use of peripheral dopa-decarboxylase inhibitors allows up to an eightfold reduction in the dose of L-dopa, which helps to reduce the peripheral adverse effects of L-dopa. A number of sustained-release preparations are available that contain both L-dopa and either carbidopa or benserazide. The beneficial effects of L-dopa may result from either augmenting the release of dopamine from the remaining dopaminergic neurones or the direct stimulation of dopamine receptors following conversion to dopamine by extraneuronal dopa decarboxylase (Fig 15.3).

Initial treatment with L-dopa can have a dramatic effect on the symptoms of Parkinson's disease with almost complete improvement in rigidity, tremor, and bradykinesia. However, the effectiveness of treatment decreases with several years of therapy, probably due to the progressive loss of dopaminergic neurones. The adverse effects of treatment with L-dopa are listed below:

- Anorexia, and nausea and vomiting, although the latter effects are minimized by the administration of the peripherally acting, dopamine antagonist domperidone.

- Hypotension and cardiac dysrhythmias.

- Confusion, insomnia, nightmares and occasionally a schizophrenia-like syndrome is present.

- Dyskinesias that are characterized by involuntary movements of the face and limbs, may be severe and as disabling

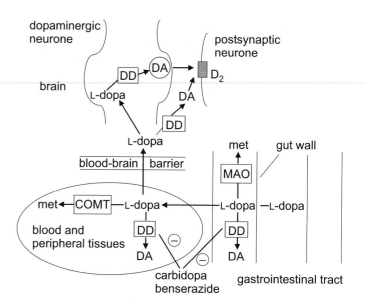

Fig 15.3 Mechanism of action and metabolism of L-dopa following oral administration. L-dopa can be metabolized by either dopamine decarboxylase (DD), monoamine oxidase (MAO), or catechol-*o*-methyltransferase (COMT) present in the gut wall, or blood and peripheral tissues. Inhibition of peripheral DD by carbidopa or benserazide increases the fraction of a dose of L-dopa that enters the brain. In the brain, L-dopa is either converted to dopamine (DA) by extraneuronal DD or taken up by neurones, augmenting dopaminergic transmission. Both routes result in increased stimulation of postsynaptic dopamine D_2 receptors. met, metabolites.

as the symptoms of Parkinson's disease. These effects disappear with a reduction in the dose of L-dopa, although rigidity can reappear.

- The 'on/off effect' where the symptoms of the disease suddenly deteriorate for minutes or hours and then improve. These fluctuations in symptoms may be due to the decline in dopamine concentrations prior to the next dose of L-dopa although, in some patients, the on/off effect is not related to the dosage regimen.

Selegiline

This compound is a selective inhibitor of MAO-B, the type of MAO found in the dopamine-containing regions of the brain. In contrast to inhibitors of MAO-A, selegiline does not produce an interaction with indirectly acting sympathomimetics (the cheese reaction). Selegiline is frequently given in combination with L-dopa to enhance its effects; however, it can also be used alone in the early stages of the disease to enhance existing dopaminergic transmission.

Amantidine

Amantidine was originally introduced into the clinic as an antiviral agent (see Chapter 12) and, by chance, was found to have beneficial effects in Parkinsonism. Its mode of action is uncertain but possible mechanisms are dopamine release or the direct stimulation of dopamine receptors. The beneficial effects of amantidine are modest. It can be used as initial treatment in the early stages of the disease or in more severe disease when used in combination with L-dopa. The adverse effects of amantidine are qualitatively similar to those of L-dopa but less severe.

Dopamine receptor agonists

An alternative to L-dopa, the precursor of dopamine, is the use of direct dopamine agonists such as bromocriptine and pergolide. Both compounds are orally active, dopamine D_2-receptor agonists that cross the blood–brain barrier and have a longer duration of action than L-dopa—plasma half-lives of 6–8 hours compared to 1–2 hours for L-dopa. They need to be administered less frequently than L-dopa, which lessens the incidence of on/off effects. Since enzymatic conversion is unnecessary for the action of bromocriptine and pergolide, it was hoped that these drugs would be more effective than L-dopa in the later stages of Parkinson's disease where there is a substantial loss of dopaminergic neurones. Whilst there is no clear evidence for this, dopamine agonists are normally used in conjunction with L-dopa in patients for whom L-dopa alone is inadequate or who are experiencing on/off effects. The adverse effects of bromocriptine and pergolide are similar to L-dopa and these drugs can also induce retroperitoneal fibrosis.

Muscarinic antagonists

The symptoms of Parkinson's disease are a result of the unrestrained action of cholinergic nerves acting via muscarinic receptors (Fig 15.2) Moreover, presynaptic muscarinic receptors are present on dopaminergic neurones, exerting an inhibitory effect on dopamine release. Blockade of muscarinic receptors will therefore help to restore the balance between dopaminergic and cholinergic nerves in the control of motor function. However, the beneficial effects of muscarinic antagonists in Parkinson's disease are moderate and limited in comparison to L-dopa; muscarinic antagonists diminish tremor and rigidity but with little effect on hypokinesia. Muscarinic antagonists also produce dry mouth, constipation, urinary retention, and blurred vision, although muscarinic antagonism is useful in patients who suffer from excessive salivation. The muscarinic antagonists used in the treatment of Parkinson's disease include benzatropine, trihexyphenidyl (benzhexol) and procyclidine, all of which have reduced peripheral antimuscarinic effects compared to antagonists such as atropine. Muscarinic antagonists are used as monotherapy in patients with mild symptoms, particularly where tremor predominates, and in combination with L-dopa in more severe forms of the disease. They have a particular use in controlling neuroleptic-induced parkinsonism, although tardive dyskinesia may be made worse.

Key facts
Parkinson's disease and its drug treatment

- Parkinson's disease is due to the degeneration of dopaminergic nerves running from the substantia nigra to the corpus striatum. Symptoms include muscle rigidity, tremor, hypokinesia, and bradykinesia. Control of symptoms can be achieved by increasing the influence of dopaminergic nerves and/or reducing the influence of cholinergic nerves.

- The precursor of dopamine, L-dopa, which crosses the blood–brain barrier, is the most effective treatment although its beneficial effects diminish after 2 years.

- L-dopa is normally given in combination with an inhibitor of peripheral dopa decarboxylase, e.g. carbidopa, which increases L-dopa effectiveness and reduces its peripheral adverse effects.

- The adverse effects of L-dopa are nausea and vomiting, anorexia, a schizophrenia-like syndrome, hypotension, involuntary movements (dyskinesias), and the on/off effect—which is a sudden deterioration in symptoms for minutes or hours followed by improvement.

- Muscarinic antagonists, such as trihexyphenidyl and procyclidine, have moderate beneficial effects with a reduction in tremor and rigidity but little effect on hypokinesia.

- Other drugs useful in Parkinson's disease are:
  - amantidine, may act by augmenting dopamine release;
  - selegiline, a selective inhibitor of monoamine oxidase B which enhances dopaminergic transmission;
  - dopamine receptor agonists, such as bromocriptine and pergolide.

  These drugs are normally used as adjuncts to treatment with L-dopa.

Hypnotics and anxiolytics
Hypnotics

Hypnotics are literally drugs which induce sleep. However, the type of sleep they produce is not physiological sleep. There are two types of sleep recognized, these vary in depth and are marked by characteristic changes most noticeably in eye movements. A non-rapid eye movement type (NREM) initiates sleep and makes up about 75% of the sleep cycle. During the NREM phase, heart rate, blood pressure, and respiratory rate are reduced. The remainder of sleep is rapid eye movement (REM) sleep—this occurs a number of times throughout the sleep cycle and just before waking. Dreams occur during REM sleep, and the rate and depth of respiration is increased. Drug-induced sleep has a reduced REM component compared to physiological sleep. When hypnotics are withdrawn there is a compensatory rise in the proportion of REM sleep, which can lead to nightmares.

Hypnotics are used to treat insomnia. However, the long-term use of drugs to manage insomnia is not recommended. As with other conditions the cause should be addressed rather than merely treating the symptoms. Nevertheless, the use of hypnotics to correct short-term sleep disturbances is useful. The indications for the prescription of a hypnotic to prevent insomnia include:

- prior to surgery;
- during a life-crisis (such as the death of a close relative).

Insomnia can present as two distinct patterns of sleep disturbance: initial insomnia (where the patient cannot get to sleep); and early morning wakening (where the duration of sleep is curtailed). The management of these conditions requires the use of drugs with different properties. A number of different categories of drug have been used as hypnotics and they may be classified as follows:

- barbiturates
- benzodiazepines
- miscellaneous.

As well as being hypnotics most of these drugs are sedatives (see later), the difference in effect being dose-dependent.

Barbiturates

Barbiturates are rarely used as hypnotics these days although they were popular in the past. They should be avoided in most cases and only prescribed for patients already taking this group of drugs who have intractable insomnia. Barbiturates are generalized CNS depressants and have a reputation for use in suicide. They have a relatively low therapeutic index and although most cases of barbiturate overdose are deliberate these drugs can produce the state known as automatism. This is drug-induced confusion where the patient cannot remember taking the medication and takes some more, leading to an overdose. Death due to barbiturate overdose is caused by respiratory depression, especially due to a decrease in responsiveness to CO_2 concentration. There is no chemical antidote to the actions of barbiturates and treatment of overdose is supportive and symptomatic: oxygen is administered, blood pressure is maintained, and any remaining drug is removed by gastric lavage and dialysis.

Barbiturates are classified in relation to their duration of action. They are categorized as:

- ultrashort acting;
- short acting;
- long acting.

MECHANISM OF ACTION Barbiturates depress the activity of all brain cells, but their effect is most pronounced in the reticular activating system (RAS). The RAS is a polysynaptic pathway in the medulla and mid-brain and activity in this system produces the conscious alert state that makes perception possible. Barbiturates exert their effects by various mechanisms, some of which are not fully understood. The actions that have been elucidated include:

(1) enhancement of CNS inhibitory activity;

(2) inhibition of CNS excitatory activity.

The most understood action of the barbiturates is the effect on the enhancement of the action of the inhibitory neurotransmitter gamma-aminobutyric acid (GABA).

GABA binds to two types of receptor—$GABA_A$ and $GABA_B$. $GABA_A$ receptors are found at the chloride channel (Fig. 15.4), which also contains receptors for barbiturates and benzodiazepines (see later). At this channel, GABA causes an influx of chloride ions into the cell thus causing hyperpolarization. Barbiturates enhance the affinity of GABA for its receptor site. In addition, barbiturates prolong the duration of GABA-activated chloride influx. At high concentrations, barbiturates influence the chloride channel in the absence of GABA. Barbiturates reduce excitatory activity in the CNS by inhibiting glutamate-induced depolarizations.

PHARMACOKINETICS Unlike most other drugs, the duration of action of barbiturates is not governed by the rate of metabolic breakdown and excretion but by the fact that they equilibrate in organs at different rates. Barbiturates are extremely soluble in lipid and there is virtually no barrier to their diffusion into tissue. The chief factor governing tissue uptake of barbiturates is the amount of blood flow to the particular organ. As the brain is well perfused, concentrations within the CNS quickly equate with the plasma concentration. As other less-well perfused tissues remove drug from the plasma, the concentration in the brain decreases and recovery occurs due to redistribution of the drug (see Chapter 1). The ultrashort-acting barbiturates are the

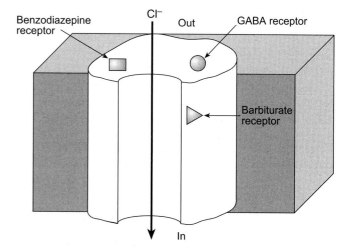

Fig. 15.4 The chloride channel showing the sites of action of GABA, barbiturates, and benzodiazepines.

most lipid-soluble and thus act quickly but, because they are redistributed widely, their duration is short-lived. Ultrashort-acting barbiturates such as methohexital (methohexitone) and thiopental (thiopentone) are not used as hypnotics but are used as general anaesthetic induction agents (see Chapter 9). The long-acting barbiturate phenobarbital (phenobarbitone) is used as an anticonvulsant (see later). Those barbiturates that have been used as hypnotics are the short-acting agents such as amylobarbital (amylobarbitone). The usual dose of amylobarbital (amylobarbitone) is 100–200 mg at bedtime. Hypnotic barbiturates are administered orally in the UK, although in other parts of the world they are available as a suppository. Redistribution is not as rapid as with the ultrashort-acting barbiturates and termination of action relies upon metabolic activity in the liver and excretion in urine.

UNWANTED EFFECTS An important aspect of barbiturate therapy is that this group of drugs induces the production of liver enzymes. This can lead to a reduction in the activity of any concurrent medication. An example of this is the reduction in the anticoagulant effects of the coumarins (such as warfarin—see Chapter 13) during simultaneous therapy. More serious, however, is the rebound increase in anticoagulant activity on withdrawal of the barbiturate.

In addition to enzyme induction, barbiturates may cause dependence and produce allergies. Barbiturates may also cause a drop in blood pressure; although this is not a concern when used as oral hypnotics, it may be a problem when using intravenous barbiturates in hypertensive patients. As mentioned above, barbiturates can produce respiratory depression but not at the doses used as a hypnotic. Occasionally barbiturates cause CNS excitation. Importantly, they have no analgesic action and some patients may overreact to painful stimuli.

CONTRAINDICATIONS TO USE Contraindications to the use of barbiturates include:

- allergy;
- severe liver disease;
- severe respiratory depression;
- history of porphyria.

Porphyria is a condition that may be inherited or acquired, and represents a deficiency in porphyrin synthesis. Barbiturates are one of many drugs capable of precipitating an attack of acute intermittent porphyria. The symptoms of this condition are varied as it appears as a result of damage to any part of the nervous system. The most common finding is abdominal pain.

Benzodiazepines

The benzodiazepines are the most commonly prescribed hypnotics at present. They are a very useful group of drugs in that as well as possessing hypnotic qualities they also exhibit anxiolytic, anticonvulsant, muscle relaxant, and amnesic properties. Compared to the barbiturates these drugs represent a minimal

suicide risk. Some have only a minimal effect on REM sleep and do not cause REM rebound. The therapeutic index is much higher than that for the barbiturates, although they do enhance the CNS depressant effects of other drugs (such as alcohol) and serious respiratory depression can occur with combined intake. Unlike the case with barbiturates, the action of the benzodiazepines can be reversed by the use of the drug flumazenil (this agent is a benzodiazepine but antagonizes the actions of the rest of the group (see Chapter 9)). The benzodiazepines used as hypnotics are flurazepam, temazepam, and nitrazepam.

MECHANISM OF ACTION Benzodiazepine receptors have been identified in many tissues and, like the barbiturates, the benzodiazepines affect activity in the RAS. In addition, they also interfere with activity in the limbic system in the cerebral cortex. This is the area concerned with the emotions and this action explains why the benzodiazepines are anxiolytic. Other receptors within the cerebral cortex account for their anticonvulsant activity.

Like the barbiturates, the benzodiazepines affect GABA activity by increasing the affinity of receptors for GABA. They potentiate the action of GABA on chloride influx by increasing the frequency of the opening of the $GABA_A$ receptor-mediated chloride channel.

PHARMACOKINETICS Benzodiazepines are taken orally when used as hypnotics. The times for different drugs to reach peak plasma concentration varies within the group, ranging from 30 minutes to 8 hours. In addition, duration of effect varies between drugs. It is important to note that the half-life does not always give an indication as to the duration of activity because some benzodiazepines (such as diazepam) have active metabolites.

Benzodiazepines are metabolized in the liver where they are conjugated to glucuronic acid, prior to urinary excretion.

UNWANTED EFFECTS When used as hypnotics benzodiazepines should be prescribed for short periods of time as they can produce dependence. The particular drug chosen is governed by the type of sleep disturbance being treated. If the problem is one of initial insomnia then a drug with a short half-life such as temazepam should be used; if the problem is early morning wakening then a medicament with a longer half-life such as nitrazepam is required. Another important factor related to the half-life of the drug is the phenomenon of rebound insomnia and rebound anxiety. These are related to the rate of elimination of the drug and to the rate of change of occupancy of benzodiazepine receptors. These conditions are more likely after acute withdrawal of short-acting benzodiazepines. This is because replacement with endogenous, benzodiazepine receptor-binding compounds does not occur immediately as their synthesis is decreased during benzodiazepine therapy.

Unlike barbiturates, the incidence of allergy with benzodiazepines is low. However, like barbiturates, benzodiazepines can occasionally produce excitation and some patients may become aggressive.

Miscellaneous

The miscellaneous hypnotics include zolpidem, zopiclone, chloral hydrate, and antihistamines.

ZOLPIDEM AND ZOPICLONE

Both zolpidem and zopiclone, although not benzodiazepines, act at benzodiazepine receptors. Zopiclone is a cyclopyrrolone and zolpidem an imidazopyridine. They are both used in the short-term treatment of insomnia. Zolpidem is taken as a 10 mg oral dose at bedtime and zopiclone as a 7.5 mg tablet.

CHLORAL HYDRATE AND TRICLOFOS

Chloral hydrate was the first synthetic hypnotic. Although it has been used for many years the mechanism of its action is still unknown. It is available as a capsule and an elixir. The usual dose is 500–1000 mg at bedtime. It is quite irritant to skin, mucous membranes, and especially gastric mucosa. Gastric irritation is reduced by dilution. Although chloral hydrate can be used in adults its main use at present is in children. Triclofos is an ester of trichloroethanol which shares the properties of chloral hydrate but is less potent. It is available as an elixir, the dose ranges from 100 mg at bedtime for a child under 1 year of age to 2 g in adults.

PHARMACOKINETICS Chloral hydrate is rapidly absorbed after oral administration. The onset of action is around 30 minutes, the duration of action is 4–8 hours, and the half-life is 8 hours. Chloral hydrate is metabolized in the liver and kidney to its active form, namely trichloroethanol. Trichloroethanol is further metabolized by conjugation with glucuronic acid and excreted in urine.

UNWANTED EFFECTS Prolonged use is not encouraged as chloral hydrate can produce tolerance and is addictive. Like the barbiturates, chloral hydrate induces the production of liver drug-metabolizing enzymes and decreases the effects of coumarin anticoagulants. The effects of other CNS depressants, such as alcohol and barbiturates, are increased during concurrent therapy with chloral hydrate.

CONTRAINDICATIONS TO USE Contra-indications to the use of chloral hydrate include:

- allergy;
- severe hepatic disease;
- severe renal disease;
- severe cardiac disease (chloral hydrate is a cardiac depressant at high dose);
- gastritis;
- nursing mothers (chloral hydrate is excreted in breast milk).

Antihistamines

The histamine H_1 antagonists are mainly used as antiallergy drugs; however, as anyone who has used them in combination with analgesics in 'cold remedies' will realize, they can produce drowsiness due to CNS depression. Antihistamines are occasionally used as hypnotics in children and the drug employed is promethazine. This is one of the phenothiazines, and its primary use is the prevention of nausea and vomiting associated with travel sickness. When it is used as a hypnotic up to 25 mg (depending upon age) is given at bedtime.

Key facts
Hypnotics

- Hypnotics are used to treat insomnia in the short-term.
- Drug-induced sleep has a lesser REM component than physiological sleep.
- Nightmares can occur on withdrawal of hypnotics due to REM rebound.
- Barbiturates have been superseded by benzodiazepines in the treatment of insomnia.
- Barbiturates and benzodiazepines achieve their effect by influencing GABA activity at the chloride channel.
- Chloral hydrate is useful in children.

Anxiolytics

Anxiolytics or sedatives have a number of uses, including:

(1) as a 'pre-med' to aid relaxation prior to dental surgery;

(2) to provide sedation (oral, transmucosal, intramuscular, or intravenous) for dental surgery (see Chapter 9);

(3) as muscle relaxants, for example in the management of temporomandibular joint (TMJ) pain or in the reduction of mandibular dislocations;

(4) to produce anxiolysis during severe pain, such as that experienced during myocardial infarction;

(5) as emergency drugs to treat status epilepticus (see Chapter 26);

(6) to produce amnesia, to eliminate the memory of a distressing event.

Not all anxiolytics produce all these effects. Among the agents used as anxiolytics are alcohol, the benzodiazepines, buspirone, and beta-adrenergic blockers.

Alcohol

Alcohol is often used as a self-prescribed anxiolytic by dental patients. It was prescribed in the past as a sedative prior to dental treatment but is not used much these days. If it is used it is best taken around 30 minutes prior to the stressful event and 60 mL of 40% alcohol will provide some degree of sedation for about 1 hour.

Benzodiazepines

The pharmacology of this group was described above. At present, these are the 'gold standard' anxiolytics. The variation in half-life and the possibility of active metabolites offers a range of duration of action. The agents most commonly used as oral anxiolytics are diazepam (2–10 mg three times daily), chlordiazepoxide (10 mg three times daily), lorazepam (1–4 mg daily in divided doses (2 doses)) and oxazepam (15–30 mg three to four times daily).

Buspirone

Buspirone is one of a group of drugs known as azapirones. It exerts its effect by acting as an agonist at 5-HT$_{1A}$ receptors. However, the entire mode of action is unclear as the onset of the effect can take weeks. Like benzodiazepines, buspirone interacts with other CNS depressants. However, unlike the benzodiazepines, sedation is not produced and withdrawal effects have not been reported. Dry mouth can occur as an unwanted effect. The usual dose range is 15–30 mg daily in divided doses (2 to 3 doses).

Beta-blockers

Beta-blockers are used to treat somatic anxiety where the effects of sympathetic overstimulation lead to problems such as tremor or palpitations. They are not used to treat anxiety in dental patients.

Key facts
Anxiolytics

- Anxiolytics have a number of uses in dentistry.
- In addition to reducing anxiety, anxiolytics are used as muscle relaxants and in the treatment of medical emergencies.
- Oral benzodiazepines are the most useful and widely used group in dental practice.
- The variation in half-lives of the different benzodiazepines allows a range in duration of action.
- Beta-adrenergic blocking drugs are used to treat somatic anxiety—they are not used in dentistry.

Epilepsy, facial neuralgias, and anticonvulsants

Anticonvulsants have two uses:

(1) to treat epilepsy; and

(2) to treat neuralgias.

Epilepsy

Epilepsy is a term used to describe a number of disorders resulting from the excessive firing of intracranial neurones. This results in transient seizures, which can be either localized or generalized. The commonest convulsive disorder is generalized epilepsy and three states are described:

(1) *petit mal*—transient brief pauses in activity, e.g. the patient may stop talking in mid sentence;

(2) *grand* mal—loss of consciousness with stiffening and jerking of joints (tonic–clonic activity);

(3) *status* epilepticus—a medical emergency where seizures follow on, one from another, with no intervening periods of consciousness, which, if left untreated, can be fatal (see Chapter 26).

No single drug controls all types of seizure and there are variations in response between patients. Indeed, combination therapy may be required for some patients to obtain satisfactory control.

Drugs used in the management of epilepsy include:

- phenytoin
- sodium valproate
- carbamazepine
- ethosuxamide
- benzodiazepines
- barbiturates.

MECHANISM OF ACTION Anticonvulsants achieve their effect by one of the following mechanisms (Table 15.1):

(1) by reducing membrane excitability by ion-channel blockade (Na$^+$ or Ca^{2+} channels);

(2) by increasing inhibitory neurotransmitter (GABA) activity.

Phenytoin and carbamazepine, like the barbiturates, induce liver microsomal enzymes and can increase the metabolism of other drugs such as oral contraceptives. Thus an anticonvulsant such as sodium valproate is preferred in women taking oral contraceptives.

Phenytoin

Phenytoin (Epanutin®) belongs to the group of drugs known as hydantoins. It is an antiepileptic drug and is also occasionally used to treat trigeminal neuralgia. It is effective against both partial seizures and generalized tonic–clonic seizures.

MECHANISM OF ACTION Phenytoin prevents excessive firing of central neurones by stabilizing sodium channels in the nerve cell membrane. At high concentrations it also affects calcium-channel function, decreasing the availability of calcium which inhibits neurotransmitter release.

PHARMACOKINETICS Phenytoin may be administered orally or by intramuscular or intravenous injection. The normal route is orally; however, absorption is slow and there is considerable variation in absorption between patients. The normal dose is 300–500 mg daily with a view to obtaining a plasma level of 10–20 μg mL^{-1}. However, as absorption is so variable individual plasma levels must be assayed. At concentrations above 10 μg mL^{-1} phenytoin exhibits saturation (zero-order) kinetics,

Table 15.1 Mechanism of action of the different anticonvulsant drugs*

Drug	Sodium-channel blockade	Calcium-channel blockade	GABA-dependent chloride-channel effect	Increase in effective GABA concentration
Phenytoin	+	+		
Valproate	+	+		+
Carbamazepine	+	+		
Ethosuxamide		+		
Benzodiazepines			+	
Barbiturates			+	
Lamotrigine	+			
Vigabratin				+
Gabapentin				+

*+ Indicates the drug acts by that particular mechanism.

which can result in large increases in plasma concentration for small increases in dose (see Chapter 1). This further emphasizes the importance of monitoring plasma concentrations. Once absorbed, the drug is rapidly distributed and is 90% protein-bound. Metabolism occurs in the liver and excretion is via bile and urine.

UNWANTED EFFECTS Phenytoin has a number of unwanted effects, including:

- allergy;
- gingival overgrowth;
- CNS effects;
- GI tract effects;
- haematological effects;
- hirsutism.

Allergic reactions to phenytoin are fairly common and affect up to 5% of individuals prescribed the drug.

Gingival overgrowth is a common finding in patients receiving phenytoin. Approximately 50% of dentate patients taking phenytoin experience gingival overgrowth, ranging from a slight enlargement of an interdental papilla to a massive overgrowth covering all dental surfaces. Clinically, the gingival tissues are pink and have a firm consistency. The tissues may be inflamed since the distorted contour can impede mechanical plaque removal. Histologically, the gingival tissues comprise dense bundles of collagen fibres. The degree of vascularization depends upon the level of inflammation.

The pathogenesis of phenytoin-induced gingival overgrowth, together with overgrowths induced by cyclosporin and nifedipine, remains uncertain. The target cell is the gingival fibroblast. In simple terms, gingival overgrowth may arise as a result of an interaction between the drug (and/or its metabolite) and the gingival fibroblast, which causes an increase in collagen production. The interaction appears to be enhanced by plaque-induced gingival inflammation. There is also evidence to suggest that a geneti-

cally determined population of gingival fibroblasts (high-activity fibroblasts) are more sensitive to phenytoin or its parahydroxyphenyl derivative. Thus patients with a large proportion of high-activity fibroblasts may be more at risk from phenytoin-induced gingival overgrowth than other patients.

Phenytoin-induced gingival overgrowth is often treated by gingival surgery (gingivectomy) and attention to oral hygiene. Regular use of a chlorhexidine mouth rinse (0.2%) can help to reduce recurrence in the early phase after gingival surgery. There is also evidence that topical folic acid mouthwash (1 mg mL^{-1}) can help to reduce the severity of this effect.

In spite of these measures, some epileptic patients on phenytoin therapy have recurrent problems with gingival overgrowth, and often undergo repeated gingival surgery. For such patients, it may be appropriate to consider a change in their anticonvulsant therapy through consultation with their physician.

The unwanted CNS effects include behavioural changes, such as irritability, confusion, and drowsiness. Disturbances in balance and tremors can also occur.

GI tract upsets include nausea, vomiting, and epigastric pain. These effects are reduced by taking the drug with food.

The haematological problems encountered with phenytoin are:

- megaloblastic anaemia;
- aplastic anaemia;
- agranulocytosis;
- thrombocytopenia.

As mentioned earlier, phenytoin induces the production of drug-metabolizing enzymes in the liver and this can interfere with concurrent therapy; for example the effects of corticosteroids are reduced.

Sodium valproate

Sodium valproate is used to treat generalized tonic–clonic seizures.

MECHANISM OF ACTION Valproate interferes with central neurotransmission by an action at sodium and calcium channels similar to that of phenytoin. In addition, valproate has a dual action on GABA: it stimulates the production and inhibits the degradation of this neurotransmitter.

PHARMACOKINETICS It is taken orally and peak plasma levels occur at about 4 hours. Like phenytoin, it is highly protein-bound (90%). The half-life is 15 hours and the drug is metabolized in the liver. The usual dose is 1–1.5 g daily and the therapeutic plasma level is 40–100 μg mL^{-1}.

UNWANTED EFFECTS Like phenytoin, valproate has a number of unwanted effects including:

* allergy;
* CNS effects;
* GI tract effects;
* haematological effects;
* hepatitis.

The CNS and GI tract effects are similar to those described for phenytoin.

The haematological effects are of interest to dental surgeons as postextraction haemorrhage may occur. Valproate can cause thrombocytopenia, interfere with platelet aggregation, and increase the prothrombin time (INR). Thus it is important not to prescribe aspirin to patients taking valproate.

The hepatitis caused by valproate may lead to liver failure.

Carbamazepine

Carbamazepine is sometimes used in the treatment of the more severe forms of epilepsy; however, it is of little use in the management of petit mal. It is of considerable interest to dentists as it is the 'gold standard' treatment for trigeminal and postherpetic neuralgias.

MECHANISM OF ACTION Carbamazepine has a membrane-stabilizing action similar to that of phenytoin, in that it reduces sodium and calcium ion fluxes.

PHARMACOKINETICS Carbamazepine is given orally and it is slowly absorbed, peak plasma levels occurring in 4–8 hours. It is 75% protein-bound, and one of its metabolites (10,11-epoxide) also has anticonvulsant properties. Metabolism occurs in the liver and excretion is in urine. The dose needed to treat epilepsy is 800–1200 mg daily; the regimen for treating trigeminal neuralgia is described below.

UNWANTED EFFECTS As with the other anticonvulsants, side-effects are common. These are:

* CNS effects;
* GI tract effects;
* haematological effects;
* water retention.

The CNS effects are visual disturbances and drowsiness. The GI upsets are nausea and vomiting.

The haematological effects of carbamazepine are of especial interest to dentists as this is probably the only anticonvulsant medication a dentist is likely to prescribe on a long-term basis (to treat trigeminal neuralgia). It produces aplastic anaemia and agranulocytosis and it is essential that patients prescribed carbamazepine for an extended time have a routine blood count performed regularly; usually every 3 months. A white blood cell count below 3×10^9 L^{-1} necessitates discontinuation of the drug.

In a manner similar to phenytoin, carbamazepine induces liver microsomal enzyme production and hence it will decrease the efficacy of other drugs (such as oral contraceptives) during concurrent therapy.

Ethosuxamide

Ethosuxamide is given orally to treat petit mal.

MECHANISM OF ACTION Ethosuxamide acts by inhibiting calcium fluxes.

PHARMACOKINETICS Ethosuxamide is well absorbed and peak plasma levels occur in 3 hours. It has a half-life of 45 hours. Ethosuxamide is metabolized in the liver; however, 25% is excreted unchanged in the urine. The normal dose is 500 mg four times daily.

UNWANTED EFFECTS Unwanted effects of ethosuxamide therapy include:

* allergy;
* CNS effects;
* GI tract effects;
* haematological effects (a leucopenia).

Benzodiazepines

The benzodiazepines have anticonvulsant properties resulting from their effect on GABA activity; however, they are not the drugs of choice for anticonvulsant prophylaxis due to their tendency to produce tolerance as well as psychological dependence (see Chapter 25). The benzodiazepines used in the management of epilepsy are clobazam and clonazepam. Clobazam is used intermittently as an additional drug. Clonazepam is rarely used but may be administered as a supplementary drug in children.

Although not commonly used in the day-to-day management of epilepsy, benzodiazepines are very important in the management of the medical emergency of status epilepticus (see Chapter 26). The drug used to treat this condition is diazepam. which is administered intravenously at a rate of 5 mg min^{-1} up to a maximum of 20 mg.

Barbiturates

The barbiturates have an anticonvulsant action since they reduce neural activity; however, their major disadvantage is that they produce incapacitating drowsiness, as well as having a high incidence of allergies. The members of this group used to treat epilepsy are phenobarbital (phenobarbitone) and its pro-drugs (methylphenobarbital (methylphenobarbitone) and primidone). Phenobarbital is given orally but is slowly absorbed, with peak plasma levels occuring at about 6 hours. It is 50% bound to protein and has a half-life of 100 hours. It is metabolized in the liver and, like ethosuxamide, 25% is excreted unchanged in the urine.

In some centres, 200–400 phenobarbital is injected IV following the use of diazepam to treat status epilepticus; however, it is important to point out that other barbiturates (such as methohexital (methohexitone)) have convulsant properties and should not be used in such a condition.

Supplementary drugs in the treatment of epilepsy

The use of the benzodiazepines clonazepam and clobazam as additional drugs in the management of epilepsy was mentioned above. Other drugs used as supplementary treatments include lamotrigine (which acts at the sodium channel in a manner similar to phenytoin and carbamazepine) and the GABA analogues vigabatrin and gabapentin. Vigabatrin irreversibly inhibits GABA transaminase thus increasing GABA concentration. Gabapentin appears to act by increasing the release of GABA.

ANTICONVULSANT OSTEOMALACIA

It was noted above that many anticonvulsants (especially phenytoin, carbamazepine, and phenobarbital) are hepatic enzyme inducers; they enhance the activity of certain enzymes, especially the mixed-function oxidases. These hepatic oxidases also increase the catabolism of dietary and endogenously produced vitamin D. If there is enhancement of the oxidase enzyme system there will be reduced serum concentrations of 25-hydroxycholecalciferol and, in turn, decreased renal production of the active 1,25-dihydroxycholecalciferol (see Chapter 21). Vitamin D deficiency can therefore occur in patients on anticonvulsant therapy and, if severe, may manifest itself as either rickets or osteomalacia. The problem is more common in institutionalized elderly patients, who may be on a restricted diet and not often exposed to sunlight. Vitamin D deficiency may also increase the tendency for fits. Patients on anticonvulsant therapy should receive dietary advice and be encouraged to enjoy sunlight.

Key facts
Epilepsy

- Generalized epilepsy is of three types—petit mal, grand mal, and status epilepticus.
- Status epilepticus is a medical emergency.
- Epilepsy is treated with anticonvulsants.
- Anticonvulsants are also used to treat neuralgias (see next section).

- Anticonvulsants achieve their effect by one of two mechanisms. The first mechanism is the blockade of sodium or calcium channels. The second is an increase in the activity of the inhibitory neurotransmitter GABA.
- Most anticonvulsants have important unwanted effects, including the production of haematological defects.
- Many anticonvulsants—including phenytoin, carbamazepine and barbiturates—are enzyme inducers.
- Phenytoin produces gingival hyperplasia.

Trigeminal neuralgia (Tic douloureux)

This condition is characterized by unilateral electric shock-like, brief stabbing pains confined to the distribution of the trigeminal nerve. There is little or no associated sensory loss. The pain is triggered by non-nociceptive stimuli, for example touch or a current of air.

Treatment of trigeminal neuralgia

Trigeminal neuralgia can be treated either surgically or with drugs.

SURGICAL TREATMENT

Surgical treatment can be either peripheral or central. Peripheral modalities involve exposure of the nerve trunk involved and treatment by cryotherapy or injection of a neurotoxic agent such as alcohol.

Central approaches are highly specialized areas of neurosurgery but, in essence, two main types of treatment are in vogue: (1) gangliolysis; and (2) suboccipital craniectomy with decompression of the trigeminal nerve. Gangliolysis is a destructive procedure and the aim is to produce pain relief with minimal loss of sensation in the region affected by pain. The results indicate that 80% of patients will obtain pain relief for 1 year and in over 50% relief will last for 5 years.

Suboccipital craniectomy is based on the observation that in trigeminal neuralgia the trigeminal nerve is often compressed by a blood vessel or very occasionally by some other local anatomical abnormality. The operation has an 85% long-term success rate.

DRUG TREATMENT

Two anticonvulsant drugs, carbamazepine and phenytoin (see above), have been shown to be effective for this condition. Carbamazepine controls the severe pains in about 60% of patients. However, it commonly produces unwanted effects including nausea, dizziness, ataxia, somnolence, and slurring of speech; rarely, a fall in the white or red cell count of the blood may occur. The starting dose is 100 mg twice daily; this is increased slowly thereafter until, if necessary, a maximum total daily dose of 1200 mg is reached. It is useful to check the plasma concentration, the therapeutic range is 5 to 10 $\mu g\,mL^{-1}$ (20–40 $\mu mol\,L^{-1}$).

As this drug has a long half-life and also produces autoinduction of drug-metabolizing enzymes, it is necessary to wait 14 days after any change in dosage before attempting to measure the plasma concentration if meaningful values are to be obtained. To detect any bone marrow changes, the haematological picture should be examined monthly during the first 3 months of treatment and thereafter at regular 3-monthly intervals; the plasma concentration can also be measured. Bone marrow suppression is most likely to occur within the first 3 months of treatment, but whenever it occurs it is an absolute indication for immediate withdrawal of the drug.

Phenytoin is the drug of second choice and is usually less effective than carbamazepine. As mentioned above side-effects are common. The starting dose is 100 mg three times daily and, as with carbamazepine, the plasma concentration should be checked; the therapeutic range is between 10 and $20\,\mu g\,mL^{-1}$ (40–$80\,\mu mol\,L^{-1}$) and the $t_{0.5}$ is 12–24 hours.

When necessary, other anticonvulsant drugs are occasionally used either alone or in combination with carbamazepine or phenytoin.

The skeletal muscle relaxant baclofen has also been used in the treatment of trigeminal neuralgia. Baclofen is a GABA analogue and its principal indication is for relief of spasticity due to multiple sclerosis or spinal cord section.

Postherpetic neuralgia

This condition follows a herpes zoster infection (shingles). Pain is a feature of the initial infection but usually only lasts for the duration of the rash. However, some patients experience severe pain for many years after the initial infection, the older age groups being especially susceptible. This postherpetic neuralgia frequently has a burning quality and may be spontaneous.

Treatment of post-herpetic neuralgia
This can be physical or pharmacological.

PHYSICAL
Transcutaneous electrical nerve stimulation (TENS), which involves the application of electrical shocks at either low (5–10 Hz) or high (100–150 Hz) frequencies, may produce very effective analgesia in some patients. A pair of carbon rubber (or other) electrodes are applied either directly on or adjacent to the painful area, and the strength of shocks adjusted to produce a tingling sensation. The patient is instructed how to use this form of treatment and can then treat him/herself on a regular basis several times daily. For TENS, patients should be referred to a pain relief clinic where, in the UK, the stimulators are likely to be provided on loan by the National Health Service.

PHARMACOLOGICAL
Selected psychotropic drugs, including anticonvulsants, may be used alone or in combination. A well-tried regimen is as follows:

1. Start carbamazepine 100 mg, 12 hourly, orally (for example 0800 h and 2000 h), increasing at intervals of several days up to a daily maximum of 1600 mg if required. As detailed earlier, the plasma concentration should be measured to confirm that it lies within the therapeutic range of 5 to $10\,mg\,L^{-1}$. The concentration should then be checked at 3-monthly intervals, together with the white cell count.

2. If carbamazepine at a therapeutic plasma concentration fails to control the pain, it should be stopped and replaced by amitriptyline, 25–75 mg, at night. This may control the pain on its own or may do so only when combined with sodium valproate (200 mg, twice daily). The plasma concentration of these drugs should be checked every 3 months; amitriptyline (100–$200\,\mu g\,mL^{-1}$), sodium valproate (40–$100\,\mu g\,mL^{-1}$). Adverse effects include: *amitriptyline*—antimuscarinic, CNS (sedation, paraesthesiae), CVS (tachycardia and other disorders of rate and rhythm), and allergic (skin, cholestatic jaundice, agranulocytosis); *sodium valproate* (see earlier).

3. If the combination of amitriptyline with sodium valproate fails to relieve postherpetic neuralgia then the sodium valproate should be withdrawn and replaced by a neuroleptic such as perphenazine, 4 mg, three times a day. Adverse effects include sedation, antimuscarinic effects, extrapyramidal signs and symptoms, hypersensitivity reactions, cholestatic jaundice, endocrine disturbances, and blood dyscrasias.

Key facts
Neuralgias

- Trigeminal neuralgia is an acutely painful condition.
- Trigeminal neuralgia can be treated surgically or pharmacologically.
- The first-line drug treatment is carbamazepine starting at a dose of 100 mg twice daily.
- Due to the effects of carbamazepine on red and white blood cells, blood samples should be taken every 3 months during therapy to monitor the haematological status.
- The second drug of choice for the treatment of trigeminal neuralgia is phenytoin.
- Postherpetic neuralgia may occur after infection with the herpes zoster virus (shingles).
- The drug treatment of choice for postherpetic neuralgia is carbamazepine.
- An alternative treatment for postherpetic neuralgia involves the use of amitriptyline with or without sodium valproate.

Migraine

This common condition affects about 5% of the adult population. The characteristic features are periodic headaches (typically unilateral), visual disturbances, and vomiting. Attacks are often preceded by visual disturbance (an aura). During a severe migraine attack, sufferers are usually prostrate and photophobic, which necessitates going to bed in a darkened room.

The aetiology of this condition is still obscure. There is clearly some disturbance in cerebral blood flow. In certain patients, food substances rich in tyramine or dopamine may precipitate an attack. Attention has focused on the role of 5-HT in migrainous headaches. Prophylaxis against migraine can be achieved with drugs that inhibit the reuptake of 5-HT by platelets. Several types of drugs have been tried; these can be classified as those used in acute attacks and those used for prophylactic purposes.

Treatment of migraine

Analgesics

Aspirin, paracetamol, and various combination analgesics are frequently used in the treatment of migraine. However, they are more effective in the early stages of a migraine since an attack is frequently associated with gastric stasis and therefore absorption of these drugs will be poor. This problem can be overcome by the use of metoclopramide, which will increase the rate of gastric emptying. There is no place for the opioids in the treatment of an acute attack of migraine because of the risk of dependence and their action on gastrointestinal function (see Chapter 7).

Antiemetics

The nausea and vomiting that often accompany an attack of migraine may respond to an antiemetic. Metoclopramide is the treatment of choice because of the absence of sedative effects.

Ergotamine

Ergotamine is an alkaloid derived from ergot, produced by a fungus (*Claviceps purpurea*) that grows on rye and other cereals. It is used to relieve an acute attack of migraine. Ergotamine interacts with 5-HT$_1$ and 5-HT$_2$ receptors as well as adrenergic and dopaminergic receptors. It can be given orally, parenterally, rectally, sublingually, or by inhalation. The usual dose regime is 2 mg as soon as the headache starts, followed by 2 mg at half-hourly intervals. The total dose per attack should not exceed 10 mg.

Unwanted effects from ergotamine include nausea and vomiting after oral administration and peripheral vasoconstriction and paraesthesiae. Gangrene of the fingers has occurred in patients taking this drug. Ergotamine should not be used during pregnancy because it causes contraction of the uterus. Although ergotamine is still used by some migraine sufferers, it has been superseded by newer drugs (see below).

Cyproheptadine

This is a potent H$_1$ and 5-HT receptor antagonist used prophylactically. Its mode of action is uncertain. It also has tranquillizing properties The usual dosage is 4 mg, followed by a further 4 mg, 30 minutes later. Cyproheptadine also has mild anticholinergic properties, and causes dry mouth and blurred vision.

Sumatriptan

Sumatriptan is a relatively new compound which is chemically related to 5-HT. It can be given orally or subcutaneously and is used for the relief of acute migraine. The drug has an elimination half-life of approximately 2 hours and is predominately metabolized by monoamine oxidases. Sumatriptan is a 5-HT agonist, and stimulates a subtype of 5-HT$_1$ receptors found in the cranial blood vessels causing vasoconstriction. The usual dose regime is 100 mg orally, followed by one or two further doses if symptoms return. Unwanted effects include malaise, fatigue, dizziness, vertigo, and sedation. The drug is contraindicated in patients with ischaemic heart disease and those with a previous history of myocardial infarction since it causes vasospasm of the coronary arteries.

Many migraine sufferers are treated adequately with simple analgesics with or without an antiemetic. Clinical trials suggest that sumatriptan is effective, but it is expensive. It should perhaps be reserved for migraine attacks that do not respond to other therapies.

Prophylactic treatment of migraine

Methysergide

Methysergide is a powerful 5-HT antagonist; it also has anti-inflammatory and vasoconstrictor properties. For the prevention of migraine, methysergide 1–2 mg should be taken three times a day with meals. The incidence of unwanted effects is high, and includes gastrointestinal problems, CNS disturbances, weight gain, oedema, and fibrotic changes in the thorax and abdomen. Retroperitoneal fibrosis limits the use of methysergide and it is mainly used if all else fails.

Other prophylactic agents

Other drugs used for the prophylaxis of migraine are pizotifen, which is structurally similar to cyproheptadine, and propranolol, a β-blocker which prevents vasodilatation of the cerebral arteries. Tricyclic antidepressants, aspirin-like drugs, and calcium-channel blockers have also been used.

Occlusal splints

There is also evidence that occlusal splints may be a useful preventative measure for certain types of migraine. The group of patients that appear to benefit from such a splint are those that awake with migraine. These patients wear a splint at night and this seems to reduce the incidence of attacks. Whilst the mechanism of occlusal splints in the prevention of migraine remains uncertain, it would suggest that a tooth grinding habit and perhaps some aberration in the blood flow arising from clenching the teeth may be an important aetiological factor for this type of migraine.

Key facts
Migraine and treatment

- Migraine is a common condition which may be vascular, neuronal, or peptidergic in origin.

- 5-HT is intimately involved in the pathogenesis of migraine, although it precise role in headache production remains uncertain.

- Simple analgesics such as aspirin and paracetamol are useful in the early phases of a migraine attack, but thereafter their efficacy is limited due to gastric stasis.

- Ergotamine is useful in the treatment of an acute attack of migraine, and can be given orally, sublingually, and rectally.

- Sumatriptan, which is a 5-HT agonist, is highly effective in aborting an acute attack, but the drug is expensive.

- Other drugs used in either the treatment or prophylaxis of migraine include cyproheptadine, methysergide, pizotifen, propanolol, calcium-channel blockers, and tricyclic antidepressants.

Further reading

Albin, R. L., Young, A. B., and Penney, J. B. (1989). The functional anatomy of basal ganglia disorders. *Trends in Neuroscience*, 12, 366–75.

Felpel, L. P. (1998). Antianxiety drugs and centrally acting muscle relaxants (Chapter 13). Sedative-hypnotics and central nervous system stimulants (Chapter 14). In *Pharmacology and therapeutics for dentistry* (4th edn) (ed. J. A. Yagiela,, E. A. Neidle, and J. J. Dowd). Mosby, St Louis.

Hassell, T. M. (1981). Epilepsy and the oral manifestations of phenytoin therapy. Karger, Basle.

Hollister, L. E. and Claghorn, J. L. (1993). New antidepressants. *Annual Review of Pharmacology and Toxicology*, 33, 165–77.

Potter, W. Z. and Hollister, L. E. (1998). Antipsychotic drugs and lithium. In *Basic and clinical pharmacology* (7th edn) (ed. B. G. Katzung), pp. 464–80. Appleton and Lange, Stamford, Connecticut.

Quinn, N. (1995). Drug treatment of Parkinson's disease. *British Medical Journal*, 310, 575–9.

16

Drugs used in the treatment of cardiovascular disease

- Hypertension
- Angina pectoris
- Heart (myocardial) failure
- Normal cardiac rhythm
- Cardiac dysrhythmias
- Further reading

Drugs used in the treatment of cardiovascular disease

Cardiovascular disease is the most common cause of mortality and morbidity in industrialized societies, consequently the dental practitioner will frequently encounter patients who have been prescribed drugs to treat such diseases. This chapter concentrates on the mode of action, clinical use, and adverse effects of drugs used in the treatment of the more common cardiovascular disorders, which are hypertension, angina pectoris, heart failure, and cardiac dysrhythmias.

Hypertension

The main elements that contribute to the control of blood pressure are:

- cardiac output;
- blood volume;
- peripheral vascular resistance (the degree of constriction of arterioles).

These elements are subject to control by the activity of: the heart, vascular smooth muscle, kidney, sympathetic nervous system, and circulating factors such as angiotensin. These systems act in an integrated manner to maintain normal blood pressure at <130/85 mmHg, i.e. a systolic pressure of <130 mmHg and a diastolic pressure of <85 mmHg. Hypertension, i.e. high blood pressure, has been defined as a sustained diastolic blood pressure greater than 90 mmHg. The various degrees of severity of hypertension have been defined and these are shown in Table 16.1.

Hypertension is classified as essential (primary) hypertension or secondary hypertension. Essential hypertension, for which no obvious cause has been identified, accounts for approximately 90% of all cases of hypertension. Secondary hypertension—which

accounts for the remaining 10% of cases—has identifiable causes, including: renal artery stenosis; phaeochromocytoma; and primary aldosteronism. Whilst the majority of patients with hypertension exhibit no symptoms, a sustained elevated blood pressure increases the risk of a range of cardiovascular and renal diseases such as heart failure, myocardial infarction, angina, stroke, and nephrosclerosis. In light of these consequences, it is important to reduce blood pressure to an acceptable level, a diastolic pressure of ≤90 mmHg. Reductions in blood pressure can be achieved by changes in lifestyle, such as taking exercise and reducing body weight; however, for the majority of patients, drug treatment is also required. A relatively large number of drugs with a variety of different mechanisms have proved effective in lowering an elevated blood pressure. The following sections describe the mode of action and adverse effects of each major category of antihypertensive drug.

Diuretics

Diuretic drugs increase the renal excretion of Na^+ and water and are used in the treatment of hypertension, to reduce oedema which can arise as a consequence of heart failure (see below), and in the treatment of oliguria (urine output of <400 mL day^{-1}). They are divided into the following groups:

- thiazide diuretics;
- loop diuretics;
- potassium-sparing diuretics;
- osmotic diuretics.

Osmotic diuretics apart, these drugs act directly on the renal tubule cells at distinct regions within the nephron (Fig. 16.1) to reduce the reabsorption of Na^+ following its filtration at the glomerulus. Diuretic drugs also increase water loss, this being secondary to the increased excretion of Na^+. With the exception of the potassium-sparing diuretic spironolactone, diuretic drugs act at carrier or ion-channel proteins on the luminal membrane (see Fig. 16.2) following filtration at the glomerulus and secretion in the proximal tubule. Spironolactone acts at an intracellular site gaining access to the tubule cells by diffusing across the basolateral membrane. An increase in Na^+ excretion produced by diuretics leads to a fall in extracellular fluid volume and plasma

Table 16.1 Definitions of the various degrees of hypertension

Category	Systolic (mmHg)	Diastolic (mmHg)
Mild	140–159	90–99
Moderate	160–179	100–109
Severe	180–209	110–119
Very severe	≥210	≥120

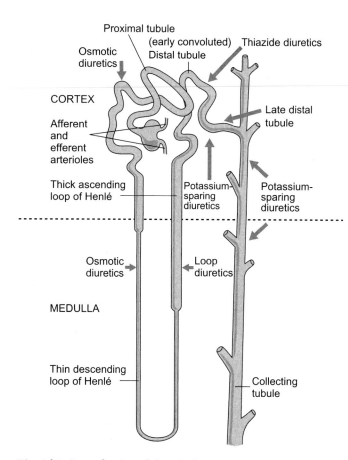

Fig. 16.1 Sites of action of diuretic drugs.

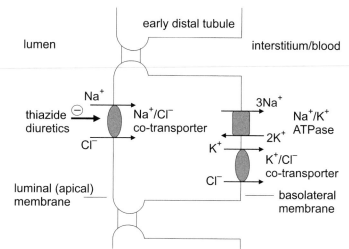

Fig. 16.2 Transport mechanisms in the early distal tubule. Thiazide diuretics increase the excretion of Na^+ and Cl^- by inhibiting the Na^+/Cl^- co-transporter in the luminal membrane.

volume, which, in turn, produces a reduction in filling pressure in the heart. The reduction in cardiac filling pressure will produce a fall in cardiac output and therefore a fall in blood pressure since:

blood pressure = cardiac output × peripheral resistance.

However, a diuretic action alone, at least for thiazide drugs, may not fully account for the antihypertensive effect of diuretic drugs (see below).

Thiazide diuretics

These diuretics, which include bendroflumethiazide (bendrofluazide), hydrochlorothiazide, and thiazide-like drugs such as chlortalidone (chlorthalidone), inhibit the Na^+/Cl^- co-transporter in the early distal convoluted tubule (co-transport is carrier-mediated transport with substances transported in the same direction) (Fig. 16.2) This action produces a moderate diuresis in which 5% of Na^+ filtered at the glomerulus is excreted (≤ 1% of filtered Na^+ is normally excreted by someone ingesting a typical diet). Thiazides also have a direct vasodilator action resulting from the activation of K^+ channels in vascular smooth muscle cells, which produces movement of K^+ out of cells. This action results in membrane hyperpolarization, and this has an inhibitory affect on L-type voltage-dependent Ca^{2+} channels such

that the opening probability of these channels is reduced. Thus, the effect of K^+ channel activation is a reduction in intracellular Ca^{2+} levels that produces relaxation of vascular smooth muscle, leading to a reduction in peripheral resistance. The anti-hypertensive effect of thiazides is therefore a combination of their diuretic and vasodilator actions.

Of the various types of diuretic drug, thiazides are the most effective antihypertensive agents and are commonly used in the treatment of essential hypertension, particularly in the elderly. They are administered orally since they are well absorbed from the gastrointestinal tract with high oral bioavailability. However thiazides are not without adverse effects, as detailed below.

Unwanted effects

- **Hypokalaemia and alkalosis:** As a result of inhibition of Na^+ reabsorption in the early distal tubule, increased delivery of Na^+ to the late distal tubule and collecting ducts promotes K^+ and H^+ secretion. This can result in hypokalaemia, which predisposes to cardiac dysrhythmias, and a metabolic alkalosis. One strategy for avoiding hypokalaemia is to give potassium supplements (oral potassium chloride) or to administer thiazides in combination with a potassium-sparing diuretic (see below).

- **Hyperuricaemia:** This effect can precipitate gout and is due to an enhanced absorption of uric acid in the proximal tubule, as a result of volume depletion produced by diuresis, or decreased secretion of uric acid due to competition between uric acid and thiazides at the organic acid secretory mechanism.

- **Impaired carbohydrate tolerance:** Thiazides may induce hypoglycaemia or aggravate existing diabetes mellitus as a result of reduced insulin secretion and diminished tissue utilization of glucose.

- **MALE SEXUAL DYSFUNCTION:** Thiazides may produce impotence, which is reversible on withdrawal of treatment.

Loop diuretics

These diuretic agents, which include furosemide (frusemide), bumetanide, and etacrynic acid (ethacrynic acid), inhibit the $Na^+/K^+/2Cl^-$ co-transporter in the thick ascending limb of the loop of Henle. They are the most powerful of all diuretic drugs, leading to the excretion of 15–25% of filtered Na^+. The thick ascending limb of the loop of Henle is impermeable to water and enables the kidney to concentrate urine by producing hypertonic conditions in the interstitium of the medulla. The high osmotic pressure in the medulla is responsible for water reabsorption from the collecting tubules in the presence of vasopressin (antidiuretic hormone). Loop diuretics reduce the tonicity of the medullary interstitium and therefore inhibit reabsorption of water in the collecting ducts. This results in a profound diuresis. Loop diuretics, which can be administered orally, are not used in the routine treatment of essential hypertension but in hypertensive patients who have not responded to other diuretics or antihypertensive drugs, usually in the presence of renal insufficiency. A major use for loop diuretics is the treatment of oedema associated with heart failure, as discussed later. The adverse effects of loop diuretics are hypokalaemia, metabolic alkalosis, and hyperuricaemia, which occur by the same mechanisms as for thiazide diuretics. Loop diuretics and particularly etacrynic acid can also produce hearing loss and tinnitus.

Potassium-sparing diuretics

These diuretics produce a mild diuresis, resulting in the excretion of 2–3% of filtered Na^+, by an action on the late distal tubule and collecting ducts. Potassium-sparing diuretics can be divided into two groups, both of which are orally active:

- the Na^+-channel blockers, triamterene and amiloride, which block channels in the luminal membrane;
- spironolactone, an aldosterone antagonist, which blocks mineralocorticosteroid receptors.

The late distal tubule and collecting ducts are the major locations for K^+ secretion in the kidney, and the transport of both K^+ and Na^+ across the luminal membrane occurs via ion channels rather than carriers. The movement of Na^+ into the cell creates a lumen-negative potential difference that facilitates movement of K^+ out of the cell and into the lumen, with subsequent excretion in the urine. Blockade of the Na^+ channels with drugs such as amiloride reduces Na^+ reabsorption and decreases K^+ secretion, hence the term potassium-sparing diuretics.

Aldosterone enters the cells of the late distal tubule and collecting duct and binds to DNA-linked receptors for mineralocorticosteroids, which leads to increased synthesis of Na^+ and K^+ channels. As a result, the net effect of aldosterone is to increase Na^+ reabsorption and K^+ secretion. Spironolactone binds to these receptors and blocks the effect of aldosterone, producing a reduction in Na^+ reabsorption and K^+ secretion.

In the treatment of hypertension, potassium-sparing diuretics are not used alone but in combination with potassium-losing diuretics, e.g. loop and thiazide diuretics. These combinations have two advantages: (1) synergistic diuretic and antihypertensive effects, i.e. maximum effects of the combination are greater than the combined maximum effect of either diuretic given alone; and (2) avoidance of the hypokalaemia produced by potassium-losing diuretics. However, potassium-sparing diuretics are not routinely given in the treatment of hypertension with thiazide diuretics unless hypokalaemia develops. In such cases, thiazides are used in combination with triamterene or amiloride, which are available combined in one tablet. Spironolactone is not used in the treatment of essential hypertension but in secondary hypertension resulting from primary aldosteronism. One disadvantage to the use of spironolactone is that, in addition to mineralocorticosteroid receptors, it has affinity for other steroid receptors, which can result in gynaecomastia (development of breasts in men), menstrual disorders, and male sexual dysfunction.

Osmotic diuretics

Osmotic diuretics, such as mannitol which is administered intravenously, are freely filtered at the glomerulus and undergo little if any reabsorption. They increase the osmotic pressure of the tubular fluid, thereby reducing the reabsorption of water and lowering luminal Na^+ concentration. A reduction in luminal Na^+ concentration results in a decrease in Na^+ reabsorption in the proximal tubule and descending loop of Henle. Osmotic diuretics are of no use in the treatment of hypertension or in the reduction of oedema, but are used to overcome oliguria and to extract water out of the eye and brain. Oliguria is a feature of some forms of acute renal failure, and the increase in urine flow produced by osmotic diuretics helps to maintain tubule patency by eliminating debris from the tubule lumen. Osmotic diuretics, by increasing the osmotic pressure of plasma, produce short-term reductions in intraocular pressure—and for this reason are used to treat acute attacks of glaucoma. Maxillofacial surgeons use osmotic diuretics to reduce ocular pressure during the management of retrobulbar haemorrhage, which is a rare complication of a fractured zygoma. In addition, they are also used to reduce cerebral oedema and brain mass before and after neurosurgery.

Key facts
Diuretic drugs

- Diuretic drugs increase the renal excretion of Na^+ and water and are used mainly in the treatment of hypertension and to reduce oedema.

(cont.)

- Thiazide diuretics, such as bendroflumethiazide, block the Na^+/Cl^- co-transporter in the early distal tubule, resulting in the excretion of 5% of the filtered Na^+. The antihypertensive action of thiazides is due to their diuretic action and a vasodilator effect resulting from the activation of potassium channels in vascular smooth muscle.

- Loop diuretics, e.g. furosemide, block the $Na^+/K^+/2Cl^-$ co-transporter in the thick ascending loop of Henle, resulting in the excretion of 15–25% of the filtered Na^+. Loop diuretics are not used in the routine treatment of essential hypertension but in hypertensive patients who have not responded to other diuretics or antihypertensive drugs. Loop diuretics are mainly used in the treatment of oedema.

- Potassium-sparing diuretics increase Na^+ excretion by 2–3% and decrease K^+ excretion by acting on the late distal tubule and collecting duct.

- Potassium-sparing diuresis is produced by blockade of luminal Na^+ channels with amiloride or triamterene, or by blockade of cytoplasmic mineralocorticosteroid receptors with spironolactone.

- Potassium-sparing diuretics are rarely used alone but in combination with thiazide and loop diuretics to counteract their potassium-losing effects.

- Osmotic diuretics, such as mannitol, reduce water reabsorption resulting in a subsequent decrease in Na^+ reabsorption in the proximal tubule and descending loop of Henle. They are used to overcome oliguria, and in the treatment of acute glaucoma and cerebral oedema.

β-Adrenoceptor antagonists (β-blockers)

These drugs were originally introduced for the treatment of angina, but an unexpected finding was a lowering of blood pressure in patients who also had hypertension. This lowering of blood pressure, which does not occur in normotensive individuals, takes days to develop. The initial cardiovascular response is a fall in cardiac output with a compensatory rise in peripheral resistance such that there is no change in blood pressure. The antihypertensive effect results from a delayed fall in peripheral resistance in conjunction with a reduced cardiac output. The fall in peripheral resistance occurs with all β-adrenoceptor antagonists despite blockade of vasodilator β_2-adrenoceptors. The exact mechanism underlying this fall in peripheral resistance is uncertain but may be due to:

- a reduction in renin release from the kidney. Stimulation of sympathetic nerves to the kidney causes the release of renin via stimulation of β_1-receptors in the wall of the afferent arteriole. Renin catalyses the production of angiotensin, which causes a rise in blood pressure (see below);

- a central action reducing sympathetic activity;

- blockade of presynaptic β-adrenoceptors on noradrenergic nerve terminals. These receptors, in contrast to presynaptic α-adrenoceptors, increase the release of norepinephrine (noradrenaline).

β-Adrenoceptor antagonists such as labetalol—which also possess α-adrenoceptor blocking activity therefore producing vasodilatation—have an additional antihypertensive mechanism of action. These drugs have particular uses in the treatment of phaeochromocytoma and hypertensive emergencies when they are administered intravenously.

The adverse effects of β-adrenoceptor antagonists have been described in Chapter 14; although, if avoided in patients with asthma, diabetes mellitus, and heart failure, the incidence of adverse effects is low. Problems can arise when β-adrenoceptor antagonists are abruptly withdrawn, resulting in sympathetic hyperactivity that can precipitate angina and rebound hypertension to blood pressure levels higher than those existing prior to treatment. Consequently, if treatment with β-adrenoceptor antagonists is to be discontinued, the dosage should gradually be reduced over a period of up to 14 days.

Calcium channel-blocking drugs (calcium antagonists)

These drugs bind to voltage-dependent, L-type calcium channels in vascular smooth muscle, producing a reduction in their probability of opening. This reduces Ca^{2+} influx and results in lower levels of intracellular Ca^{2+} available to activate contractile proteins. The antihypertensive effect of calcium channel blockers is therefore due to vasodilatation and a fall in peripheral resistance. There are three main groups of calcium-channel blocking drugs:

- dihydropyridines, of which there are a number of examples including nifedipine, nicardipine and felodipine;

- phenylalkylamines, e.g. verapamil;

- benzothiazepines, e.g. diltiazem.

In contrast to the dihydropyridines, which are 'vascular selective', verapamil and diltiazem also bind to L-type calcium channels in the heart, resulting in reductions in heart rate and contractility (negative chronotropic and inotropic effects), and a reduction in conduction at the AV-node. As a result of their negative inotropic effects, verapamil and diltiazem are contraindicated in patients with heart failure. Dihydropyridines do not have a depressant effect on cardiac function but can elicit increases in cardiac rate and force of contraction produced by a reflex increase in sympathetic activity. The vasodilator effect of calcium channel blockers accounts for the adverse effects of flushing and headache, whilst constipation can result from the use of verapamil. An unusual adverse effect of calcium-channel blockers, which is of direct interest to dental surgeons, is that of gingival overgrowth.

Angiotensin-converting enzyme inhibitors and angiotensin receptor antagonists

These drugs interfere with the renin–angiotensin system that contributes to the maintenance of blood pressure and extracellular fluid volume. Renin is secreted from the cells in the wall of the afferent arteriole in the kidney in response to:

- a fall in blood pressure;
- an increase in the activity of sympathetic nerves that innervate these cells (a β_1-adrenoceptor-mediated effect);
- a reduction in the sodium concentration of fluid in the early distal tubule detected by specialized epithelial cells known as the macula densa.

The afferent arteriole, at a point just prior to entering the glomerulus, is in close apposition to the macula densa and this area of the nephron is referred to as the juxtaglomerular apparatus.

Renin acts on angiotensinogen, a plasma globulin synthesized by the liver, splitting off a decapeptide, angiotensin I (Fig. 16.3). A second proteolytic enzyme, angiotensin-converting enzyme (ACE), removes two amino acids from angiotensin I to form the octapeptide angiotensin II. ACE is a membrane-bound enzyme present in the brain, kidney, heart, and vascular smooth muscle and endothelial cells. It is particularly abundant in the lung which has an extensive area of vascular endothelium. Angiotensin II, via stimulation of a G-protein-coupled angiotensin (AT) receptor, has a number of actions, of which vasoconstriction and stimulation of aldosterone secretion from the adrenal cortex are the most important in relation to the control of blood pressure. Constriction of blood vessels increases peripheral resistance, whilst aldosterone, as discussed above, promotes sodium reabsorption in the kidney thereby increasing plasma volume. The vasoconstrictor and sodium-retaining effects of angiotensin both contribute to an increase in blood pressure. Consequently, interruption of the renin–angiotensin system will result in an antihypertensive effect. This is achieved by β-adrenoceptor antagonists (as discussed above), inhibitors of ACE, and angiotensin-receptor antagonists.

The first ACE inhibitor to be introduced into the clinic was captopril followed by a number of other compounds including enalapril, lisinopril, and quinapril, all of which are orally active. In addition to inhibiting the production of angiotensin II, these compounds cause the accumulation of bradykinin since ACE catalyses the metabolism of this peptide. Bradykinin has a vasodilator action and therefore its accumulation will contribute to the antihypertensive effect of ACE inhibitors.

A number of the adverse effects of ACE inhibitors have been attributed to the accumulation of bradykinin. These are cough, due to the elevation of bradykinin levels in the bronchial mucosa, which occurs in 5–20% of patients, and angioneurotic oedema— a rapid swelling of the nose, throat, mouth, glottis, larynx, lips and/or tongue. This latter effect, which occurs in only a small proportion of patients (0.1–0.2%), produces airway obstruction and respiratory distress, and may be fatal. Other adverse effects are hypotension following the first dose (particularly in patients who

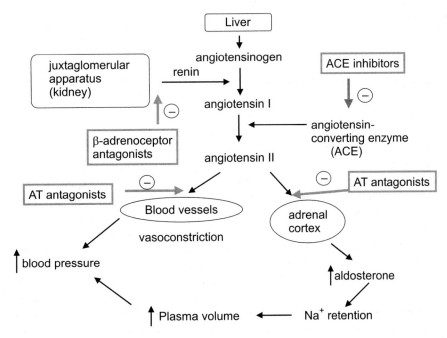

Fig. 16.3 The formation and actions of angiotensin II. β-Adrenoceptor antagonists inhibit the sympathetically mediated release of renin; ACE inhibitors prevent the conversion of angiotensin I to angiotensin II; and angiotensin receptor antagonists (AT antagonists) block the actions of angiotensin II.

are also taking diuretic drugs), hyperkalaemia, skin rash, altered sense of taste, and acute renal failure in patients with bilateral renal artery stenosis.

Angiotensin antagonists are recent additions to the armoury of antihypertensive agents, examples of which are losartan and valsartan. Both drugs are reversible competitive antagonists at the AT_1-receptor and are active orally. The adverse effects of losartan are similar to those of ACE inhibitors except the incidence of cough and angioneurotic oedema, which are probably due to bradykinin accumulation, is lower than with ACE inhibitors.

Treatment of hypertension

The main groups of drugs used to treat hypertension are thiazide diuretics, β-adrenoceptor antagonists, calcium channel-blocking drugs, and ACE inhibitors. In the event of failure to control hypertension satisfactorily with one drug, combinations of drugs with different modes of actions are employed to produce additive effects. Suitable combinations are:

- β-adrenoceptor antagonists and thiazide diuretics;

- β-adrenoceptor antagonists and dihydropyridine calcium-channel blocking drugs (note: the combination of a β-blocker with verapamil or diltiazem is *dangerous* since this may produce cardiac failure and conduction block at the AV-node since each drug has cardiac depressant effects);

- thiazide diuretics and ACE inhibitors.

However, when blood pressure has not been controlled by the main groups of antihypertensive drugs or in hypertensive emergencies, then other categories of drugs with antihypertensive actions are used, either alone or in combination. These drugs are described below. The sites of action of antihypertensive drugs are shown in Fig 16.4.

- α-ADRENOCEPTOR ANTAGONISTS (see Chapter 14).

- SODIUM NITROPRUSSIDE: This is administered intravenously to produce a rapid lowering of blood pressure in a hypertensive emergency. It spontaneously degrades to release nitric oxide (NO) which produces vasodilatation (see nitrates used in the treatment of angina).

- HYDRALAZINE: Lowers blood pressure by acting directly on smooth muscle to produce vasodilatation, therefore lowering peripheral resistance, although its mechanism of action is unknown. When given alone, hydralazine produces tachycardia and fluid retention. To counteract these effects, hydralazine is given with a β-adrenoceptor antagonist and a thiazide diuretic. Hydralazine has low oral bioavailability (on average 25%) due to first-pass metabolism. It is metabolized in part by acetylation and therefore has a lower bioavailability, with a reduced antihypertensive effect, for a given dose in fast acetylators compared to slow acetylators (see Chapter 1). An adverse effect of this drug, if used in doses exceeding 200 mg daily, is an autoimmune syndrome resembling systemic lupus erythematosus in which damage occurs to joints, lungs, and kidneys.

- TRIMETAPHAN: This is a ganglion blocker administered intravenously to treat hypertensive emergencies (see Chapter 14).

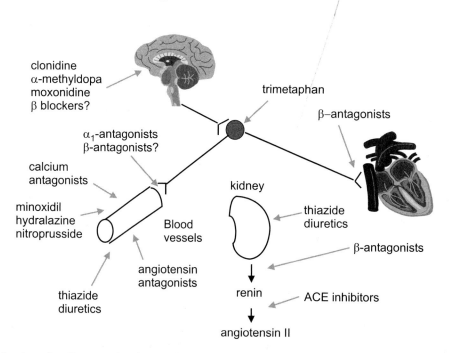

Fig. 16.4 Sites of action of antihypertensive drugs. The nerves shown are sympathetic nerves. The question mark indicates possible sites of action of β-adrenoceptor antagonists. Note that angiotensin antagonists also block the angiotensin receptor-mediated release of aldosterone from the adrenal cortex.

- MINOXIDIL: It is used to control severe hypertension resistant to other drugs. This drug produces hyperpolarization, which reduces Ca^{2+} influx via L-type calcium channels, by activating ATP-sensitive potassium channels. The reduction of Ca^{2+} influx into vascular smooth muscle cells produces vasodilatation and is a result of the action of monoxidil sulfate, the active metabolite. Similar to hydralazine, vasodilatation produced by minoxidil is accompanied by tachycardia and fluid retention and is therefore always administered with a β-adrenoceptor antagonist and a loop diuretic. A common adverse effect is stimulation of hair growth (hypertrichosis) on the face, arms, and legs which limits its use in women, although this drug is also marketed for topical use in the treatment of male baldness.

- CENTRALLY ACTING ANTIHYPERTENSIVES: Drugs such as α-methyldopa, clonidine, and moxonidine produce falls in cardiac output and peripheral resistance as a result of a reduction in sympathetic and an increase in parasympathetic outflows from the brain. These effects are due to stimulation, within the brainstem, of either postsynaptic $α_2$-adrenoceptors and/or a recently identified class of receptors termed imidazoline receptors. Inhibition of norepinephrine release from sympathetic nerves in the periphery, by stimulation of presynaptic $α_2$-adrenoceptors, may also contribute to the antihypertensive effect of these drugs. α-Methyldopa, which is metabolized within noradrenergic nerve terminals to the α-agonist, α-methylnorepinephrine (α-methylnoradrenaline), is recommended for use in hypertensive pregnant women since it has no adverse effects on the fetus. The use of clonidine is limited by the production of sedation and dry mouth, and the potential to cause rebound hypertension.

Key facts
Hypertension and antihypertensive drugs

- Hypertension, i.e. high blood pressure, has been defined as a sustained diastolic blood pressure greater than 90 mmHg. Essential hypertension, the cause of which is unknown, accounts for 90% of all cases of hypertension.

- The main groups of drugs used to treat hypertension are the thiazide diuretics, β-adrenoceptor antagonists, calcium antagonists, and angiotensin-converting enzyme (ACE) inhibitors.

- The antihypertensive effect of β-adrenoceptor antagonists results from a delayed fall in peripheral resistance in conjunction with a reduced cardiac output.

- Calcium channel-blocking drugs, such as verapamil and nifedipine, lower blood pressure by a vasodilator action that produces a fall in peripheral resistance.

- ACE inhibitors inhibit the production of angiotensin II and cause the accumulation of bradykinin, this latter effect producing cough. The antihypertensive effect of ACE inhibitors is due to vasodilatation and inhibition of the secretion of aldosterone, a steroid hormone that promotes Na^+ reabsorption in the kidney.

Angina pectoris

Angina pectoris is characterized by pain in the chest that can radiate to the arm, lower jaw, and neck, and is the result of ischaemic heart disease. The pain is caused by the accumulation of metabolites, such as adenosine, released from myocardium that has become ischaemic due to an imbalance in oxygen supply relative to oxygen demand. The most frequent cause of angina is atheromatous obstruction of the large coronary vessels, which is termed atherosclerotic, classical, or stable angina. In this form of angina, pain occurs when myocardial oxygen demand increases such as during exercise—it is therefore 'angina of effort'. Angina can also result from the transient spasm of localized sections of coronary vessels. This form of angina is classified as Prinzmetal's or variant angina and can occur at rest. Unstable angina is angina that occurs suddenly at rest or with minimal physical activity and increases in severity and frequency. This form of angina heralds the occurrence of myocardial infarction (death of an area of myocardium due to blockage or prolonged occlusion of a coronary artery) and results from platelet aggregation at a site of a ruptured atheromatous plaque. Treatment with aspirin, which inhibits platelet aggregation (see Chapter 6), has been found to reduce the risk of myocardial infarction by approximately 50% in patients with unstable angina.

Drugs used in the treatment of angina pectoris

To correct the imbalance between oxygen supply and demand, drugs used in the treatment of angina should either increase oxygen supply, by increasing coronary blood flow to the ischaemic myocardium, or decrease oxygen demand by reducing cardiac work. Both approaches are used, although a reduction in cardiac work is the easier of the two to achieve. Three main categories of drug are used in the treatment of angina, namely:

- nitrates;
- β-adrenoceptor antagonists;
- calcium channel-blocking drugs.

Nitrates

Glyceryl trinitrate/nitroglycerin is widely used in the treatment of angina, either for the relief of an anginal attack once started or prophylactically, when taken prior to exertion. It is normally administered sublingually either as a tablet held under the tongue or by means of a multidose spray. Whilst expensive, the multidose spray has an indefinite shelf life, in contrast to the tablets that degrade once the bottle is opened. Glyceryl trinitrate cannot be taken orally because of a pronounced first-pass effect. The duration of action of glyceryl trinitrate when taken sublingually is 30 minutes and, since it is well absorbed through the skin, can be administered by means of a transdermal patch to prevent anginal attacks occurring. The transdermal patch, which is replaced every 24 hours, is useful for patients who suffer anginal attacks at rest, particularly at night. Longer acting nitrates have been developed and include isosorbide mono- and dinitrate, and pentaerithrityl tetranitrate (pentaerythritol tetranitrate). These longer acting compounds have good oral bioavailability and therefore can be administered by mouth, although isosorbide dinitrate can also be taken sublingually in tablet form or as a spray.

The basis for the beneficial effects of nitrates in angina is a vasodilator action. This effect is a result of the generation of nitric oxide (NO) from a reaction with tissue-SH groups. NO activates guanylyl cyclase, which increases the formation of cyclic guanosine monophosphate (cGMP) so activating protein kinases (Fig. 16.5). cGMP-dependent protein kinases phosphorylate—thereby inactivating—myosin light-chain kinase. They also activate potassium channels, which results in the hyperpolarization of vascular smooth muscle. Both actions contribute to a vasodilator effect. It is important to note that NO is an endogenous compound that contributes to the control of vascular tone following its release from vascular endothelial cells in response to shear stress and mediators such as bradykinin and 5-HT.

Nitrates preferentially dilate large veins as opposed to arteries

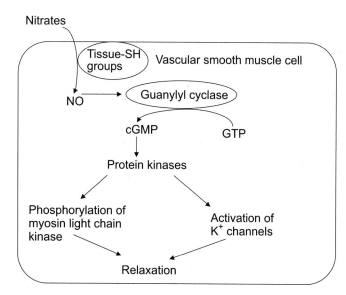

Fig. 16.5 Mode of action of nitrates. Nitrates generate nitric oxide (NO) which stimulates guanylyl cyclase with the formation of cyclic guanosine monophosphate (cGMP) from guanosine triphosphate (GTP). cGMP produces relaxation of vascular smooth muscle via activation of cGMP-dependent protein kinases.

and arterioles. This venodilator action reduces venous return to the heart, which decreases the pressure at diastole and therefore distension of the ventricle (ventricular end-diastolic pressure), i.e. a decrease in 'preload' A reduction in preload leads to a fall in cardiac output and a reduction in myocardial oxygen demand. A further beneficial effect of a reduced preload is an increase in the pressure gradient for perfusion across the ventricle wall. This improves perfusion of the subendocardium (ventricular muscle adjacent to the ventricular chamber)—i.e. the area of the myocardium most vulnerable to ischaemia. Nitrates may produce some dilatation of arterioles, so reducing peripheral resistance and decreasing 'afterload', that is to say the impedance to the output from the left ventricle. This reduction in afterload will also reduce cardiac work and oxygen consumption. In addition to systemic vasodilator effects, nitrates can also affect the coronary circulation resulting in an improvement in blood flow to the ischaemic myocardium. The exact mechanism responsible for this action is unclear, but it may involve dilatation of obstructed epicardial arteries and dilatation of collateral vessels—'bypass tracts' which circumvent partially blocked vessels. Nitrates are used in the treatment of both stable and variant angina; in the latter form, a relaxant effect on coronary arteries opposes the vascular spasm. Glyceryl nitrate can also be administered intravenously and is given by this route to relieve the pain of unstable angina.

The adverse effects of nitrates are also a result of their vasodilator actions and include:

- headache due to the dilatation of meningeal vessels,

- postural hypotension leading to dizziness and possibly fainting if the patient is standing;

- tachycardia as a compensatory sympathetic reflex to any fall in blood pressure.

Repeated administration of nitrates results in a diminished vasodilator effect, possibly as a result of depletion of free -SH groups. This tolerance to the antianginal effects of nitrates does not occur with glyceryl trinitrate (which has a short duration of action) unless it is administered by a skin patch, but this tolerance can arise with longer acting nitrates such as isosorbide mononitrate. A strategy to avoid the problem of tolerance is to allow a 'nitrate-free' period of 8–12 hours each day.

β-Adrenoceptor antagonists

These drugs are useful in the treatment of angina since they reduce myocardial oxygen consumption by reducing heart rate and contractility. This is the principal beneficial effect, but other actions may also contribute to their usefulness in angina. The subendocardial regions of the left ventricle only receive blood flow during diastole, as during systole the pressure inside the ventricle compresses the blood vessels that supply this part of the heart. The reduction in heart rate produced by β-blockers increases the time the heart is in diastole and therefore increases the time that the subendocardial regions of the heart are perfused. β-

Adrenoceptor antagonists have antihypertensive actions, as discussed above, and if a patient suffers from both hypertension and angina, the reduction in peripheral resistance produced by these drugs will reduce afterload and therefore decrease cardiac oxygen demand.

β-Blockers are not used for the symptomatic relief of an anginal attack, as are sublingual nitrates, but are administered orally to prevent or reduce the incidence of these attacks. Nitrates and β-blockers may be given in combination, this has the added useful effect that any increase in heart rate produced by nitrates will be reduced by the presence of the β-blocker. Whilst useful in the treatment of stable angina, β-blockers have no role in variant angina since they may increase vasospasm and worsen the pain. This effect in variant angina is probably due to antagonism of the β-adrenoceptor-mediated vasodilator effects of circulating epinephrine (adrenaline). Such an action would enhance the α-adrenoceptor-mediated constrictor effects of epinephrine, exacerbating coronary artery spasm. The properties and adverse effects of β-adrenoceptor antagonists are discussed in Chapter 14.

Calcium channel-blocking drugs

As described above, calcium-channel blockers reduce Ca^{2+} entry into cardiac muscle and vascular smooth muscle by binding to L-type calcium channels and reducing their probability of opening. Their beneficial effects in angina result from a decrease in cardiac oxygen demand due to negative inotropic and chronotropic actions, although these actions are only produced by calcium-channel blockers such as verapamil and diltiazem, and not by the dihydropyridines. All calcium channel blockers lower blood pressure, thereby reducing cardiac afterload with an associated fall in cardiac oxygen consumption. These drug also increase coronary blood flow by a dilatory action on epicardial arteries, which increases blood flow to the inner ischaemic subendocardium. In contrast to β-adrenoceptor antagonists, calcium-channel blocking drugs are useful in the prophylaxis of both stable and variant angina; their use in the latter, rarer form of angina is particularly effective in preventing coronary artery spasm. In the treatment of angina, calcium channel-blocking drugs can be used in combination with either nitrates or β-adrenoceptor antagonists although, as outlined above, the combination of a β-blocker with verapamil or diltiazem is to be avoided.

Key facts
Drugs used in the treatment of angina

- Angina pectoris occurs when coronary blood flow is insufficient to meet cardiac oxygen demands. Drugs used in the treatment of angina either improve oxygen supply by increasing blood flow to the ischaemic areas of the myocardium and/or decrease oxygen demand by reducing cardiac rate and contractility.

- Nitrates, such as glyceryl trinitrate, decrease cardiac contractility by reducing ventricular end-diastolic pressure as a result of a venodilator action. These drugs also increase coronary blood flow to the ischaemic myocardium, in part, by dilating collateral vessels. Their cellular mechanism of action is the generation of nitric oxide that then stimulates guanylyl cyclase.

- Glyceryl trinitrate is normally administered sublingually, either as a tablet or spray, for the acute relief of an anginal attack, or as transdermal patch which produces a longer effect for preventing episodes of angina.

- Nitrates are used in the treatment of both stable (fixed coronary artery narrowing due to atheroma) and variant angina (coronary artery spasm).

- The beneficial effects of β-adrenoceptor antagonists in angina are due to a reduction in cardiac rate and contractility that decreases oxygen demand. They are used in the prophylaxis of stable but not variant angina.

- Calcium channel-blocking drugs, such as verapamil and diltiazem, reduce cardiac oxygen demands by reducing heart rate and contractility. All calcium channel-blocking drugs, including dihydropyridines such as nifedipine, increase coronary blood flow and lower blood pressure thus reducing cardiac afterload, which decreases myocardial oxygen consumption.

- Calcium channel-blocking drugs are used in the treatment of both stable and variant angina

Heart (myocardial) failure

Heart failure can be defined as a state in which an abnormality of cardiac function leads to a failure of the heart to supply sufficient blood to meet the metabolic needs of the body. This state has a number of causes, including: myocardial infarction; cardiac valve disease; cardiomyopathies (diseases of the myocardium); and hypertension. Heart failure usually begins with left ventricular failure resulting in breathlessness due to pulmonary congestion and oedema (an increase in the volume of interstitial fluid), and decreased exercise tolerance. Left ventricular failure then causes the right ventricle to fail, although the exact mechanisms underlying this relationship are unclear. Failure of the right ventricle produces distended neck veins, hepatic engorgement, and peripheral oedema such as swelling of the ankles and legs. The combination of left and right ventricular failure associated with pulmonary and peripheral oedema is referred to as congestive heart failure. In heart failure, both cardiac output and blood pressure are reduced, which triggers compensatory reflexes to help maintain adequate organ and tissue perfusion. These compensatory reflexes include the activation of the sympathetic nervous system and the renin–angiotensin system, together with an increase in cardiac muscle mass (myocardial hypertrophy). However, these compensatory mechanisms are not well maintained and progressively fail to sustain an adequate cardiac output. Congestive heart failure can be acute, such as the sudden drop in cardiac output produced by myocardial infarction, or chronic, with a progressive deterioration in cardiac function as a consequence of hypertension or ischaemic heart disease.

There are three main approaches to the treatment of congestive heart failure:

- the use of diuretics to relieve oedema;
- drugs with a positive inotropic action resulting in an increase in cardiac output;
- drugs that produce vasodilatation and thereby decrease cardiac preload and afterload.

Diuretics in congestive heart failure

Diuretics increase renal Na^+ and water excretion, which reduces plasma volume and thereby venous pressure. The reduction in venous pressure reduces oedema and its symptoms, such as breathlessness resulting from pulmonary oedema. The lowering of venous pressure reduces preload (ventricular filling pressure) although, in patients with heart failure, this does not significantly lower cardiac output. Thiazide diuretics, such as bendroflumethiazide, are used in the treatment of mild congestive

heart failure, albeit at higher doses than required to treat hypertension. Loop diuretics, for example furosemide, are used in more severe congestive heart failure or in patients who no longer respond to thiazides. Loop diuretics may be given intravenously to produce rapid relief of acute pulmonary oedema. In order to limit the K^+ loss produced by thiazide and loop diuretics, these drugs can be given in combination with potassium-sparing diuretics (see above).

Drugs with a positive inotropic action

β-adrenoceptor agonists

Stimulation of cardiac β_1-receptors produces positive inotropic and chronotropic effects, although the two agonists used in the treatment of heart failure, dopamine and dobutamine, produce greater inotropic than chronotropic effects. These drugs can only be given intravenously and their use is restricted to the emergency situation of acute heart failure, such as that resulting from myocardial infarction.

Dopamine, whilst a neurotransmitter in its own right and a precursor in the synthesis of norepinephrine, is also a β-adrenoceptor agonist. Its positive inotropic effect is a result of directly stimulating β_1-adrenoceptors (Fig. 16.6) and an indirect sympathomimetic effect, i.e. the release of endogenous norepinephrine. Dopamine also stimulates specific dopamine receptors in the kidney that mediate increases in renal blood flow and urine

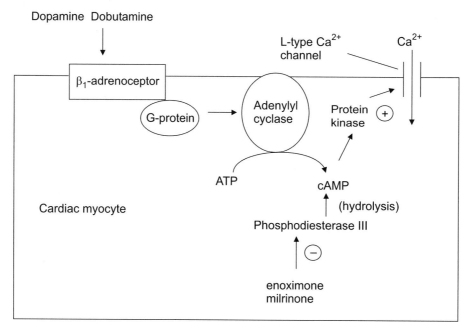

Fig. 16.6 The positive inotropic action of β-adrenoceptor agonists (dopamine and dobutamine) and phosphodiesterase inhibitors (enoximone and milrinone). Dopamine and dobutamine stimulate β_1-adrenoceptors, which results in an increase in the concentration of cyclic adenosine monophosphate (cAMP). cAMP activates cAMP-dependent protein kinases which phosphorylate L-type calcium channels resulting in an enhanced influx of Ca^{2+}. Enoximone and milrinone increase the concentration of cAMP by inhibiting phosphodiesterase III which hydrolyses cAMP.

output. This effect is useful since the reduction in renal blood flow resulting from a lowered cardiac output can lead to an impairment of renal function. Dobutamine is a relatively selective β_1-adrenoceptor agonist although, compared to dopamine, it does not directly affect renal blood flow. One hazard associated with the use of dopamine and dobutamine is that stimulation of cardiac β-adrenoceptors, particularly in the presence of myocardial ischaemia, can precipitate cardiac dysrhythmias. In addition, at high concentrations these agonists can also stimulate α-adrenoceptors producing vasoconstriction, which may exacerbate heart failure.

Phosphodiesterase inhibitors

Phosphodiesterase enzymes hydrolyse and therefore inactivate the cyclic nucleotides cGMP and cAMP. Inhibitors of phosphodiesterase used in the treatment of heart failure, such as enoximone and milrinone, are selective inhibitors of the type III family of phosphodiesterase isoenzymes that selectively hydrolyse cAMP. These drugs cause a rise in the intracellular concentration of cAMP, leading to an increase in the amount of Ca^{2+} that enters the cell during an action potential (Fig. 16.6). This produces an increase in the force of contraction of the heart resulting in a rise in cardiac output. Type III phosphodiesterase inhibitors also cause vasodilatation and therefore reduce peripheral resistance with no change in blood pressure or heart rate. However, they are only used in the short-term management of severe congestive heart failure, when they are administered intravenously, and not in the longer term treatment of patients with heart failure as clinical trials have shown that they can actually increase mortality.

Cardiac glycosides

The most widely used cardiac glycoside is digoxin, which is extracted from the purple (*Digitalis purpurea*) and white (*Digitalis lanata*) foxglove plant. Another example of a cardiac glycoside is digitoxin, also obtained from foxglove plants. Both cardiac glycosides have high oral bioavailability (70–100%), and whilst digoxin is primarily eliminated unchanged by renal excretion with a half-life of 36–48 hours, digitoxin is extensively metabolized in the liver with a half-life of 4–7 days. The longer half-life of digitoxin is, in part, a result of enterohepatic cycling following biliary excretion. Both drugs have a similar structure, consisting of a steroid nucleus, a lactone group, and a series of sugar residues.

Cardiac glycosides increase cardiac contractility and thus cardiac output by inhibiting membrane-bound Na^+/K^+ ATPase. This enzyme pumps three Na^+ ions out of the cell and two K^+ ions into the cell, and therefore inhibition results in an increase in the cytoplasmic Na^+ concentration. The increase in Na^+ concentration leads to an increase in Ca^{2+} concentration as a result of inhibition of the Na^+/Ca^{2+} exchanger (countertransporter) (Fig. 16.7). During diastole, this carrier protein normally moves Ca^{2+} out of the cell in exchange for Na^+. An increase in Na^+ concentration, due to inhibition of Na^+/K^+ ATPase, reduces the concentration gradient for Na^+ across the cell membrane, which, in turn, reduces the activity of the Na^+/Ca^{2+} exchanger, with the result that less Ca^{2+} is extruded. The elevated intracellular Ca^{2+} is actively pumped into the sarcoplasmic reticulum where it is available for release by subsequent action potentials; the net result being an increase in contractility.

In addition to affecting contractility, cardiac glycosides also

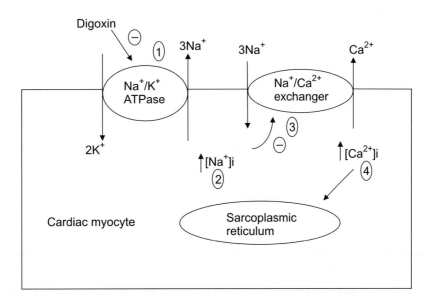

Fig. 16.7 The positive inotropic action of cardiac glycosides. Inhibition of Na^+/K^+ ATPase by cardiac glycosides such as digoxin (1) results in an increase in intracellular Na^+ concentration (2), which reduces the activity of the Na^+/Ca^{2+} exchanger (3). Less Ca^{2+} is transported out of the cell and the resulting increased levels of Ca^{2+} (4) are sequestered by the sarcoplasmic reticulum. This increases Ca^{2+} available for release by action potentials, enhancing cardiac contractility.

alter the electrical activity of the heart. They produce a reduction in heart rate, a decrease in conduction velocity, and an increase in refractory period at the atrioventricular (AV) node. These effects are the result of an increase in parasympathetic activity in the vagus nerve due, in part, to an action of cardiac glycosides in the CNS. The effect of cardiac glycosides on the AV node is responsible for their use in the treatment of supraventricular dysrhythmias (see below).

Cardiac glycosides have a low therapeutic index and therefore a narrow margin between concentrations that are effective compared to concentrations that produce toxic effects. The adverse effects of these drugs are nausea, vomiting, disturbed colour vision, confusion (especially in the elderly), and cardiac dysrhythmias ranging from AV block to ventricular tachycardia. The risk of cardiac glycoside overdose in patients can be minimized by monitoring their blood concentrations. Should overdose occur, treatment is available in the form of intravenous digoxin antibody fragments (Fab fragments). The high affinity of these fragments for cardiac glycosides prevents their binding to Na^+/K^+ ATPase, enabling the drugs to be cleared from the circulation. The potential of cardiac glycosides to produce cardiac dysrhythmias is increased if plasma K^+ decreases (hypokalaemia), since cardiac glycosides and K^+ ions compete for the same binding site on Na^+/K^+ ATPase. This effect is important since thiazide and loop diuretics, which are also used in the treatment of congestive heart failure, are liable to produce hypokalaemia.

Cardiac glycosides are widely used in the treatment of cardiac failure associated with atrial fibrillation, although their use in heart failure patients in sinus rhythm has declined with the increased use of ACE inhibitors (see below).

Vasodilators in the treatment of heart failure

The use of vasodilators in the treatment of heart failure is an alternative approach to prescribing drugs with a positive inotropic effect. The beneficial effects of vasodilators are due to reductions in preload and afterload produced by dilatation of veins and arterioles, respectively. A reduction in preload lowers venous pressure leading to a fall in ventricular filling pressures thereby relieving pulmonary oedema and oedema in the periphery (swelling of ankles and legs). Preload reduction also reduces myocardial oxygen demand with minimal effects on cardiac output in patients with congestive heart failure. A reduction in afterload reduces the impedance to emptying of the left ventricle and therefore results in an increase in cardiac output.

Angiotensin-converting enzyme (ACE) inhibitors

These drugs are the first-line treatment for congestive heart failure since they have been shown to prolong survival. ACE inhibitors, such as captopril and enalapril, produce dilatation of veins and arterioles, which leads to reductions in both preload and afterload. In addition, ACE inhibitors diminish the angiotensin II-mediated release of aldosterone from the adrenal cortex (see

Fig. 16.3), a hormone that promotes Na^+ reabsorption in the collecting tubules of the kidney. This action reduces plasma volume, which, together with venodilatation, contributes to the fall in preload. Local generation of angiotensin II within in the heart has been implicated in myocardial hypertrophy—i.e. a compensatory response to heart failure. Myocardial hypertrophy initially helps to maintain cardiac output but with time the ventricles become less compliant, an effect that eventually contributes to the reduction in cardiac output. In addition, myocardial hypertrophy is a risk factor for the development of ventricular dysrhythmias. ACE inhibitors therefore have the advantageous effect of reducing the development of myocardial hypertrophy. A summary of the beneficial actions of ACE inhibitors in congestive heart failure is shown in Fig. 16.8, whilst their adverse effects have been detailed above. Angiotensin (AT_1) receptor antagonists, such as losartan, would be expected to have similar beneficial effects in congestive heart failure as ACE inhibitors, but this remains to be established.

Nitrovasodilators and hydralazine

Nitroprusside is equally effective as a dilator of veins or arteries, and as a result produces falls in both preload and afterload. This drug has a role in the short-term management of acute heart failure when given by IV infusion, with the infusion rate titrated to produce optimum haemodynamic effects.

Glyceryl trinitrate and longer acting nitrates, such as isosorbide dinitrate, preferentially dilate veins and therefore reduce preload, whilst hydralazine lowers afterload since it selectively dilates arterioles. A combination of hydralazine and nitrates therefore reduces both preload and afterload, an effect similar to ACE inhibitors, and such combinations have been shown to reduce mortality in patients with congestive heart failure. This combination is useful for the treatment of patients who are unable to tolerate ACE inhibitors.

Key facts
Drugs used in the treatment of congestive heart failure

- Congestive heart failure is characterized by a reduced cardiac output associated with pulmonary and peripheral oedema.

- Diuretic drugs such as thiazide and loop diuretics are used to reduce oedema.

- Stimulation of cardiac β_1-adrenoceptors by dopamine and dobutamine produces a positive inotropic effect. These drugs are administered IV to elevate cardiac output in the short-term management of acute heart failure following myocardial infarction.

- Phosphodiesterase inhibitors, such as enoximone and milrinone, cause a rise in cAMP levels thereby producing a positive inotropic effect. They are given IV in the short-term treatment of severe congestive heart failure.

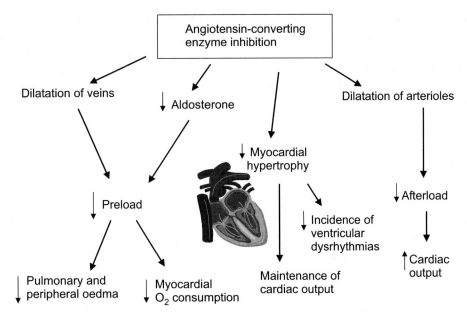

Fig. 16.8 The beneficial effects of angiotensin-converting enzyme inhibition in congestive heart failure. Inhibition of the production of angiotensin II reduces both preload and afterload and reduces myocardial hypertrophy.

- Cardiac glycosides, for example digoxin, produce a positive inotropic effect by inhibiting Na^+/K^+ ATPase, which indirectly elevates intracellular Ca^{2+} concentration. The principal use of these drugs is for the treatment of heart failure in patients who also suffer from atrial fibrillation.

- Angiotensin-converting enzyme (ACE) inhibitors, such as captopril, are the first-choice treatment for congestive heart failure and have been shown to reduce mortality. These drugs reduce preload, which reduces oedema, and lower afterload, which produces an increase in cardiac output.

- A combination of hydralazine and nitrates is an alternative to the use of ACE inhibitors.

Normal cardiac rhythm

The resting membrane potential of normal cardiac muscle is about −80 mV and, similar to other excitable tissue such as nerves, cardiac muscle depolarizes in response to a transient increase in Na^+ permeability via opening of voltage-dependent Na^+ channels. This increase in sodium permeability represents phase 0 of the action potential, which, along with other phases of the action potential, is shown in Fig. 16.9. The heart possesses specialized pacemaker cells, such as in the sinoatrial (SA) and AV nodes, that undergo spontaneous depolarization (phase 4 of the action potential) resulting in the generation of action potentials. Other differences between cardiac muscle and other excitable tis-

sues are: (1) an action potential of long duration and a long refractory period; and (2) a large influx of Ca^{2+} during the plateau of the action potential (phase 2) that triggers the release of Ca^{2+} from the sarcoplasmic reticulum.

The action potentials generated by the SA node are rapidly conducted throughout the heart by specialized conducting tissues such as the Purkinje fibres. During normal function, the atria contract a fraction of a second prior to ventricular contraction, which allows adequate filling of the ventricles. The conducting systems of the heart also produce a co-ordinated contraction of the ventricle—this is necessary for generating effective pressures in the ventricles in order to propel blood through the pulmonary and peripheral circulations. The pacemaker cells in the heart and the conducting system are influenced by the autonomic nervous system. Stimulation of parasympathetic vagal nerves reduces heart rate, by reducing the rate of spontaneous depolarization at the SA node, and decreases excitability at the AV node, thereby slowing transmission of impulses to the ventricles. Stimulation of sympathetic nerves produces essentially opposite effects. Conducting tissue and pacemaker cells are susceptible to damage, especially by ischaemia, leading to abnormalities of cardiac rhythm that can the affect the pumping efficiency of the heart.

Cardiac dysrhythmias

Cardiac dysrhythmias or arrhythmias, the two terms being interchangeable, refer to an abnormal heart rhythm and their classification is based on electrocardiographic recordings (a normal electrocardiogram (ECG) is shown in Fig. 16.9). Their origin may be supraventricular, i.e. in the atria or AV node, or

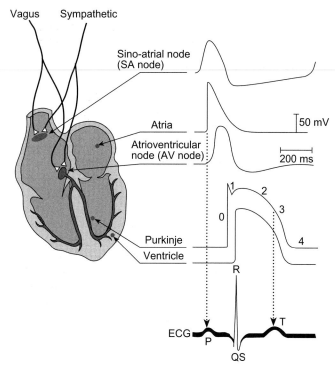

Fig. 16.9 The cardiac action potential in various regions of the heart in relation to a normal electrocardiogram (ECG). The different phases of the action potential for a Purkinje fibre are: phase 0, rapid depolarization due to the influx of Na^+ via voltage-dependent sodium channels; phase 1, partial repolarization due inactivation of Na^+ channels; phase 2, the plateau phase resulting from slow Ca^{2+} influx via L-type voltage-sensitive Ca^{2+} channels; phase 3, the repolarization phase due to inactivation of the Ca^{2+} current and efflux of K^+ due to activation of K^+ channels (delayed rectifier K^+ channels); and phase 4, the pacemaker potential (shown clearly for the SA node) which is a gradual depolarization during diastole resulting from a number of currents including inward movement of Na^+ and Ca^{2+}.

ventricular. The characteristics of the main dysrhythmias are outlined below:

- *Atrial tachycardia* (atrial rate: 120–250 beats min^{-1}). The AV node may conduct all the abnormal impulses to the ventricles, or there is an element of AV block where only some impulses are conducted.

- *Atrial flutter* (atrial rate: 250–350 beats min^{-1}) is associated with a degree of AV block. Usually 1 in 2 impulses generated in the atria are conducted to the ventricle, giving a ventricular rate of 150 beats min^{-1}.

- *Atrial fibrillation* (atrial rate 350–600 beats min^{-1}) in which beating of the atria is irregular. The pumping function of the atria is minimal and the ventricular rate is also irregular. Thrombosis may occur in the left atrium and thrombi

may leave to produce systemic emboli that can result in a stroke.

- *Ventricular premature beats* (ventricular ectopic beats) are defined as discrete premature QRS complexes.

- *Ventricular tachycardia* is defined as a run of four or more consecutive ventricular premature beats.

- *Ventricular fibrillation* is a rapid totally uncoordinated contraction of ventricular muscle that is fatal within minutes; 90% of all deaths following myocardial infarction are caused by ventricular fibrillation.

- *Torsade de points*, is a French term meaning twisting of points; it is a life-threatening form of ventricular tachycardia with an undulating baseline on the ECG usually associated with a prolonged QT interval.

A major cause of dysrhythmias, particularly ventricular, is myocardial ischaemia resulting from arteriosclerosis or coronary artery spasm that may eventually lead to myocardial infarction. The link between myocardial ischaemia and the generation of dysrhythmias has not been clearly identified, but it may be due to the accumulation of extracellular K^+ and/or the release of inflammatory mediators. Stimulation of cardiac β-adrenoceptors, as a result of high levels of cardiac sympathetic nerve activity or elevated circulating levels of epinephrine (adrenaline), may also trigger dysrhythmias. Myocardial ischaemia can also lead to stimulation of cardiac β-adrenoceptors since the release of norepinephrine from sympathetic nerves occurs during ischaemia. A further cause of dysrhythmias are drugs, the major group of which are paradoxically those used to treat dysrhythmias (see below).

Mechanisms of dysrhythmias

Dysrhythmias can arise as a result of two basic mechanisms:

(1) abnormal impulse generation due to:

- abnormal pacemaker activity,
- triggered abnormal impulse generation;

(2) abnormal impulse conduction due to:

- heart block,
- re-entry.

Abnormal impulse generation

ABNORMAL PACEMAKER ACTIVITY

Pacemaker activity (automaticity) occurs in the SA and AV nodes and conducting tissue such as Purkinje fibres. In a normal heart, the SA node discharges at the fastest rate and dominates the heart rhythm whilst other pacemakers, referred to as subsidiary pacemakers, discharge at a slower rate and are suppressed by the faster rate of the SA node. Partial depolarization due to ischaemia and/or the release of norepinephrine can produce an increase in the rate of discharge of subsidiary pacemakers or induce pacemaker activity in parts of the heart that are normally quiescent. Such conditions trigger dysrhythmias such as atrial tachycardias or ventricular premature beats.

TRIGGERED ABNORMAL IMPULSE GENERATION

This form of abnormal impulse generation is due to either early or delayed after-depolarizations triggered by the previous 'normal' impulse. Early after-depolarizations occur during the repolarization of the action potential (phase 3, Fig. 16.9). This form of triggered activity occurs during an abnormally prolonged action potential that can be produced by class III antidysrhythmic drugs (see below) resulting in *torsade de points*. Delayed after-depolarizations occur after the preceding action potential has finished. They appear to be a result of an elevated intracellular Ca^{2+} concentration that produces a transient inward current due to the activity of the Na^+/Ca^{2+} exchange mechanism. Delayed after-depolarizations are thought to underlie the production of ventricular tachycardia.

Abnormal impulse conduction

HEART BLOCK

Nodal tissue such as the AV node may become damaged, for example as a result of myocardial infarction, so that it fails to conduct normally, i.e. heart block. The extent of the block varies depending on the extent of damage to the AV node. The block may be partial and regular, such as 2:1 or 3:1 as indicated on the ECG with more than one P wave for each QRS–T complex. Alternatively, the heart block may be complete and here the atria and ventricles beat independently at rates determined by their own pacemakers with no relationship between P waves and QRS–T complexes. Heart block may occur 'physiologically' such as in atrial flutter when the rate of impulse generation in the atria exceeds the maximum rate of conduction of impulses at the AV node (see characteristics of dysrhythmias above).

RE-ENTRY

This type of abnormal impulse conduction occurs when there is a unidirectional block in an area of cardiac tissue; conduction fails in the normal direction (anterograde) but can occur in the reverse direction (retrograde conduction) (Fig. 16.10). This situation can arise when there is damage to an area of cardiac tissue, such as that produced by ischaemia, resulting in partial depolarization. Retrograde conduction through the damaged area is slow but, when the action potential emerges, it is able to re-excite the area beyond the block since this tissue has passed through its refractory period. The action potential then continuously circulates around this pathway (circus movement) to create a dysrhythmia. Re-entry is considered to be involved in a range of dysrhythmias including atrial fibrillation, ventricular tachycardia, and ventricular fibrillation. One mechanism by which antidysrhythmic drugs can terminate re-entry activity is to prolong the refractory period, such that when the retrograde action potential emerges from the area of unidirectional block, the adjacent tissue is still in its refractory period and will fail to propagate the action potential.

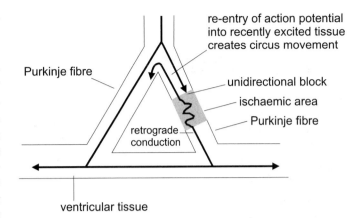

Fig 16.10 An example of re-entry activity in Purkinje fibres and ventricular tissue. An area of ischaemia produces a unidirectional block in which conduction in the anterograde direction is blocked, but conduction is allowed in the retrograde direction. Retrograde conduction through the ischaemic areas is slow (as indicated by the wavy line), and when the action potential emerges from this area it is able to re-excite the adjacent tissue producing continuous circulation of the action potential (circus movement).

Classification of antidysrhythmic drugs

Antidysrhythmic drugs were originally classified by Vaughan Williams on the basis of their predominant antidysrhythmic action (Table 16.2). This classification system defines the principal type of antidysrhythmic drug action, although some drugs have an antidysrhythmic profile of action that incorporates properties from more than one class.

Class 1 antidysrhythmic drugs

These drugs exert their actions by blocking cardiac sodium channels. Their sodium-channel blocking action is identical to that of local anaesthetics (see Chapter 8) but higher concentrations are required for a block of neuronal conduction than for antidysrhythmic actions. Sodium channels can exist in three states: open; closed; and inactivated (refractory). Class I antidysrhythmic drugs only bind to the channel when it is in the open or inactivated state, and once bound they stabilize the inactivated state. Therefore, these drugs show the property of use-dependence, i.e. the more frequently the channels are activated, the greater the degree of block. This is a useful characteristic as it results in channel blockade at the high excitation frequencies that occur in dysrhythmias, with little effect on cardiac function at normal rates of beating. Sodium-channel block produced by class I drugs results in a number of antidysrhythmic effects, including: a decrease in pacemaker activity; inhibition of early and delayed after-depolarizations; and abolition of re-entry activity. The effect on re-entry is due to either an increase in refractory period (see above) or a depression of conduction in ischaemic tissue such that unidirectional block is converted to bidirectional block.

Table 16.2 The classification of antidysrhythmic drugs and their adverse effects

Class	Action	Examples	Uses	Adverse effects
Ia	Block of Na$^+$ channels	Quinidine, procainamide and disopyramide	Supraventricular and ventricular dysrhythmias	Negative inotropic effects *Torsade de points* Atropine-like effects Quinidine—thrombocytopenia, dizziness, tinnitus, nausea, vomiting, and diarrhoea Procainamide—systemic lupus erythematosus
Ib	Block of Na$^+$ channels	Lidocaine (IV only), mexiletine and tocainide	Ventricular dysrhythmias following myocardial infarction	CNS effects: drowsiness, disorientation, and convulsions
Ic	Block of Na$^+$ channels	Flecainide and encainide	Ventricular tachycardias	Increased mortality after myocardial infarction
II	β-Adrenoceptor antagonism	Atenolol, metoprolol, and esmolol (IV only)	Control of ventricular rate in atrial fibrillation. Prevention of ventricular dysrhythmias following myocardial infarction	See Chapter 14
III	Prolongation of action potential duration (blockade of delayed rectifier K$^+$ channels)	Amiodarone, sotalol	Supraventricular and ventricular dysrhythmias	*Torsade de points* Amiodarone—photosensitive skin rashes; hypo- or hyperthyroidism due to iodine content; pulmonary fibrosis and corneal deposits Sotalol—see Chapter 14
IV	Calcium channel-blocking drugs	Verapamil, diltiazem	Supraventricular tachycardias and control of ventricular rate in atrial fibrillation	Negative inotropic effects Verapamil—constipation
V*	Cardiac glycosides	Digoxin	Control of ventricular rate in atrial fibrillation	Ventricular premature beats, ventricular tachycardia, ventricular fibrillation (also see under treatment of heart failure)

* This group is not always included in classification of antidysrhythmic drugs.

Class I antidysrhythmic drugs can be subclassified according to the kinetics of their binding to sodium channels.

- Class Ia agents, such as quinidine, procainamide, and disopyramide, were the earliest examples of class I drugs, and their rates of association and dissociation at the sodium channel are intermediate between classes 1b and 1c. They are used in the treatment of both supraventricular and ventricular tachycardias although, as a result of adverse effects, the use of quinidine and procainamide is very limited.

- Class 1b drugs, for example lidocaine (lignocaine), mexiletine, and tocainide, associate and dissociate rapidly. They dissociate from the channels in time for the next action

potential if the cardiac rhythm is normal, but they will prevent premature beats because the channels will still be blocked. These drugs also bind selectively to sodium channels in the refractory state, which are present in ischaemic tissue where the cells are depolarized. This subclass is therefore particularly useful in the control of ventricular dysrhythmias following myocardial infarction. Lidocaine is an exception amongst antidysrhythmic drugs in that it cannot be given orally due to a large first-pass effect, and therefore is only administered intravenously.

- Class Ic drugs, such as flecainide and encainide, associate and dissociate much more slowly than those of the class Ia group and, in contrast to other class 1 drugs, do not prolong the refractory period. They are used for ventricular tachycardias, although with caution since clinical trials have shown that these drugs cause an increase, as opposed to an expected decrease, in sudden death associated with ventricular fibrillation when given to patients who have already suffered a myocardial infarction.

Class II antidysrhythmic drugs (β-adrenoceptor antagonists)

Increased sympathetic activity and elevated circulating levels of epinephrine resulting from exercise or emotional stress can trigger cardiac dysrhythmias. This effect is mediated by stimulation of cardiac β_1-adrenoceptors, which increases Ca^{2+} influx (see Fig 16.6). An increase in Ca^{2+} influx has a number of dysrhythmogenic effects including: enhanced pacemaker activity; an increase in the probability of delayed afterdepolarizations; and an increase in the rate of conduction at the AV node. β-Adrenoceptor antagonists therefore have antidysrhythmic actions and are used to reduce the occurrence of ventricular dysrhythmias following myocardial infarction, which are, in part, due to increased sympathetic activity. Such use of β-adrenoceptor antagonists has been shown to reduce mortality. β-Adrenoceptor antagonists are also used to reduce the ventricular rate in supraventricular tachycardias as a consequence of slowing conduction within the AV node. All β-blockers have antidysrhythmic properties: the selective β_1-blockers atenolol and metoprolol being the most frequently used for the longer term treatment of dysrhythmias, whilst intravenous esmolol is used for immediate treatment, such as the control of ventricular rate in atrial fibrillation.

Class III antidysrhythmic drugs

This class of antidysrhythmic drugs induce prolongation of the action potential duration, which increases the refractory period of the myocardium. This effect is most probably a result of the blockade of delayed rectifier K^+ channels that open during repolarization (phase 3 of the action potential). One example of a drug in this class is amiodarone, which is used to treat both supraventricular and ventricular dysrhythmias. In addition to class III actions, amiodarone also blocks Na^+ channels and β-adrenoceptors—i.e. class I and II actions, which may contribute to its antidysrhythmic actions. Amiodarone is extensively bound to tissues and has a very long half-life of over 50 days such that its action normally takes days or weeks to develop. Consequently, an intravenous loading dose (see Chapter 1) is used in the treatment of life-threatening dysrhythmias. Sotalol, as its name indicates, is a β-adrenoceptor antagonist although this is a property of the *l*-isomer only, whilst class III activity is shared by both *d*- and *l*-isomers. Sotalol has similar antidysrhythmic actions to amiodarone but lacks its adverse effects (see Table 16.2) and is useful in patients in whom β-adrenoceptor antagonists are not contraindicated. As discussed above, prolongation of the action potential produced by both sotalol and amiodarone is liable to produce *torsade de points*.

Class IV antidysrhythmic drugs (calcium channel-blocking drugs)

Antidysrhythmic actions are possessed by the calcium channel-blocking drugs verapamil and diltiazem, but not by dihydropyridine compounds, such as nifedipine, which predominately act on vascular smooth muscle. The predominant electrophysiological effects of the blockade of L-type, voltage-dependent calcium channels in the heart is a slowing of the SA node pacemaker, and slowing of conduction and prolongation of refractory period at the AV node. In addition, conduction through ischaemic tissue is also slowed since such tissues are partially depolarized, with inactivation of sodium channels, so that the upstroke of the action potential is more dependent on the slower Ca^{2+} current. This effect may terminate re-entry activity by converting unidirectional to bidirectional block. Verapamil and diltiazem are used to terminate supraventricular tachycardias and to control ventricular rate in atrial fibrillation when such control has not been achieved with digoxin (see below). These drugs are not used in the treatment of ventricular dysrhythmias.

Class V antidysrhythmic drugs (cardiac glycosides)

Digoxin, in addition to having positive inotropic effects, has antidysrhythmic properties. As discussed above, digoxin slows conduction and increases the refractory period at the AV node, which is useful in reducing ventricular rate in atrial fibrillation. This action does not abolish the fibrillation but improves pumping efficiency by increasing the time available for ventricular filling.

Key facts
Cardiac dysrhythmias and antidysrhythmic drugs

- Cardiac dysrhythmias arise as a result of either abnormal impulse generation or abnormal impulse conduction. Abnormal impulse generation is produced by abnormal pacemaker activity or triggered impulse generation, whilst abnormal impulse conduction is a result of heart block or re-entry that produces circus movement of an action potential.

- Class I antidysrhythmic drugs produce a use-dependent block of cardiac Na^+ channels and are divided into three groups depending upon their rate of association and dissociation at the Na^+ channel. Class Ia drugs, such as disopyramide, are used in the treatment of supraventricular and ventricular dysrhythmias. Lidocaine is an example of a class Ib drug and is used to control ventricular dysrhythmias following myocardial infarction. Class Ic drugs, such as flecainide, are used in the treatment of ventricular tachycardias.

(cont.)

- Class II antidysrhythmic drugs are β-adrenoceptor antagonists, used to prevent ventricular dysrhythmias following myocardial infarction and to control the ventricular rate in supraventricular tachycardias.

- Class III antidysrhythmic drugs prolong the action potential duration as a result of blockade of K^+ channels. Examples are amiodarone and sotalol that are used in the treatment of both supraventricular and ventricular dysrhythmias.

- Class IV drugs are calcium-channel blocking drugs, such as verapamil and diltiazem, which are used to terminate supraventricular tachycardias and to control ventricular rate in atrial fibrillation.

- Class V drugs are cardiac glycosides, for example digoxin, which increase the refractory period and slow conduction at the AV node. This effect is useful in reducing ventricular rate in atrial fibrillation.

Further reading

Cohn, J. N. (1996). The management of chronic heart failure. *New England Journal of Medicine*, **335**, 490–8.

Moncada, S. and Higgs, A. (1993). The L-arginine–nitric oxide pathway. *New England Journal of Medicine*, **329**, 2002–12.

Roden, D. M. (1996). Antiarrhythmic drugs. In *Goodman and Gilman's the pharmacological basis of therapeutics* (9th edn) (ed. J. G. Hardman, L. E. Limbird, P. B. Molinoff, R. W. Ruddon, and A. G. Gilman), pp 839–74. McGraw Hill, New York.

Rutherford, J. D. (1993). Pharmacologic management of angina and myocardial infarction. *American Journal of Cardiology*, **72**, 16C–20C.

World Health Organisation (1993). The 1993 guidelines for the treatment of mild hypertension. *Hypertension*, **22**, 392–403.

Yates, M. S. and Bowmer, C. J. (1997). Drugs and the renal system. In *Integrated pharmacology* (ed. C. P. Page, M. J. Curtis, M. C. Sutter, M. J. A. Walker, and B. Hoffman), pp. 215–30. Mosby, London.

17

Drugs acting on the respiratory system

Drugs acting on the respiratory system

Regulation of the airway glands and smooth muscle

Normal function of the airways is controlled by:

- the parasympathetic nervous system (via the vagus nerve);
- the sympathetic nervous system;
- circulating epinephrine (adrenaline);
- an inhibitory, non-adrenergic, non-cholinergic (NANC) nervous system.

In addition, in respiratory diseases such as asthma and bronchitis, inflammatory mediators such leukotrienes and NANC contractile mediators also influence airway function.

The parasympathetic nervous system releases acetylcholine, which stimulates muscarinic M_1 and M_3 receptors mediating glandular secretion and the contraction of smooth muscle in the larger airways. Sympathetic nerves innervate glands, producing inhibition of secretion, but do not innervate bronchial smooth muscle. However, β_2-adrenoceptors are present in bronchial smooth muscle and are stimulated by circulating epinephrine which produces relaxation, leading to increased airway patency in both large and small airways (bronchi and bronchioles). The NANC nervous system can be regarded as a further division of the autonomic nervous system. The inhibitory component involves nitric oxide or vasoactive intestinal peptide (VIP) as neurotransmitters that mediate the relaxation of airway smooth muscle. Stimulant NANC mediators are excitatory neuropeptides, such as substance P, that can be released from sensory nerves by an axon reflex, producing contraction of bronchiolar smooth muscle and an increase in mucus secretion. An axon reflex is a local neural mechanism whereby a response in a sensory nerve is relayed down other branches of the sensory nerve to adjacent tissues. A summary of the factors that control the tone of bronchial smooth muscle is shown in Fig. 17.1.

Bronchial asthma

Bronchial asthma is a recurrent reversible airway obstruction, which results in cough, wheezing, and dyspnoea (disorder of breathing) characterized by difficulty in breathing out. Whilst acute attacks are reversible, the underlying inflammatory changes may not be reversible but progressive. Asthma is not

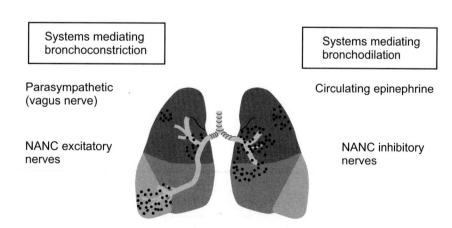

Fig. 17.1 Systems which control the tone of bronchial smooth muscle. Bronchial smooth muscle tone is a balance between the constrictor effects of the parasympathetic nervous system and non-adrenergic, non-cholinergic (NANC) excitatory nerves as opposed to the dilator effects of circulating epinephrine and NANC inhibitory nerves.

simply an anaphylactic reaction to allergens, such as pollen and proteins from the house dust mite, but a condition of bronchial hyper-responsiveness in which there is an abnormal airway response to other stimuli such as respiratory infections, cigarette smoke, cold air, and exercise. In many cases of asthma it is possible to distinguish two phases: an immediate phase consisting mainly of bronchospasm lasting for 1–2 hours; and a delayed, more protracted, inflammatory phase occurring 4–5 hours after the initial irritant stimulus. The incidence of asthma is increasing, ranging from 5 to 10% of the population in industrialized countries, and in a small proportion of cases proves fatal.

The initial stimulus in asthma activates mast cells and monocytes to release a range of inflammatory mediators, including: histamine; prostaglandins; platelet-activating factor (PAF); and leukotrienes LTB_4, LTC_4, and LTD_4 (Fig. 17.2). These mediators produce bronchospasm, of which the most important are LTC_4 and LTD_4, whilst LTB_4 and PAF act as chemotaxins attracting T-cells and eosinophils to the area. These cells release further inflammatory mediators, including cytokines, which activate axon reflexes and release NANC excitatory peptide neurotransmitters. These peptides, in conjunction with the other mediators, cause mucus production and oedema, in addition to bronchospasm. Epithelial damage is also produced by the release from eosinophils of major basic protein (MBP), eosinophil peroxidase (EP), and eosinophil cationic protein (ECP). Epithelial damage produces bronchial hyper-responsiveness due, in part, to the exposure of sensory nerves; this hyper-responsiveness makes them more easily stimu-

Key facts
Bronchial asthma

- Asthma is recurrent, reversible airway obstruction resulting in cough, wheezing, and difficulty in breathing out due to the contraction of bronchial smooth muscle and increased mucus secretion.

- It is an inflammatory disease associated with the release of a range of inflammatory mediators such as PAF, leukotrienes, cytokines, and neuropeptides released by axon reflexes, whilst histamine plays only a minor role in the inflammatory response.

- Asthma is characterized by bronchial hyper-responsiveness —an abnormal airway response to a range of stimuli including allergens, exercise, and respiratory infections. Bronchial hyper-responsiveness is due to damage to the bronchial epithelium produced by proteins released from eosinophils.

lated by irritants, with the further release of NANC excitatory peptides.

Drugs used in the treatment of asthma

The treatment of asthma involves two categories of drugs: bronchodilators to directly counteract bronchospasm; and anti-inflammatory drugs to inhibit the underlying inflammatory process.

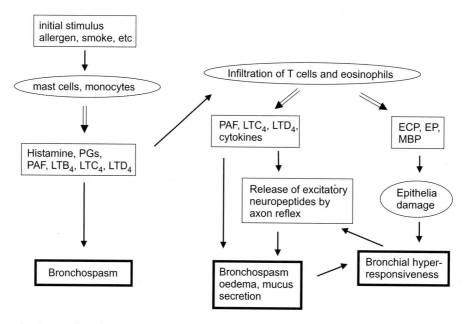

Fig. 17.2 The mechanisms and mediators involved in asthma. PGs, prostaglandins; PAF, platelet-activating factor; LTB_4, LTC_4, and LTD_4, leukotrienes B_4, C_4, and D_4; ECP, eosinophil cationic protein; EP, eosinophil peroxidase; MBP, major basic protein.

Brochodilators

β₂-ADRENOCEPTOR AGONISTS

Stimulation of β₂-adrenoceptors, via activation of adenylyl cyclase, produces dilatation of bronchial smooth muscle. Agonists at these receptors act as physiological antagonists (see Chapter 2) of the bronchoconstriction produced by inflammatory mediators. β₂-Adrenoceptor agonists also inhibit the release of inflammatory mediators from mast cells. They are normally given by inhalation in the form of an aerosol, powder, or nebulized solution, although some β₂-adrenoceptor agonists may be administered orally or, in the treatment of severe acute asthma (status asthmaticus), by subcutaneous injection.

β₂-Adrenoceptor agonists available for the treatment of asthma are divided into short- and longer acting agents. Drugs such as salbutamol, terbutaline, and fenoterol have a short duration of action of 3–4 hours with a maximum effect within 30 minutes. Longer acting drugs, which include salmeterol and eformoterol, have a duration of action of 12 hours or longer, although salmeterol has a delayed onset of action compared with short-acting agents. The prolonged duration of action, at least of salmeterol, is due to the presence of a long lipophilic tail in the molecule that binds to an 'exoreceptor' adjacent to the β₂-adrenoceptor in bronchial smooth muscle. Short-acting β₂-adrenoceptor agonists are used for the acute relief of bronchospasm, whilst the longer acting drugs are used for the prevention of asthmatic attacks, which is of particular use in nocturnal asthma. The adverse effects associated with the use of β₂-adrenoceptor agonists are tremor and occasionally hypokalaemia when used in conjunction with xanthines and glucocorticoids.

XANTHINES

The main xanthine used in the treatment of asthma is theophylline, which is given orally. It is also available for intravenous use in attacks of severe asthma as aminophylline (theophylline combined with ethylenediamine), which is 20 times more soluble than theophylline. The mechanism of the bronchodilator action of theophylline is unclear, but it may result from the inhibition of phosphodiesterases (enzymes which hydrolyse cyclic nucleotides). Such an action causes a rise in the level of cAMP, which—similar to the effects of β₂-adrenoceptor agonists—produces relaxation of bronchial smooth muscle. Theophylline is also a competitive antagonist at receptors for adenosine. This could also account for its bronchodilator action since adenosine produces bronchoconstriction in asthmatic subjects.

Theophylline has a low therapeutic index with adverse effects of nausea vomiting, nervousness, and tremor, and may also evoke cardiac dysrhythmias and convulsions. The incidence of these effects is lower with the use of oral sustained-release preparations that also prolong the duration of action for up to 12 hours.

Nevertheless, oral theophylline is not the first-line treatment of asthma, but is used in addition to β₂-adrenoceptor agonists and anti-inflammatory drugs when these have failed to produce adequate control of asthma.

MUSCARINIC ANTAGONISTS

The muscarinic antagonist with a role in the treatment of asthma is ipratropium; this drug is given by aerosol inhalation. Bronchodilatation is produced by antagonism of the bronchoconstrictor effect of acetylcholine released from parasympathetic nerves. Ipratropium also reduces mucus secretion, which is stimulated by the parasympathetic system. Inhalation of ipratropium produces a bronchodilator effect for up to 5 hours, with minimal systemic effects since it is poorly absorbed from the lung into blood. The principal adverse effect is a dry mouth. Ipratropium is not as effective a bronchodilator in asthma compared with the β₂-adrenoceptor agonists, but is used in combination with β₂-adrenoceptor agonists and glucocorticoids when these have not controlled asthma. In contrast to its limited role in asthma, ipratropium is more effective in relieving bronchoconstriction in chronic bronchitis (see below).

Anti-inflammatory drugs

These drugs do not have a bronchodilator action and therefore do not relieve the immediate response of an asthmatic attack. However, they do reduce the underlying inflammatory processes in asthma and it is now accepted that early treatment with anti-inflammatory drugs results in better long-term control of asthma than relying only on symptomatic relief produced by bronchodilators.

GLUCOCORTICOIDS

These drugs have a well-established role in the management of asthma and are recommended for use in all but the mildest forms of asthma, which are defined as the need for an inhaled β₂-adrenoceptor agonist once daily only. The anti-inflammatory properties of glucocorticoids are described in Chapter 4 and their anti-inflammatory actions and other beneficial effects in asthma are summarized below:

- They inhibit phospholipase A₂ by inducing lipocortin synthesis. This action reduces the production of prostaglandins, leukotrienes, and PAF, which have direct inflammatory effects as well as attracting and activating inflammatory cells such as eosinophils.

- They inhibit the production of cytokines, which have both direct inflammatory effects and chemotactic actions.

- They bring about a reduction in mast-cell production.

- They cause an upregulation of β₂-adrenoceptors, which may prevent the development of tolerance to bronchodilator β₂-agonists.

Glucocorticoids such as beclometasone (beclomethasone), budesonide, and fluticasone are commonly administered by inhalation, either in the form of an aerosol, powder, or nebulized solution. When given by this route, adverse effects are uncommon but oral or pharyngeal candidiasis and dysphonia (hoarseness) can occur. These effects can be minimized if an aerosol inhaler is used in conjunction with a spacing device—this reduces the deposition of particles in the buccal cavity and pharynx, whilst increasing the deposition of particles in the airways. Large doses of inhaled steroids, particularly in children, can cause systemic effects such as adrenal suppression. In chronic or deteriorating asthma, oral glucocorticoids, for example prednisolone, may be necessary although this may produce the adverse effects associated with the systemic use of glucocorticoids, as described in Chapter 20. Treatment of acute severe asthma requires intravenous hydrocortisone or oral prednisolone together with oxygen and nebulized salbutamol.

SODIUM CROMOGLICATE (SODIUM CROMOGLYCATE) AND SODIUM NEDOCROMIL

The anti-inflammatory effects of these drugs in asthma was originally attributed to stabilization of mast cells, thus preventing the release of inflammatory mediators. However, it is now clear that this does not explain their beneficial effects, but a mechanism of action has not been clearly identified. Evidence has emerged suggesting these drugs depress the axon reflexes that release excitatory neuropeptides in response to the stimulation of irritant receptors. Such an effect would suppress the development of bronchial hyper-reactivity. In addition, these drugs also inhibit the release of cytokines from T cells.

Sodium cromoglicate and sodium nedocromil are given by inhalation, either as an aerosol, powder, or nebulized solution. These drugs are less effective in adults than inhaled glucocorticoids since it is difficult to predict which patients will benefit from treatment. However, they provide a useful alternative in adult patients who experience adverse effects with inhaled glucocorticoids. Children respond better than adults to these drugs and they are an alternative first-line anti-inflammatory treatment in younger patients. Sodium cromoglicate is also useful in the prophylaxis of exercise-induced asthma when it is given 30 minutes beforehand. The adverse effects of these drugs are limited, consisting mainly of irritation to the respiratory tract, producing cough and transient bronchospasm.

LEUKOTRIENE ANTAGONISTS

Since leukotrienes are important inflammatory mediators in asthma, they represent a logical target for the development of novel antiasthma drugs—recently, montelukast and zifirlukast, which are potent orally active leukotriene antagonists, have become available. Their exact role in the management of asthma remains to be established, although they improve respiratory function in patients with mild–moderate asthma when used to supplement treatment with glucocorticoids. In addition, leukotriene antagonists reduce the severity of exercise-induced asthma.

Key facts
Treatment of asthma

- Drugs used to treat asthma are either bronchodilators or anti-inflammatory drugs.

- Bronchodilatation is produced by β_2-adrenoceptor agonists such as salbutamol or salmeterol, ipratropium (a muscarinic antagonist), and theophylline:
  - β_2-Adrenoceptor agonists are normally given by inhalation. and produce physiological antagonism of the bronchoconstriction produced by inflammatory mediators.
  - Ipratropium is also given by inhalation, and is used in combination with β_2-adrenoceptor agonists and glucocorticoids when these have not controlled asthma. Ipratropium is a more effective bronchodilator in patients with chronic bronchitis.
  - Theophylline produces bronchodilatation by either inhibiting phosphodiesterase and/or blocking adenosine receptors. It is a second-line drug, of use when patients have not responded to β_2-adrenoceptor agonists.

- Anti-inflammatory drugs used to treat asthma include glucocorticoids, such as beclometasone, sodium cromoglicate, and nedocromil, as well as leukotriene antagonists, e.g. montelukast. These drugs reduce the underlying inflammatory process in asthma.
  - Glucocorticoids reduce the production of inflammatory mediators such as prostaglandins, leukotrienes, cytokines, and PAF. Glucocorticoids such as beclometasone are administered by inhalation, but in deteriorating or severe acute asthma are given orally (prednisolone) or intravenously (hydrocortisone).
  - Cromoglicate and nedocromil depress axon reflexes, which release inflammatory neuropeptides and inhibit the release of cytokines from T cells. They are given by inhalation and are an alternative to glucocorticoids.
  - Leukotriene antagonists can be used to supplement treatment with glucocorticoids.

Chronic bronchitis

The airway obstruction in chronic bronchitis is due to narrowing of the lumen of the airways and mucus plugs, predisposing to secondary infection that may accelerate the progress of the disease. It is characterized by cough, excessive production of sputum, and breathlessness on exertion. Chronic bronchitis and emphysema, characterized by destruction of the alveolar walls, often occur together in heavy smokers, and is referred to as chronic obstructive pulmonary (airway) disease, COP(A)D.

Drug treatment of chronic bronchitis involves the use of bronchodilators and antibacterial drugs. β_2-Adrenoceptor agonists, theophylline, and ipratropium can all provide relief of airway obstruction. Ipratropium is the first choice since it reduces mucus production, caused by the stimulation of muscarinic receptors, and limits the bronchospasm produced by the stimulation of irritant receptors by smoking. Patients with chronic bronchitis are prone to secondary bacterial respiratory infections, these are normally treated with amoxicillin (amoxycillin), trimethoprin, or tetracycline.

Rhinitis

Rhinitis is inflammation of the nasal mucosa, resulting in nasal congestion and difficulty in breathing through the nose. The congestion is due to increased nasal mucosal blood flow and increased vascular permeability. Rhinitis is often associated with rhinorrhea, i.e. excessive watery secretions produced by the nasal mucosa. The common causes of rhinitis and rhinorrhea are:

- a viral infection of the nasal mucosa, i.e. the common cold;

- an allergic response, involving reaction of an allergen with tissue-bound IgE antibodies in the nasal mucosa; a common example is hayfever.

Nasal congestion can be alleviated by sympathomimetic drugs (see Chapter 14), which produce vasoconstriction of the nasal blood vessels as a result of stimulation of α-adrenoceptors. In addition, α-adrenoceptor stimulation also produces an inhibitory effect on excessive nasal secretion. Sympathomimetic drugs such as pseudoephedrine and oxymetazoline are available to the public without a prescription and are commonly used to relieve the symptoms of a common cold.

The inflammatory response in allergic rhinitis can be suppressed by the use of glucocorticoids such as beclometasone (beclomethasone) and sodium cromoglicate, which are administered via a nasal spray. In addition, histamine H_1-receptor antagonists (see Chapter 4) are also of use since, in contrast to asthma, histamine is an important inflammatory mediator in allergic rhinitis. The histamine H_1-receptor antagonists most frequently used in the treatment of allergic rhinitis are drugs, such as cetirizine and loratidine, that poorly penetrate the blood-brain barrier and therefore produce little if any sedation. These drugs are classed as non-sedative antihistamines, limited supplies of which are available without prescription from pharmacists. Sedative antihistamines, for example chlorphenamine (chlorpheniramine) and diphenhydramine, are also effective in allergic rhinitis, but their sedative effects enhance the effects of alcohol and may impair activities such as driving.

Cough suppressants (antitussives)

Coughing is a useful reflex that acts as a protective mechanism to expel unwanted material from the airways. It is normally trig-

gered by mechanical or chemical stimulation of receptors in the upper respiratory tract, 'cough receptors'. The afferent nerves from cough receptors relay in the cough centre in the brain and activate efferent nerves that produce the sudden contraction of respiratory muscles which results in coughing. In some situations, cough suppression is warranted such as the sleep disturbance due to a dry unproductive cough or in the palliative care of terminal lung cancer.

A popular remedy for a persistent cough is lozenges impregnated with menthol or eucalyptus oil. The vapour from these lozenges provides temporary relief from coughing by reducing the sensitivity of cough receptors. A depressant action on the cough centre is produced by opioid receptor agonists. A painful and unproductive cough can be suppressed by drugs such as codeine, pholocodine, and dextromethorphan. The latter two drugs are opiate derivatives, but have no analgesic properties, whilst codeine produces cough suppression at doses below those required for analgesia. The main adverse effect of such drugs is constipation, which is more likely to occur with codeine. Preparations for coughs and colds frequently contain codeine, pholcodine, or dextromethorphan in combination with either nasal decongestants, paracetamol or, if relief is required at night, sedative antihistamines. The stressful cough in terminal lung cancer requires the use of drugs with greater efficacy at opioid receptors such as morphine, diamorphine/heroin/diacetylmorphine, or methadone (see Chapter 7).

Further reading

Barnes, P. J. (1993). Anti-inflammatory therapy for asthma. *Annual Review of Respiratory Medicine*, 44, 229–49.

Israel, E. and Drazen, J. M. (1994). Treating mild asthma—when are inhaled steroids indicated? *New England Journal of Medicine*, 331, 737–9.

Naclero, R. M. (1991). Allergic rhinitis. *New England Journal of Medicine*, 325, 860–9.

Page, C. P., Curtis, M. J., Sutter, M. C., and Walker, M. J. A. (1997). Drugs and the respiratory system. In *Integrated pharmacology* (ed. C. P. Page, M. J. Curtis, M. C. Sutter, M. J. A. Walker, and B. B. Hoffman), pp. 231–51. Mosby, London.

Serafin, W. E. (1996). Drugs used in the treatment of asthma. In *Goodman and Gilman's the pharmacological basis of therapeutics* (9th edn) (ed. J. G. Hardman, L. E. Limbird, P. B. Molinoff, R. W. Ruddon, and A. G. Gilman), pp. 659–82. McGraw Hill, New York.

Drugs and gastrointestinal tract

18

Drugs and the gastrointestinal tract

Almost everyone will, at some stage, suffer from a disturbance of gastrointestinal function. In many cases, such upsets produce only temporary discomfort and inconvenience although in a significant proportion of individuals the problem may be more protracted. This chapter describes the properties of drugs used to treat the most common gastrointestinal problems, i.e. peptic ulcers, diarrhoea, constipation, and vomiting.

The control of gastric acid secretion

Gastric acid (HCl) is produced by parietal cells in the stomach and its secretion is regulated by three pathways.

1. Parasympathetic stimulation occurs via the vagus nerve, the preganglionic fibres of which synapse at ganglia where muscarinic M_1 receptors play an important role in neurotransmission.

2. Gastrin is released from G cells in the antrum of the stomach.

3. There is a local release of histamine from enterochromaffin-like (ECL) cells.

Stimulation of muscarinic or gastrin receptors on ECL cells causes the release of histamine, which activates histamine H_2-receptors on parietal cells (Fig. 18.1). Histamine H_2-receptors are positively coupled to adenylyl cyclase and stimulation therefore results in an increase in the intracellular concentration of cAMP. Parietal cells also possess muscarinic (M_2 and M_3) as well as gastrin receptors, and when these are stimulated they produce an increase in intracellular Ca^{2+}. An increase in cAMP or Ca^{2+} in parietal cells causes cytoplasmic vesicles containing the enzyme H^+/K^+-ATPase to migrate to the apical membrane. The enzyme is inserted into the membrane with the subsequent secretion of H^+ into the stomach lumen. Associated with the activation of H^+/K^+-ATPase is stimulation of a K^+/Cl^- co-transporter that results in the secretion of Cl^-, whilst K^+ is taken back into the cell by H^+/K^+-ATPase. These mechanisms for the control of gastric acid secretion can be interrupted by:

- histamine H_2-receptor antagonists that will not only block the effect of histamine but also, in part, the effects of stimulation of muscarinic and gastrin receptors;

- muscarinic receptor antagonists: the selective M_1-antagonist pirenzepine was used in the treatment of peptic ulcers but has been discontinued;

- inhibitors of H^+/K^+-ATPase (proton-pump inhibitors).

In addition to mechanisms that promote gastric acid secretion, the stimulation of prostanoid receptors by prostaglandin E_2 (PGE_2) and prostacyclin (PGI_2) exerts an inhibitory effect on gastric acid secretion. Stimulation of prostanoid receptors results in inhibition of adenylyl cyclase which opposes stimulation of the enzyme by histamine H_2-receptor activation. Prostaglandins also stimulate mucus and bicarbonate secretion from superficial epithelial cells adjacent to parietal cells (Fig. 18.1). The mucus and bicarbonate form a gel-like layer that protects the mucosa from the erosive actions of pepsin and gastric acid. The proteolytic enzyme pepsin is secreted from peptic cells in the stomach and, if secreted in excess, can digest the mucosa. Inhibition of the synthesis of prostaglandins by non-steroidal anti-inflammatory drugs (NSAIDs), such as aspirin, results in the loss of an inhibitory effect on gastric acid production and a reduction in mucus and bicarbonate secretion, both effects contributing to their ulcerogenic action (see Chapter 6).

Peptic ulcer disease (erosions of the gastric and duodenal mucosa) can be considered an imbalance between factors that may produce ulcers (gastric acid, pepsin, and infection with *Helicobacter pylori*—see below) and the protective actions of prostaglandins, and mucus and bicarbonate secretions. Treatment therefore consists of reducing gastric acid secretion, eradicating *H. pylori* infection, and augmenting the protective mucosal barrier.

Key facts
Gastric secretions

- Acid is secreted from parietal cells by a proton pump (H^+/K^+-ATPase).

- Acid secretion is stimulated by acetylcholine, histamine, and gastrin.

(cont.)

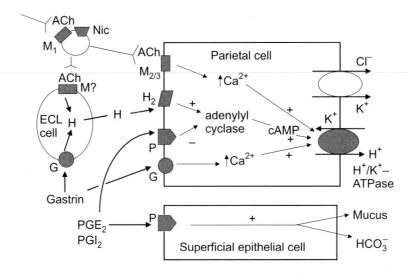

Fig. 18.1 Mechanisms involved in the control of gastric secretions. Na^+/K^+-ATPase (proton pump) on the apical membrane of parietal cells secretes H^+ into the stomach lumen when activated by: (1) stimulation of muscarinic receptors and gastrin receptors on parietal cells; and (2) stimulation of muscarinic and gastrin receptors on enterochromaffin-like (ECL) cells which release histamine (H) that in turn stimulates histamine H_2 receptors on parietal cells. Stimulation of prostanoid receptors on parietal cells by prostaglandin E_2 (PGE_2) and prostacyclin (PGI_2) inhibits adenylyl cyclase which reduces histamine-stimulated acid secretion. In addition, activation of prostanoid receptors also stimulates mucus and bicarbonate (HCO_3^-) secretion from superficial epithelial cells. ACh, acetylcholine; G, gastrin receptor, H_2, histamine H_2 receptor; M, muscarinic receptor; Nic, nicotinic receptor; P, prostanoid receptor.

- PGE_2 and PGI_2 inhibit acid secretion and stimulate mucus and bicarbonate secretion.

- Peptic ulcer disease (erosions of the gastric and duodenal mucosa) is the result of an imbalance between:
  - factors that damage the mucosa (acid, pepsin, and *Helicobacter pylori*);
  - mucosal protective factors (PGE_2 and PGI_2; mucus and bicarbonate).

Inhibitors of gastric acid secretion

Histamine H_2 receptor antagonists

Drugs such as cimetidine, ranitidine, famotidine, and nizatidine are competitive antagonists at histamine H_2 receptors with little or no effect at H_1 receptors. These drugs inhibit both basal and food-stimulated acid secretion that promotes the healing of gastric and duodenal ulcers. In addition to reducing H^+ secretion, H_2 antagonists also reduce the volume of gastric juice, resulting in a parallel reduction in pepsin secretion. Ulcers may recur when treatment is discontinued and, as a result, some patients are on long-term treatment with H_2 antagonists. All drugs are well absorbed from the gastrointestinal tract and are taken once or twice daily. Adverse effects are rare although there are reports of dizziness, nausea, and skin rashes. Cimetidine may cause sexual dysfunction and gynaecomastia in men, and confusion in the elderly. Cimetidine is also an inhibitor of cytochromes P450, inhibiting the metabolism, and therefore prolonging the action, of drugs cleared by this pathway.

Proton pump inhibitors

This category of drugs includes omeprazole and lansoprazole, which irreversibly inhibit H^+/K^+-ATPase and produce a marked inhibition of both basal and food-stimulated acid secretion. Proton pump inhibitors are pro-drugs, in that they need to be activated in the acid environment of the stomach before producing inhibition. At neutral pH they are lipid-soluble but devoid of any inhibitory activity. Following their diffusion from blood into the secretory canaliculi of parietal cells, proton pump inhibitors become protonated to produce a sulfenamide that is lipid-insoluble and trapped in the canaliculi. Sulfenamide covalently binds to sulfydryl groups on the enzyme, with full inhibition occurring when two molecules of drug are bound per molecule of enzyme.

Proton pump inhibitors are administered orally as capsules containing enteric-coated grains to prevent generation in the stomach lumen of sulfenamide, which would not be absorbed due to its poor lipid-solubility. Since proton pump inhibitors are irreversible, their action persists after the drug has disappeared from plasma and, on withdrawal of the drug, pretreatment levels of acid secretion are not achieved until 4–5 days later. This delay reflects the time needed for synthesis of H^+/K^+-ATPase and its insertion in the apical membrane. Proton pump inhibitors promote healing of gastric and duodenal ulcers and are useful when such healing has not been achieved with histamine H_2 antagonists. They are also particularly useful in the treatment of the Zollinger–Ellison syndrome (peptic and oesophageal ulceration associated with gastrin-producing tumours) and as one component in the eradication of *H. pylori* (see below). Similar to histamine H$_2$ antagonists, proton pump inhibitors are well tolerated with only a small proportion of patients (1.5–3%) experiencing gastrointestinal problems such as diarrhoea, nausea, and abdominal colic. Other reported adverse effects include headache, dizziness, and skin rashes.

Antacids

These drugs are weak bases that react with gastric hydrochloric acid to form a salt and water thus raising gastric pH. Administration of antacids will inhibit the activity of pepsin if pH is increased to >2, and pepsin is inactivated if sufficient antacid is taken to raise the pH to >5 (normal gastric pH ranges from 1 to 2). The elevation in pH produced by antacids is dependent on whether the stomach is empty or full, since these compounds pass through an empty stomach in 30 min whilst the presence of food prolongs the effects by about 2 hours. Antacids are commonly taken for the relief of symptoms of non-ulcer dyspepsia. Moreover, if given in sufficient quantities and for a long enough period (4–8 weeks), treatment with antacids will promote the healing of duodenal ulcers to a similar extent as histamine H$_2$ antagonists. However, antacids are less effective than H$_2$ antagonists in healing gastric ulcers.

Antacids in common use are salts of magnesium and aluminium such as magnesium hydroxide, magnesium carbonate, magnesium trisilicate, and aluminium hydroxide, available as tablets, gels, or suspensions. Antacids in combination with alginates are used in the treatment of gastroesophageal reflux (see below), since alginates foam in the presence of acid and form a protective layer on the stomach contents which reduces reflux of gastric contents into the oesophagus. Antacids can produce adverse gastrointestinal effects, with magnesium salts producing diarrhoea whilst aluminium salts can produce constipation. Some antacid preparations contain both types of salts in an attempt to maintain normal bowel function. Both aluminium and magnesium salts may reduce the bioavailability of other drugs present in the gastrointestinal tract, such as tetracycline, phenytoin, and ranitidine. The mechanisms underlying these interactions are a reduction in dissolution and absorption of other drugs—due to elevation of gastric pH—or the formation of insoluble complexes. These interactions can generally be avoided by taking antacids 2 hours before or after the ingestion of other drugs.

Agents that protect the mucosa

Bismuth chelate (tripotassium dicitratobismuthate)

This compound, taken as tablets or liquid, has a number actions that protect the mucosa in the stomach and duodenum, including coating the surface of the ulcer, adsorbing pepsin, and stimulating mucus and bicarbonate secretion. In addition, it also has a direct toxic effect on *H. pylori* (see below). Bismuth chelate has been shown to be as effective as histamine H$_2$ antagonists in promoting the healing of gastric and duodenal ulcers. The adverse effects of bismuth chelate include nausea and vomiting, and blackening of the tongue and faeces.

Sucralfate

Sucralfate is a complex of aluminium hydroxide and sulfated sucrose, although with minimal antacid properties. It reacts with gastric acid, acquiring a negative charge that facilitates binding to positively charged groups on proteins and glycoproteins. It binds to both damaged and normal mucosa, providing a protective layer against gastric acid. Other protective actions include inhibition of the action of pepsin and stimulation of mucus and bicarbonate secretion. It also reduces the adherence of *H. pylori* to gastric mucosa. Sucralfate promotes the healing of both gastric and duodenal ulcers, although it is more effective in the latter when used as maintenance treatment. Antacids reduce the effectiveness of sucralfate since it requires an acid environment for activation. The incidence of adverse effects with sucralfate is very low with constipation, due to its aluminium content, the most common (in 2% of patients) although dry mouth, nausea, rashes, and headache may also occur.

Misoprostol

Misoprostol is a stable analogue of prostaglandin E$_2$ which is administered orally. Prostaglandins have a protective action on the gastric mucosa due to stimulation of mucus and bicarbonate secretion, and inhibition of gastric acid production (Fig. 18.1), although higher doses are required to inhibit acid production than to stimulate protective secretions. Misoprostol is only moderately effective at promoting the healing of gastric and duodenal ulcers, although it has a particular use in preventing the gastric damage that may arise from treatment with NSAIDs. Treatment with misoprostol is therefore useful in patients with arthritis who cannot be withdrawn from treatment with NSAIDs. Adverse effects of misoprostol are mainly those on the gastrointestinal tract such as diarrhoea, which may be severe, abdominal cramps, and nausea and vomiting.

Eradication of *Helicobacter pylori*

Helicobacter pylori is a Gram-negative rod that colonizes mucus covering the gastric epithelium. Infection with *H. pylori* is an important factor in the development of peptic ulcers. Whilst the majority of the adult population may be infected with *H. pylori*, only 10–20% develop peptic ulcer disease. However, virtually all patients with duodenal ulcers and 80–90% of patients with gastric ulcers are infected with *H. pylori*. Eradication of *H. pylori* infection is recommended in patients with peptic ulcer who test positive for the presence of the bacterium, since such treatment, combined with drugs that inhibit gastric acid secretion, results in a greater rate of ulcer healing than the use of antisecretory agents alone. In addition, successful treatment of *H. pylori* infection reduces the recurrence of duodenal ulcers to 5% within a year, compared to a rate of recurrence of up to 80% if *H. pylori* is not eradicated.

There are a number of treatment regimens for the eradication of *H. pylori*, but with no consensus on the ideal combination of drugs. Treatments always include antibacterial drugs (see Chapter 12) usually combined with an inhibitor of gastric acid secretion and sometimes in conjunction with bismuth chelate. Inclusion of an inhibitor of gastric acid production (usually omeprazole), which raises gastric pH, improves the ability of antibacterial drugs to eliminate *H. pylori*. Examples of treatment regimens are given below.

- *Triple therapy* (one-week treatment): amoxicillin (amoxycillin) or clarithromycin + metronidazole + omeprazole;

- *Triple therapy* (two-week treatment): tetracycline + metronidazole + bismuth chelate;

- *Dual therapy* (two-week treatment): amoxicillin or clarithromycin + omeprazole.

Triple therapy regimens are more successful in eradicating infection, but patient compliance may be a problem due to the possible adverse effects resulting from three drugs and complex dosing schedules. Consequently triple therapy treatment involving one week of treatment is preferable. A summary of drugs effective against *H. pylori* infection and the mechanisms of action of other drugs used in the treatment of peptic ulcers are shown in Fig. 18.2.

Key facts
Treatment of peptic ulcers

- This can involve a range of different categories of drug.
- Inhibitors of gastric acid secretion:
  - histamine H_2 receptor antagonists, e.g. ranitidine;
  - proton pump inhibitors, e.g. omeprazole.

- Antacids such as aluminium hydroxide that neutralize gastric acid. These agents provide symptomatic relief in peptic ulcers and may promote healing if taken for a long enough period. They are also used to treat non-ulcer dyspepsia.

- Agents that protect the mucosa:
  - bismuth chelate;
  - sucralfate;
  - misoprostol used to prevent gastric damage that may arise from treatment with non-steroidal anti-inflammatory drugs.

- Eradication of *H. pylori* infection:
  - recommended in patients with peptic ulcers who test positive for the presence of the bacterium;
  - involves a combination of drugs, for example amoxicillin or clarithromycin + metronidazole + omeprazole.

Gastroesophageal reflux disease

This is a common problem in which the contents of the stomach reflux into the oesophagus causing 'heartburn', i.e. an inflammation of the oesophageal mucosa. If the problem becomes chronic, it may progress to erosive oesophagitis. Occasional instances of reflux are normally treated by self-medication with antacids or limited supplies of histamine H_2 antagonists which are available without a prescription. The relief provided by antacids may be greater with those that contain alginates (see above). Should gastroesophageal reflux become a persistent problem, long-term maintenance treatment with an inhibitor of gastric acid production may be required; in this regard proton pump inhibitors appear to be more effective than histamine H_2 antagonists. In addition to treatment with an inhibitor of gastric acid secretion, metoclopramide may be useful in controlling gastroesophageal

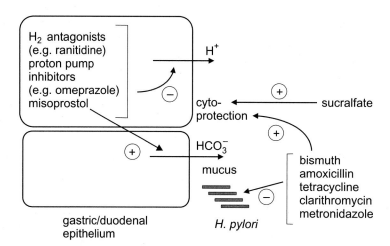

Fig. 18.2 Mechanisms of action of drugs used in the treatment of peptic ulcers. Negative signs indicate an inhibitory effect whilst positive signs indicate a stimulant action.

reflux. This drug has a range of pharmacological actions, including antagonism at dopamine D_2 receptors and 5-hydroxytryptamine$_3$ (5-HT$_3$) receptors as well as stimulant actions at 5-HT$_4$ receptors. One mechanism for its beneficial effects is the ability to stimulate gastric motility, which increases the rate of gastric emptying therefore reducing the time available for any reflux of stomach contents. A further action is to enhance the tone of the lower oesophageal sphincter, an effect that will help to prevent reflux. Cisapride, a drug with similar actions on the gastrointestinal tract as metoclopramide, is also used to reduce gastroesophageal reflux. In addition to its effects on gastrointestinal motility, metoclopramide has antiemetic actions which are described below.

Laxatives

Laxatives promote defaecation and are used to relieve constipation. Laxatives are widely overused due to self-medication by a public that has rigid views on what frequency of bowel movements are normal and in eating disorders when used to reduce calorie intake. Constipation can be frequently relieved by increasing the fibre and water content of the diet and taking regular exercise. In some situations a laxative may be necessary, for example in drug-induced constipation and when straining should be avoided, as in patients with angina or haemorrhoids. Laxatives are divided into the following categories:

- *Dietary fibre and bulk-forming laxatives* including bran, methylcellulose, ispaghula husk, and sterculia. These agents relieve constipation by increasing faecal mass which stimulates peristalsis. They take 1–3 days to work.
- *Stimulant laxatives* such as bisacodyl, danthron, and senna, which stimulate the mucosa of the gut, activating local reflexes that produce contraction of intestinal smooth muscle. They act within hours and should be restricted to short-term use.
- *Osmotic laxatives* which include the disaccharides lactulose and lactitol, magnesium sulfate or hydroxide, and polyethylene glycol-electrolyte solutions. They act by retaining fluid in the gut by their osmotic properties, and as a result stimulate peristaltic activity. Magnesium salts are effective within hours and are of use when rapid bowel evacuation is necessary, such as prior to abdominal radiography or surgery, whilst lactulose and lactitol may take up to 48 hours to produce the desired effect.
- *Faecal softeners*, for example docusate and liquid paraffin, that penetrate and soften the stool, reducing straining during defaecation.

Drugs used for the treatment of diarrhoea

Diarrhoea can result from viral or bacterial infections, anxiety, and the effect of drugs. Its consequences can be life-threatening, particularly in undernourished children in developing countries, or inconvenient and uncomfortable in a healthy adult. Diarrhoea comprises an increase in gastrointestinal motility and a decrease in the absorption of fluid, both contributing to a loss of water and electrolytes The treatment of diarrhoea involves the following approaches:

- the maintenance of fluid and electrolyte balance;
- the use of antibacterial agents;
- the use of drugs that reduce gastrointestinal motility.

Oral rehydration therapy

Oral rehydration therapy is the priority in the management of diarrhoea. Such treatment does not produce an initial reduction in the volume of diarrhoea, but the absorption of water and salts in the gut corrects fluid and electrolyte imbalance. In adults suffering from traveller's diarrhoea, rehydration can be achieved with sports drinks or flavoured mineral water (containing glucose in a hypotonic solution). For the treatment of diarrhoea in infants, powdered formulations are available for oral rehydration that must be dissolved in the appropriate volume of uncontaminated drinking water. All formulations include sodium chloride and glucose along with other salts such as sodium citrate and potassium chloride. Inclusion of glucose in such formulations promotes Na^+ and water absorption in the gut since there is a co-transport system for Na^+ and glucose across the gastrointestinal epithelium. In many cases of diarrhoea, oral rehydration therapy is the only treatment required and this can be life-saving particularly in children in developing countries. However, intravenous therapy may be needed if there is a severe electrolyte imbalance.

Antibacterial treatment

Treatment with antibacterial agents is usually unnecessary since most cases of gastroenteritis are of viral origin, and those in which bacteria are involved normally resolve without antimicrobial therapy. Certain bacterial infections that produce gastroenteritis do require specific antibacterial treatment, for example severe infections with *Campylobacter* spp. should be treated with either erythromycin or ciprofloxacin. Drug treatment may lead to bacterial infections that produce diarrhoea. The use of antibacterial agents such as ampicillin and clindamycin can destroy the normal gut flora with overgrowth of organisms such as *Clostridium difficile*. Superinfection with this bacterium can lead to pseudomembranous colitis that requires treatment with metronidazole or vancomycin (see Chapter 12).

Drugs that reduce intestinal motility

Opiate drugs increase tone in smooth muscle of the intestinal tract but reduce peristaltic activity, actions that increase transit time and therefore reduce diarrhoea. These effect are the result of an inhibitory action on intramural nerve plexuses in the gut wall produced by the stimulation of μ-opioid receptors. The opiate drugs used to treat diarrhoea include codeine, diphenoxylate, and loperamide, the latter two agents being congeners of pethidine used only for their actions on the gut. Diphenoxylate is available in combination with a low dose of the muscarinic antagonist atropine which also reduces gut motility. Loperamide undergoes enterohepatic cycling which prolongs its action in the gut, whilst codeine and loperamide, in addition to their effects on intestinal motility, have antisecretory actions which will reduce diarrhoea. These drugs can reduce the duration of diarrhoea in viral gastroenteritis and traveller's diarrhoea, normally resulting from infection with enterotoxin-producing *Escherichia coli*. Adverse effects that may arise with the use of codeine, diphenoxylate, and loperamide are abdominal cramps and paralytic ileus, whilst the inclusion of atropine with diphenoxylate can produce typical antimuscarinic effects such as blurred vision and dry mouth.

Key facts
Laxatives and drug used to treat diarrhoea

- Laxatives promote defaecation and are used to relieve constipation. They are frequently overused.

- A laxative action is produced by:
  - dietary fibre and bulk-forming laxatives, which include bran and ispaghula husk;
  - stimulant laxatives such as danthron and senna;
  - osmotic laxatives, such as the disaccharides lactulose and lactitol, which act by retaining fluid in the gut by their osmotic properties and as a result stimulate peristaltic activity.
- Treatment of diarrhoea involves:
  - oral rehydration therapy, which is the priority and is particularly important in infants;
  - drugs which reduce gastrointestinal motility such as loperamide;
  - on rare occasions antibacterial treatment may be necessary, e.g. in severe infections with *Campylobacter* spp.

Vomiting

Vomiting (emesis), which is invariably preceded by nausea, is a result of the complex co-ordinated activity of somatic abdominal and respiratory muscles, and smooth muscle of the gastrointestinal tract. Nausea and vomiting are produced by a range of stimuli including:

- pain;
- emotional factors;
- repulsive smells or sights;
- drugs, e.g. cytotoxic drugs used in cancer chemotherapy, morphine, and digoxin;
- gastrointestinal irritation such as that produced by radiation, bacteria and viruses, cytotoxic drugs, and excessive alcohol;
- morning sickness during the first trimester of pregnancy;
- migraine;
- raised intracranial pressure;
- metabolic disorders such as uraemia and hypoglycaemia;
- disturbance of balance (e.g. motion sickness).

Nausea and vomiting may be multifactorial in origin. Postoperative nausea and vomiting is due to a number of different factors such as the general anaesthetic agent, pain, anxiety, and postoperative drug treatments, e.g. opioid analgesics. The type of surgery may be also be a factor, as in abdominal surgery when there may irritation to the gastrointestinal tract due to distension and tissue damage.

The central regulation of vomiting involves two centres: (1) the vomiting centre in the medulla, which co-ordinates the activity of the relevant somatic and smooth muscle; and (2) the chemoreceptor trigger zone (CTZ) located in the area postrema on the floor of the fourth ventricle. The blood–brain barrier is poorly developed in the area postrema and the CTZ is therefore accessible to emetic substances in the blood. Irritation of the gastrointestinal tract produces the release of 5-HT, prostaglandins, and kinins—these stimulate afferent vagal fibres that activate the vomiting centre via relay in the CTZ or solitary tract nucleus. In addition, 5-HT released in the gut may enter the blood and directly stimulate the CTZ. Motion sickness, such as sea sickness, is produced by certain kinds of movement that generate nervous impulses in the labyrinth of the vestibular apparatus, which are then relayed to the vomiting centre via the vestibular nucleus, cerebellum, and the CTZ. Figure 18.3 shows the various pathways involved in producing vomiting, together with the receptors for the associated main neurotransmitters, namely acetylcholine, dopamine, histamine, and 5-HT. The location of these transmitters and their receptors provides a rationale for the use of antiemetic drugs.

Antiemetic drugs

Muscarinic antagonists

The muscarinic antagonist used to treat vomiting is hyoscine, which is effective in motion sickness and against vomiting resulting from local irritation in the stomach. However, it is ineffective against substances that directly stimulate the CTZ. The principal use of hyoscine is for the prophylaxis of motion sickness, being less effective when vomiting has started. It can be taken orally or by means of a skin patch. The adverse antimuscarinic effects associated with doses of hyoscine required for an antiemetic effect are dry mouth and sedation. Consequently, in the treatment of travel sickness, hyoscine is suitable for passengers but not the driver!

Histamine H$_1$ antagonists

Histamine antagonists with useful antiemetic actions include cinnarizine, cyclizine, dimenhydrinate, and promethazine.

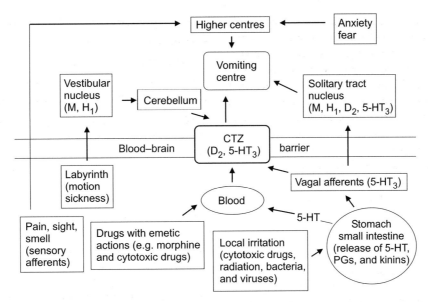

Fig. 18.3 The factors and pathways involved in the control of vomiting. The receptors for the main neurotransmitters that control vomiting are shown in parentheses. M, muscarinic; H_1, histamine H_1; D_2, dopamine D_2; 5-HT_3, 5-hydroxytryptamine$_3$; CTZ, chemoreceptor trigger zone; PGs, prostaglandins.

Histamine H_1 and muscarinic receptors are present in the same pathways that control vomiting (Fig. 18.3) and antagonists at these receptors have similar antiemetic uses. Consequently, histamine antagonists, which are administered orally, are an alternative to the use of hyoscine in the treatment of motion sickness. Histamine antagonists are slightly less effective than hyoscine but are better tolerated. In addition, promethazine is of use in the acute treatment of severe vomiting in pregnancy, on the rare occasions when this is considered necessary. Most histamine antagonists that are effective antiemetics are also muscarinic antagonists, a pharmacological property which will contribute to their antiemetic actions. Similar to hyoscine, histamine antagonists are more effective if taken before the onset of nausea and vomiting, but may produce a dry mouth and sedation.

Dopamine antagonists

Dopamine, via activation of dopamine D_2 receptors (see Chapter 15 for a description of the classification of dopamine receptors), is involved in transmission in emetic pathways in the CTZ and solitary tract nucleus (Fig. 18.3). Dopamine antagonists, whilst generally ineffective in motion sickness, are useful for combating the effects of agents that directly stimulate the CTZ. Some are also active against emetic stimuli in the gut. They can be given orally, rectally, or parenterally—the latter routes allowing drug administration after a patient starts to vomit. The different categories of dopamine antagonists and their antiemetic uses are described below.

- Phenothiazines are neuroleptic drugs (see Chapter 15); however, in relatively low doses they can act as antiemetic agents. In addition to dopamine antagonism, phenoth-

iazines also have a blocking action at muscarinic and histamine H_1 receptors thus adding to their antiemetic action. Phenothiazines used as antiemetics include chlorpromazine, prochlorperazine, perphenazine, and trifluoperazine. These drugs are of use in treating nausea and vomiting produced by gastroenteritis, radiation, as well as drugs such as cytotoxic agents, opioid analgesics, and general anaesthetics. The adverse effects of phenothiazines are sedation and dystonias (muscle spasm), which are more likely to occur in children. A more complete description of the adverse effects of neuroleptic drugs is given in Chapter 15.

- Neuroleptic butyrophenones such as haloperidol and droperidol also possess an antiemetic action that is useful in combating vomiting produced by the anticancer agent cisplatin.

- Metoclopramide is dopamine D_2 antagonist that at high doses will also block 5-HT_3 receptors, a property particularly useful in reducing nausea and vomiting resulting from cancer treatment involving radiation or cytotoxic drugs (see below). In addition to its use in cancer chemotherapy, at lower doses it is used to treat vomiting produced by gastrointestinal disorders and migraine where its ability to promote gastric emptying (see above) contributes to its antiemetic actions. Similar to the phenothiazines and butyrophenones, the adverse effects of metoclopramide are those associated with blockade of dopamine receptors in the CNS, i.e. sedation and disorders of movement (dyskinesias).

- Domperidone is a dopamine antagonist that does not readily cross the blood–brain barrier and therefore is less likely to cause the central effects seen with the use of other dopamine antagonists. It is used for the relief of nausea and vomiting caused by cytotoxic drugs and the dopamine receptor-stimulating drugs levodopa and bromocriptine used in the treatment of Parkinson's disease. Domperidone is also used to control postoperative nausea and vomiting.

5-HT$_3$-receptor antagonists

Ondansetron, granisetron, and tropisetron are 5-HT$_3$-receptor antagonists that produce relief of nausea and vomiting by blockade of receptors in the CTZ, solitary tract nucleus, and on vagal afferent fibres in the gut (Fig. 18.3). They are the drugs of choice in preventing vomiting resulting from cytotoxic drugs used in cancer chemotherapy, of which the most emetic agent is cisplatin. Cytotoxic drugs, in addition to any direct stimulation of the CTZ, cause the release of 5-HT from enterochromaffin cells within gastrointestinal mucosa. 5-HT$_3$-receptor antagonists—which can be administered orally or by intravenous infusion—are effective in preventing nausea, retching, and vomiting in 70% of patients receiving their first cancer chemotherapy, with a reduction in the severity of symptoms in the remaining patients. However, their effectiveness diminishes on subsequent treatments with cytotoxic agents. To prevent this reduction in effectiveness and to improve the control of vomiting on first treatment with cytotoxic drugs, 5-HT$_3$-receptor antagonists are administered in combination with a glucocorticosteroid, either dexamethasone or methylprednisolone. The mechanism of the antiemetic action of glucocorticosteroids is unknown. They are used to supplement the antiemetic action of other drugs since, when given alone, their ability to control vomiting is only moderate.

In addition to antagonizing vomiting produced by cytotoxic drugs, 5-HT$_3$-receptor antagonists are also useful in relieving radiation-induced emesis and postoperative nausea and vomiting. In the latter, 5-HT$_3$-receptor antagonists are as effective as dopamine antagonists. The adverse effects of 5-HT$_3$-receptor antagonists are mild, consisting of occasional reports of headache, constipation, and a sensation of warmth.

Key facts
Antiemetic drugs

- The main neurotransmitters in the pathways that produce vomiting are acetylcholine acting via muscarinic receptors, histamine interacting with H$_1$ receptors, 5-HT acting via 5-HT$_3$ receptors, and dopamine which stimulates D$_2$ receptors.

- The muscarinic receptor antagonist hyoscine and histamine H$_1$ antagonists, such as cinnarizine and promethazine, are used to treat motion sickness. Their adverse effects are sedation and dry mouth.

- Neuroleptic phenothiazines, for example prochlorperazine, have antiemetic actions due to the blockade of dopamine D$_2$ receptors. These drugs also block muscarinic and histamine H$_1$ receptors, actions that may contribute to their antiemetic effects. They are used to relieve nausea and vomiting resulting from gastroenteritis, radiation, and drugs such as cytotoxic agents, opioid analgesics, and general anaesthetics. Adverse effects of phenothiazines are sedation and disorders of movement.

- Metoclopramide is a dopamine D$_2$ antagonist which, at high doses, will also block 5-HT$_3$ receptors. It is used to treat vomiting produced by cytotoxic drugs, gastroenteritis, and migraine.

- 5-HT$_3$-receptor antagonists, such as ondansetron, are the drugs of choice in relieving vomiting produced by cytotoxic agents used in cancer chemotherapy. Their antiemetic effects are enhanced if given in combination with a glucocorticosteroid, e.g. dexamethasone. They are also effective in radiation sickness and postoperative nausea and vomiting.

Further reading

Dupont, H. L. and Ericsson, C. D. (1993). Prevention and treatment of traveler's diarrhea *New England Journal of Medicine*, **328**, 1821–7.

Langman, M. J. S. (1991). Omeprazole, for resistant ulcers and severe oesophageal reflux disease. *British Medical Journal*, **303**, 481–2.

Mitchelson, F. (1992). Pharmacological agents affecting emesis, a review (Parts I and II). *Drugs*, **43**, 295–315, 443–63.

Walsh, J. H. and Peterson, W. L. (1995). The treatment of *Helicobacter pylori* infection in the management of peptic ulcer disease. *New England Journal of Medicine*, **333**, 984–91.

Wolfe, M. M. and Soll, A. H. (1988). The physiology of gastric acid secretion. *New England Journal of Medicine*, **319**, 1707–15.

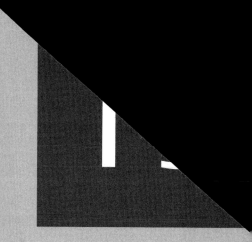

Chemotherapeutic agents in neoplastic disease

- The cell cycle
- Principles of chemotherapy
- Classification of chemotherapeutic agents
- Oral and dental problems associated with chemotherapy
- Further reading

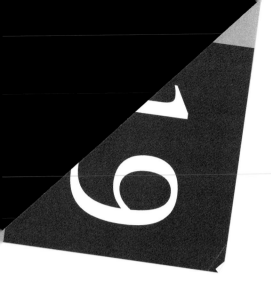

Chemotherapeutic agents in neoplastic disease

Chemotherapeutic agents are widely used in the treatment of cancer and other neoplastic conditions. In addition, some of these drugs are used as immunosuppressants, for example in transplant rejection and autoimmune diseases such as rheumatoid arthritis. They are often the treatment of choice for some types of neoplasia, such as Hodgkin's disease and acute leukaemia. These agents are either used on their own, or as an adjunct to surgery or radiotherapy. The precise treatment will depend upon the type of neoplasia, its rate of growth, and its capacity to metastasize. All chemotherapeutic agents block various stages in the cell cycle. Therefore, knowledge of the normal cell-growth cycle is necessary for an understanding of their mechanism of action.

The cell cycle

Cells progress through stages of development while they are synthesizing, growing, and dividing. However, most cells in the body are fully developed and differentiated, and are no longer cycling or replicating. A portion of normal cells in tissues undergoing cellular turnover are in the process of controlled growth and division (for example, skin, bone marrow, and the lining of the gastrointestinal tract). In contrast, tumour cells continue to grow and divide beyond the normal control of the host.

The stages of cell growth and division are called the cell cycle. Cells begin the cycle in the intermitotic phase (G_1). Substances necessary for cell growth and division are produced in the synthetic phase (S), during which DNA, RNA, and major protein synthesis occurs. At the cessation of S phase, the premitotic or G_2 phase occurs, followed by mitosis (M phase). Cells that are not in the replicating cycle move into the non-proliferating phase (G_0), from which they may return to the active proliferating phase. As the S phase is the period when the cell carries out intensive metabolic and synthetic activities, it is also the phase when it may be most sensitive to agents that interfere with DNA, RNA, and protein synthesis.

Principles of chemotherapy

The following factors govern the success or otherwise of chemotherapy in the treatment of neoplastic disease.

1. *Tumour susceptibility*: Different tumours will respond to different drugs at varying rates. To achieve optimal results, the tumour cells must be susceptible to the chemotherapeutic agent.

2. *Drug/tumour contact*: It is essential that the drug comes into contact with the tumour cells in sufficient concentrations during the critical period of cell division.

3. *Size of tumour*: Chemotherapeutic agents destroy a constant percentage of cells, rather than a constant number. This is referred to as first-order kinetics (see Chapter 1). If a drug destroys 99.99% of tumour cells, this will still leave a substantial number of cells, especially if the initial tumour mass was large. Even if a few tumour cells remain, there is the possibility of relapse and metastasis.

4. *Tumour cell resistance*: If a tumour becomes unresponsive to a chemotherapeutic agent, it may be due to a build-up of tumour cell resistance. A number of factors can cause this resistance; for example, poor penetration of the tumour due to an impaired blood supply, enzyme alteration, and tumour cell mutation.

5. *Immunotherapy*: The host tissues will possess some measure of defence against the tumour cells. Appropriate immunotherapy may enhance this defence mechanism and, given in conjunction with chemotherapy, may increase the tumour-killing potential of the drugs.

6. *Combination therapy*: Different chemotherapeutic agents act at different stages in the cell cycle. The administration of different drugs will increase their range of activity against the tumour. Furthermore, combination therapy reduces the possibility of development of tumour resistance.

7. *Unwanted effects*: The drugs chosen should not cause severe unwanted effects that may prevent the completion of treatment. For a given drug, altering the route of administration may reduce the incidence of these effects.

Classification of chemotherapeutic agents

Chemotherapeutic agents can be conveniently divided into seven groups:

(1) alkylating agents, which release alkyl radicals that react with organic compounds essential for cell metabolism; they also prevent cell division by crosslinking strands of DNA;

(2) antimetabolites, which act as competitive antagonists for folic acid, purine, and pyrimidine bases, and are essential for the synthesis of DNA, RNA, and certain co-enzymes;

(3) natural products, including the vinca alkaloids;

(4) cytotoxic antibiotics;

(5) hormones;

(6) radioactive isotopes and implants;

(7) enzymes.

Details of the various drugs in each of the categories, together with their mode of action, indications, and unwanted effects are described in Table 19.1.

Oral and dental problems associated with chemotherapy

Nearly all the chemotherapeutic agents cause unwanted effects that manifest themselves in the mouth and related structures. The oral epithelium has a rapid cell turnover and is therefore very susceptible to the cell destructive properties of these drugs. A mucositis often develops within 3–7 days of starting chemotherapy. Also, many of the chemotherapeutic agents cause bone-marrow suppression resulting in a leucopenia and thrombocytopenia. The oral mucosa and gingival tissues are very sensitive to these changes, and thus chemotherapeutic agents can have an additional indirect effect on the mouth. Any breach of the oral mucosa is likely to become infected, since the oral bacterial flora is large. Hence the mouth can be important as a potential portal of entry for infective agents, especially in patients with suppressed bone-marrow activity.

Table 19.1 Synopsis of the pharmacological properties of the various chemotherapeutic agents used in the management of malignant diseases

		Pharmacodynamics	Indications	Unwanted effects
1	*Alkylating agents*			
1a	Nitrogen mustards, e.g. cyclophosphamide, chlorambucil	Alkylating agents target DNA (forming crosslinks) and disrupt mitotic activity, cell growth, and differentiation. They are particularly effective for rapidly growing tumours	Cyclophosphamide: Hodgkin's disease, leukaemia, and lymphosarcoma. Chlorambucil: chronic leukaemias and lymphomas. Busalfan: chronic granulocytic leukaemia.	Bone-marrow suppression is the main unwanted effect of the alkylating agents. This is rapid and occurs 6–8 days after commencement of therapy. Amenorrhoea and impaired spermatogenesis usually follow a course of treatment. Other unwanted effects include alopecia, nausea, and vomiting
1b	Busulfan			
1c	Nitrosureas, e.g. lomustine, carmustine		Nitrosureas: brain tumours.	
1d	Cisplatin	Not an alkylating agent, but has a similar action (forms intrastrand links in DNA)	Cisplatin: germ-cell tumours	Cisplatin causes nephrotoxicity and deafness
2	*Antimetabolites*			
2a	Folic acid analogues, e.g. methotrexate	Folic acid analogues destroy cells during the S phase of the cycle. Methotrexate's action is reversed by folinic acid, the so-called 'rescue technique'	Methotrexate: acute leukaemias, cancer of the breast, tongue, pharynx, and lung; also used in the treatment of Wegener's granulomatosis	Leucopenia and thrombocytopenia secondary to bone-marrow suppression. Troublesome oral ulceration and diarrhoea
2b	Pyrimidine analogues, e.g. fluorouracil, cytarabine	Fluorouracil interferes with thymidylate synthesis and hence DNA synthesis; cytarabine inhibits DNA polymerase	Fluorouracil: palliative treatment for a variety of malignant conditions. Topical/fluorouracil: premalignant keratosis and basal cell carcinoma of the skin	Anorexia, nausea, diarrhoea, and severe stomatitis with sloughing and ulceration; bone-marrow suppression
2c	Purine analogues, e.g. mercaptopurine, thioguanine	Purine analogues are converted into 'fraudulent' nucleotides which in turn inhibit purine synthesis	Mercaptopurine: most types of leukaemia	Bone-marrow suppression, damage to epithelial lining of gut, pancreatitis and rarely liver damage

Table 19.1 (*cont.*)

		Pharmacodynamics	Indications	Unwanted effects
3	*Natural products*			
3a	Vinca alkaloids, e.g. vincristine, vinblastine	Vinca alkaloids block mitosis at the metaphase by binding to tubulin, an essential protein component of cellular microtubules	Vincristine: Hodgkin's disease leukemias, breast cancer. Vinblastine: neuroblastomas Letterer–Siwe disease	Leucopenia, neurological disturbances, mood changes
3b	Epipodophyllotoxins, e.g. etopside	May inhibit mitrochondrial function and nuceloside transport	Lung cancer, testicular tumours, Hodgkin's disease, lymphoma and Kaposi's sarcoma	Nausea, vomiting, hair loss, myelosuppression, stomatitis, and diarrhoea
3c	Pactitaxel (Taxol)	'Freezes' microtubules in the polymerized state	Ovarian cancer and drug-resistant breast cancer	Bone-marrow suppression, paraesthesia
4	*Cytotoxic antibiotics*			
4a	Anthracyclines, e.g. doxorubicin	Binds to DNA and inhibits both DNA and RNA synthesis	Leukaemias, lymphomas, and various solid tumours	Bone-marrow suppression, dose-related cardiac damage, hair loss
4b	Bleomycin	Fragments DNA by chain scission	Squamous cell carcinoma of head and neck, oesophagus, skin, and genitourinary tract	Pulmonary fibrosis, vesiculation of the skin, hyperpyrexia
5	*Hormones*			
5a	Glucocorticoids	Inhibitory effect on lymphocyte proliferation	Leukaemias, lymphomas	See Chapter 20
5b	Oestrogens, e.g. fosfestrol	Block the effect of androgens in androgen-dependent prostatic tumours	Tumours of the prostate and breast cancer in postmenopausal women	Impotence and gynaecomastia
5c	Progestogens, e.g. megestrol	ibid	Endometrial neoplasms, breast cancer in postmenopausal women	Nausea, vomiting, diarrhoea, hypercalcaemia
5d	Gonadotrophin-releasing hormone analogues, e.g. goserelin	Inhibits gonadotrophin release	Prostate cancer and advanced breast cancer in postmenopausal women	
5e	Antioestrogens, e.g. tamoxifen	Competes with oestrogen and inhibits the transcription of oestrogen-responsive genes. Also induces production of transforming growth factor-β	Hormone-dependent breast cancer and endometrial cancer	Hot flushes, nausea, and vomiting
6	*Radioactive isotopes*			
6a	Radioactive iodine (^{131}I)	Emits both γ-rays and β particles. The β radiation exerts a local cytotoxic effect to the thyroid follicular cells	Follicular cell carcinoma of the thyroid, and metastatic thyroid cancer	Hypothyroidism
7	Enzymes, e.g. crisantaspase	Breaks down asparigine to aspartic acid and hence inhibits cell protein synthesis	Acute lymphoblastic leukaemia	Nausea and vomiting, CNS depression, and anaphylactic reactions

Common problems that accompany chemotherapy are oral ulceration, mucositis and stomatitis (due to atrophic thinning of the oral mucosa), xerostomia, infection, gingivitis, pain, and haemorrhage. In addition, radiotherapy applied to the head and neck area will damage the salivary glands and cause xerostomia. In dentate patients this will increase the risk of caries, especially root surface caries, whilst in edentulous patients the poor salivary flow will give rise to significant problems of denture retention and an increased risk of mucosal infections.

Management

Many of these oral and dental problems can be reduced or alleviated by certain pretreatment measures. Oral hygiene should be meticulous in these patients to reduce the incidence of gingival problems. All potential sources of infection, such as periapical inflammatory lesions, impacted third molars that have caused pericoronitis, periodontal pockets, and carious cavities, should be treated. Sharp cusps or restorations should be smoothed to avoid trauma to the oral mucosa. It is thus important that patients who are about to undergo a course of chemotherapy have a thorough dental screening, and where possible treatment completed before therapy. All too often this aspect of the patient's care is overlooked or the urgency of the chemotherapy takes precedence. In many of these instances, significant dental and oral problems arise either during or immediately after a course of chemotherapy, and the dental surgeon is then faced with the problem of treating an often debilitated patient. The successful management of patients undergoing chemotherapy requires a team approach, with the dental surgeon ensuring that oral and dental problems during or after treatment are kept to a minimum.

Mucositis, stomatitis, and oral ulceration

Benzocaine lozenges or lidocaine (lignocaine) gel may provide enough surface analgesia to make eating more comfortable, although some patients find these topical anaesthetics unacceptable. Other remedies used to alleviate mucosal pain include sucking ice cubes or the topical application of vitamin E. Secondary infection of the ulcers can be reduced by using a chlorhexidine mouthwash 0.2%, although some patients may find this concentration too irritant to the oral mucosa. A 0.12% solution is available which may cause less discomfort without reducing efficacy. Many mouthrinses contain alcohol or phenols. These constituents can further damage an already compromised mucosa and thus cause further pain and discomfort. If the ulcers become infected, a tetracycline mouthbath together with an antifungal agent should be used topically and then swallowed.

Diluted hydrogen peroxide (0.5%) may be useful in removing the thick mucus and slough that often covers ulcerated oral mucosa. Such treatment may be particularly useful if there is an underlying fungal infection that is being treated with topical antifungals.

Xerostomia

Saliva substitutes (such as Glandosane, Saliva Orthana, and Luborant) may be of some use in those with xerostomia, or the regular use of lemon drops (provided the patient is edentulous) may encourage salivary flow. Artificial saliva seldom relieves symptoms for more than an hour or two, and by no means do all patients derive benefit greater than that afforded by frequent sips of water. There should also be treatment with a topical fluoride to prevent xerostomia-induced dental caries. Angular cheilitis often accompanies xerostomia and should be treated with an appropriate antifungal agent, such as nystatin ointment or miconazole cream. If the cheilitis is secondarily infected with *Staphylococcus aureus* then topical sodium fusidate should applied together with the antifungal treatment.

Oral infection

Infection is a problem that frequently occurs with cancer chemotherapy. Ulcerated areas become infected and organisms involved include *Pseudomonas* species, *Serratia* species, *Klebsiella* species, and *Escherichia* coli. Multiple antimicrobial combinations may have to be given parenterally in order to prevent systemic spread of the infection, as no single drug is likely to be effective against all potential pathogens.

Candidal infections are common in such patients and the prophylactic use of antifungals should be considered to prevent the spread of an oral infection to the oesophagus or bronchi. The use of nystatin pastilles can help to prevent candidiasis. The pastille should be held in the mouth near the lesion 4–6 times per day and allowed to dissolve. Other remedies to treat candidal infections are discussed in Chapter 11.

Patients on cancer chemotherapy may also be susceptible to oral herpetic infections. Acyclovir is the antiviral agent of choice for the treatment of infections due to herpes simplex type 1 and 2, and varicella zoster.

The management of infections that may arise in patients receiving cancer chemotherapy should be undertaken in consultation with the patient's medical supervisor. Regular monitoring of the patient's white blood cell count will help to serve as a marker for the risk and response to infection.

Gingival and mucosal bleeding

Haemorrhage associated with chemotherapy is invariably due to bone-marrow suppression and the resultant thrombocytopenia. Mild cases of bleeding may respond to systemic aminocaproic acid. Severe haemorrhage should be treated by platelet transfusion.

Gingival bleeding in patients on chemotherapy is most likely to be due to an exacerbation of an existing periodontal problem. Extensive periodontal therapy is uncalled for in these patients since they will be unable to cope with vigorous oral hygiene therapy or other forms of non-surgical management. The use of a soft toothbrush will remove most plaque and not cause significant trauma to the gingival tissues and excessive bleeding. A chlorhexidine mouth rinse will reduce plaque formation and also the inflammatory component in the gingival tissues. Again the extent of the gingival bleeding and the response to treatment will depend upon the patient's haematological. profile.

Pain

Patients on chemotherapy often complain of pain in the teeth and jaws. It is essential to eliminate any causative dental factors; if there is no dental cause, the pain will resolve on cessation of treatment. Pain associated with chemotherapy may respond to a peripherally acting analgesic, the type and dosage of which should be tailored to the individual patient.

Further reading

Beck, A. (1979). Impact of a systematic oral care protocol on stomatitis after chemotherapy. *Cancer Nursing*, 2, 185–99.

Nikoskelainen, J. (1990). Oral infections related to radiation and immunosuppressive therapy. *Journal of Clinical Periodontology*, 17, 504–7.

Toth, B. B., Martin, J. W., and Fleming, T. J. (1990). Oral complications associated with cancer therapy. *Journal of Clinical Periodontology*, 17, 508–515.

20

The endocrine system

The endocrine system

Endocrine glands secrete hormones, which regulate cellular metabolism and maintain homeostasis. Hormones are defined as substances secreted by specific tissues and transported to a distant tissue where they exert their effect. The endocrine system is mostly regulated by the pituitary gland (hypophysis), which comprises a glandular component (the anterior pituitary or adenohypophysis) and a neural component (the posterior pituitary or neurohypophysis). Both parts of the pituitary have a direct relationship with the hypothalamus, the neurones of which consist of two distinct systems influencing both parts of the gland respectively. Trophic hormones are produced by the anterior pituitary, and in turn they regulate the activity of other endocrine glands. The secretion of trophic hormones is controlled by specific releasing factors from the hypothalamus. Production of these factors and of trophic hormones is controlled by a feedback mechanism from circulating hormones. The posterior pituitary stores and releases hormones that are produced in the hypothalamus.

Posterior pituitary hormones

The posterior pituitary secretes two polypeptide hormones: antidiuretic hormone (ADH; vasopressin) and oxytocin. Both are synthesized in the hypothalamus and transported in combination with carrier proteins along nerve fibres to be stored as secretory granules in the nerve endings in the posterior pituitary. When action potentials are transmitted down nerve fibres, the hormones are immediately released from the secretory granules by exocytosis and absorbed into the surrounding capillaries.

Antidiuretic hormone (ADH; vasopressin)

Antidiuretic hormone is synthesized in the supraoptic and paraventricular nuclei of the hypothalamus and passes via the hypothalamiconeurohypophyseal tract to be stored and released from the posterior pituitary. The main property of ADH is fluid preservation, and its site of action is the collecting ducts of the kidney.

Secretion is controlled by hypothalamic neurones that act as osmoreceptors. A high plasma osmolality and a low blood volume (which causes the release of renin and angiotensin from the kidney), stimulate the secretion of ADH. Drugs may affect the secretion of ADH; for example ethanol inhibits secretion whilst lithium and the tetracycline derivative, demeclocycline blocks the action of ADH on the collecting tubules. Depressed patients treated with lithium (see Chapter 15) may develop nephrogenic diabetes insipidus (resistance to the action of ADH), which is usually reversible on stopping the drug. Demeclocycline is used to treat the hyponatraemia that is associated with the syndrome of inappropriate (excess) secretion of ADH.

The actions of ADH are mediated by two types of G-protein-coupled receptors, designated V_1 and V_2. Stimulation of V_2 receptors in the basolateral membrane of the collecting duct of the kidney results in the insertion of preformed water channels (aquaporins) into the apical membrane, with a consequent increase in water permeability. ADH also produces contraction of smooth muscle, particularly in blood vessels, via a stimulation of V_1 receptors. However, since these receptors have a lower affinity for ADH than V_2 receptors, vasoconstriction only occurs at ADH concentrations higher than those which effect water reabsorption in the kidney. In addition to renal and cardiovascular effects, ADH has additional actions including:

- platelet aggregation and degranulation (V_1);
- an increase in the concentration of clotting factor VIII (V_2);
- release of adrenocorticotrophic hormone (ACTH);
- release of cortisol (hydrocortisone) from the adrenal cortex (V_1);
- acceleration of glycogen breakdown in the liver;
- antipyretic activity.

ADH or the selective V_2 agonist desmopressin are used to treat central diabetes insipidus, a condition characterized by the excessive production of a dilute urine due to failure to produce sufficient ADH. Desmopressin can be given orally, intranasally, or by subcutaneous injection. ADH cannot be given orally, since it is broken down by trypsin in the alimentary tract, and is thus administered by injection. It is a potent vasoconstrictor and, at high dose, ADH is sometimes used to arrest haemorrhage from oesophageal varices. A derivative of vasopressin is felypressin, which is used as a vasoconstrictor with the local anaesthetic agent, prilocaine (see Chapter 8). Desmopressin increases circulating factor VIII and is sometimes used to prevent bleeding in haemophiliacs. It is also used in the management of nocturnal enuresis (bed-wetting).

Oxytocin

This octapeptide is synthesized in the paraventricular nucleus of the hypothalamus. It is released from the posterior pituitary gland following suckling of the breast or uterine stretching. Oxytocin acts on the myoepithelial cells of the mammary glands, causing contraction and milk ejection. It also acts on the smooth muscle of the uterus, initiating contraction; it is widely believed that oxytocin initiates labour and parturition. The main therapeutic use of oxytocin is in obstetrics to stimulate contraction of the uterus and induce labour.

Key facts
Posterior pituitary hormones

- ADH (vasopressin) and oxytocin are the two polypeptide hormones secreted by the posterior pituitary.

- Secretion of ADH is influenced by plasma osmolality and blood volume, and actions of the hormones are mediated by V_1 and V_2 receptors.

- ADH actions are mainly on the kidney, where the hormone increases the water permeability of the collecting ducts.

- ADH is used in the treatment of central diabetes insipidus, and derivatives of the hormone are used as vasoconstrictors (felypressin) and to control haemorrhage in haemophiliacs. Desmopressin, a selective V_2 agonist, is also used to treat central diabetes insipidus.

- Oxytocin acts on the mammary glands to cause milk ejection; it is also used in obstetrics to induce labour.

Anterior pituitary hormones

The anterior pituitary gland (adenohypophysis) secretes three groups of hormones:

(1) the somatomammotrophic hormones, i.e. growth hormone, prolactin, and placental lactogen;

(2) the glycoprotein hormones, i.e. luteinizing hormone, follicle-stimulating hormone, and thyroid-stimulating hormone;

(3) peptides derived from pro-opiomelanocortin, i.e. corticotropin (ACTH), α-, β-, and γ-melanocyte-stimulating hormones, and β-lipotrophin.

The trophic hormones are discussed under the section related to the glands upon which they act. The somatomammotrophins are discussed in the next section.

Growth hormone (somatotrophin)

Growth hormone is a small protein molecule that is synthesized and stored in cells, known as somatotrophs, in the anterior pituitary gland. The secretion of growth hormone is controlled by two regulating factors produced in the hypothalamus—growth hormone-releasing factor and growth hormone-inhibiting factor (somatostatin). Secretion of the hormone is pulsatile, with six to eight bursts per day. In growing children, most of the bursts occur during sleep. Plasma concentrations of growth hormone are reduced by food, and increased by fasting, during sleep, and physical exercise, and at times of stress and emotional excitement.

Pharmacological and physiological actions
Growth hormone affects growth, protein synthesis, and carbohydrate metabolism.

GROWTH
The hormone is essential for normal growth and development. A lack of production during the growth period will cause dwarfism; excessive production in a child will cause gigantism and, in an adult, acromegaly (a condition characterized by enlarged hands and feet, coarse facial features, and mandibular prognathism). Many of the actions of growth hormone on tissue size are mediated by its effects on sulfation factors or somatomedins.

Somatomedins are growth-promoting factors produced by the liver and kidneys. The major somatomedins are identical to polypeptides that have been termed insulin-like growth factors 1 and 2 (IGF-1, IGF-2). These polypeptides appear be the principal mediators for the action of growth hormone. When IGFs are injected into hypophysectomized rats, there is an increase in proteoglycan, protein, RNA, and DNA synthesis. IGFs also increase lipolysis and the transport of amino acids and glucose into muscle. Plasma IGF levels are low in African pygmies.

PROTEIN SYNTHESIS
Growth hormone increases the transport of amino acids into tissues, and accelerates their incorporation into proteins. This results in a reduction of blood urea levels due to a diversion of amino acids into anabolic pathways.

CARBOHYDRATE AND LIPID METABOLISM
Growth hormone, insulin and, to a lesser extent, glucocorticoids, glucagon, and catecholamines play important roles in carbohydrate and lipid metabolism. Insulin and growth hormone have opposite metabolic effects, with insulin promoting glucose as a source of energy and growth hormone facilitating the use of fat. Hence it may appear that growth hormone has an antagonistic effect with insulin. The increased production of growth hormone during fasting may be an adaptation to lack of food. Growth hormone causes an increase in free fatty acids in the blood due to its lipolytic action on adipose tissue. This action may explain the increased secretion of the hormone that occurs during exercise, when fat deposits are used as an alternative source of energy.

Uses
Growth hormone is used to correct pituitary dwarfism. There are two commercial preparations of growth hormone available, somatropin and somatrem.

Prolactin

This has a similar structure to growth hormone and is synthesized, stored, and secreted by lactotrophic cells in the anterior pituitary gland. Secretion of prolactin is controlled by a prolactin release-inhibiting hormone, which is produced in the hypothalamus and is now considered to be dopamine.

The principal action of prolactin is on the development of the mammary glands and the production of milk. It is also produced by the placenta. The plasma concentration of prolactin increases throughout pregnancy. During breast-feeding, prolactin levels are increased, and production is controlled by the sucking stimulus. The hormone also inhibits gonadotrophin release and hence suppresses ovulation. This explains why breast-feeding can constitute a natural contraceptive mechanism.

Pharmacological and physiological properties

Prolactin is essential for the development of the mammary glands and their preparation for milk production. It promotes the proliferation and subsequent differentiation of mammary ductal and alveolar epithelium. In preparation for milk production, prolactin increases the synthesis of RNA, milk proteins, and the enzymes necessary for lactose synthesis. Like growth hormone, production of prolactin is influenced by sleep, fasting, and stress.

Key facts
Anterior pituitary hormones

- The anterior pituitary secretes three groups of hormones: somatomammotrophic (e.g. growth hormone and prolactin), glycoproteins (e.g. luteinizing hormone), and peptides derived from pro-opiomelanocortin.

- Growth hormone affects growth (mediated by somatomedins), protein synthesis, and carbohydrate metabolism.

- A lack of growth hormone production will cause dwarfism in children, whereas excessive production will result in gigantism and acromegaly.

- Growth hormone is used to correct pituitary dwarfism.

- Prolactin acts on the mammary glands and facilitates milk production; the hormone also suppresses ovulation by inhibiting the release of gonadotrophins.

Thyroid gland

The thyroid gland secretes three hormones: levothyroxine (thyroxine) (T_4); tri-iodothyroxine (T_3); and calcitonin, which is dealt with in Chapter 21. Secretion of levothyroxine and tri-iodothyroxine are under the control of the anterior pituitary peptide, thyroid-stimulating hormone (TSH). Secretion of TSH is stimulated by the hypothalamic peptide, thyrotrophin-releasing hormone (TRH). The pituitary TSH increases the vascularity, cellularity, and size of the thyroid gland, and accelerates the synthesis and release of thyroid hormones. The production of TSH is inhibited by circulating levels of levothyroxine and tri-iodothyroxine.

Levothyroxine (thyroxine) and tri-iodothyroxine

These thyroid hormones are synthesized and stored as thyroglobulin in the thyroid gland. The synthesis and release of thyroid hormones involve the following processes:

(1) uptake of iodide ions by the gland;

(2) oxidation of iodide, and iodination of *p*-tyrosyl groups of thyroglobulin;

(3) proteolysis of thyroglobulin, and release of levothyroxine and tri-iodothyronine into the bloodstream;

(4) conversion of levothyroxine to tri-iodothyronine in the tissues.

Thyroid hormones are strongly bound to plasma proteins (globulin and albumin). They are broken down in the liver, conjugated with glucuronic acid and sulfate, and excreted in the bile. In health, these hormones are slowly eliminated from the body and have a half-life of 6–7 days.

Physiological and pharmacological properties

Thyroid hormones have four main functions: (1) they regulate growth and development—they also have (2) calorigenic, (3) metabolic, and (4) cardiovascular effects. The pharmacodynamics of thyroid hormones relate to their ability to enter a cell and bind with a specific receptor protein associated with DNA. Once bound, the hormones induce a conformational change in the receptor protein that leads to the synthesis of specific mRNA and protein. The effects produced by the conformational change will depend upon the cell type. Within cells, T_3 is three to five times more active than T_4; and as a proportion of T_4 is converted to T_3, levothyroxine (thyroxine) can be considered a prohormone.

GROWTH AND DEVELOPMENT

These hormones exert their effect on growth and development by directly controlling DNA transcription and protein synthesis, and indirectly by influencing growth hormone production and actions. They are also essential for the development of the nervous system, in particular, cell differentiation, proliferation, and myelinization.

CALORIGENIC EFFECTS

Thyroid hormones stimulate oxygen consumption and heat production, consequently they regulate body temperature (calorigenic effect) by controlling basal metabolic rate. They have a particular effect on the heart, lungs, liver, and kidneys.

METABOLIC EFFECTS

These hormones stimulate the metabolism of cholesterol to bile salts, and accelerate the utilization of carbohydrate for increased calorific demand.

CARDIOVASCULAR EFFECTS

Thyroid hormones cause an increase in cardiac output due to an increase in heart rate and force of contraction. These effects may arise as a direct action of the hormones on the heart, or as a consequence of the increased metabolic and calorigenic effects arising from increased thyroid function. In hyperthyroidism, an increase in myocardial β-adrenoceptors has been observed. Consequently, β-adrenoceptor antagonists are of value in its management (see Chapter 14).

Iodine

This element is essential for the formation of the thyroid hormones. Dietary iodine, in the form of iodide oripdate, is absorbed from the stomach and small intestine, transported in the blood, and taken up by the thyroid gland. Within the gland, iodide is oxidized to iodine and utilized to form levothyroxine (thyroxine) and tri-iodothyroxine. A deficiency of iodine causes non-toxic goitre, which usually responds to potassium iodide. Iodized salt is used to prevent this type of goitre, especially in areas of iodine deficiency.

Radioactive isotopes of iodine are used in the management of hyperthyroidism. Excessive intake of iodine can cause swelling of the salivary glands (the so-called iodine mumps).

Disorders of thyroid gland function

Hypofunction of the thyroid gland at birth results in cretinism and, in adults, causes myxoedema. Hypothyroidism is often associated with impairment of the normal immune response and those affected may be susceptible to oral candidiasis. Both cretinism and myxoedema are treated with levothyroxine (thyroxine).

Hyperfunction of the thyroid gland (hyperthyroidism) can take the form of a diffuse toxic goitre (Graves' disease) or toxic nodular goitre (Plummer's disease). Signs and symptoms of hyperthyroidism include an intolerance to heat, muscle weakness, tremor, insomnia, anxiety, and an increased heart rate. The cardiovascular changes in hyperthyroidism may be due to an increased sensitivity of the heart to catecholamines.

In cases of uncontrolled hyperthyroidism, local anaesthetic solutions containing epinephrine (adrenaline) should be avoided.

Antithyroid drugs

These are used to treat hyperthyroidism and the most widely used are the thioureylenes. These compounds inhibit the formation of thyroid hormones by interfering with the incorporation of iodine into levothyroxine (thyroxine) and tri-iodothyroxine. Examples include carbimazole and propylthiouracil; both drugs can cause a leucopenia, so monitoring of white blood cells is important during therapy.

Potassium perchlorate is also used to treat hyperthyroidism by preventing the uptake and storage of iodine in the thyroid gland.

Key facts
Thyroid hormones

- The thyroid gland secretes 3 hormones: levothyroxine (thyroxine) (T_4), tri-iodothyroxine (T_3), and calcitonin.

- Iodine is essential for the formation of the thyroid hormones, which are stored as thyroglobulin in the lumen of the gland.

- Levothyroxine (thyroxine) and tri-iodothyroxine regulate growth and body temperature, have metabolic actions, and increase cardiac output.

- Hypofunction of the thyroid gland causes myxoedema in adults and cretinism in children; it is treated with levothyroxine.

- Hyperfunction of the thyroid gland (hyperthyroidism) can be treated with either thioureylenes, radioactive iodine, or potassium perchlorate.

- The β-adrenoceptor blocker propranolol is useful in reducing the cardiac effects and tremor that accompany hyperthyroidism.

The adrenal cortex

This part of the adrenal gland synthesizes and secretes mainly glucocorticoids and mineralocorticoids, together with small amounts of testosterone, oestrogen, and progesterone. Secretion of glucocorticoids is under the control of ACTH, whereas the secretion of mineralocorticoids is controlled by the renin–angiotensin system (see Chapter 16).

Adrenocorticotrophic hormone (ACTH)

This peptide, secreted by the anterior pituitary gland, stimulates the adrenal cortex to secrete glucocorticoids (cortisol and corticosterone). It also stimulates the synthesis of adrenocortical hormones by increasing the concentration of the substrate for steroid synthesis, i.e. cholesterol. The release of ACTH is under dual control. One controlling element is the hypothalamus, which produces a peptide known as corticotropin-releasing factor (CRF). This travels via the hypophyseal–portal vessel to the anterior pituitary and there stimulates the production of ACTH. The release of CRF is under neural control (Fig. 20.1).

The second element controlling the production and secretion of ACTH and CRF is a negative-feedback regulatory influence from cortisol and other glucocorticoids. High levels of glucocorticoids suppress the secretion of both ACTH and CRF, and the converse applies with low levels. Production of ACTH also shows diurnal variation, with maximum levels occurring in the early morning and minimal levels at midnight.

An analogue of ACTH (tetracosactrin) is used as a diagnostic agent in adrenal insufficiency (see later).

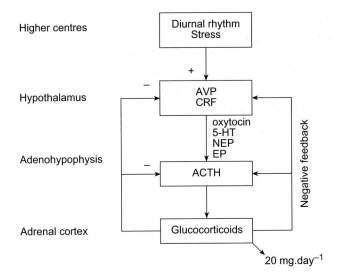

Fig. 20.1 Factors that control the release of adrenocorticotrophic hormone (ACTH). AVP, arginine vasopressin; CRF, corticotropin-releasing factor; 5-HT, 5-hydroxytryptamine; NEP, norepinephrine; EP, epinephrine.

Physiological and pharmacological properties of corticosteroids

There are two types of steroids synthesized in the adrenal cortex—the 19-carbon androgens and the 21-carbon corticosteroids. Both are derived from cholesterol. The 21-carbon corticosteroids can be further classified into: (1) *glucocorticoids* (hydrocortisone, also known as cortisol and corticosterone), because of their action on carbohydrate metabolism; and (2) *mineralocorticoids* (aldosterone), because of their effect on sodium retention. These actions are not mutually exclusive as glucocorticoids have considerable effects on electrolyte balance.

Aldosterone production is under the control of angiotensin acting on the adrenal cortex. The synthesis and secretion of all other corticosteroids is under the control of ACTH. The corticosteroids are continuously synthesized and secreted, so there is minimal storage in the adrenal cortex. Under normal conditions, the adrenal cortex produces 20–30 mg of cortisol per day.

Corticosteroids, via an interaction with DNA-linked receptors, have a diverse range of properties and functions. They are involved in carbohydrate, fat, and protein metabolism; they affect electrolyte and water balance; and they are essential for the normal function of the cardiovascular system, kidney, skeletal muscle, and nervous system. They also enable the organism to withstand changes in the environment and cope with stressful events. The many different properties of the corticosteroids are due to their action on protein synthesis, especially DNA transcription and the production of specific proteins.

CARBOHYDRATE AND PROTEIN METABOLISM

Corticosteroids have the following effects on carbohydrate metabolism:

- They stimulate the formation of glucose.
- They reduce the utilization of glucose in the peripheral tissues (perhaps by antagonizing the action of insulin).
- They promote the storage of glucose as glycogen.

These actions ensure that the brain always has sufficient glucose for the essential glucose-dependent functions. Corticosteroids act on the liver and stimulate the synthesis of glucose from amino acids. They also inhibit protein synthesis in muscles and connective tissue, thus mobilizing additional amino acids. Therefore, the overall effect of corticosteroids is to cause an increase in blood sugar and liver glycogen content, and an increase in urinary nitrogen excretion. Hence long-term corticosteroid administration (see the section below entitled 'Other unwanted effects') or high output from the adrenal cortex will cause protein wasting, resulting in an increase in capillary fragility, muscle wasting, and a reduction in the protein matrix of bone (osteoporosis). The actions on glucose metabolism can induce a diabetic-like state.

LIPID METABOLISM

Corticosteroids have several actions on lipid metabolism. They inhibit fatty acid synthesis, but facilitate the mobilization of fatty acids from adipose tissue by lipolytic enzymes. They also have an effect on the distribution of body fat, with excessive production causing an increase in fatty acid deposits in the face (moon face) and on the back of the neck (buffalo hump).

ELECTROLYTE AND WATER BALANCE

Corticosteroids, in particular aldosterone, affect this balance through a direct action on the kidney. They cause an increase in the urinary excretion of potassium and hydrogen ions, and enhanced reabsorption of sodium ions from the tubular fluids. These actions result in an increase in sodium retention, hypokalaemia, alkalosis, and an increase in extracellular fluid. Hence, excessive corticosteroid production or long-term use will cause oedema and hypertension. In patients with a pre-existing cardiac problem, long-term corticosteroid therapy will increase the incidence of left ventricular hypertrophy and congestive heart failure. Conversely, a deficiency of endogenous corticosteroids will cause sodium loss, a reduction in extracellular fluid, and cellular hydration.

EFFECTS ON BLOOD

Excess corticosteroids cause an increase in red blood cells and their haemoglobin content, and an increase in polymorphonuclear neutrophils. Other white blood cells are reduced in number. A reduction in corticosteroid production will cause a normochromic, normocytic anaemia.

IMMUNE SYSTEM

Corticosteroids suppress both immune and inflammatory reactions (see Chapter 4) and their immunosuppressive properties are extensively used after transplant surgery to prevent graft rejection. They interfere with several stages of the immune response (see Chapter 4), and these are listed below:

- They decrease the production of interleukin (IL)-2, which subsequently decreases the action of T-helper cells and the clonal proliferation of T cells.
- They decrease synthesis of the cytokines IL-1, IL-2, IL-3, IL-4, IL-5, IL-6, IL-8, and tumour-necrosis factor-α (TNF-α).
- They decrease the complement proteins in plasma.
- They reduce the efficacy of cytokine-activated macrophages.

When used clinically to suppress or prevent graft rejection, corticosteroids suppress the initiation and generation of a 'new' immune response more efficiently than a response that is already established. The anti-inflammatory properties of corticosteroids are discussed in Chapter 4.

Pharmacokinetics

Synthetic corticosteroids can be administered orally, topically, parenterally, and rectally. Some preparations are given into the synovial fluid. Corticosteroids are well absorbed from any site of administration, and are transported in the plasma extensively bound to plasma protein. Most are metabolized in the liver to 11-oxy-17-ketosteroids, a large proportion of which are conjugated with sulfate or glucuronic acid prior to excretion in the urine. The rate of steroid metabolism is dependent upon the preparation. Steroids with a double bond (e.g. methylprednisolone), or with a fluorine atom (e.g. betamethasone), are metabolized slowly when compared to hydrocortisone.

Unwanted effects of corticosteroids

Adrenocortical suppression

Long-term administration of corticosteroids can cause suppression of the anterior pituitary–adrenal cortex axis, with a reduction in the production and release of ACTH. As a result, there is atrophy of the adrenal cortex, therefore the cortex cannot produce sufficient endogenous corticosteroids to cope with stress, so an adrenal crisis may develop. After cessation of corticosteroids, the return of adrenal function may take 9 months. During this recovery period, and for an additional 1–2 years, patients with adrenocortical suppression may need to be protected with supplementary corticosteroids during stressful situations, such as dental surgical procedures and severe infections (see below). The features and treatment of an adrenal crisis are dealt with in Chapter 26.

The extent of adrenocortical suppression will depend upon the type of steroid, its potency, dose, and duration of treatment. Adrenocortical suppression is not observed when corticosteroids are used for just a few weeks.

Abrupt cessation of corticosteroid therapy can result in acute adrenal insufficiency, characterized by fever, joint and muscle pain, and malaise. Therefore, corticosteroid therapy should be reduced slowly.

Assessing adrenocortical function

Occasions may arise when a clinician needs to ascertain the viability of the adrenal cortex and its ability to synthesize and secrete glucocorticoids. Examples would include patients on long-term steroid therapy, or those with any form of adrenal gland pathology. Adrenocortical function is assessed by the ACTH challenge test.

The test involves giving the patient an intramuscular injection of 250 µg of tetracosactrin, which is the synthetic 1–24 N-terminal of ACTH. Then, 45 minutes after the injection, a venous blood sample is withdrawn and assayed for plasma cortisol. In people with normal adrenal function, this challenge will result in a plasma cortisol concentration of $600 \, nmol \, L^{-1}$. Values less than this are consistent with primary or secondary adrenocortical suppression.

Corticosteroid cover in dentistry

There is now considerable debate as to whether patients on long-term steroid therapy require supplementary corticosteroids prior to certain dental procedures. Factors that need to be considered include the steroid preparation (potency), dose, duration of treatment, the dental procedure to be undertaken, and the level of the patient's anxiety. In general, most dental procedures (this includes restorative work, soft-tissue surgery, and simple extractions) will not require additional steroids over and above the patient's normal steroid medication. For dental surgical procedures under general anaesthesia (and the insertion of implants), steroid supplementation may be required to cover these operations. If a steroid patient is very anxious about dentistry, then the procedure can be completed under sedation. In such cases reducing the patient's anxiety by pharmacological means also reduces the need for supplementary steroids. It is desirable that all patients on long-term corticosteroids have their blood pressure monitored before, during, and after their dental treatment, irrespective of whether supplementary steroids have been administered. If the blood pressure (BP) falls by more than 25% of the preoperative reading, then hydrocortisone 100 mg IV should be given immediately.

Other unwanted effects

Alterations in carbohydrate metabolism can cause glycosuria, but this is usually controlled by diet. Altered protein metabolism may lead to an increase in capillary fragility causing ecchymosis, muscle wasting, and poor wound healing. Osteoporosis is a common unwanted effect of long-term corticosteroid therapy, especially in the elderly. Steroids produce hypocalcaemia by inhibiting calcium absorption and increasing urinary calcium excretion. The hypocalcaemia causes an increase in parathyroid hormone secretion, which in turn stimulates osteoclastic activity. Thus, there is both increased resorption and decreased formation of bone. Steroid-induced osteoporosis commonly affects the spinal column and sometimes the mandible; spontaneous fractures of these and other bones may occur.

The actions of corticosteroids on lipid metabolism cause the characteristic moon face and buffalo hump (see the section entitled 'Lipid metabolism' above). Disturbances in electrolyte and water balance cause hypokalaemia, oedema formation, hypertension, and alkalosis.

Immunosuppressive effects render the patient more susceptible to opportunistic infections such as candidiasis, and to postoperative infections, the incidence of which can be reduced by prophylactic antibiotic cover prior to surgery. Topical or systemic corticosteroids should not be used for their anti-inflammatory properties if the underlying cause of the inflammation is infective. If corticosteroids are erroneously used in the presence of infection, they will mask its signs and permit it to spread.

Peptic ulceration is an occasional complication of corticosteroid therapy; it may be due to alterations in mucosal cell defence mechanisms.

Administration of corticosteroids can cause a feeling of well-being; however, long-term corticosteroid administration can cause certain behavioural disturbances, including insomnia, anxiety, mood changes, and even suicidal tendencies, the mechanisms of which are unknown.

Corticosteroids cause inhibition or arrest of growth in children. Although the mechanism for this effect is unknown, some studies have shown normal growth can be maintained with growth hormone treatment.

Uses

They are particularly used for their anti-inflammatory, anti-allergic, and immunosuppressive properties in various medical conditions exemplified by rheumatoid arthritis, nephrotic syndrome, collagen disease, allergic states, ocular disease, skin disease, asthma, ulcerative colitis, and certain malignancies. Corticosteroids are also used in substitution therapy in patients with adrenal insufficiency. Their use in dentistry is discussed in Chapter 4.

Key facts
Adrenocortical hormones

- The adrenal cortex synthesizes and excretes glucocorticoids (e.g. cortisol) and mineralocorticoids (e.g. aldosterone).

- Synthesis and secretion of glucocorticoids is under the control of ACTH, whereas angiotensin controls the secretion of aldosterone.

- Release of ACTH is under dual control: corticotropin-releasing factor (CRF); and circulating levels of glucocorticoids.

- Glucocorticoids have a variety of effects on carbohydrate, lipid, and protein metabolism, whereas mineralocorticoids affect water and electrolyte balances.

- Corticosteroids have a significant effect upon the immune and inflammatory responses by inhibiting the synthesis and actions of several cytokines.

- Unwanted effects of corticosteroids include adrenocortical suppression, glycosuria, muscle wasting, poor wound healing, osteoporosis, hypertension, moon face, increased susceptibility to infection, and mood changes.

- Corticosteroids are used extensively in medicine for their anti-inflammatory and immunosuppressive actions; they are widely used to treat diseases that have an autoimmune or allergic component.

The pancreas

The islets of Langerhans are made up of distinct cell groups designated α, β, and δ. The α-cells synthesize and secrete glucagon, whilst the β-cells synthesize and secrete insulin and amylin. All three hormones are essential for glucose metabolism and their production is controlled by the level of blood glucose. A high glucose concentration stimulates the secretion of insulin, whereas a low concentration stimulates the release of glucagon. Amylin opposes the action of insulin by stimulating the breakdown of glycogen in striated muscles and inhibits insulin secretion. The results of the activities of the various pancreatic hormones is to maintain a blood glucose concentration of $100 \, mg \, mL^{-1}$.

The δ-cells in the pancreas secrete somatostatin, which has an inhibitory action on both insulin and glucagon secretion.

Insulin

This was first isolated in 1921 and used to treat diabetes (see below) in the following year. The insulin molecule is made up of two chains of amino acids, an acidic or A-chain, and a basic or B-chain. Insulin is synthesized in β-islet cells from the precursor pro-insulin, which in turn is derived from prepro-insulin. Proteolytic enzymes convert the pro-insulin to insulin, which is then released from the Golgi complex together with any unconverted pro-insulin and a superfluous C-peptide. Insulin secretion is stimulated by many factors including carbohydrates, fatty acids, amino acids, growth hormone, ACTH, levothyroxine (thyroxine), and glucagon. Secretion of insulin is inhibited by insulin itself, somatostatin, and α_2-adrenoceptor agonists.

The β-cells respond to both the actual glucose concentration and also to the rate of change of blood glucose. Glucose metabolism within β-cells increases the ratio of ATP/ADP, which blocks ATP-sensitive K^+-channels that control the resting membrane potential. Blockade of these channels, through which K^+ moves out of cells, produces depolarization, opening voltage-dependent Ca^{2+} channels. The resulting influx of Ca^{2+} triggers the release of insulin by exocytosis from secretory granules. There is a steady basal release of insulin and also a response to a rise in blood glucose concentrations. This response has two phases: (1) an initial rapid response due to the release of stored hormone; and (2) a slower, delayed phase reflecting both the release of stored insulin and new synthesis. In diabetes mellitus this response is abnormal.

Under fasting conditions, the islets produce about 40 μg of insulin per hour, resulting in a systemic concentration of $0.5\,ng\,mL^{-1}$. Food intake results in a rise in insulin synthesis and secretion.

Pharmacokinetics

Insulin preparations were once of either bovine or porcine origin. More recently, human insulins have become available and are now the most commonly used forms of insulin. Human insulin is produced either by micro-organisms using recombinant DNA technology or semi-synthetically by the substitution of one amino acid in porcine insulin. Insulin is broken down in the gastrointestinal tract and hence can only be given parenterally, usually by subcutaneous injection. In emergency situations, the drug can be given intramuscularly or intravenously. Insulin has a half-life of 6–9 minutes and is metabolized in the liver to inactive peptides. A wide range of insulin preparations are available with differing pharmacokinetic properties, some of which are listed below.

SHORT/RAPIDLY ACTING INSULINS

- *Soluble insulin*: This is the only preparation that can be given intravenously when used to treat diabetic emergencies; for example, ketoacidosis and hyperglycaemia. When given subcutaneously, it has a short duration of action (5–8 hours).

INTERMEDIATE-ACTING INSULINS

Compared to soluble insulins, these preparations dissolve more slowly resulting in a slower onset and longer duration of action (18–24 hours).

- *Isophane insulin preparation*: This is a suspension of insulin complexed with zinc and protamine in a phosphate buffer.
- *Lente insulin (insulin zinc suspension)*: This is a mixture of crystallized (ultralente) and amorphous (semilente) insulin in an acetate buffer.

LONG-ACTING INSULINS

These preparations have a very slow onset and prolonged duration of action (20–36 hours) due to their low solubility.

- *Ultralente insulin* (extended insulin zinc suspension): This is crystallized insulin in an acetate buffer.

A common regimen for insulin-dependent diabetics is to inject a combination of short and intermediate acting insulins twice daily, before breakfast and before the evening meal. New tech-niques for insulin administration are being evaluated, these include intranasal administration, and the incorporation of insulin into biodegradable microspheres.

Pharmacological and physiological properties

Insulin controls the blood concentration of glucose by acting via tyrosine kinase-linked receptors (glycoproteins) on cell membranes. Activation of receptors causes the following:

- an increase in the glucose uptake due to insertion of glucose transporters into cell membranes;
- an increase in the rate of glucose utilization;
- an increase in the rate of glycogen deposition;
- inhibition of hepatic gluconeogenesis.

Insulin also causes increases in cellular amino-acid uptake, DNA and RNA synthesis, and oxidative phosphorylation.

Insulin requirements increase during pregnancy, prolonged exercise, severe infections, and stress.

Unwanted effects of insulin

The most serious of these is hypoglycaemia, which can be fatal if not promptly recognized and treated. The clinical features and management of hypoglycaemia are discussed in Chapter 26.

Insulin derived from pigs or cows is a foreign protein and so antibodies can develop against it and impurities present in the preparations, which will give rise to insulin resistance or local or systemic allergic reactions. However, the incidence of such reactions is falling due to the development of very pure insulin preparations. The use of human insulins has further reduced the incidence of resistance and allergic reactions, although these may still occur due to immune responses from contaminants, or aggregated or denatured insulin.

Repeated insulin injections at the same site can cause lipodystrophy and swelling. This problem can be overcome by regularly changing the site of injection.

Rebound hyperglycaemia can follow excessive insulin use. This is due to the release of compensatory hormones from the pancreas.

Diabetes mellitus

Diabetes mellitus is the term used for a group of metabolic disorders that are clinically and genetically heterogeneous, but share the characteristic of glucose intolerance. There are two types of diabetes:

1. *Type I*, or insulin-dependent diabetes mellitus (also referred to as juvenile-onset diabetes), is characterized by an abrupt onset of symptoms, decreased insulin in the serum, dependence on exogenous insulin, and the tendency for ketosis.

2. *Type II*, or non-insulin-dependent diabetes mellitus (also referred to as maturity-onset diabetes), presents with few or no symptoms of metabolic imbalances. This condition is not prone to ketosis, is often associated with obesity, and

can be controlled by diet alone or a combination of diet and oral hypoglycaemic drugs.

A lack of insulin causes a rise in blood glucose levels due to increased gluconeogenesis and decreased glucose uptake. Fat metabolism is also altered. There is an increase in lipase activity and a decrease in triglyceride synthetase activity, both of which lead to an increase in blood levels of unesterified fatty acids. The excess fatty acids are metabolized by acetyl coenzyme A, which results in the formation of ketone bodies, so causing the metabolic acidosis that often accompanies hyperglycaemia. The increase in blood glucose, fatty acids, and their metabolites contributes to the polyuria and dehydration that is often an early sign of the disease.

Diabetics are prone to a variety of systemic complications, which appear to be related to the degree of diabetic control. Many of these complications are due to vascular changes (change in the basement membrane and accelerated atheroma formation), and include hypertension, retinopathy, kidney damage, and peripheral vascular disease.

DENTAL PROBLEMS ASSOCIATED WITH DIABETES

The dental problems associated with diabetes mellitus include periodontal disease, increased susceptibility to caries and oral infections, and salivary gland disorders.

Epidemiological studies suggest that diabetics are more prone to periodontal breakdown than non-diabetics. The group most at risk appears to be the poorly controlled Type I diabetics who also suffer from complications such as nephropathy and retinopathy. Vascular changes in the gingival tissues, impaired polymorphonuclear leucocyte chemotaxis and increased collagenase activity may all be contributory factors.

Type I diabetics are also more susceptible to dental caries, especially in the early stages of the disorder. In part, this may be due to the reduced salivary flow found in these patients. The caries incidence decreases when they are placed on a reduced carbohydrate diet.

Xerostomia is a common symptom in diabetic patients, and salivary gland enlargement—which is seen in 10–20% of patients—may be a compensatory change in the glands in order to increase salivary flow. The reduced salivary flow and impairment in polymorphonuclear leucocyte function may account for the increased susceptibility of diabetics to oral infections such as candidiasis.

The main problem with diabetic patients in dentistry is that dental treatment may interrupt their food intake and insulin requirements, especially if a general anaesthetic is to be administered. Several dental infections may also cause hazards for the insulin-controlled diabetic, leading to loss of diabetic control and the potential for the spread of infection. Thus, such infections should be treated promptly. Monitoring blood and urine sugar levels is essential to ensure that diabetics do not become hypo- or hyperglycaemic as a consequence of the infection.

Dental procedures and simple oral surgical procedures under local anaesthesia are usually well tolerated by diabetic patients. Treatment should ideally take place in the morning and not interfere with mealtimes.

Management of diabetic patients before a general anaesthetic will depend upon their current therapy. Those controlled by diet alone can usually tolerate a general anaesthetic for minor oral surgical procedures. Regular monitoring of their urine and blood sugar levels is essential, and soluble insulin should be available if hyperglycaemia develops. If the diabetic is controlled by oral hypoglycaemic drugs (see below), they should be admitted to hospital before the procedure and placed on insulin. Those on insulin therapy should also be admitted to hospital before the procedure and placed on soluble insulin. During surgery, patients are infused with 3 units of soluble insulin per hour and glucose solution at the rate of $6\,g\,hour^{-1}$. This regimen is continued until normal feeding and soluble insulin control can be resumed.

All diabetic patients must be treated in hospital if general anaesthetics are being administered. Changes in their insulin regimen should only be made in consultation with their physician. Poorly controlled diabetics are more prone to infection and they may require prophylactic antibiotic cover for minor oral surgical procedures.

Oral hypoglycaemic drugs

Oral drugs used to control hypoglycaemia are of two types: the sulfonylureas and the biguanides.

SULFONYLUREAS

These drugs stimulate islet tissues to secrete insulin by causing degranulation in the β-cells. They also increase the sensitivity of the peripheral tissues to insulin. Their action therefore depends upon the pancreas having some ability to synthesize and secrete insulin, and their effects are due to a blockade of ATP-sensitive K^+-channels on the surface of β-cells which regulate insulin secretion in response to glucose (see above). Examples of sulfonylureas include chlorpropamide, glibenclamide, glipizide, gliclazide, and tolbutamide.

PHARMACOKINETICS All sulfonylureas are well absorbed from the gastrointestinal tract, and differences between individual drugs relate to their duration of action. Tolbutamide is taken every 6–8 hours, whereas chlorpropamide is given only once a day.

SULFONYLUREA-INDUCED HYPOGLYCAEMIA Hypoglycaemia is the most common and serious unwanted effect associated with the sulfonylureas. Its incidence and severity varies between the different drugs. On the basis of the incidence of hypoglycaemic episodes, it was estimated that if the standardized incidence ratio for hypoglycaemia was 100 for chlorpropamide, that for glibenclamide would be 111, glipizide 46, and tolbutamide 21. Other factors that affect sulfonylurea-induced hypoglycaemia include age, duration of treatment, concurrent medications, and impaired renal and hepatic function.

OTHER UNWANTED EFFECTS Other unwanted effects include skin rashes, gastrointestinal disturbances, jaundice, and haemopoietic changes. Alcohol and non-steroidal anti-inflammatory drugs, including aspirin, interact with the sulfonylureas, enhancing their hypoglycaemic effect. In addition, chlorpropamide causes flushing after alcohol ingestion by a similar mechanism as metronidazole (see Chapter 11). This sulfonylurea also enhances the action of antidiuretic hormone on the collecting tubules of the kidney which can result in hyponatraemia. As a result of these adverse effects and its potential to cause hypoglycaemia, the use of chlorpropamide is declining in comparison to other sulfonylureas.

BIGUANIDES

It is not clearly established how the biguanides exert their hypoglycaemic effect. They may reduce glucose absorption from the gastrointestinal tract or facilitate glucose entry into tissues (especially skeletal muscle), thus increasing glucose uptake by the peripheral tissues. The biguanides are rarely used as hypoglycaemic agents because of their high incidence of unwanted effects. These include nausea, vomiting, anorexia, and a metallic taste in the mouth. Metformin, is the only biguanide in clinical use.

GLUCAGON

This is a single-chain polypeptide secreted by the α_2-cells of the islets. Secretion is mainly controlled by the plasma glucose concentration, with a rise in plasma glucose inhibiting secretion and a fall facilitating secretion. A further stimulus to glucagon release is the plasma amino-acid level, with secretion being increased after a high-protein meal. Glucagon is broken down in the plasma, liver, and kidney; it has a plasma half-life of 3–6 minutes.

PHYSIOLOGICAL AND PHARMACOLOGICAL PROPERTIES Glucagon antagonizes the actions of insulin; whereas insulin acts as a hormone of glucose storage, glucagon is a hormone of glucose utilization. It acts on the liver to stimulate glycogen breakdown and gluconeogenesis, and to inhibit glycogen synthesis and glucose oxidation. During fasting or starvation, there is an increase in glucagon secretion and an inhibition of insulin secretion. Glucagon secretion is also increased after severe trauma and injury (for example, after burns). In such instances, glucagon stimulates gluconeogenesis and provides an essential supply of glucose.

USES Glucagon (1 mg) can be used as an emergency drug in the treatment of hypoglycaemia, especially in diabetic patients where intravenous glucose is unavailable. The drug can be given intravenously, intramuscularly, or subcutaneously. Clinical improvement is rapid, but must be followed by oral glucose since the hyperglycaemic action of glucagon is transient. If there is no response to glucagon, the patient must be treated with an intravenous glucose solution. Nausea and vomiting are the most frequent adverse effects.

Key facts
Pancreatic hormones

- The islet cells of the pancreas secrete insulin, glucagon, somatostatin, and amylin; all four hormones effect glucose homeostasis.

- The release of insulin is primarily controlled by blood glucose levels; once released in response to a rise in blood glucose, the hormone facilitates cellular glucose uptake and utilization. It also increases glycogen synthesis and decreases gluconeogenesis.

- Various types of insulin are used in the management of Type I diabetes mellitus (a metabolic disorder characterized by high blood glucose levels).

- Unwanted effects of insulin are hypoglycaemia, allergic reactions, and rebound hyperglycaemia.

- The sulfonylureas (e.g. chlorpropamide and tolbutamide) and the biguanides (metformin) are oral hypoglycaemic drugs used in the treatment of Type II diabetes.

- Glucagon is produced by the α_2 cells of the islets and secretion is mainly controlled by plasma glucose concentrations.

- Glucagon antagonizes the actions of insulin and is used in the management of hypoglycaemia.

- Somatostatin and amylin have inhibitory effects on the action of insulin.

Reproductive organs

Hormonal production from the ovaries and testes is under the control of gonadotrophic hormones synthesized and secreted by the anterior pituitary. The release of these hormones is controlled by gonadotrophin-releasing hormone, which is secreted in a pulsatile fashion from peptidergic neurones in the hypothalamus. The gonadotrophic hormones are follicle-stimulating hormone (FSH) and luteinizing hormone (LH). The placenta also produces two gonadotrophins, chorionic gonadotrophin (CG) and chorionic follicle-stimulating hormone (CFSH). The function of CFSH is unknown.

FSH and LH

These are glycoproteins produced and secreted by cells (gonadotrophs) in the anterior pituitary. The plasma concentrations of these hormones are low in infancy, but increase at puberty. Postpubertal concentrations of gonadotrophins vary in women according to the phase of their menstrual cycle. Although concentrations vary, the secretion of FSH and LH is controlled via negative feedback effects on the hypothalamus and anterior pituitary, with estrogen decreasing the secretion of FSH and progesterone inhibiting LH secretion. Gonadotrophins are mainly used to treat infertility.

Action on the ovary

FSH controls the development of ovarian follicles, stimulates granulosa cell proliferation, and increases oestrogen production. In addition, FSH stimulates the Graafian follicle to secrete the glycoprotein inhibin, which has a negative feedback on FSH secretion. LH induces ovulation and initiates and maintains the progesterone-secreting corpus luteum.

Action on the testes

FSH is responsible for spermatogenesis, whereas LH acts on Leydig cells to produce the hormone testosterone—essential for the maturation of spermatocytes and the development of male secondary sexual characteristics.

The actions of both FSH and LH on the ovaries are mediated via receptors on the corpus luteum, and those on the testes are mediated by receptors on the Leydig cells.

Chorionic gonadotrophin

This is produced by syncytiotrophic cells of the placenta shortly after implantation; it maintains the corpus-luteum phase of the ovary, which forestalls the next menstrual cycle. CG is detectable in the urine in the very early stages of pregnancy, and this forms the basis of commercial pregnancy tests.

Estrogens and progesterone

Estrogens

These steroids are synthesized in the ovary from acetate and cholesterol. There are three types of estrogens: estradiol (oestradiol)-17β; estrone (oestrone); and estriol (oestriol). The oestrogens are metabolized in the liver, and excreted as glucuronide and sulfate conjugates in the bile and urine. Estrone and estriol are derived from the potent estradiol-17β by oxidation and hydration reactions, respectively.

PHYSIOLOGICAL AND PHARMACOLOGICAL PROPERTIES

Estrogens control the secondary female sexual characteristics that occur from puberty onwards. Estrogens induce the early proliferative phase of the endometrium, an increase in thickness and vascularity, which occurs from day 5 or 6 until day 14 of the menstrual cycle. They also stimulate the production of an alkaline cervical mucus that facilitates the passage of spermatozoa.

High concentrations of estrogens block bone resorption. The osteoporosis often seen in postmenopausal women may be partly due to reduced estrogen levels.

Many of the actions of estrogens in the development of secondary sexual characteristics, the menstrual cycle, and pregnancy are complementary with those of progesterone.

Progesterone

This is structurally similar to estrogen; it is secreted by the ovary, mainly from the corpus luteum, during the second half of the

menstrual cycle. Production of progesterone is under the control of LH.

PROPERTIES

Progesterone secretion causes the development of the secretory endometrium; abrupt cessation of progesterone from the corpus luteum determines the onset of menstruation. Progesterone is also important for the maintenance of pregnancy and in preparing the breast for milk production.

Uses

The main use of estrogens and progesterone is the oral contraceptive pill and in hormone replacement therapy (see below). Estrogen is also used where there is hypofunction of the ovaries, and to treat certain neoplastic conditions, such as carcinoma of the prostate and breast (see Chapter 19). Progesterone is used for certain gynaecological conditions; however, these are beyond the scope of this book.

Women suffering from menstrually related, oral aphthous ulceration have shown an improvement in their symptoms when treated with the contraceptive pill or progesterone.

THE CONTRACEPTIVE PILL

There are two main types of contraceptive pill: the combination pill and the progesterone-only pill. The combination pill contains a mixture of an estrogen (normally ethinylestradiol (ethinyloestradiol)) and a progesterone (e.g. norethisterone). The oestrogen component suppresses the development of the ovarian follicle by inhibiting the release of FSH, whilst progesterone inhibits the release of LH and thus prevents ovulation. Progesterone also produces changes in the endometrium that discourage implantation, it also has a thickening effect on cervical mucus making it impenetrable to sperm. This latter mode of action is the basis of the progesterone-only contraceptive pill (mini pill).

The combination pill is taken daily for 21 days. Medication is then stopped for 7 days and the withdrawal of oestrogen produces uterine bleeding; the pill is restarted on day 28. The progesterone-only pill is taken continuously.

Another type of hormonal oral contraceptive is the postcoital or 'morning-after pill' which only contains an estrogen. Long-term depot hormonal contraceptives are popular in the Third World and in patients who show poor compliance with pill taking. Intramuscular medroxyprogesterone provides effective contraception for 2–3 months. Progesterone implants and hormonal impregnated vaginal rings are further methods of long-term, depot hormonal contraceptives.

UNWANTED EFFECTS
It is estimated that some 60 million women world-wide take the contraceptive pill, and many epidemiological studies have outlined the risks associated with this very effective method of contraception. The incidence of unwanted effects increases with age (especially in women over the age of 35), the length of time on the pill, and whether there is a

history of smoking. Problems that have been associated with use of the pill include:

- *Increased risk of cardiovascular disease*: Estrogen increases blood coagulability; however, the low doses of oestrogen currently used are unlikely to pose a risk. Indeed, there is evidence that low-dose oestrogens protect the arterial wall against atheromatous changes, whilst progesterone increases the level of high-density lipoproteins that have a protective effect against cardiovascular disease. Despite this evidence, certain women who take the pill may be at risk from cardiovascular disease. These include smokers, women where there is a clear history of heart disease, and those over the age of 35. Some degree of hypertension can occur in women who take the combined pill, and obviously this will exacerbate any existing blood pressure problems.

- *Increased risk of breast and cervical cancer*: There is conflicting evidence with respect to breast cancer, with some studies showing a slight increased risk, whilst others have failed to show any association. With cervical cancer, the evidence is again equivocal. Oral contraceptives may promote, rather than initiate, cervical neoplasia.

- *Other unwanted effects associated with the pill*: These include weight gain, nausea, flushing, depression, and skin changes such as increased pigmentation and acne.

The unwanted effects of the pill need to be balanced against the beneficial effects including the problems of unwanted or unplanned pregnancies. Clinically there is a reduced risk of iron deficiency anaemia, benign breast disease, ovarian cysts, and uterine fibroids.

Of dental significance are the effects of the contraceptive pill on the gingival tissues—an enhancement of plaque-induced inflammation and an increase in gingival crevicular fluid. It has also been reported that women taking the contraceptive pill are more susceptible to 'dry socket' after tooth extraction. There is also an increased incidence of radiopacities in the mandible.

DRUG INTERACTIONS The widespread use of the contraceptive pill has implicated this drug in a number of interactions. Of concern to the dental surgeon is that between the pill and antibiotics, although there is now evidence (see below) that suggests the problem has been overstated. Estrogen is conjugated with glucuronide and extensively excreted in the bile. Once excreted, it may, in part, undergo enterohepatic circulation, whereby the conjugates are broken down (hydrolysed) by bacteria in the gut. Estrogen is released from the conjugate and absorbed through the bowel wall. Any antibiotic therapy that destroys the gut flora will subsequently impair the breakdown of the conjugated hormone; hence it will not be absorbed and the conjugate will be excreted in the faeces. Plasma levels of oestrogen may be considerably reduced and the pill may be ineffective as a contraceptive.

Antibiotics implicated in destruction of the gut flora and reduction of the pill's effectiveness include penicillin, ampicillin, co-trimoxazole, and the tetracyclines. Indeed, many animal studies substantiate the reduction in gut flora with a fall in plasma contraceptive steroid concentration.

However, in human studies the situation is less clear. Controlled studies with tetracycline, ampicillin, and co-trimoxazole in women taking the pill have failed to show a significant reduction in the plasma concentrations of the sex hormones. Large amounts of the ethinylestradiol conjugate were found in the bile of one of the women studied in this investigation, this was because she was unable to form other conjugates. Such patients who show abnormal metabolism of the contraceptive steroids may be more at risk from an interaction with broad-spectrum antibiotics. Since there is no means of readily detecting these patients in a population, it may be prudent to warn patients of the risks of pill failure when prescribing a broad-spectrum antibiotic. The woman should use an alternative contraceptive method for the remainder of her menstrual cycle.

Rifampicin and anticonvulsants (such as carbamazepine) also cause failure of oral contraceptives: both drugs induce hepatic microsomal enzymes, thereby decreasing the plasma concentration of the steroids.

Oral contraceptives also interact with antihypertensive and antidepressant drugs which becomes less effective in pill takers; the mechanism for these interaction is uncertain.

HORMONE REPLACEMENT THERAPY (HRT) HRT is used to reduce menopausal symptoms associated with a decline in estrogen production. These include hot flushes, palpitations, atrophic vaginitis, mood changes, etc. Estrogen is the main hormone used in HRT. Other benefits of HRT include a reduction in the prevalence of both coronary heart disease and postmenopausal osteoporosis.

HRT can be given orally, by transdermal patches or by subcutaneous implant.

The unwanted effects of HRT include an increased risk of endometrial and breast cancer, uterine bleeding, and minor gastrointestinal upsets. As with the contraceptive pill, it would seem that the benefits of HRT outweigh the risks.

The effect of female sex hormones on the oral mucosa

It is well documented that puberty and pregnancy are associated with an increase in the incidence of gingival inflammation. Menopausal women also frequently complain of sore mouths, which may be due to thinning (atrophy) of the epithelial lining of the oral mucosa.

The gingival changes in puberty and pregnancy may be due to progesterone causing an increase in vascular permeability. The action of progesterone on vessel walls is uncertain, although it has been suggested that this hormone affects the nature of the carbohydrate fraction associated with the vessel wall and ground substance. Alternatively, progesterone may enhance pore formation in the vessel wall, causing an increase in permeability and oedema formation. These gingival changes usually resolve after puberty and parturition.

Male sex hormones

The principal male sex hormone is testosterone, produced by the Leydig cells of the testes (90%) and, to a lesser extent, by the adrenal cortex (10%). Secretion of testosterone is stimulated by LH, which in males is also called interstitial-cell stimulating hormone (ICSH). Testosterone acts on a variety of tissues and, in most target tissues, is converted by the enzyme 5α-reductase to the more active hormone, dihydrotestosterone. Both testosterone and dihydrotestosterone are extensively bound to plasma proteins and are inactivated in the liver.

Properties

Testosterone is essential for the development of the male secondary sexual characteristics. It is also required for spermatogenesis, the maturation of sperm, and the production of seminal fluid. Testosterone has marked anabolic effects by causing the retention of nitrogen and an increase in protein synthesis. Hence, this hormone has been used by some sportspeople to encourage muscle development.

Uses

Testosterone is used in replacement therapy in cases of hypogonadism, and to initiate puberty in patients where it is delayed. When used injudiciously in women, testosterone will cause the development of male characteristics.

Key facts
Sex hormones

- Gonadotrophic hormones (follicle-stimulating hormone and luteinizing hormone) secreted by the anterior pituitary stimulate the ovaries to produce estrogen and progesterone, whilst luteinizing hormone stimulates the testes to produce testosterone.

- Secretion of gonadotrophic hormones is under the control of gonadotrophin-releasing hormone from the hypothalamus.

- Estrogen controls female sexual characteristics and induces the early proliferative phase of the endometrium.

- Progesterone is secreted by the corpus luteum and is mainly responsible for the development of the secretory endometrium; cessation of progesterone secretion causes the onset of menstruation.

- Both estrogen and progesterone are used in contraceptive pills, whereas oestrogen is the main constituent of HRT.

- Although the unwanted effects of the pill include an increased risk of cardiovascular disease, breast and cervical cancer, the benefits as a contraceptive outweigh the risks.

- The contraceptive pill is involved in several drug interactions; of concern to the dental surgeon is the potential for pill failure if the patient is prescribed broad-spectrum antibiotics and carbamazepine.

- HRT is used to treat menopausal symptoms; other benefits include a reduced risk for coronary heart disease and osteoporosis.

- The main male sex hormone is testosterone, which is produced by the Leydig cells in the testes.

- Testosterone is essential for the development of male sexual characteristics and spermatogenesis.

Further reading

Alberti, K. G. M. M. (1993). Preventing insulin dependent diabetes mellitus. *British Medical Journal*, 307, 1435–6.

Baird, D. T. and Glassier, A. F. (1993). Hormonal contraception. *New England Journal of Medicine*, 328, 1543–9.

Barnes, P. J. and Adcock, I. (1993). Anti-inflammatory actions of steroids; molecular mechanisms. *Trends in Pharmacological Sciences*, 14, 436–42.

Belchetz, I. (1994). Hormonal treatment of postmenopausal women. *New England Journal of Medicine*, 330, 1062–71.

Evans, R. M. (1988). The steroid and thyroid hormone superfamily. *Science*, 240, 889–95.

Krane, S. M. (1993). Some molecular mechanisms of glucocorticoid action. *British Journal of Rheumatology*, 32, 3–5.

Williams, G. (1994). Management of non-insulin-dependent diabetes mellitus. *Lancet*, 343, 95–100.

Vitamins and minerals

Vitamins and minerals

Vitamins are organic substances that must be provided in small quantities in the diet for the synthesis, by tissues, of co-factors essential for a variety of metabolic reactions. Vitamins can be classified as either water-soluble (B and C) or fat-soluble (A, D, E, and K). Normal human requirements and sources of the vitamins are shown in Table 21.1. Vitamin D is considered in Chapter 22, whilst vitamin K is discussed in Chapter 13.

Iron is essential for many of the body's functions and occurs in a variety of forms in the earth's crust. It plays an essential role in haemopoiesis, and this function is linked with some of the vitamins described in this section.

Vitamin A

A night blindness that could be corrected by diet was first described about 1500 BC; however, it was not until 1923 that this type of night blindness was associated with a deficiency of vitamin A. There are several variants and sources of vitamin A. Retinol (vitamin A_1) is present in fish and meat. The plant pigment, carotene, is a pro-vitamin that is rapidly converted to vitamin A in the body.

Table 21.1 Daily requirements and food sources of vitamins

Vitamin	Daily requirements	Food sources
A	2 mg	Dairy products, fish liver oils
B_1 (thiamine)	2 mg	Cereals, meat, kidneys, eggs
B_2 (riboflavin)	3 mg	Cereal germ, meat, liver, kidney, milk
Nicotinic acid	20 mg	Liver, yeast
B_6 (pyridoxine)		Cereals, liver
Folic acid	5 mg	Green vegetables, salad, yeast
B_{12}	1 μg	Liver, lean meat
C	10–30 mg	Citrus fruits, potatoes, green vegetables
D	500 IU	Dairy products Action of sunlight on skin
K	Adequate supply from gut bacterial flora	Green vegetables, salads

Properties and functions

Vitamin A has many important diverse properties: it is essential for the normal function of the retina and the immune system; for the growth and differentiation of epithelial tissues; and for bone growth and embryonic development. These different functions are mediated by different forms of the vitamin A molecule, which are collectively known as the retinoids (retinal, retinol, and retinoic acid). Most of the actions are mediated by DNA-linked receptors similar to those for steroid and thyroid hormones (see Chapter 2). Retinal is essential for normal vision, whereas retinol is important in the reproductive process.

A variety of food substances contain vitamin A, and ideal sources are shown in Table 20.1. Supplementary doses of vitamin A are given orally in the form of halibut liver-oil capsules. The vitamin is well absorbed from the gastrointestinal tract, and any excess is stored in the liver. The storage of vitamin A is enhanced by vitamin E.

Vitamin A and epithelial development

Vitamin A is essential for the induction and control of epithelial cell differentiation and the production of keratin and mucus. In the absence of vitamin A, goblet mucous cells disappear and are replaced by a stratified, keratinized epithelium. Thus the protective mucus layer is depleted and the underlying tissues are more prone to infection and irritation. The effect of vitamin A on epithelial development has led to a considerable interest in its use in the prevention and treatment of certain malignant conditions.

Animal experiments have shown that a deficiency of vitamin A can result in marked epithelial hyperplasia and reduced cellular differentiation, changes that may be associated with premalignancy. The administration of retinol reverses these changes, thus the progression of premalignant cells to cells with invasive malignant characteristics is slowed, delayed, or arrested.. The mechanisms of this 'anticarcinogenic' effect remain unclear. It may be related to changes in cellular function or an action of the vitamin on the host's immune system.

Deficiency

Dietary deficiency of vitamin A leads to retarded growth and development. The first sign of this is often impaired vision in dim light, a condition known as nyctalopia (night blindness). Other signs include hyperkeratosis of the skin, impaired renal function, and urinary calculi. Severe deficiency results in faulty modelling of bone; diarrhoea also occurs due to alteration in the epithelial lining of the gastrointestinal tract.

Deficiency of vitamin A is commonly seen in undernourished populations from the Third World. Deficiency also occurs in patients with chronic diseases that affect fat absorption, such as colitis, sprue, Crohn's disease, and disease of the biliary tract.

Hypervitaminosis A

Acute poisoning with vitamin A has been reported following the consumption of polar-bear liver, but is more commonly associated with accidental overdose in children. Signs and symptoms include drowsiness, headache, vomiting, papilloedema, and peeling of the skin. Chronic overdose can result in vomiting, loss of appetite, dryness of the skin, gingivitis, and angular cheilitis. Hyperostoses (bony swellings) of the skull can occur with long-term consumption of excess vitamin A. Congenital abnormalities can occur in infants whose mothers have consumed >7.5 mg of vitamin A during the first trimester of pregnancy. Hypervitaminosis A can be overcome by increasing the intake of vitamin E.

Uses

Vitamin A is used to correct deficiency states and as a prophylaxis during periods of increased requirements, which may occur in pregnancy, lactation, and infancy. Retinoic acid derivatives such as tretinoin and isotretinoin are used topically in the treatment of acne to promote healing. Retinoids are also administered orally in the treatment of other skin diseases, such as psoriasis, Darier's disease, and keratosis follicularis. The use of vitamin A as an anti-cancer drug still remains experimental.

Key facts
Vitamin A

- Vitamin A occurs in meat and fish, and the plant pigment carotene is a pro-vitamin.
- It is essential for normal function of the retina, embryonic development and growth, and differentiation of epithelial tissue.
- A deficiency of vitamin A leads to night blindness, hyperkeratosis of the skin, and renal impairment.
- Uses of vitamin A include correction of deficiency states, treatment of certain skin diseases, and perhaps as an anti-cancer drug.

The vitamin B complex

This comprises 11 different compounds, all of which are found in yeast and liver. Dietary deficiency often involves several components of the B complex in the same patient.

Thiamine (vitamin B_1)

This occurs in numerous plants and animal foods (Table 21.1), especially in the husks and coatings of many grain cereals. In the body, thiamine is converted to thiamine pyrophosphate, which then acts as an important co-enzyme in carbohydrate metabolism. Thiamine requirements are directly related to carbohydrate utilization and metabolic rate. The body is unable to store thiamine and a poor diet will lead to signs of deficiency within 2 weeks.

Deficiency

Thiamine deficiency causes beriberi, a disease mainly confined to the Far East, where it is due to the consumption of polished rice. In Western countries, thiamine deficiency is often seen in alcoholics and, occasionally, in pregnancy and infancy. Early signs of deficiency include a peripheral neuritis with areas of hyperaesthesia and anaesthesia, and a reduction in muscle strength. Severe deficiency will lead to cardiovascular changes, which include dyspnoea on exertion, palpitations, and tachycardia.

Uses

Thiamine is only used to correct deficiency states. If the deficiency is severe, then it should be given intravenously; however most cases can be corrected by giving the vitamin orally.

Riboflavin (vitamin B_2)

This occurs naturally as the yellow respiratory enzyme found in yeast. In the body, riboflavin is converted into two enzymes, flavine mononucleotide and flavine adenine dinucleotide, both of which are essential for the proper functioning of the electron transport chain in the process of oxidative phosphorylation.

Deficiency

Early signs of riboflavin deficiency include sore throat and angular cheilitis. These are followed by glossitis and cheilosis (sore and red lips). In extreme cases there is a generalized dermatitis, anaemia, and neuropathy. Deficiency states can be corrected by an oral dose of 5–10 mg daily.

Nicotinic acid

This is found mainly in liver and yeast, and functions in the body after it has been converted to the co-enzymes, nicotinamide adenine dinucleotide (NAD) and nicotinamide adenine dinucleotide phosphate (NADP). Both co-enzymes catalyse a variety of oxidation–reduction reactions that are essential for respiration.

Deficiency

Lack of nicotinic acid causes pellagra, a disease found in countries where large quantities of maize are eaten. Early signs of deficiency include generalized dermatitis and stomatitis; severe deficiency causes enteritis and dementia. Deficiency states can be corrected by a daily oral dose of 50 mg of nicotinic acid.

Pyridoxine (vitamin B$_6$)

Pyridoxine, pyridoxal, and pyridoxamine are the three naturally occurring forms of vitamin B$_6$. All three forms are converted in the body to pyridoxal phosphate, which acts as a co-enzyme in the various stages of amino acid metabolism. Pyridoxine occurs naturally in various cereals and liver.

Deficiency

Vitamin B$_6$ deficiency is common in alcoholics, and produces glossitis, seborrhoea, fits, and peripheral neuropathy. Signs of deficiency can also occur in tuberculosis patients taking isoniazid, and patients taking hydralazine, as both drugs interfere with the pyridoxine metabolism. Prolonged use of penicillamine can also cause a deficiency of vitamin B$_6$.

Biotin

The organic acid is found in egg yolk and yeast. Like most of the vitamins in the B complex, biotin is also a co-enzyme and catalyses several carboxylation reactions. It also plays an important role in carbon dioxide fixation. Hence it is essential for carbohydrate and fat metabolism.

Deficiency

Signs of biotin deficiency include dermatitis, atrophic glossitis, hyperaesthesia, and muscle pain. Biotin deficiency can occur in newborn babies, and is readily corrected by daily oral doses of 5–10 mg.

Key facts
Vitamin B complex

- The vitamin B complex comprises 11 different compounds, which are all found in yeast and liver.

- These vitamins are involved in a variety of enzymatic reactions and often act as co-enzymes.

- Deficiencies of the various vitamin B constituents can affect the mouth and cause glossitis, angular cheilitis, and cheilosis.

Vitamin B$_{12}$ and folic acid

These two dietary components are essential for the synthesis of DNA and hence for chromosomal replication and cell division. Tissues with a high cellular turnover, such as haemopoietic tissue, are very sensitive to a deficiency of these two vitamins.

Vitamin B$_{12}$ represents a group of compounds known as the cobalamins. in which the cobalt ion is linked to cyanide (cyanocobalamin), or a hydroxyl group (hydroxycobalamin), or a methyl group (methylcobalamin). Cobalamins are synthesized by micro-organisms in the intestines, but in humans they are not absorbed. Hence humans depend upon a dietary source to meet their requirements. Foods rich in vitamin B$_{12}$ include liver, kidneys, and shellfish.

Properties and functions of vitamin B$_{12}$

Vitamin B$_{12}$ is essential for cell growth and division, and for the normal myelination of nerve fibres. It is necessary for folic acid metabolism, and is also involved in the metabolism of lipids and carbohydrates. Deficiency of vitamin B$_{12}$ causes pernicious anaemia.

Absorption of vitamin B$_{12}$ from dietary sources is dependent upon an intrinsic factor (a glycoprotein) produced by the parietal cells of the stomach. Gastric acid causes the release of dietary B$_{12}$ from proteins. The released vitamin is immediately bound to the intrinsic factor, and the combination reaches the ileum, where it combines with specific receptors on the ileal mucosal cell. The vitamin B$_{12}$ and intrinsic factor are then transported into the circulation. Total body stores of vitamin B$_{12}$ are approximately 3 mg.

Deficiency

This affects both the haemopoietic system and the nervous system. Vitamin B$_{12}$ is essential for cell growth and replication, so the high rate of cell turnover in the bone marrow makes it very susceptible to vitamin B$_{12}$ deficiency states. The result is pernicious anaemia, which is characterized by a hypochromic, macrocytic anaemia. Clinical signs of pernicious anaemia include a sore red tongue, angular cheilitis, and premature greying of the hair. Severe vitamin B$_{12}$ deficiency can result in irreversible damage to the nervous system due to demyelination of neurones. Early signs of such changes are paraesthesia of the extremities and decreased tendon reflexes. Those affected can become confused, disorientated, and suffer visual disturbances.

Vitamin B$_{12}$ deficiency can result from a poor intake, as could occur in strict vegetarians. More commonly, the deficiency arises in those who lack intrinsic factor, including patients with gastritis or who have undergone gastric surgery. Various types of ileal disease (i.e. Crohn's disease and coeliac disease) can affect the absorption of the vitamin B$_{12}$–intrinsic factor complex, and result in signs and symptoms of deficiency. Certain drugs, for example para-aminosalicylic acid and neomycin, affect the absorption of vitamin B$_{12}$. If these drugs are used for prolonged periods, a deficiency state can arise.

Uses

Vitamin B$_{12}$ (cyanocobalamin) is used to treat pernicious anaemia and other signs of deficiency. It is usually given by intramuscular injection, and mild forms of pernicious anaemia usually respond to 500 μg every 2 months.

Folic acid

This is a weak organic acid (pteroylglutamic acid) present in yeast, liver, and green vegetables. Folic acid is essential for the normal production of red blood cells, and a deficiency results in a megaloblastic anaemia. In the body, folic acid is reduced to tetrahydrofolate by the enzyme dihydrofolate reductase. This enzyme is inhibited by various chemotherapeutic agents (see

Chapter 19). Dietary folic acid is absorbed in the small intestines and mainly stored in the liver. These stores will last for about 4 months.

Deficiency

Folic acid deficiency is a common occurrence in patients with disease of the gastrointestinal tract, where there is impaired absorption. Deficiency is also found in alcoholics, in pregnancy, and in patients taking phenytoin and phenobarbital (phenobarbitone)—drugs that affect the absorption of folic acid. Folic acid deficiency causes a megaloblastic anaemia identical to that produced by vitamin B_{12}. However, unlike vitamin B_{12} deficiency, there are no neurological symptoms with folic acid deficiency.

A deficiency of folic acid is thought to be linked with spina bifida. Thus women are advised to take folic acid supplements before conception and throughout pregnancy.

Key facts
Vitamin B_{12} and folic acid

- Vitamin B_{12} (cobalamins) is essential for cell growth and division and for the myelination of nerve fibres.

- Absorption of B_{12} is dependent upon binding with an intrinsic factor (a glycoprotein) produced in the stomach.

- A deficiency of B_{12} causes pernicious anaemia.

- Folic acid is essential for the production of red blood cells, and a deficiency causes megaloblastic anaemia.

- Deficiency is found in alcoholics, in pregnancy, and in patients taking the phenytoin and phenobarbital (phenobarbitone)-drugs that affect the absorption of folic acid.

- Lack of folic acid is also linked with spina bifida and hence is taken during pregnancy.

Vitamin C (ascorbic acid)

The dietary value of fresh lemons in the prevention of scurvy was first established by Lind in 1747. However, the identification of vitamin C and its link with scurvy did not occur until 1907.

Ascorbic acid is structurally related to glucose, and some species can synthesize their own vitamin C from this carbohydrate. Vitamin C is involved in a number of body functions, including the synthesis of collagen, corticosteroids, and lysine chains in certain proteins. The major function of vitamin C is in the synthesis of intercellular substances, including collagen, the matrices of teeth and bone, and the intercellular cement of the capillary endothelium. Vitamin C is well absorbed when taken orally, and widely distributed throughout all tissues in the body.

Deficiency

This causes scurvy, which is associated with a defect in collagen synthesis. Clinical features include poor healing of wounds, rup-

ture of capillaries leading to petechiae and ecchymoses, loosening of the teeth, and bleeding from the gingival tissues. Scurvy is sometimes seen in alcoholics, drug addicts, children, and the elderly.

Uses

Vitamin C is used in the treatment of scurvy. It is also widely used as a prophylaxis against the common cold. There is no firm evidence to suggest that vitamin C reduces either the chances of catching a cold or shortens its course. Indeed, excessive use of vitamin C can predispose the individual to oxalate renal calculi.

Key facts
Vitamin C

- Vitamin C is found in citrus fruits and is essential for collagen synthesis.

- A deficiency of vitamin C leads to scurvy, which is characterized by poor wound healing, bleeding gums, and loosening of the teeth.

- In addition to treating deficiency states, vitamin C is also used to prevent the common cold; the latter is of questionable efficacy.

Vitamin E

This vitamin, which occurs in wheatgerm oil, was first isolated in 1936. Its pharmacological and physiological functions in humans are not established. Animal experiments have shown that deficiency of vitamin E causes spontaneous abortion and impaired spermatogenesis. The role of vitamin E in the human reproductive system is uncertain. Evidence suggests that it may protect the red blood cell against haemolysis. The vitamin is widely consumed as part of multiple vitamin therapy; fortunately, large doses of vitamin E have no serious unwanted effects.

Vitamin K

This is essential for the synthesis of several factors required for blood clotting (II, VII, IX, and X). The vitamin (K_1) is concentrated in chloroplasts and in vegetable oils. Vitamin K_2 is synthesized by gut bacteria.

Deficiency of vitamin K causes hypoprothrombinaemia and hence an increased tendency to bleed. Patients will suffer from ecchymoses, epistaxis, haematuria, and gastrointestinal bleeding. Vitamin K is used to treat symptoms of deficiency, drug-induced hypoprothrombinaemia, and the hypoprothrombinaemia of the newborn (see Chapter 13).

Iron

This is the fourth most abundant element in the earth's crust and is essential for the normal function of many living species. In humans, iron is used for the synthesis of haemoglobin, myoglobin, and certain enzymes. Iron not used for these purposes is stored as ferritin or haemosiderin (aggregation of ferritin) mainly in the liver, spleen, and bone marrow. A shortage of iron results in iron-deficiency anaemia. There is also evidence that iron deficiency can lead to behavioural and learning difficulties in children.

Pharmacokinetics

Although iron is absorbed throughout the small intestine, the main site of absorption is the duodenum. Absorption of iron, either from the diet or from a variety of iron preparations, can be affected by many factors. Certain foods, particularly cereals, reduce iron absorption. Certain drugs, such as tetracyclines, chelate iron and there is impaired absorption of the chelate. Thus, patients on iron therapy should not be prescribed tetracyclines. Similarly, antacids reduce iron absorption. Iron in the ferrous form is more readily absorbed than ferric iron. In addition, vitamin C and intrinsic factor facilitate iron absorption. Control of absorption appears to be related to the capacity of the intestinal mucosa to transport iron into the bloodstream.

On absorption into the mucosal cell, iron combines with the protein apoferritin to form ferritin. However, in patients with iron deficiency, the formation of ferritin does not occur and the iron passes straight into the plasma. Free iron in the plasma, or iron released from ferritin, is transported in the bloodstream attached to the glycoprotein transferrin, from where it is delivered and stored in the bone marrow. Total body stores of iron are 3–4 g.

Small quantities of iron are lost via shedding of the mucosal cell in the small intestine, from the bile, and via the kidneys. Iron requirements increase during pregnancy and lactation.

Uses

Iron is given to correct or prevent iron-deficiency anaemia (see below). Usually it is given orally in the form of either ferrous sulfate, gluconate, or fumarate. The response to iron replacement therapy usually occurs 5–10 days after commencement of dosage, and treatment should continue for 6 months after haemoglobin levels have reached the normal range.

Iron can also be given via the parenteral route (in the form of iron dextran), if stores are to be rapidly and completely replenished.

Unwanted effects of iron replacement therapy

When given orally, ferrous salts can produce nausea, epigastric pain, constipation, and diarrhoea. Iron dextran can produce staining of the skin.

Iron-deficiency anaemia

This is a common disease, and is especially prevalent in the Third World. The incidence is higher in menstruating and pregnant women. The anaemia is either due to an inadequate diet, impaired iron absorption, or chronic blood loss. Thorough investigation of those with iron deficiency is essential to elucidate the underlying cause. Early signs of deficiency often occur in the mouth; these include ulceration, angular cheilitis, candidiasis, and glossitis. The patients may have cardiovascular problems, such as dyspnoea and angina, and they will appear pale. Their nails may be brittle and spoon-shaped (koilonychia).

Examination of the blood film is a useful diagnostic procedure for confirming iron-deficiency anaemia; the red blood cells are microcytic and hypochromic. The mean corpuscular volume (MCV), mean corpuscular haemoglobin concentration (MCHC), and serum ferritin levels are also significantly reduced.

Key facts
Iron

- Iron is essential for the synthesis of haemoglobin, myoglobin, and certain enzymes.

- On absorption from the duodenum, iron combines with apoferritin to form ferritin; iron released from ferritin is transported attached to the glycoprotein transferrin.

- A deficiency of iron causes iron-deficiency anaemia.

- Ferrous salts (sulfate and gluconate) are used as iron replacement therapy; in severe iron deficiency, intravenous iron dextran is used.

Further reading

Beck, W. S. (1988). Cobalamin and the nervous system. *New England Journal of Medicine*, **318**, 1752–4.

Finch, C. A. and Hueber, S. H. (1982). Perspective in iron metabolism. *New England Journal of Medicine*, **306**, 1520–8.

Levine, M. (1986). New concepts in the biology and biochemistry of ascorbic acid. *New England Journal of Medicine*, **314**, 892–902.

Wald, N. J. and Bower, C. (1994). Folic acid, pernicious anaemia, and neural tube defects. *Lancet*, **343**, 307.

Calcification

Calcification

Salts of calcium and phosphate comprise the major inorganic portion of bone. Both compounds have several important physiological roles to play in normal body function. This chapter deals with the pharmacological and physiological properties of calcium and phosphate, together with the endocrine factors (parathyroid hormone, calcitonin, and vitamin D) that control their metabolism.

Calcium

Nearly all the body's calcium is found in the skeletal tissues; although small quantities occur in cell cytoplasm and in the extracellular fluid. Ionized calcium is involved in nerve conduction, muscle contraction, cardiac function, and blood clotting. The body's calcium requirements vary with the demands of age, growth spurts, pregnancy, and lactation (dietary requirements are in the range 360–1200 mg day^{-1}). The concentration of calcium in plasma is 2.5 mM, and the calcium is present in three fractions:

1. 40% of Ca^{2+} ions are bound to plasma proteins.

2. 10% are diffusable, but complexed with citrate and phosphate ions.

3. 50% are diffusable as ionic calcium. It is this fraction that exerts the physiological effects.

Pharmacokinetics

Soluble, ionized calcium is mainly absorbed in the proximal segment of the small intestine; absorption is augmented by vitamin D and parathyroid hormone. Transport of calcium across the gut mucosal cells is probably by means of a calcium-binding protein (calcitriol). Glucocorticoids will depress this transport system. Absorption of calcium is also affected by phytate, oxalate, and phosphate ions in the bowel, which form insoluble salts with calcium. Patients with chronic diarrhoea and steatorrhoea suffer from decreased calcium absorption. Calcium ions are excreted into the gastrointestinal tract, bile, saliva, and pancreatic juices; calcium is also lost in sweat, and in significant amounts during lactation. Calcium is excreted via the kidney under the control of parathyroid hormone and vitamin D. Parathyroid hormone stimulates calcium reabsorption by an action on the distal tubule, whereas vitamin D stimulates reabsorption from the proximal tubule. Calcitonin inhibits the proximal tubular reabsorption of calcium and thus facilitates excretion.

Pharmacological and physiological properties

Calcium is essential for the normal functioning of the neuromuscular system. A rise in extracellular calcium concentration will cause a rise in the threshold for excitation of nerve fibres and muscle. This will result in muscle weakness, lethargy, and eventually coma. Calcium is involved in the activation of muscle contraction, in both skeletal and cardiac muscle. It is also involved in the release of catecholamines from the adrenal medulla. In addition, calcium ions are essential for the release both of neurotransmitters from synapses and of autocoids from various sites and tissues in the body. The integrity of mucosal membranes, cell-adhesion processes, and the functions of individual cell membranes are all calcium-dependent.

In blood coagulation, Ca^{2+} (factor V) is essential for the action of thromboplastin on prothrombin to form thrombin (see Chapter 13). Calcium salts, especially calcium chloride, cause irritation and sloughing of tissues if given subcutaneously. Hence this drug should only be given intravenously.

Abnormalities of calcium metabolism

Blood calcium levels can be affected by a variety of factors: these can give rise to either a hypocalcaemic or hypercalcaemic state.

Hypocalcaemia

The signs and symptoms of hypocalcaemia include tetany, paraesthesia, laryngospasm, muscle cramps, and convulsions. Hypocalcaemia is associated with the following:

- Poor intake of calcium and vitamin D: the resultant hypocalcaemia gives rise to an increased production of parathyroid hormone, which mobilizes Ca^{2+} from bone; in adults, this leads to osteomalacia, whereas in infants it causes rickets.

- Hypoparathyroidism.
- Renal insufficiency accompanied by hyperphosphatasia: the high plasma concentrations of phosphate inhibit the conversion, in the kidney, of 25-hydroxycholecalciferol to 1,25-dihydroxycholecalciferol.
- Overdose of sodium fluoride: the fluoride forms a complex with calcium ions leading to reduced calcium absorption.
- Massive transfusions with citrated blood: the citrate ions will chelate calcium to form an insoluble complex, thus reducing plasma concentrations of calcium ions.

Hypocalcaemic states are corrected by a dietary increase in calcium. In severe cases of tetany associated with hypocalcaemia, treatment is with intravenous calcium chloride.

Hypercalcaemia

High plasma concentrations of calcium principally affect the kidney, causing pathological changes in the collecting ducts and distal tubules. The net result is a reduction in renal function if left untreated, and hypercalcaemia will cause renal failure. Hypercalcaemia is associated with the following conditions:

- Diet: especially the milk–alkali syndrome caused by the excessive consumption of milk and antacids, which contain soluble calcium salts—massive amounts of antacids need to be regularly consumed to produce this syndrome.
- Excessive intake of vitamin D.
- Hyperparathyroidism.
- Sarcoidosis: patients with this granulomatous disorder may have a hypersensitivity to vitamin D.
- Neoplasms: metastatic deposits in bone can activate osteoclasts and cause bone resorption. In addition, the deposits can cause the release of prostaglandins, which also stimulate bone resorption.
- Disuse atrophy: as occurs when a limb has been immobilized for a long time.
- Following renal transplantation: owing to secondary hyperparathyroidism, which is a consequence of previous chronic renal failure.

TREATMENT OF HYPERCALCAEMIA

Hypercalcaemia can usually be corrected by the body's homeostatic mechanisms. These mechanisms can be facilitated by an infusion of saline with a diuretic such as furosemide (frusemide) which increases the secretion of Ca^{2+}. Corticosteroids also reduce hypercalcaemia but large doses are required (30–50 mg of prednisone a day). Furthermore, the response to therapy is slow. Other agents used to treat hypercalcaemia include calcitonin (see later), the chelation agent edetate disodium, and the chemotherapeutic agent mithramycin. However, these drugs are not without unwanted effects and should be considered the last line of treatment.

Key facts
Calcium

- Calcium is a key element in the skeleton and is essential for a diverse range of cellular functions.
- Serum calcium concentrations (2.5 mM) are controlled by the actions of vitamin D, parathyroid hormone, and calcitonin.
- Disorders of calcium homeostasis are referred to as hypercalcaemia or hypocalcaemia; the latter is characterized by tetany, muscle cramps, paraesthesia, and convulsions.
- Causes of hypocalcaemia include a poor intake of vitamin D and calcium, hypoparathyroidism, renal insufficiency, an overdose of sodium fluoride, and a massive infusion of citrated blood.
- Hypercalcaemia can cause renal failure; causes include diet, excessive intake of vitamin D, hyperparathyroidism, sarcoidosis, bone neoplasms, disuse atrophy, and following renal transplantation due to secondary hyperparathyroidism.
- The treatment of hypercalcaemia is dependent upon the cause; drugs used to lower serum calcium include furosemide (frusemide), corticosteroids, calcitonin, and edetate disodium.

Phosphate

Phosphate is present in extracellular fluids, collagen, and bone. A balance exists between plasma concentrations of calcium and phosphate. There is also an inverse relationship between plasma phosphate concentration and the rate of renal hydroxylation of 25-hydroxy-vitamin D_3. A reduction in plasma phosphate leads to an increase of calcium in the blood, which in turn inhibits the deposition of new bone salts. An increase in plasma phosphate facilitates the effect of calcitonin on the deposition of calcium in bone.

Phosphate ions are absorbed from the bowel, and absorption is enhanced by vitamin D and regulated by calcitriol. Large quantities of calcium and aluminium in the bowel will reduce the absorption of phosphate. Like calcium, phosphate requirements vary with age, growth, pregnancy, and lactation.

Vitamin D (calciferol)

Although referred to as a vitamin, calciferol (or more precisely the metabolite 1,25-dihydroxy-vitamin D_3 or calcifediol) is now considered to be a hormone secreted by the kidney. The metabolism of vitamin D is shown in Fig. 21.1. The precursor of vitamin D is

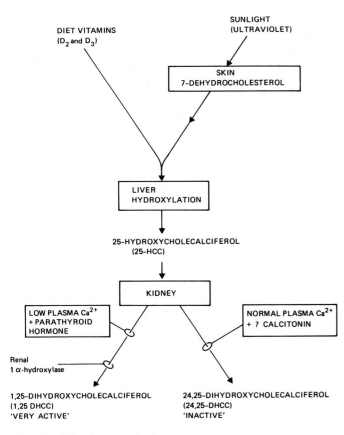

Fig. 22.1 Vitamin D synthesis.

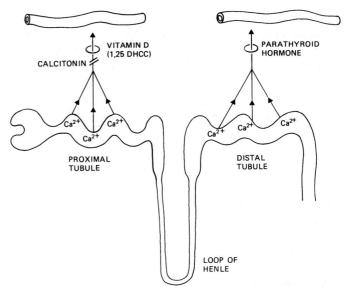

Fig. 22.2 Calcium homeostasis and the renal tubule.

from the proximal tubule (Fig. 22.2). Both 1,25-DHCC and parathyroid hormone mobilize calcium from bone.

Uses

Vitamin D is used to correct deficiency states (see below), and is available in three forms: ergocalciferol (vitamin D₂), alfacalcidol, and calcitriol. Ergocalciferol is the most widely used vitamin D preparation.

Unwanted effects

The main adverse effect associated with vitamin D preparations is hypervitaminosis D, characterized by hypercalcaemia, osteoporosis, soft-tissue calcification, and renal calculi.

Deficiency

A deficiency of vitamin D, either from dietary sources or a lack of sunlight, results in rickets or osteomalacia. Both conditions are characterized by a pathological defect in the mineralization of new bone. Rickets presents clinically during growth, whereas osteomalacia is the adult form of the disease. Oral manifestations of vitamin D deficiency depend upon the severity and age of onset. During growth, vitamin D deficiency will affect the mandibular condylar cartilage, causing retarded development of the mandibular ramus. There is often delayed eruption of the teeth and hypoplasia of tooth enamel. In both rickets and osteomalacia, the jaw bones are weak and prone to fracture.

Patients with chronic renal failure may suffer from renal rickets due to impaired synthesis of 1,25-DHCC. This will result in calcium malabsorption, hypocalcaemia, and a secondary rise in parathyroid hormone production. Hence such patients will have the signs and symptoms of osteomalacia and (secondary) hyperparathyroidism.

7-dehydrocholesterol, which is synthesized in the skin. The action of ultraviolet light converts this precursor to cholecalciferol. Further hydroxylation of cholecalciferol occurs in the liver to form 25-hydroxy-vitamin D₃ (25(OH)D₃). This hydroxylation process is controlled by circulating levels of cholecalciferol, with high levels inhibiting the hydroxylation. The 25(OH)D₃ is finally activated in the kidneys by the enzyme, renal 1α-hydroxylase, and the product depends upon the calcium needs.

In the presence of low calcium concentrations, 25(OH)D₃ is hydroxylated to 1,25-dihydroxy-vitamin D₃ (calcitriol), and the hydroxylation is facilitated by parathyroid hormone.

The actions of vitamin D (1,25-dihydroxycholecalciferol; 1,25-DHCC) are mediated via specific cytosolic receptors in target tissues. The receptor–hormone complex interacts with certain genes, and either enhances or inhibits their transcription. The net result of receptor activation is an increase in plasma Ca²⁺.

With normal or high calcium concentrations, 25(OH)D₃ is hydroxylated to the relatively inactive 24,25-dihydroxycholecalciferol. This hydroxylation may be facilitated by calcitonin.

Thus 1,25-DHCC enhances the absorption of calcium from the small intestine, and it also facilitates reabsorption of calcium ions

Vitamin D-resistant rickets

This is a rare, sex-linked familial disease characterized by a hypophosphataemia associated with a decreased renal tubular reabsorption of PO_4^{3-}. Patients will present with the signs and symptoms of rickets or osteomalacia depending upon their age. This form of rickets appears to respond to a metabolite of vitamin D—1α-hydroxycholecalciferol. This is an example of a disease due to a receptor abnormality.

Key facts
Vitamin D

- Vitamin D (calciferol) is now considered to be a hormone, and is synthesized from the precursor 7-dehydrocholesterol.

- The active metabolite of vitamin D (calcitriol) enhances the absorption of calcium from the small intestines and decreases its secretion by the kidney; the production of this metabolite is determined by serum calcium concentrations.

- A deficiency of vitamin D causes rickets in children and osteomalacia in adults.

- Ergocalciferol is the most widely used vitamin D preparation and is used to correct deficiency states.

Parathyroid hormone (PTH)

The parathyroids are small, yellow glandular bodies, usually attached to the undersurface of the thyroid gland. They were first discovered in 1880, but their physiological function was not determined until the 1920s. The glands synthesize and secrete PTH.

Physiological functions

PTH controls calcium metabolism and ensures that the extracellular fluid concentration of Ca^{2+} is kept constant. It regulates the absorption of Ca^{2+} from the gastrointestinal tract, the deposition and mobilization of Ca^{2+} in bone, and the excretion of Ca^{2+} via the kidney.

The secretion of PTH is inversely related to the plasma concentration of calcium. When the concentration of Ca^{2+} is low there is an increased secretion of PTH; with normal or high concentrations of Ca^{2+}, secretion is reduced.

Parathyroid hormone increases bone resorption, especially from the older portion of mineralized bone, leading to an increase in the plasma concentration of Ca^{2+}. It acts directly on the osteolytic cells (osteoclasts and osteocytes), and increases the rate of mesenchymal cell differentiation to osteoblasts. Osteoclastic activity is evident some 20 minutes after an infusion of PTH.

The hormone has a dual action in the kidney: it increases tubular reabsorption of Ca^{2+}; and it inhibits tubular reabsorption of PO_4^{3-} (Fig. 22.2), which results in increased renal excretion of inorganic phosphate. The overall effect of PTH on the kidney is to retain Ca^{2+} and maintain the plasma concentration.

Calcium and phosphate ions, as described earlier, are absorbed in the gastrointestinal tract, and parathyroid hormone has an indirect effect on their absorption. The absorption of Ca^{2+} is dependent upon the active metabolite of vitamin D (1,25-DHCC); PTH enhances the renal hydroxylation of 25(OH)D$_3$ to 1,25-DHCC (Fig 22.1). The increase in the production of 1,25-DHCC increases Ca^{2+} absorption.

Disorders of parathyroid function

There are two such disorders: hypo- and hyperparathyroidism.

Hypoparathyroidism

This can result from either hypofunction of the parathyroid glands, surgical removal of the glands following thyroidectomy, or the rare genetic disorder of pseudohypoparathyroidism, in which target organs do not respond to PTH. This genetic disorder is another example of a disease due to a receptor abnormality. In all varieties of hypoparathyroidism, the clinical symptoms are those of hypocalcaemia, and include paraesthesia of the extremities, muscle twitching and, if severe, tetany. In chronic cases of hypoparathyroidism, there are various ectodermal changes including loss of hair, grooved and brittle fingernails, and enamel hypoplasia. Hypoparathyroidism is treated with vitamin D and, where necessary, calcium supplements.

Hyperparathyroidism

This is characterized by excessive production of parathyroid hormone. Three forms of the disease are recognized: primary, secondary, and tertiary. Primary hyperparathyroidism is associated with hyperplasia or neoplasia of the parathyroid glands. In secondary hyperparathyroidism, the underlying cause is a hypocalcaemia associated with chronic renal failure, which stimulates excessive production of PTH. Patients with long-standing renal disease and secondary hyperparathyroidism may develop an apparent autonomous hypersecretion of PTH, and this is known as tertiary hyperparathyroidism.

CLINICAL FEATURES

Primary hyperparathyroidism has an incidence of 1:1000 of the population, with females being more affected than males. Excessive PTH activity will cause hypercalcaemia and hypophosphataemia. The presenting symptoms are those of hypercalcaemia, and include anorexia, thirst, polyuria, renal colic, and renal stones. Approximately one-third of patients show evidence of bone disease, including the bone disorder known as osteitis fibrosa cystica. This condition is characterized by foci of bone destruction leaving spaces filled with vascular and cellular connective tissue and containing large numbers of osteoclastic giant cells. Such lesions often occur in the jaws, especially the mandible. Primary hyperparathyroidism is treated by surgical excision of the parathyroid glands. In secondary or tertiary hyperparathyroidism, the underlying renal disease must be corrected.

Key facts
Parathyroid hormone (PTH)

- The secretion of PTH from the parathyroid glands in the neck is controlled by plasma calcium levels, with low concentrations stimulating secretion.
- PTH regulates the absorption of Ca^{2+} from the gut, the deposition and mobilization of Ca^{2+} from bone, and the excretion of Ca^{2+} from the kidney.
- Hypoparathyroidism causes hypocalcaemia and is treated with vitamin D and calcium supplements.
- Hyperparathyroidism causes hypercalcaemia and hypophosphataemia, both of which can predispose to the formation of renal calculi.
- The presence of localized areas of bone destruction is also a feature of hyperparathyroidism (osteitis fibrosa cystica), and such lesions often affect the mandible.

Calcitonin

This was first described in 1964, and is a hormone secreted by the parafollicular ('C') cells of the thyroid gland. Like PTH, calcitonin secretion is controlled by plasma levels of calcium: it lowers plasma calcium and phosphate levels by an alteration in intracellular cyclic AMP. Calcitonin has two effects on calcium homeostasis. First, it inhibits osteoclastic resorption, thus reducing the release of Ca^{2+} and PO_4^{3-} from the skeletal tissues. This inhibition is more pronounced when there is a high turnover of bone, as occurs in Paget's disease and thyrotoxicosis. Second, it has a minor effect on the kidneys, enhancing the excretion of phosphate, calcium, and sodium (Fig. 22.2).

Calcitonin (porcine or salmon varieties) is used to treat Paget's disease, and the hypercalcaemia secondary to malignancy or vitamin D excess. The hormone can only be given parenterally because it is destroyed by gastric secretions. Patients with Paget's disease usually show a response to calcitonin therapy within 2 months. Unwanted effects are pain at the site of injection, nausea, and flushing of the face.

Key facts
Calcitonin

- Calcitonin is secreted by the parafollicular cells of the thyroid gland, and secretion is controlled by plasma calcium levels.
- Calcitonin lowers plasma calcium and phosphate levels.
- Calcitonin effects calcium homeostasis by inhibiting osteoclastic bone resorption and enhancing the renal excretion of calcium, phosphate, and sodium.
- Porcine and salmon derivatives of calcitonin are used in the management of Paget's disease and hypercalcaemia.

Bisphosphonates

Bisphosphonates reduce bone turnover by inhibiting osteoclast activity. The main bisphophonate in clinical use is disodium etidronate, which is used in the management of Paget's disease, hypercalcaemia, and osteoporosis.

Further reading

Chestnut, C. H. (1992). Osteoporosis and its treatment. *New England Journal of Medicine*, 326, 406–8.

Reichel, H., Koeftler, H. P., and Norman, A. W. (1989). The role of the vitamin D endocrine system in health and disease. *New England Journal of Medicine*, 320, 980–91.

23

Adverse effects of drugs

- Classification
- Prevention of the unwanted effects of drugs
- Oral reactions to drugs
- References
- Further reading

Adverse effects of drugs

Unwanted effects due to drugs are fairly common in medical practice and information about their prevalence is increasing. However, the overall picture is still not clear. This is partly because unwanted effects may not be recognized as such either by the patient, the doctor, or the dentist. Moreover, it will only be possible to calculate the incidence of such effects for a particular drug when accurate information about the numbers of patients exhibiting adverse effects is available, together with accurate returns that indicate the total number of patients receiving the drug.

In dental practice, unwanted effects due to drugs appear to be less common than in medical practice, but they can still represent a significant problem in both diagnosis and management. They are likely to arise in two different ways. The dentist may be the first to observe an unwanted effect produced by a drug prescribed by the patient's medical practitioner; for example, ulceration in the mouth that accompanies agranulocytosis. On the other hand, as part of dental treatment, the dentist may prescribe a drug to which the patient reacts adversely. To obtain accurate information about the incidence of unwanted drug effects in dental practice, it is most important for all practitioners in the UK to report any suspected unwanted drug effect to the Medical Assessor (Adverse Reactions), Committee on Safety of Medicines, Freepost, London SW8 5BR. (Special yellow-coloured report cards with prepaid postage are available for this purpose from the Committee on Safety of Medicines).

Classification

It is difficult to classify unwanted effects satisfactorily because very often the mechanism is not clear. However, it is useful to have some form of classification for reference. One broad classification has divided unwanted effects into two classes: type A reactions and type B reactions (see Rawlins and Thompson 1991).

Type A reactions are reactions that would be expected, or could be expected, from the known pharmacology of the drug or mixtures of drugs. Such reactions are relatively common and usually not serious, although they may be unpleasant. An example of this sort of reaction arises from the use of antihistamines (H_1 blockers) to prevent histamine access to receptors involved in allergic responses. In addition to this blocking property, the antihistamines have, in general, an intrinsic sedative effect, and this may be unwanted.

Type B reactions cannot be predicted or explained by the known pharmacology of the drug. They are relatively uncommon and are often much more serious than the type A reaction. Allergic reactions to drugs generally come under this heading.

Another useful classification, a modified version of that proposed by Rosenheim and Moulton is given below. Both classifications fit well into each other.

(1) overdosage;

(2) intolerance;

(3) side-effects;

(4) secondary effects;

(5) idiosyncrasy;

(6) teratogenic effects;

(7) hypersensitivity;

(8) drug interactions.

These effects will now be considered in detail, except for drug interactions. These have been mentioned under individual drugs and will also be discussed in Chapter 24.

Overdosage

Unwanted effects due to an excess of drug will be related to the amount of drug in the body. It is important to realize that all drugs are potentially poisonous, although some are more poisonous than others. The safety of a drug depends upon the size of the margin between the effective dose (ED) and the lethal dose (LD), as discussed in Chapter 1. This cannot be measured in humans but can be determined in animals where, in order to allow for biological variation, a series of different doses are given to two groups of animals. The results are then drawn on two graphs: one for effectiveness and one for lethality. From these graphs the amount of drug required to produce the desired effect in 50% of animals (ED_{50}) can be read, and also the amount required to kill 50% of them (LD_{50}). The safety, or therapeutic index, can be obtained by determining the ratio LD_{50}/ED_{50} (see Chapter 1). The larger the value of this ratio, the safer is the drug, although it is important to relate the route of administration used in these determinations to that which may be used in humans, and to make allowance for species differences.

Absolute overdosage

This may be immediate, due to too much drug being taken in error or deliberately with suicidal intent. Alternatively, it may be a cumulative effect brought about by slow excretion of the drug, with the result that there is a steady increase in the amount of drug in the body. For example, digoxin and levothyroxine (thyroxine) take more than a week to be half-excreted; they therefore accumulate in the body unless steps are taken to reduce the initial dosage when an adequate therapeutic effect has been achieved. By contrast, penicillin is half excreted in less than an hour and is therefore not liable to accumulate.

Relative overdosage

This occurs when the mechanisms for metabolism and/or excretion of a drug are impaired. Under these circumstances, normal or even subnormal doses of the drug may causes signs of overdosage. In hepatic failure, drugs may be metabolized more slowly than normal, with the result that the amount of active drug in the body declines more slowly than usual, leading to an increased and prolonged effect. For example, the duration of apnoea after a normal dose of the short-acting muscle relaxant suxamethonium may be greatly prolonged in patients with low plasma cholinesterase levels due to liver disease (Fig. 23.1). Similarly, renal failure will result in a diminished rate of excretion of a drug such as digoxin where this is the main route of excretion from the body.

Intolerance

This is said to occur when there is a lowered threshold to the normal pharmacological action of the drug. It is a phenomenon attributable to biological variation. Thus, whereas the normal therapeutic dose produces the desired effect in the majority of individuals, in a minority it may produce too large or too small an effect. The former is due to intolerance, the latter to tolerance. Put the other way round, the dose required to produce the desired effect in an intolerance patient is less than the normal dose, whilst the requisite dose for a tolerance patient is greater than the normal, as illustrated in Fig. 23.2. It follows that it is the intolerance patient who is liable to exhibit unwanted effects when the normal dose is used; the tolerant patient shows little or no effect.

Side-effects

These effects are therapeutically undesirable but pharmacologically unavoidable actions due to a drug. Side-effects can be subdivided into two main groups:

Extension of main action

Some side-effects are due to an extension of the main action of the drug at sites additional to those required for therapeutic purposes. For example, atropine given in order to produce a dry mouth may also interfere with the accommodation of the eye, and the normal functioning of the bladder and bowels. On the other hand, a patient given atropine to relieve the spasms associated with irri-

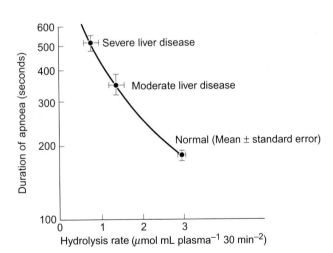

Fig. 23.1 The effect of liver disease on the rate of destruction (by hydrolysis) of the short-acting neuromuscular blocking drug suxamethonium. Plasma cholinesterase, which is manufactured by the liver, is responsible for the hydrolysis of suxamethonium. Since the presence of liver disease reduces the production of cholinesterase, it also affects the rate of breakdown of suxamethonium and hence the duration of neuromuscular block including apnoea after a dose of this drug. (Drawn from data of Foldes *et al.* 1956.)

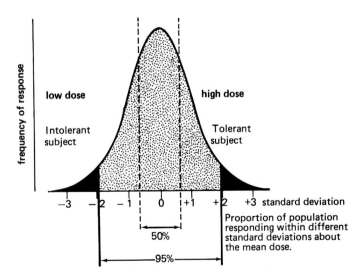

Fig. 23.2 Idealized frequency distribution curve for the responses of a population to a drug. The areas under the curve that represent 50% and 95% of the population are shown, and subjects who are considered to be intolerant or tolerant have been arbitrarily shown as belonging to the remaining 5% of the population (black areas). (Standard deviation is a measure of scatter; numerically the value will vary from drug to drug. Where the value is small, the range of doses required about the mean dose will be small, and vice versa.)

table bowel syndrome may complain of a dry mouth, which under these circumstances becomes the side-effect. Although this drug produces widespread effects they are all due to a common mechanism—atropine competes with acetylcholine released from the postganglionic parasympathetic nerve endings for muscarinic receptors situated on parasympathetic effector organs.

Additional actions

Other side-effects are due to one or more additional actions that are inherent in the particular drug. For example, some histamine H_1-receptor antagonists also possess hypnotic effects. In some circumstances, such as an itching urticarial rash that prevents sleep, these effects may be an added therapeutic benefit; in other situations, such as when used to treat hay fever in a bus driver, they may be highly undesirable. A further example is the neuroleptic drug chlorpromazine (see Chapter 15). Its beneficial effects in schizophrenia are attributed to a blockade of dopamine receptors. However, it also has affinity for muscarinic and α-adrenoceptors resulting in the adverse effects of a dry mouth and postural hypotension, respectively.

Secondary effects

These are not due to the direct pharmacological action of a drug but are the indirect consequences of it. For example, the prolonged use of broad-spectrum antibiotics may result in superinfection. Under these conditions, the normal bowel flora is altered by the antibiotic so that pathogenic organisms gain a hold and a new infection supervenes. A patient who was originally being treated for a simple infection may contract and possibly die from a very serious one, for example staphylococcal enteritis. Another example is the prolonged use of a tetracycline mouthwash, which leads to a candidal infection of the mouth.

A number of patients treated with the antibiotic clindamycin have developed a dangerous pseudomembranous colitis as a secondary effect arising from the use of this drug over several days (see Chapter 11). However, with the short-term recommended regimens for the use of clindamycin in the prophylaxis of endocarditis this is not a problem.

Idiosyncrasy

This is a qualitatively abnormal reaction to a drug, which is due to some abnormality of the individual showing the response. For example, the prolonged apnoea that may occur after the administration of the neuromuscular blocking drug suxamethonium can be due to the presence of an abnormal cholinesterase (Fig. 23.3). It has been estimated that about 1 in 2800 persons possess this atypical esterase, which hydrolyses suxamethonium much more slowly than normal cholinesterase with the result that the duration of neuromuscular block is greatly prolonged.

Another example is the precipitation of acute porphyria by the administration of barbiturates. This can only occur in patients who are qualitatively different in that they suffer from latent porphyria.

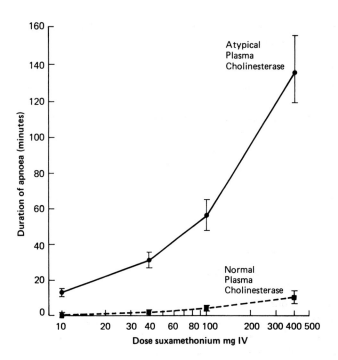

Fig. 23.3 The duration of apnoea after a single intravenous injection of different doses of suxamethonium in adult males with normal and atypical cholinesterase. The greatly reduced rate at which atypical cholinesterase hydrolyses suxamethonium is evident from the prolonged duration of apnoea (upper graph). (Drawn from data of Kalow and Gunn1957; reproduced by courtesy of Williams and Wilkins Co., Baltimore, MD.)

Teratogenic effects

Drugs that damage the embryo, but do not kill it, so abnormalities are observable postnatally, are called teratogens. There are some drugs that have been positively identified as being teratogenic, thalidomide being the obvious example. Others include androgens and tetracyclines (the latter produce discoloured teeth). Yet other drugs are suspected as being potentially teratogenic, whilst others are possibly teratogenic. For instance, the anticonvulsant phenytoin is suspected as a potential teratogen.

Key facts
Classification of unwanted effects

- Unwanted effects from drugs can be classified as either type A or type B.

- Type A reactions can be predicted from the known pharmacological properties of the drug, whereas the converse applies to type B reactions.

- Unwanted effects of drugs can also be classified according to the following criteria:
  - overdose
  - intolerance
  - side-effects
  - idiosyncrasy
  - teratogenic effects
  - hypersensitivity (see below)
  - drug interactions (see Chapter 24).

Hypersensitivity (allergy)

Allergy, a term derived from two Greek words (*allos*, other; *ergon*, work or energy), means 'altered reactivity'; it was first introduced by von Pirquet and describes an immunological phenomenon. It is well known that some unfortunate individuals are unable to eat certain foodstuffs, such as strawberries or lobster, because to do so makes them ill. Similarly, when the majority of people are enjoying summer weather, the pollen in the air causes others to suffer miserably from hay fever. These abnormal responses are examples of allergy and are attributable to an underlying antigen–antibody reaction of a particular type. Likewise, certain patients show abnormal responses to drugs, which are also due to an antigen–antibody reaction, and are examples of drug allergy.

Incidence of drug allergy

The overall incidence of drug allergy varies and appears to be range from 2 to 24%. Many of these reactions are harmless and include skin reactions and the like. The more serious, life-threatening reactions such as anaphylaxis, haemolysis, or bone-marrow depression are fortunately rare occurrences. Penicillin is the drug most frequently implicated in anaphylactic reactions. The incidence of death from this drug-induced reaction is 1:50 000 patients medicated with penicillin.

Drugs as antigens

An antigen is a substance that is able to evoke a specific immunological response, namely the production of antibodies. Antigens are substances of large molecular weight (MW), which are usually proteins but sometimes polysaccharides. Simple chemicals with MW of about 1000 or less cannot alone acts as antigens. In food allergy, the affected individual reacts immunologically to some macromolecular constituents of the offending food.

The majority of drugs consist of small molecules (MW less than 1000), which alone are unable to act as antigens. When an individual becomes hypersensitive to a drug, for example penicillin, it is believed that the antibiotic forms a covalent bond with a body protein. The penicillin–protein conjugate is antigenic; substances that combine in this way with proteins and thereby form antigens are known as haptens (or pro-antigens). The hapten, in this case penicillin, confers specificity on the antigen (that is to say the production of antibodies that will react only with penicillin or some closely related chemical compound, for example cephalosporins) whilst the protein confers antigenicity, as indicated below:

penicillin + protein → penicillin–protein conjugate.
(confers specificity)   (confers antigenicity)

It appears that readily reversible drug/protein binding, which commonly takes place between drugs and plasma proteins, is much less likely to lead to sensitization than is the irreversible conjugation that occurs when covalent bonds link a drug to a protein.

Classification of hypersensitivity reactions

There are various types of hypersensitivity reactions, and these have been classified as described below.

TYPE I—ANAPHYLACTIC TYPE REACTIONS

An initial contact with an antigen can cause activation of the various components of the immune system, and then secondary contact with the antigen leads to further boosting of the system (secondary response). However, in some individuals the secondary response may be excessive and lead to gross tissue damage. This excessive response (hypersensitivity) is exemplified by the type I reaction. In type I reactions, antigen combines with antibody (IgE) on the surface of mast cells, which degranulate bringing about the release of platelet-activation factor (PAF), serotonin, bradykinin, and eicosanoids as well as histamine. This type of reaction causes systemic anaphylaxis, allergic asthma, rhinitis, and some forms of urticaria, as well as angio-oedema. Chemical mediators of this reaction include:

1. *Histamine* (see Chapter 4), this amine, normally stored in an inactive form inside cells (in particular, mast cells), is one of the most important pharmacologically active substances released from immunologically damaged cells. It causes contraction of smooth muscle, dilatation and increased permeability of capillaries (resulting in a sudden fall of blood pressure), and weal formation.

2. *Platelet-activation factor* (see Chapter 4), this eicosanoid is generated and released from most inflammatory cells. It produces local vasodilation, increases vascular permeability and is a chemoattractant to PMNs and monocytes. PAF also causes spasm of bronchial smooth muscle and its role in asthma is discussed in Chapter 17.

3. *5-hydroxytryptamine* (5-HT, serotonin), is another amine distributed in brain, intestine, and platelets, and also stimulates a variety of smooth muscles and nerves.

4. *Bradykinin*, a nonapeptide, also causes a slow contraction of smooth muscle, vasodilatation with increased capillary permeability, and stimulates sensory nerve endings to produce pain.

5. *Eicosanoids*, these are derived by enzymatic action on phospholipids. They are important mediators of inflammation and their properties are discussed in Chapter 4.

The most dramatic and dangerous type I hypersensitivity reaction is the anaphylactic reaction following the administration of a protein or drug to which the subject has become sensitized. The clinical picture usually starts with flushing and itching of the skin, followed by severe difficulty in breathing due to laryngospasm and bronchospasm, and a severe fall in blood pressure. The pulse is rapid, weak, and may be almost imperceptible. The condition may be rapidly fatal unless immediate steps are taken to administer epinephrine (adrenaline). The earlier the onset of symptoms following administration of the drug allergen, the more severe and dangerous the reaction is likely to be; in fact, dangerous reactions are rare after the first 30 minutes. For this reason a counsel of perfection is to keep all patients who have received injections under observation for at least 30 minutes.

Penicillin is one of the drugs most likely to produce this dangerous reaction. Although anaphylactic reactions are usually associated with injection of a drug or of a foreign protein (skin test, wasp or bee stings), aspirin taken by mouth has produced this reaction in a highly susceptible subject.

Not all reactions are so dramatic; the sort of acute critical situation outlined above is unlikely to be encountered in ordinary clinical practice. Nevertheless, it must be anticipated and appropriate preparations made. What is most likely to occur is a less serious version, appearing less dramatically and not causing such concern. The management of the acute and less dramatic event is somewhat different, although the same range of drugs is used, and these should always be available.

TREATMENT OF ANAPHYLACTIC SHOCK Treatment of a severe, acute anaphylactic reaction must be immediate, and the necessary drugs should always be at hand, i.e. epinephrine (adrenaline), corticosteroid, and antihistamine (H_1 blocker) (see Fig. 23.4). The patient should be placed horizontally either by adjusting the dental chair or by placing him/her on the floor. If respiratory depression is present, oxygen should be administered or mouth-to-mouth respiration given (see Chapter 26).

Then 0.5 mL of 1:1000 (0.1 mg mL^{-1}) epinephrine (adrenaline) solution should be injected intramuscularly (NEVER INTRAVENOUSLY). This should be followed by hydrocortisone sodium succinate, 100 mg intravenously. Further doses of epinephrine (adrenaline) can be given as required at intervals of 5 minutes until the symptoms begin to subside. The maximum safe dose is about 1.5 mL over a period of 15 minutes—a substantial dose that is not without its own risks (see later). Great care must be taken to see that epinephrine (adrenaline) is not injected into a blood vessel because it may produce a fatal ventricular fibrillation if given intravenously.

The principal disturbances that occur in anaphylactic shock can be attributed to damage to the endothelial lining of blood vessels resulting in increased permeability and dilatation; and spasm of smooth muscle in the bronchial tree. Epinephrine (adrenaline) acts as a physiological antagonist to these effects by

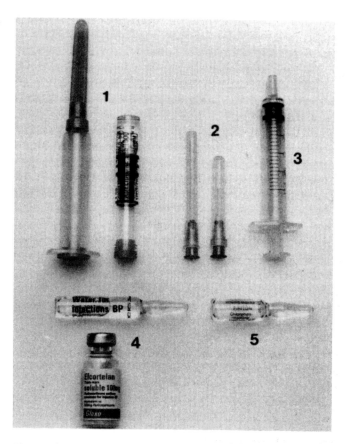

Fig. 23.4 Drugs, needles, and syringes which should always be immediately available for the treatment of drug hypersensitivity reactions.
1. Syringe and cartridge—1 ml, single dose of epinephrine (adrenaline) hydrochloride 1:1000 (1 mg mL^{-1}).
2. Needles for intravenous, intramuscular, and subcutaneous use.
3. 2 ml syringe (removed from sterile wrapper for photograph).
4. Hydrocortisone sodium succinate 100 mg, with 2 ml ampoule of water in which it is dissolved for injection.
5. Chlorphenamine (chlorpheniramine) injection BP ('Piriton'), 10 mg in 1 ml.

virtue of its vasoconstrictor and bronchodilator actions, and so opposes the potentially lethal actions that have been caused by histamine and other pharmacologically active agents explosively released during the anaphylactic reaction.

Although epinephrine (adrenaline) is the first line of defence, intravenous hydrocortisone 100 mg is also important. Glucocorticoids are antiallergic agents and this dose should ensure that an adequate amount of hydrocortisone (which is normally required and released endogenously under a variety of 'stressful' conditions) is available. Hydrocortisone does not prevent the occurrence of the antigen–antibody reaction, but acts by protecting the cells from the outcome of this immunological reaction. The reversal of the vasodepressor response by epinephrine (adrenaline) is dependent upon the presence of adequate hydrocortisone. If for any reason this is insufficient, for example in a patient who has an impaired adrenocortical response following prolonged corticosteroid therapy, then IV hydrocortisone is mandatory.

Antihistamines are usually *ineffective* in the treatment of acute anaphylactic shock for at least three reasons. First, histamine is only one of the pharmacologically active agents released; the effects of the other mediators are not antagonized by H₁ blockers. Second, these drugs may confound the situation due to their own vasodepressor action. If the reaction to the introduction of the drug allergen is not so immediate and acute as those considered so far, another line of treatment may be used. It may suffice to administer hydrocortisone as the first line of defence, followed by an H₁ blocker. The antihistamine could be administered parenterally, for example chlorphenamine (chlorpheniramine) 10–20 mg intramuscularly (in a lesser reaction, blockade of histamine receptors may well be useful). An additional benefit is that chlorphenamine (chlorpheniramine) has sedative properties and this is useful as patients are likely to be apprehensive about their condition. Of course, epinephrine (adrenaline) should always be available in this lesser situation in case the other remedies prove ineffective.

The question might be asked why epinephrine (adrenaline) is not used routinely as it seems to be effective in all situations. The answer resides in the nature of epinephrine itself; it can be a dangerous substance and so should be reserved for those life-endangering situations when other drugs will not suffice.

Other important examples of type I reactions are asthma, rhinitis (hay fever)—both conditions are discussed in Chapter 17—angio-oedema, and urticaria. These are also known as the atopic states, which are usually less severe than acute anaphylaxis.

ANGIO-OEDEMA This is a condition where leakage of fluid from vessels causes localized or more generalized swellings. It is commonly seen in the face, mouth, and upper respiratory tract, and is probably due to the release of histamine from sensitized mast cells. If the condition is very serious, the whole face may become swollen and there may be oedema of the pharynx and larynx to the degree that respiration is jeopardized. The swelling occurs suddenly and dramatically, and is often preceded by the skin becoming very itchy. Immediate relief of the swelling, especially if the larynx is involved, can be obtained by the subcutaneous injection of epinephrine (adrenaline) 1:1000 up to a total dose of 1.5 mL. The greater danger in this condition is respiratory obstruction (more likely to occur in children) and, if the epinephrine (adrenaline) fails to bring relief, then it will be necessary to bypass the supralaryngeal airway. The recommended technique is laryngotomy, which is performed by passing a fine-bore tube (cannula), or a large-gauge 'Venflon', between the thyroid and cricoid cartilages (i.e. through the cricothyroid membrane). Oxygen is then introduced through this tube and can be enough to maintain life. An emergency tracheostomy is not advocated; this is an extremely skilled procedure and, in an emergency situation, may prove a problem even to the experienced surgeon, never mind the dental surgeon unskilled in such techniques.

If the attack is less severe, an intramuscular injection of an antihistamine (H₁ blocker), such as chlorphenamine (chlorpheniramine) 10–20 mg, or promethazine 25–50 mg, followed by an adequate oral dosage may suffice.

URTICARIA This is due to the release of histamine from sensitized mast cells in the skin. It is commonly known as 'nettle rash', which is appropriate, since the lesions are very like those of a nettle sting. In urticaria there is a widespread eruption of firm, pink or white weals, accompanied by intense itching. A very characteristic feature is its effervescent nature, the lesions appearing suddenly and disappearing within hours or even minutes. It is a common manifestation of allergic hypersensitivity to foods and drugs. In many ways, urticaria is an odd phenomenon: it sometimes occurs in people who are apparently not sensitive to any food substance, but who are under some form of emotional stress. Often no cause can be found. The most common dietary causes of urticaria are the proteins of shellfish, eggs, and milk, and some fruits—especially strawberries.

Whilst histamine H1-antagonists are effective in treating urticaria, its normal transient nature may not warrant treatment. The best solution is to avoid the substance that triggered the allergic response.

It will be appreciated that any of these atopic states can be a manifestation of allergy to a drug. All are type I hypersensitivity reactions and are those most likely to be encountered by the dental practitioner.

TYPE II—CYTOXIC REACTIONS

These reactions are mediated by IgG and IgM antibodies. The antibody combines with an antigen on the cell surface, the complement system is activated, and cell lysis occurs. The principal target cells are those in the circulatory system. An example of a type II reaction is Rhesus incompatibility in the newborn child, where antibodies are produced by a Rhesus-negative mother against the Rhesus factor on the red cells of the fetus. The antibodies cross the placenta and cause haemolysis. Other examples are sulfonamide-induced granulocytopenia, and penicillin-induced haemolytic anaemia.

TYPE III—ARTHUS REACTIONS, SERUM SICKNESS

These are primarily mediated by IgG; the combination between antigen and antibody forms complexes that subsequently activate complement. The rate of formation of antigen–antibody complexes depends upon the absolute amount of antigen and antibody present and their relative proportions. In the presence of *antibody excess*, antigen–antibody complexes are readily precipitated and are localized at the site of antigen introduction. Complement factors are activated (especially C3a and C5a), and the responses occur at the site of antigen introduction. This reaction is known as the Arthus reaction and is characterized by local oedema and necrosis.

When there is *antigen excess*, soluble antigen–antibody complexes are formed that circulate and may become located in vascular endothelium, so producing a destructive inflammatory response called the serum-sickness syndrome. The clinical symptoms are fever, an urticarial rash, lymphadenopathy, and swelling of the joints (arthralgia). The condition usually lasts for about 6–12 days, and subsides on removal of the offending drug (antigen). Sulfonamides, penicillin, and streptomycin, as well as other drugs, can cause this syndrome.

The treatment of serum sickness is by steroids; corticosteroids control all its manifestations and are drugs of first choice. Although urticarial and oedematous lesions respond well to H_1 blockers, these drugs often have no effect on the fever or arthralgia.

TYPE IV—DELAYED HYPERSENSITIVITY REACTIONS

These are mediated by sensitized T-lymphocytes (cytotoxic T-cells and lymphokine-releasing cells) and macrophages, and are therefore cell-mediated reactions (see earlier). When sensitized T-lymphocytes come into contact with antigen, they undergo blast transformation and the resultant cells produce cytokines (see Chapter 4). Type IV reactions take place 1–4 days after antigen exposure; examples include contact dermatitis and organ transplant rejection. Many reactions due to drugs, chemicals, and foods belong to this group; for example, contact dermatitis due to procaine, penicillin, or metals such as mercury and nickel.

These reactions do not respond to sympathomimetic agents or to H_1 blockers; indeed, if antihistamines are applied topically, they may themselves produce a delayed hypersensitivity. Corticosteroids are the most useful group of drugs in the treatment of this type of reaction, but these cases should be referred to a dermatologist.

It is important for dental surgeons to remember that they themselves are liable to become sensitized to substances they handle regularly. Perhaps the most common offender is latex or the powder incorporated into rubber gloves.

Key facts
Hypersensitivity reactions

- Hypersensitivity reactions can be classified as follows:
  – type I, anaphylactic reaction;
  – type II, cytotoxic;
  – type III, Arthus reaction, serum sickness;
  – type IV, delayed hypersensitivity.

- Type I reactions are the most significant and can range from a life-threatening anaphylaxis to a troublesome urticarial rash.

- The reaction is mediated by antigen binding with IgE antibody on the surface of mast cells.

- Histamine, PAF, 5-HT, bradykinin, and the eicosanoids are released as a consequence of a Type-I reaction.

- The management of a Type-I hypersensitivity reaction will depend upon the severity; 0.5 mL of 1:1000 epinephrine (adrenaline) IM and hydrocortisone 100 mg IV are the treatments for an acute anaphylactic reaction; less severe reactions usually respond to corticosteroids and H_1-receptor blockers such as chlorphenamine (chlopheniramine).

- Type IV reactions are also important in dentistry and may be caused by various metals, including amalgam, and rubber gloves.

Prevention of the unwanted effects of drugs

A number of points should be noted. First, there is an increased incidence of adverse drug reactions in neonates and in the aged. For some reason, it seems that women tend to suffer more from adverse drug reactions than do men. Patients with a history of allergic responses are also more prone to adverse reactions, and this may include reactions for which there seems to be no immunological explanation—the asthmatic's reaction to aspirin may be of this nature. Clearly, the presence of renal and hepatic disease can predispose to adverse effects by causing drug accumulation. Certain drugs appear to be especially liable to produce unwanted effects; these include anticoagulants, antihypertensive drugs, non-steroidal anti-inflammatory drugs, and antimicrobials (penicillin being particularly prone, perhaps because of its extensive use).

In order to reduce the incidence of adverse reactions, the following points should be considered:

1. Medical history-taking must include a drug history; any previous untoward experiences with drugs should be noted and the drug withheld if there is a history of allergy.

2. If a patient is sensitized to one drug, he or she is likely to be sensitized to all drugs in the same group and possibly also to related drugs, for example penicillin and the cephalosporins.

3. Has the patient any underlying medical conditions such as renal failure that might predispose to a build-up of the drug and toxicity?

4. Is the drug really necessary—is the medical condition self-limiting?

5. Is the safest drug possible being used for the treatment?

6. Is there a possibility of a drug interaction?

In spite of taking into account all factors, unwanted effects still occur. However, a proper consideration of all these factors will minimize the problem.

Oral reactions to drugs

These are relatively rare considering the extent of consumption of drugs. This is a wide subject, and is dealt with fully in specialized textbooks (for example Seymour *et al.* 1996), Table 23.1 gives some examples of the sort of reaction that can occur in the mouth, but it makes no pretence to be exhaustive. In general, the mechanisms behind these oral reactions are ill-understood, although in some instances there is an immunological basis.

Table 23.1 Unwanted effects of drugs in the orofacial region, oral mucosa and tongue; drugs marked with an asterix are the compounds most frequently implicated

Type I Hypersensitivity reactions
e.g. penicillin, lidocaine (lignocaine), aspirin

Type IV hypersensitivity reactions
Stomatitis medicamentosa (fixed drug eruptions)
barbiturates, dapsone, indometacin (indomethacin), meprobamate, phenindione, phenolphthalein, salicylates, sulfonamides, tetracyclines

Stomatitis venenata (contact dermatitis)
antimicrobials, 'amalgam', antiseptic lozenges, beryllium, chewing gum, cosmetics, dental fixatives, mouthwashes, *nickel, toothpastes, topical anaesthetics

Erythema multiforme (Stevens–Johnson syndrome)
ampicillin, *barbiturates, benzodiazepines, carbamazepine, chlorpropamide, clindamycin, diflunisal, ethambutol, furosemide (frusemide), gold salts, iodine-containing mouthwashes, meprobamate, mercurials, minoxidil, penicillin, *phenylbutazone, phenothiazines, phenytoin, propranolol, quinine, rifampicin, salicylates, sulindac, *sulfonamides (long-acting), tetracylines, *thiazides

Lupus erythematosus (systemic)
e.g. carbamazepine, chlorpromazine, hydralazine, isoniazid, labetalol, penicillamine, phenylbutazone, phenytoin, primodone, procainamide, pindolol, sulfasalazine, thiouracils

A wide variety of drugs has been implicated in the production of SLE. The oral mucosa is involved in about 25% of patients. Drugs involved range from antihypertensives to anti-infective agents, e.g. tetracylines. In some instances there is convincing evidence of drug involvement, e.g. phenytoin, hydralazine, but in other cases it is less convincing.

Lichenoid eruptions
amiphenazole, β-adrenoceptor blockers, bismuth, captopril, chlorpropamide, chloroquine, gold salts, lithium carbonate, mepacrine, methyldopa, non-steroidal anti-inflammatory drugs, penicillamine, phenothiazines, quinine, quinidine, sodium aminosalicylate (PAS), spironolactone, tetracycline, thiazide diuretics

Oral ulcerations
Local irritants
aspirin, cocaine, ergotamine tartrate, gentian violet, isoprenaline, pancreatin, potassium, toothache solutions, trichloroacetic acid

Other agents, acting systemically
(occurring secondary to leucopenia)
antineoplastic drugs, e.g. actinomycin D (Dactinomycin), bleomycin, doxorubicin, fluorouracil, methotrexate, naproxen, proguanil hydrochloride

Discoloration of the oral mucosa and teeth
Teeth
*chlorhexidine, iron preparations, stannous fluoride toothpastes, *tetracyclines, minocycline

Mucosal tissues
bismuth, copper, gold, lead, mercury, silver, zinc, antimalarial drugs (e.g. chloroquine) antimicrobials (some), hydrogen peroxide, sodium perborate causes black hairy tongue
heroin—pigmented lesions of the tongue may occur in addicts who inhale the smoke
methyldopa—similar lesions to above reported
phenothiazines—bluish-grey discoloration of the oral mucosa may occur
oral contraceptives—pigmentation of oral mucosa reported
hormone replacement therapy

Table 23.1 (*cont.*)

Periodontal tissues
Gingival overgrowth
*cyclosporin, *calcium-channel blockers (e.g. nifedipine), oral contraceptives, *phenytoin

Dental structures
Xerostomia and caries
lithium carbonate, *tricylic antidepressants, antineoplastic drugs

Salivary glands
Xerostomia
atropine and related drugs, amfetamines (amphetamines), anoretic agents (e.g. fenfluramine and diethylpropion), antiarrhythmics (e.g. disopyramide), antihistamines (H$_1$ blockers), antineoplastics (occasionally), antihypertensives (e.g. guanethidine, clonidine, methyldopa, rauwolfia alkaloids), antiparkinsonian drugs (e.g. benzhexol, benztropine, orphenadrine), benzodiazepines, bromocriptine, butyrophenones (e.g. haloperidol), clonidine, levodopa, lithium, methyldopa, phenothiazines, phenylbutazone, tetracyclics, tricyclics

H$_2$-receptor antagonists (e.g. cimetidine, famotidine, and ranitidine) have been reported to cause
and exacerbate Sjogren's syndrome

Ptyalism
ACE inhibitors (e.g. captopril), anticholinesterases (e.g. neostigmine, distigmine, edrophonium), bromides, ethionamide (antileprotic drug), iodides, ketamine (intravenous anaesthetic agent), mercurial salts, niridazole, parasympathomimetics (e.g. bethanecol)

Pain and/or swelling
antihypertensives (e.g. bethanidine, clonidine, methyldopa), antiarrhythmic (e.g. bretylium), chlorhexidine, doxycycline, H$_2$-receptor blockers, iodides, nitrofurantoin, phenylbutazone, warfarin sodium

Cleft lip and palate
anticonvulsants (carbamazepine, phenytoin, sodium valproate), alcohol, benzodiazepines (?), corticosteroids, isotretinoin (vitamin A analogue), smoking, sulfasalazine

Disturbances of taste and halitosis
Disturbances of taste
*ACE inhibitors (e.g. captopril), acetazolamide, antimicrobials (e.g. metronidazole, griseofulvin, carbenicillin, lincomycin), antidiabetic drugs, (e.g. metformin), aspirin, azelastine (antihistamine), calcium-channel blockers (e.g. nifedipine, diltiazem), captopril, carbimazole, carmustine (anticancer drug), chlorhexidine, clofibrate, ethambutol, gold, imipramine, levodopa, lithium, penicillamine, phenindione, propafenone, prothionamide

If an alteration in taste occurs, this could be a blunting or decreased sensitivity in taste perception (hypogeusia), a total loss of the ability to taste (ageusia), or a distortion in perception of the taste of a substance (dysgeusia), in which, for example, sweet tastes seem sour.

Halitosis
disulfiram, isosorbide dinitrate (sublingual form)

Muscular and neurological disorders
Dyskinesias
antipsychotic drugs (e.g. phenothiazines, butyrophenones, such as haloperidol), amfetamines (amphetamines), benzodiazepines (withdrawal), carbamazepine, diazoxide, levodopa, lithium, methyldopa, metoclopramide, reserpine, tricyclics

Meige's syndrome
levodopa and carbidopa (long-term combination therapy), 'Dristan' decongestant nasal spray (contains phenylephrine, chlorphenamine (chlorpheniramine), benzalkonium chloride)

Neuropathy
acetazolamide, chlorpropamide, some antimicrobials, colistin, isoniazid, nalidixic acid, nitrofurantoin, polymyxin B, streptomycin, ergotamine, hydralazine, monoamine oxidase inhibitors, nicotinic acid (in large doses), tolbutamide, tricyclic antidepressants

Table 23.1 (*cont.*)

Oral infections induced or aggravated by drugs

antimicrobials—especially broad-spectrum—may induce secondary infections

cytotoxic drugs—nearly all cytotoxic drugs cause bone-marrow suppression and this may promote infections

corticosteroids—given in non-physiological amounts over a long period carry an increased risk of bacterial, fungal, or viral infections

oral contraceptives—their use has been associated with 'dry socket' after tooth extraction

immunosuppressive drugs—e.g. azathioprine, prednisone, cyclosporin—bacterial or fungal infections, and severe herpes simplex infections have been observed

Cervical lymphadenopathy

phenylbutazone, phenytoin, primidone,

Drug-induced aplastic anaemia, agranulocytosis, and thrombocytopenia

antibacterial drugs—e.g. cefalotin (cephalothin), chloramphenicol, penicillins, streptomycin, sulfonamides (including co-trimoxazole), tetracyclines, vancomycin

anticonvulsant drugs—e.g. carbamazepine, ethosuximide, hydantoin derivatives, sodium valproate

antihistamines—e.g. chlorphenamine (chlorpheniramine), H_2-receptor blockers

antimalarial drugs—e.g. chloroquine, pyrimethamine, quinine

antirheumatic drugs—e.g. aspirin, gold salts, ibuprofen and related drugs, indometacin (indomethacin), naproxen, penicillamine, phenylbutazone

antithyroid drugs—e.g. carbimazole, propylthiouracil

cardiotropic drugs—e.g. captopril, digoxin, disopyramide, quinidine, procainamide

cytotoxic drugs—alkylating agents (e.g. cyclophosphamide), antibiotics (e.g. doxorubicin) antimetabolites (e.g. methotrexate), vinca alkaloids (e.g. etoposide), radioactive isotopes, therapeutic X-rays (NB All cytotoxic drugs cause marrow depression apart from vincristine and bleomycin)

diuretics—e.g. acetazolamide, bendrofluazide, chlorothiazide, chlorthalidone, cyclopenthiazide, hydrochlorothiazide, hydroflumethiazide

psychotropic drugs—e.g. benzodiazepines, meprobamate, phenothiazine derivatives, tricylics and related antidepressants

sulfonylureas—e.g. chlorpropamide, tolbutamide

Blood dyscrasias frequently show oral manifestations, and the dental surgeon should be on the look out for unexplained spontaneous mucosal bleeding, sore tongue or mouth, and ulcerations in the mouth. These may point to a drug-induced haematological problem.

The occurrence of such reactions as listed in this table must be viewed in the context of the overall usage of the drug(s) concerned. The Table is unlikely to be complete, but gives enough information to indicate many unusual reactions that may occur due to drug usage. It is important for the dental surgeon to realize the possibilities, look out for any such unwanted drug effects, and to report them.

References

Foldes, F. F., Swerdlow, M., Lipschitz, E., van Hees, G. R., and Shanor, S. P. (1956). Comparison of the respiratory effects of suxamethonium in man. *Anaesthesiology*, 17, 559–68.

Kalow, W. and Gunn, D. R. (1957). The relationship between dose of succinylcholine and duration of apnoea in man. *Journal of Pharmacology and Experimental Therapeutics*, 120, 203–14.

Rawlins, M. D. and Thompson, J. W. (1991). Mechanisms of adverse drug reactions. In *Textbook of adverse drug reactions* (4th edn), pp. 10–21, (ed. D. M. Davies). Oxford University Press.

Seymour, R. A., Meechan, J. G., and Walton, J. G. (1996). *Adverse drug reactions in dentistry* (2nd edn). Oxford University Press.

Further reading

Seymour, R. A. (1991). Dental disorders. In *Textbook of adverse drug reactions* (4th edn), pp. 234–58, (ed. D. M. Davies). Oxford University Press.

24

Drug interactions (drug-drug interactions)

- Incidence and importance of drug interactions
- Classification of drug interactions
- Conclusions
- Further reading

Drug interactions (drug–drug interactions)

The use of several drugs is sometimes necessary to obtain the desired therapeutic effect. Examples include the use of a local anaesthetic and a vasoconstrictor, combinations of drugs in the treatment of hypertension and heart failure, and cancer chemotherapy which normally involves multiple drug therapy. In such instances, the use of several drugs is planned with the various drugs interacting synergistically to produce a beneficial effect.

By contrast, some drugs when given concurrently produce adverse effects that may be potentially dangerous. These interactions can arise when a number of drugs are used to treat a patient with several diseases; the result of an interaction being the potentiation or antagonism of one drug by another. Clearly the dental surgeon may, in the absence of sufficient knowledge about drug interactions, prescribe a drug to a patient who is already taking another one for some medical condition, and unwittingly precipitate a drug interaction.

Incidence and importance of drug interactions

In theory, many interactions are possible, but in practice only a relatively small number are of clinical importance. An accurate estimate of their incidence amongst out-patients is not available but, for hospital in-patients, it has been estimated to range from 2 to 3% for patients taking a few drugs to as high as 20% for patients receiving more than 10 different drugs. However, for certain drugs the potential for reaction is much higher than for others, and it is for patients taking these drugs that caution must be exercised when administering or prescribing drugs. For example, in a study of 277 patients taking oral anticoagulants, 94 were receiving other drugs with which the anticoagulants might have interacted (33.9 % of the total). Clinically significant interactions were considered to have developed in 6 patients, which represents an incidence of 6.4% in those taking drug combinations.

Drug interactions are likely to be of clinical importance if the affected drug has a steep dose–response curve or a low therapeutic index (see Chapter 2). In these instances, a relatively small quantitative change in the concentration of drug at the target protein (receptor or enzyme, etc.) or alteration in tissue responsiveness to the drug can lead to substantial changes in therapeutic or adverse effects—for example, digoxin and lithium.

In the UK, suspected adverse drug reactions, including drug interactions with recently introduced products, or serious or unusual reactions with established products should be reported to the Committee on Safety of Medicines using the 'yellow' card reporting system.

Classification of drug interactions

Drug interactions may be classified into three groups, namely: pharmaceutical; pharmacokinetic; and pharmacodynamic.

Pharmaceutical interactions

These are due to the formulation or mixing of chemically incompatible substances. Thus pharmaceutical interactions are most likely to occur when drugs interact in the same infusion solution (for example ampicillin with glucose) or when one drug interacts with the solution (for example amphotericin is unstable in a dextrose–saline solution). Details about the addition of medication to infusion fluids are included in the *British national formulary* (see Appendix 6). This form of interaction is unlikely to occur in dental practice because of the nature of the drugs and the routes of administration normally used. Nevertheless, the dental practitioner should be aware of and alert to this form of interaction.

Pharmacokinetic interactions

These result from the modification of the action of one drug (X) by another (Y) as a result of an alteration in the concentration of drug X that reaches its site of action. Such interactions are due to changes in absorption, distribution, metabolism, or excretion of one drug by another. Examples of these types of interaction and an explanation of their mechanisms are given below.

Absorption

Example of adverse interactions related to decreased absorption are those between tetracyclines and antacids that contain divalent and trivalent cations (e.g. Ca^{2+}, Al^{3+}, Mg^{2+}), dairy products, oral iron preparations, sucralfate, and zinc sulfate. These interactions result in the production of poorly soluble chelates with reduced tetracycline absorption. Therefore these combinations of drugs or products should be avoided otherwise the therapeutic effect of tetracyclines will be reduced. However, separating the dose of tetracycline from the dose of interacting drug by 2–3 hours, so that they are not present in the same part of the gastrointestinal tract, will reduce the effect of this interaction. A further example of an adverse interaction associated with absorption is the malabsorption syndrome produced by neomycin which impairs the absorption of a number of drugs including phenoxymethylpenicillin.

Distribution

In the context of drug interactions, the factor most likely to affect the distribution of a drug in the body is an alteration in the extent to which it is bound to plasma protein. The displacement of drug X from some of its binding sites on plasma protein by drug Y (Y must occupy the majority of X's binding sites) leads to an elevation of the plasma concentration of unbound drug X; if drug Y is withdrawn the reverse will occur. It is the free, unbound drug that is pharmacologically active. However, it is important to realize that for a significant alteration of the free plasma concentration to take place, two conditions must be satisfied. First, the drug to be displaced (drug X) must be highly bound to plasma protein. Second, the major part of the total dose of drug X must be distributed in plasma rather than tissues, i.e. a low apparent volume of distribution (V_d); if V_d is large, then extensive displacement from plasma binding sites produces only a small change in the unbound concentration of drug. There are three groups of drugs that fulfil these criteria: oral anticoagulants such as warfarin (99% bound, volume of distribution, V_d, 10 L); oral hypoglycaemics such as tolbutamide (96% bound, V_d 10 L); and the antiepileptic phenytoin (90% bound, V_d 45 L).

The clinical dangers of drug interactions due to displacement from protein-binding sites have turned out to be much less than originally anticipated. This is because, for drugs likely to be involved, the rate of elimination is dependent upon the fraction of unbound drug in the plasma. As a consequence, the increase in plasma concentration that follows from binding displacement is offset by a compensatory increase in elimination, so that the plasma concentration of unbound drug remains virtually unchanged once the new steady-state has been reached. Nevertheless, until this state has been reached, there will be an increase in the amount of free drug in the plasma. If this increase in free drug concentration exceeds the normal therapeutic range, a potentially adverse reaction may result; for example, haemorrhage due to excessive anticoagulation (warfarin). In practice this occurs rarely, and when it does other mechanisms are also involved, usually inhibition of drug metabolizing enzymes (see below).

Metabolism (biotransformation)

The intensity and duration of effect of many drugs depend largely upon their rate of biotransformation, chiefly in the liver, to less active or inactive metabolites. Therefore, if the rate of metabolism of one drug is altered by another drug, this will substantially modify the effect of the first drug. The altered metabolism of one drug by another is the most common cause of adverse drug interactions.

Stimulation (induction) of drug–metabolizing enzymes (DMEs)

Certain drugs such as phenytoin, barbiturates, carbamazepine, rifampicin, and ethanol (in chronic use), as well as cigarette smoking, are powerful inducers of DMEs. The result is that the half-life of some drugs may be reduced substantially. Enzyme induction develops over several weeks and takes about the same time to disappear after the inducing agent has been withdrawn. Examples of metabolized drugs likely to be altered by enzyme inducers are anticoagulants and oral contraceptives. The metabolism of warfarin may be increased by enzyme induction, so leading to a diminished anticoagulant effect and the need for an increased dosage. If the inducer is then withdrawn, the subsequent reduced metabolism will lead to an increased effect with possible haemorrhagic complications.

Inhibition of drug–metabolizing enzymes

A number of drugs may inhibit DMEs; these include metronidazole, chloramphenicol, erythromycin, cimetidine, and monoamine oxidase inhibitors. The result of this type of interaction is accumulation of the affected drug or an intermediate metabolite such that plasma concentrations may reach levels where toxicity is apparent. Examples include:

- ethanol and metronidazole with the resulting accumulation of ethanal (acetaldehyde), which produces flushing, and nausea and vomiting;

- inhibition of the metabolism of carbamazepine by erythromycin, such that patients develop signs of carbamazepine toxicity including drowsiness, dizziness, and nausea and vomiting.

Excretion

The rate of excretion of drugs that are weak electrolytes can be modified by altering the pH of the urine (see Chapter 1). The rate of excretion of weak acids, such as salicylates, can be expedited by making the urine alkaline. This increases the proportion of salicylate molecules present in the ionized form; these are more water-soluble (less lipid-soluble) than the corresponding unionized molecules, which would be reabsorbed by the tubules. This effect is exploited in the treatment of aspirin poisoning, when it is necessary to remove the drug from the body as quickly as possible.

An alternative form of interaction occurs when two drugs compete for the same transport system in the proximal tubule of the kidney. It is by this mechanism that probenecid and aspirin reduce the rate of excretion of the penicillins. No particular precautions need to be taken for these drug combinations, indeed, probenecid can be used to prolong the half-life of penicillins.

Disruption of enterohepatic cycling

A potentially important interaction of this type is that between oral contraceptive steroids and broad-spectrum antibiotics such as ampicillin and tetracycline. This is an example of an interaction involving biliary excretion and drug metabolism. There have been sporadic reports of women who have become pregnant whilst taking an antibiotic at the same time as an oral contraceptive steroid. As a consequence, the impression has gained ground that oral contraceptive steroids may fail in the presence of antibiotics (see Chapter 20). This suggestion received support from animal studies, where there is clear evidence of an enterohepatic circulation of estrogens (oestrogens) that can be modulated by broad-spectrum antibiotics. Antibiotics suppress the gut microflora, which normally deconjugate (and therefore reactivate) steroids previously inactivated by conjugation in the liver and excreted in the bile. However, human studies suggest that, in most women, enterohepatic recirculation of contraceptive steroids plays only a minor metabolic role and is most unlikely to account for contraceptive failure in the presence of broad-spectrum antibiotics. A much more likely explanation is failure of compliance. When there is special concern about a particular patient and the possible effect of an antibiotic on the contraceptive steroids, then she should be advised to use a barrier method of contraception whilst taking the course of antibiotics and for at least 7 days afterwards.

Pharmacodynamic interactions

This type of drug interaction occurs when drug Y affects the action of drug X, with no change in the concentration of drug X at its site of action. This type of interaction may result from opposing actions of drugs at the target protein; for example blockade of the bronchodilator action of the β_2-adrenoceptor agonist salbutamol by β-adrenoceptor antagonists (NB β-adrenoceptor antagonists are contraindicated in asthmatics taking bronchodilator drugs, see Chapters 14 and 17). However, the majority of pharmacodynamic interactions are the result of drugs having additive or opposing effects, which are less direct and involve different sites/mechanisms of actions.

Common interactions occur in the central nervous system. Thus, many drugs that depress the CNS will produce additive or synergistic effects when given together. A well-known, although not always heeded example, is the danger of drinking ethyl alcohol (ethanol) in the presence of benzodiazepines or neuroleptic drugs. Antihypertensive drugs may interact in a useful way; for example, thiazide diuretics and β-adrenoceptor antagonists are synergistic drug combinations in the control of high blood pressure. Conversely, combinations of the calcium-channel blocking drug verapamil and β-adrenoceptor antagonists are potentially harmful since these may result in excessive depression of cardiac function. An example of a pharmacodynamic interaction involving antibiotics is that between penicillins and tetracyclines. Tetracycline is a bacteriostatic agent, inhibiting the multiplication of bacteria, whilst penicillins are bactericidal and only kill rapidly dividing cells. The result of the interaction is that tetracyclines inhibit the bactericidal action of penicillins and therefore this combination should be avoided.

Pharmacodynamic interactions may also occur as a result of changes in fluid or electrolyte balance. An important example (although one unlikely to be of relevance to the dental practitioner) is the potentiation of the effect of cardiac glycosides as a result of hypokalaemia induced by potassium-losing diuretics.

Conclusions

It can be seen that drug interactions form a large, heterogeneous, and potentially hazardous group of problems, and it is most important for the dental practitioner to be aware of their existence. Through ignorance of this subject, a dental practitioner may prescribe a drug that interacts with one already being taken by the patient. The list of interactions is growing steadily, and dental practitioners must be prepared to keep themselves well informed. **If unsure about a possible adverse drug interaction—consult an appropriate reference text**, e.g. *British national formulary*. The following tables, organized under the major classes of drugs used or prescribed in dentistry, have been prepared as a guide to the adverse interactions that the dental practitioner is most likely to meet—but it is not exhaustive. It indicates the clinical outcome and, wherever possible, the probable mechanism of action for each example.

Key facts
Drug interactions

- Combinations of drugs may given to enhance the clinical response; for example, epinephrine (adrenaline) and a local anaesthetic—a beneficial drug interaction.

- Conversely, the administration of a drug to a patient who is already taking medication for an existing medical condition may result in an unintended potentiation or inhibition of the action of one of the drugs—an adverse drug interaction.

- Drug interactions may be classified into three groups, namely: pharmaceutical, pharmacokinetic, and pharmacodynamic.

- Pharmaceutical drug interactions are due to the formulation or mixing of chemically incompatible substances— these are unlikely to be of importance to the dental practitioner.

- Pharmacokinetic interactions result from one drug altering the concentration of another at its site of action by affecting either its absorption, distribution, metabolism, or excretion. The majority of adverse drug interactions result from one drug increasing or inhibiting the metabolism of another.

- There are many mechanisms underlying pharmacodynamic drug interactions, although the concentrations of the interacting drugs are unaffected. This type of interaction may occur when drugs have similar or opposing pharmacological effects.

Table 24.1(a) Drug interactions with antimicrobial drugs

Drug given for dental treatment	Drug given for medical treatment	Result of interaction	Action and comments	Mechanism of interaction
Ampicillin Amoxicillin (amoxycillin) Tetracyclines	Combined oral contraceptives (estrogen + progestogen)	Low risk of contraceptive failure	Patients should be advised to use an alternative form of contraception	Interruption of enterohepatic cycling of estrogens (see text)
Co-trimoxazole Fluconazole Ketoconazole Miconazole Metronidazole	Phenytoin	Increased plasma levels of phenytoin (possible toxicity)	Avoid combinations unless facilities available to monitor phenytoin levels	Inhibition of phenytoin metabolism
Co-trimoxazole Erythromycin Metronidazole Miconazole Tetracyclines	Warfarin	Enhanced anticoagulant effect of warfarin (possible haemorrhage)	Avoid combination or inform patient's doctor (dose of warfarin may need to be reduced)	Inhibition of metabolism
Erythromycin	Theophylline	Theophylline toxicity	Avoid combination	Inhibition of metabolism
Erythromycin Ketoconazole	Terfenadine, astemizole	Risk of cardiac dysrhythmias (prolonged QT interval)	Avoid combination	Increased plasma levels of H_1 antagonist due to inhibition of metabolism
Erythromycin	Midazolam*	Profound sedation	Reduce dose of midazolam	Inhibition of metabolism
Erythromycin	Carbamazepine*	Increased risk of carbamazepine toxicity	Avoid combination or inform patient's doctor (dose of carbamazepine may need to be reduced)	Inhibition of metabolism
Erythromycin Tetracycline	Digoxin	Digoxin intoxication	Avoid combination	Inhibition of digoxin metabolism by gut flora

* May also be used in dental treatment.

Table 24.1(b) Further drug interactions with antimicrobial drugs

Drug given for dental treatment	Drug given for medical treatment	Result of interaction	Action and comments	Mechanism of interaction
Fluconazole Itraconazole Ketoconazole Amphotericin	Cyclosporin	Increased risk of nephrotoxicity	Avoid combination or inform patient's doctor (dose of cyclosporine may need to be reduced)	Azole antifungal agents inhibit cyclosporin metabolism; cyclosporin + amphotericin— additive nephrotoxic effects
Metronidazole	Lithium	Increased lithium toxicity	Avoid combination	Mechanism unknown
Metronidazole	Alcohol (ethanol)	Flushing, nausea, vomiting, headache	Warn patients not to consume alcohol	Accumulation of acetaldehyde due to inhibition of its metabolism
Tetracyclines	Antacids iron supplements	Loss of antibacterial action of tetracyclines	Avoid combination or take 3 hours apart	Formation of insoluble chelates in the gut
Penicillins	Tetracyclines*	Inhibition of bactericidal action of penicillins	Avoid combination	Bacteriostatic effect of tetracyclines antagonizes action of penicillins
Phenoxymethylpenicillin	Neomycin	Impaired absorption of penicillin	Increase penicillin dose	Neomycin produces a malabsorption syndrome

*May also be used in dental treatment.

Table 24.2 Drug interactions with anti-inflammatory drugs

Drug given for dental treatment	Drug given for medical treatment	Result of interaction	Action and comments	Mechanism of interaction
Aspirin	Heparin	Risk of haemorrhage (particularly in GI tract)	Avoid combination (use paracetamol)	Both drugs prolong bleeding time; aspirin is ulcerogenic
Aspirin (possible risk with other non-steroidal-anti-inflammatory drugs)	Warfarin	Risk of haemorrhage (particularly in GI tract)	Avoid combination	Both drugs prolong bleeding time; aspirin is ulcerogenic
Aspirin	Insulin, chlorpropamide (possibly other oral hypoglycaemics)	Hypoglycaemia	Avoid combination	Additive hypoglycaemic effects; blockade of tubular secretion of chlorpropamide
Aspirin	Penicillins*	Increased plasma half-life of penicillins	Uncertain—be aware	Competition for tubular secretion
Aspirin Ibuprofen	Captopril + other ACE inhibitors	Reduction in antihypertensive effect of captopril	Avoid combination	Block of prostaglandin synthesis in kidney inhibits antihypertensive effect
Aspirin	Alcohol (ethanol)	Increased risk of damage to gastric mucosa	Warn patients not to consume alcohol	Both drugs irritant to gastric mucosa
Aspirin	Sodium valproate	Valproate toxicity (tremor, ataxia etc.); post-extraction haemorrhage	Avoid combination	Aspirin displaces valproate from protein binding sites and inhibits metabolism; both drugs inhibit platelet aggregation
Aspirin	Parenteral corticosteroids	Increased risk of damage to gastric mucosa and bleeding; risk of salicylate toxicity on corticosteroid withdrawal	Avoid aspirin in patients on long-term corticosteroid therapy	Both drugs irritant to gastric mucosa; corticosteroids increase the clearance of salicylates, and salicylates may accumulate on corticosteroid withdrawal
Ibuprofen	Digoxin	Digoxin toxicity	Avoid combination	Mechanism uncertain

* May also be used in dental treatment.

Table 24.3 Drug interactions with centrally acting drugs

Drug given for dental treatment	Drug given for medical treatment	Result of interaction	Action and comments	Mechanism of interaction
Carbamazepine	Oral contraceptives (combined and progestogen-only)	Break-through bleeding (combined preparations) and risk of contraceptive failure	Patients should be advised to use alternative form of contraception	Induction of hepatic drug-metabolizing enzymes
Carbamazepine	Warfarin, corticosteroids, amitriptyline, plus other drugs	Reduction in plasma levels of interacting drug with consequent reduction in effect	Avoid combination or inform patient's doctor (dose of interacting drug may need to be increased). Whenever carbamazepine is prescribed, check for any potential interaction	Induction of hepatic drug-metabolizing enzymes
Diazepam nitrazepam	CNS depressants: e.g. alcohol (ethanol), sedative H_1 antagonists, neuroleptics, antiepileptics, etc.	Excessive sedation, impaired psychomotor skills, possible respiratory depression	Advise patient not to consume alcohol; avoid combinations or consult patient's doctor	Combinations of CNS depressant drugs have additive effects
Diazepam Nitrazepam	Cimetidine	Increased plasma levels of diazepam and nitrazepam	Normally of no clinical importance, but occasional patient may experience increased drowsiness	Inhibition of metabolism
General anaesthetics	Antihypertensive drugs	Risk of marked hypotension particularly with ACE inhibitors	Concurrent use need not be avoided, but particular care required	Additive depressant effects on systems that control blood pressure
Halothane Enflurane Sevoflurane	Epinephrine* (adrenaline) for haemostasis	Risk of cardiac dysrhythmias particularly with halothane	Dose of epinephrine should not exceed 10 mL of 1:100 000 in 10 minutes nor 30 mL per hour	Halothane, etc. sensitize the myocardium to catecholamines

*May also be used in dental treatment.

Further reading

British national formulary No 37 (1999). British Medical Association and The Royal Pharmaceutical Society of Great Britain.

Seymour, R. A., Meechan, J. G., and Walton, J. G. (1996). *Adverse drug reactions in dentistry*. Oxford University Press, Oxford.

Stockley, I. H. (1996). *Drug interactions; a source book of adverse interactions, their mechanisms, clinical importance and management* (4th edn). Pharmaceutical Press, London.

Orme, M. L'E. and Back, D. J. (1986). Drug interactions between oral contraceptive steroids and antibiotics. *British Dental Journal*, 160, 169–70.

25

Drug abuse and dental patients

- Alcohol
- Nicotine
- Cannabis
- Opioids
- Central nervous system depressants
- Central nervous system stimulants
- Amfetamines (amphetamines) and Ecstasy
- Hallucinogens
- Solvent abuse
- Anabolic steroids and performance-enhancers
- Conclusions
- Further reading

Drug abuse and dental patients

This chapter considers the pharmacological effects of drug abuse, the influence of drug abuse on the orodental structures, and the management of dental patients who are drug abusers.

Drug abuse is defined as a pattern of pathological behaviour associated with the continued use of a drug or drugs despite persistent social, psychological, or physical problems caused by such use. In addition to being defined as a pathological state, drug abuse can produce pathological changes; for example cardiac and liver damage. Patterns of abuse vary from experimentation by the curious through to the life-style dominating condition of drug dependence. Dependence can be divided into psychological and physical. Psychological dependence is defined as a feeling of satisfaction or psychic drive that requires periodic or continuous administration of the drug to produce pleasure or avoid discomfort. Physical dependence, which is also known as neuroadaptation, is characterized by physical disturbances when the drug is suspended or when its actions are antagonized. Psychological dependence often outlasts physical dependence and is the major cause of relapse in treated addicts.

Another principle that is important in relation to drug abuse, but which is also pertinent to the action of prescribed medication, is the phenomenon of tolerance. Tolerance is the reduction in the effect of a drug due to prior exposure, and is dependent upon both the dose and frequency of exposure. The physiological basis for tolerance can be due to a decrease in the number of drug receptors, depletion of essential mediators, or a decrease in plasma concentration with prolonged usage. Tolerance may be overcome by increasing the dose of the drug.

Why do individuals abuse drugs? There are psychiatric and social considerations which are beyond the scope of this text; however, a simple explanation is that drug abuse produces pharmacological rewards. For example, many drugs such as alcohol, cocaine, opioids, and amfetamines (amphetamines) increase dopamine release. In addition there may be a genetic influence on the sensitivity to abuse. Twin studies suggest that 60% of the susceptibility to alcoholism is due to genetic factors and there is a higher frequency of a mutation in a dopamine-receptor gene in multiple drug abusers compared to control subjects.

Some signs of drug abuse and characteristics of drug abusers are given in Tables 25.1 and 25.2.

Caries and periodontal disease are common in drug abusers for a number of reasons. Those dependent upon drugs may sacrifice a normal diet to finance their habit and this will lead to nutritional deficiencies. Many drugs such as ecstasy and anabolic steroids increase caries as they induce a craving for increased carbohydrate intake. Carbohydrates are also used as bulking agents in some drug preparations. Xerostomia is also a contributory factor either as a direct result of drug action (for example barbiturates) or as a result of dehydration due to drug-induced overactivity (for example ecstasy). Another factor is that the drug may mask dental pain, thus the abuser does not seek treatment. Figures 25.1(a) and (b) show the rapid progress of dental disease over a 20-month period in a heroin addict in her mid-twenties.

Illicit drugs which are administered intravenously can produce endocardial problems due to damage from contaminants used to bulk the agent. In addition, any form of abuse that involves injection (either intramuscularly or intravascularly) exposes the abuser to blood-borne viral infections such as hepatitis and HIV.

The following drugs will be considered in this chapter:

- alcohol
- nicotine
- cannabis
- opioids
- CNS depressants
- CNS stimulants
- hallucinogens
- volatile substances
- anabolic steroids and performance-enhancers.

This list is not exhaustive, for example it does not include the commonly used drug caffeine, the consumption of which is considered an accepted social activity. Table 25.3 summarizes the effects of these drugs on the teeth and oral structures.

Table 25.1 Signs of drug abuse

Mood swings
Loss of interest in appearance
Inappropriate wearing of sunglasses
Needle tracks
Odd tattoos over veins

Table 25.2 Drug abuser characteristics

Poor historians
Lie about intake
Disproportionate demand for analgesics
Good knowledge of formulary
Inappropriate fear of needles in the hands of others
Intravenous access may be difficult due to lack of patent peripheral veins

Table 25.3 The effects of drugs of abuse on oral structures and dental management

	Teeth	Oral mucosa	Interaction with GA and sedative agents	Interaction with LA containing epinephrine (adrenaline)	Bleeding	Cardiac effects	HIV/ hepatitis	Drug interactions
Alcohol	+	+	+		+	+		+
Nicotine	+	+	+					
Cannabis		+	+	+				
Opioids		+			+	+	+	+
CNS depressants		+	+		+			+
CNS stimulants		+	+	+	+	+	+	+
Hallucinogens								+
Volatile agents			+	+		+		
Anabolic steroids/ performance enhancers			+	+	+	+	+	+

+ Means an interaction between the drug and the structure/function indicated.

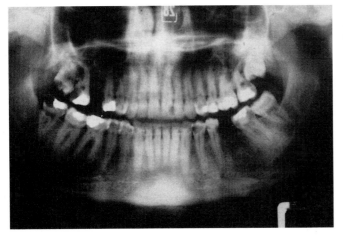 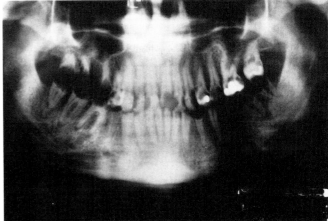

Figs 25.1(a) and (b) These orthopantomograms show the progression of caries over a 20-month period in a heroin addict in her mid-20s.

Key facts
Dental disease in drug abusers

- This can be caused by poor diet and nutrition.
- An increased carbohydrate intake can be a contributory factor.
- Carbohydrate bulking agents are used in some drug formulations.
- Xerostomia can lead to dental disease.
- Dental pain can be masked by various drugs.

Alcohol

Alcohol (ethanol) is the most widely used drug in the United Kingdom. It produces both tolerance and dependence.

Pharmacological effects

Alcohol exerts its depressant effects of the central nervous system by a combination of non-specific and specific mechanisms. The non-specific action is an alteration in membrane fluidity similar to the action of the volatile anaesthetic agents (see Chapter 9). The specific actions include calcium-channel blockade in neurones, stimulation of GABA-mediated inhibition similar to that of the benzodiazepines (see Chapter 15), and inhibition of glutamate function. The effect of alcohol on the CNS in relation to consumption is shown in Table 25.4.

Alcohol has a dual effect on blood glucose. Initially it increases blood glucose due to reduced glucose uptake by the tissues, but this leads to increased insulin output, which will cause hypoglycaemia.

Table 25.4 The effect of alcohol on the CNS

Number of units	Effect
1–2	Normal
3–4	Warmth, friendliness, digestive discomfort, lengthening of reaction to visual field
6	Diminished sense of depth, impaired driving
8	Loss of inhibition, euphoria, aggressive behaviour, visual disturbances
10	Deterioration of motor reaction and loss of precision
12	Uncertain movements, reduced ability for adaptation
14	Accommodation disturbances, loss of balance
16	Obvious drunkenness, loss of muscular co-ordination
18	Irritability, depression, nausea, loss of sphincter control
24–8	Stupor
30–6	Coma
40–60	Paralysis of respiratory centre, death

NB In the UK, 1 unit of alcohol is equivalent to 1 measure of spirits, or 1/2 pint of beer/lager, or 1 glass of wine.

Other pharmacological effects of alcohol include peripheral vasodilatation and diuresis.

Effects on orodental structures

- Alcoholic patients have a greater prevalence of pathological tooth-wear compared to control populations. There are two explanations for this effect. First, dissolution of enamel by the alcoholic drink or any mixers it contains. Second, alcohol is a gastric irritant and causes an increase in regurgitation of acidic gastric contents.
- Some of the mucosal changes caused by the chronic abuse of alcohol such as glossitis and stomatitis are due to nutritional deficiencies and anaemia. Similarly, the progress of orofacial infections suffered by alcoholics may be more severe due to the immunosuppression.
- Many orofacial injuries, such as those suffered as a result of violence or road traffic accidents, are a result of alcoholic intoxication.
- Alcohol may affect salivary gland structure and function. Sialosis, which is a painless swelling of the salivary glands (usually the parotids), is a recognized side-effect of alcohol. The consumption of alcohol initially leads to an increase in salivary flow; however, chronic use leads to the degeneration of salivary tissue causing xerostomia.
- Alcohol is a recognized risk factor for oral cancer.
- Cleft lip and palate are part of the fetal alcohol syndrome which may affect the newborn of alcoholic mothers.

Influence of alcohol on dental management

As mentioned above tooth-wear can be a problem, and satisfactory treatment of this condition may be a thankless task in the committed alcoholic. As is the case with many drug-dependent patients, regular attendance to maintain dental health is difficult due to the addict's life-style and prioritization of finances to support the habit.

A small amount of alcohol may make the management of some patients easier than normal as the drug acts as an anxiolytic. Indeed, alcohol was used to reduce anxiety in the past although it has now been superseded by the benzodiazepines. However, the drunk (not necessarily alcoholic) patient may present problems due to a lack of co-operation and some may resort to abusive and violent behaviour.

Excessive use of alcohol produces tolerance both to itself and to other CNS depressants such as sedatives and general anaesthetic agents. Therefore the required doses of drugs such as midazolam used during dental sedation are much greater in alcohol-dependent patients.

The effect of alcohol on the liver can lead to bleeding problems following dental surgery. Before performing surgery on alcohol-dependent patients it is prudent to perform clotting studies and liver function tests.

The severe alcoholic is at risk of infective endocarditis

following gingival manipulation due to their immunocompromised status. The use of prophylactic antibiotics should be considered for such individuals.

Alcohol produces interactions with some drugs that may be prescribed by dentists. Due to the increased bleeding tendency the prescription of aspirin should be avoided. There is a disulfiram-type reaction between alcohol and antimicrobial drugs. Disulfiram is a drug used to treat alcoholism. It inhibits the enzyme aldehyde dehydrogenase leading to an accumulation of aldehyde (Fig. 25.2). This produces unpleasant side-effects such as flushing, hyperventilation, and feelings of panic. The antimicrobials that can produce a disulfiram-like reaction include metronidazole, some cefalosporins, and the antifungal drug ketoconazole.

Key facts
Alcohol

- Alcohol is a central nervous system depressant.
- It increases tooth-wear.
- In addition to producing oral mucosal lesions, alcohol affects salivary gland function.
- Alcohol is an aetiological factor for oral cancer.
- It has an adverse drug interaction with metronidazole.

Nicotine

Nicotine is a pharmacologically active constituent of tobacco smoke. It is present at a concentration of about 2% in cigarettes, but is higher in cigars and pipe tobacco.

Pharmacological effects

Nicotine produces excitation of autonomic ganglia and sensory receptors (see Chapter 14). Such stimulation causes an increase in

heart rate and raises blood pressure. In addition, nicotine promotes catecholamine-release which contributes to these cardiovascular effects.

Effects on orodental structures

- The influence of smoking tobacco on periodontal disease is now well established. Smoking has been implicated in the production of acute ulcerative gingivitis and is a significant risk factor for adult periodontitis. In addition, smokers respond less well to periodontal therapy compared to non-smokers.

- The absorption of nicotine through the oral mucosa causes a localized vasoconstriction due to norepinephrine (noradrenaline) release. This means that smokers show less gingival bleeding than non-smokers and the level of blood-filling in extraction sockets is significantly lower in smokers.

- Smoking may stain the teeth but this is reversible.

- Nicotinic stomatitis is a recognized entity, and a characteristic cobblestone appearance may be found on the palate due to inflammation and hyperkeratosis of palatal minor salivary gland ducts.

- Smoking can produce oral leukoplakia and, as with alcohol, it is a recognized risk factor for oral cancer. Indeed, the effects of smoking and alcohol are more than additive in relation to the aetiology of oral malignancy.

Influence of nicotine on dental management

The successful management of periodontal disease in some patients may depend upon the cessation of smoking.

The incidence of painful (or dry) socket is increased in smokers and they should be warned of this possibility when having extractions.

Smoking induces the synthesis of liver microsomal enzymes, which can interfere with the activity of other drugs the patient may be taking. This means that smokers may require higher doses of intravenous sedatives and postoperative analgesics than non-smokers.

Key facts
Smoking

- Smoking has adverse effects on the periodontium.
- It produces oral mucosal lesions such as leukoplakia.
- Tobacco is an aetiological factor for oral cancer.
- It may increase 'dry socket' production.

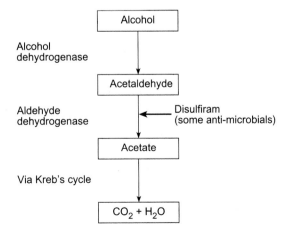

Fig. 25.2 The metabolism of alcohol showing the influence of disulfiram on the activity of aldehyde dehydrogenase.

Cannabis

Cannabis is the most widely abused drug in the United Kingdom other than nicotine and alcohol.

Pharmacological effects

The active ingredient of cannabis is Δ^1 tetrahydrocannabinol (Δ^1THC). There are endogenous G-protein-coupled receptors for Δ^1THC in the central nervous system and the periphery. The endogenous mediator for these receptors is anandamide, which is a derivative of arachidonic acid. The physiological function of these receptors is not known. At the cellular level the actions of cannabis are similar to those of the opioids; adenylyl cyclase is inhibited and calcium-channel function is blocked. In addition cannabis shows some sympathomimetic activity. Cannabis is also an antiemetic and its use to counter the emetic effects of anti-cancer treatments is being investigated.

Effects on orodental structures

- Cannabis can cause gingival hyperplasia.
- Leukoplakia has also been noted in cannabis smokers. This is not surprising as cannabis burns at a much higher temperature than cigarette smoke.
- Cannabis smoke contains more carcinogens than cigarette smoke and, although there is no association with lung cancer in cannabis users, there are reported cases of lingual carcinoma.

Influence of cannabis on dental management

Due to its sympathomimetic action it may be wise to warn cannabis users to avoid using the drug prior to any dental visit that involves the use of local anaesthetics containing epinephrine (adrenaline).

Key facts
Cannabis

- Cannabis has adverse effects on oral mucosa such as the production of gingival hyperplasia and leukoplakia.
- It interacts synergistically with epinephrine.

Opioids

The archetypal opioid of abuse is heroin. There is a high incidence of physical dependence to this drug. Methadone is widely used in rehabilitation from opioid addiction.

Pharmacological effects

The pharmacological effects of the opioids were described in Chapter 7.

Effects on orodental structures

The use of methadone in the rehabilitation of opioid addicts can produce rampant caries. This is due to the fact that oral methadone is supplied as a sugary syrup to prevent intravenous abuse of the drug.

Influence of opioid abuse on dental management

Heroin addicts will have poor pain tolerance and may demand excessive postoperative analgesia.

Intravenous heroin abuse can produce endocardial damage and thus abusers should be protected against the possibility of infective endocarditis subsequent to gingival crevice manipulation by the use of appropriate prophylactic antibiotics (see Chapter 11). The endocardial damage is produced by contaminants in the injected material and the risk of endocarditis is increased by the use of shared needles.

Postoperative bleeding is also a concern in those who abuse heroin as the drug can produce a thrombocytopenia. It is therefore appropriate to request a full blood count prior to any surgical intervention.

Heroin interacts with some drugs that dentists may prescribe. The absorption of paracetamol and orally administered diazepam are delayed and reduced due to delayed gastric emptying.

Some of the drug interactions of methadone are worth noting. Carbamazepine reduces serum methadone levels due to enzyme induction and this is clinically important. The degree of drowsiness produced by diazepam is increased in those taking methadone. The serum levels of tricyclic antidepressants is increased in those taking methadone probably due to interference with metabolic hydroxylation.

Key facts
Opioids

- Opioids produce physical dependence.
- They lead to decreased pain tolerance and increased analgesic demands.
- Intravenous abuse produces cardiac damage that may lead to endocarditis.
- They can increase bleeding due to thrombocytopenia.

Central nervous system depressants

The central nervous system depressants that may be abused include barbiturates and benzodiazepines.

Pharmacological effects

The pharmacological effects of the barbiturates and benzodiazepines have been described in Chapter 15.

Effects on orodental structures

Barbiturates can produce a xerostomia and fixed drug eruptions on the oral mucosa.

Influence of central nervous system depressants on dental management

Patients taking benzodiazepines over an extended period of time (longer than 1 month) will develop tolerance to this group of drugs. This will interfere with the use of benzodiazepines in dental sedation. Whereas it is unusual to exceed a dose of 10 mg of midazolam during intravenous sedation in most dental patients it is sometimes necessary to give up to 50 mg of this drug to achieve satisfactory sedation in a patient tolerant to benzodiazepines.

Central nervous system stimulants

Included in this category are cocaine, the amfetamines (amphetamines), and ecstasy (3,4-methylenedioxymetamfetamine).

Cocaine

Cocaine is a local anaesthetic agent (see Chapter 8) but is rarely used for this purpose now because of the problems of addiction. Cocaine is a widely abused substance particularly in North America. Although there is no clear-cut physical dependence, there is a strong psychological dependence with this drug.

Pharmacological effects

Cocaine is a sympathomimetic agent. It inhibits the uptake of catecholamines at nerve terminals thus prolonging their action. Centrally, this produces a feeling of well-being. Effects on the cardiovascular system include tachycardia, vasoconstriction, and increased blood pressure.

Effects on orodental structures

The purity of a batch of cocaine is often tested by users by rubbing the substance on the gingival margin (usually in the maxillary premolar region). This can cause a localized vasoconstriction that is sufficiently profound to produce localized gingival and alveolar bone necrosis. In addition, this habit can produce localized dental caries due to the fact that the cocaine may be bulked out with cariogenic carbohydrates. Cases of spontaneous gingival bleeding as a result of thrombocytopenia have been reported in those who abuse cocaine. The newborn of mothers who abuse cocaine have a higher incidence of ankyloglossia (tongue-tie) than control populations.

Influence of cocaine on dental management

Full blood counts are appropriate prior to surgery, as cocaine addicts may bleed due to thrombocytopenia.

Among the recognized drug interactions of cocaine that may affect dental management are the following:

- Carbamazepine reduces the cocaine 'high' making the illicit drug less pleasurable.

- The combination of cocaine and propofol have produced opisthotonus (arching of the body with hyperextension of the neck) and grand mal seizures.

- Due to its sympathomimetic action patients should be advised to refrain from abusing cocaine prior to dental treatment involving the use of epinephrine (adrenaline)-containing local anaesthetics.

Key facts
Cocaine

- Cocaine can cause localized gingival and alveolar bone necrosis.
- This drug can produce gingival bleeding due to thrombocytopenia.
- It enhances the effects of epinephrine (adrenaline).

Amfetamines (amphetamines) and Ecstasy

Around 5% of those who abuse amfetamines become physically dependent upon the drug and there is a strong psychological dependence. Ecstasy (3,4-methylenedioxymethamfetamine; MDMA) is related to amfetamine although, as well as being a stimulant, it also acts as a 'feeling enhancer' but without the effects of the major hallucinogens (see below).

Pharmacological action

Amfetamines (amphetamines) stimulate the release of catecholamines from nerve terminals in the central nervous system. This causes an increase in blood pressure, increased motor activity, and a decrease in gut motility. Ecstasy has a similar action to LSD (see below).

Effects on orodental structures

Amfetamines and Ecstasy produce a xerostomia. This, together with the increased carbohydrate intake stimulated by these drugs, increases the risks of dental caries.

These drugs, due to increased motor activity, can encourage bruxism which may lead to trismus.

Influence of amfetamines (amphetamines) and ecstasy on dental management

These drugs can increase bleeding following surgery because they produce a thrombocytopenia and interfere with coagulation. Chronic abusers should therefore have a full blood count and clotting screen before surgical procedures.

Monoamine oxidase inhibitors and tricyclic antidepressant drugs should not be prescribed for those taking amfetamines since a hypertensive crisis may be precipitated.

Key facts
Amfetamines (amphetamines) and Ecstasy

- Both can increase caries due to xerostomia and increased carbohydrate intake.
- They can produce TMJ problems due to muscle overactivity.
- Amfetamines and ecstasy interact adversely with antidepressant medication.

Hallucinogens

Included in this group of drugs are LSD (lysergic acid diethylamide), mescaline, and phencyclidine (angel dust). These drugs do not usually produce dependence although a high degree of tolerance occurs.

Pharmacological properties

LSD acts as a 5-HT receptor agonist in the central nervous system, whereas phencyclidine is thought to stimulate opioid σ-receptors.

Effects on orodental structures

As was the case with amfetamines (amphetamines) the hallucinogens can encourage bruxism and trismus. Hallucinogenic trips may also lead to orofacial injuries.

Influence of hallucinogens on dental management

Stressful situations can encourage the phenomenon of flashback in those abusing hallucinogenic drugs. Flashback is the recurrence of some of the hallucinogenic effects of the drug which may be unpleasant, cause panic attacks, and lead to management problems. The combination of LSD and selective serotonin-reuptake inhibitors (see Chapter 15) increases the incidence of flashback and can lead to grand mal seizures.

Opioids should not be prescribed for patients taking phencyclidine as there is a danger of respiratory depression.

Key facts
Hallucinogens

- This group of drugs can lead to TMJ problems due to bruxism.
- They can adversely affect management if 'flashback' occurs.
- Hallucinogens interact adversely with opioids.

Solvent abuse

Various substances are contained in this group, including fluorinated hydrocarbons, chlorinated solvents, inert gases, and nitrous oxide.

Pharmacological effects

The diverse agents in this group all produce effects on the central nervous system that are similar to those produced by alcohol. However, there is a more rapid onset.

Effects on orodental structures

A characteristic circumoral erythema ('glue-sniffer's rash') may be noted in solvent abusers. Oral frost-bite has been reported following inhalation from an aerosol.

As is the case with alcohol and the hallucinogens orofacial injuries may occur during periods of intoxication.

Influence of solvent abuse on dental management

The main adverse effects of solvent abuse in dentistry relate to anaesthesia. The provision of general anaesthesia may be hazardous as solvent abuse can produce liver disorders, anaemia, and cardiac arrhythmias. In addition, some abused solvents are chemically similar to the halogenated, inhalational anaesthetic agents and this can increase the risks of anaesthetic toxicity.

Solvents may sensitize the myocardium to the actions of epinephrine (adrenaline) in a manner similar to that produced by the halogenated hydrocarbon, general anaesthetic agents. Therefore the avoidance or sensible dose reduction of epinephrine-containing local anaesthetics must be considered in those abusing solvents.

Those who abuse solvents are at risk of convulsions and the possibility of status epilepticus must be considered in this group.

Key facts
Solvents

- Solvents may produce circumoral erythema.
- They can adversely affect general anaesthesia due to cardiac, haematological, and liver damage as well as due to their similarity with general anaesthetic agents;
- They can sensitize the myocardium to the effects of epinephrine (adrenaline).

Anabolic steroids and performance-enhancers

Anabolic steroids are abused by many who are not professional athletes. They are used to increase muscle bulk and not surprisingly can produce physical dependence. Performance-enhancing drugs include ephedrine and clenbuterol.

Pharmacological effects

Anabolic steroids are modified androgens and achieve their effects by stimulating protein synthesis. Ephedrine and clenbuterol are sympathomimetic agonists.

Effects on orodental structures

The use of anabolic steroids and performance-enhancers can lead to the consumption of a diet high in carbohydrate and this increases the risk of dental caries in this population.

Influence of anabolic steroids and performance enhancers on dental management

- General anaesthesia can be a problem for individuals abusing anabolic steroids. Coronary artery disease can lead to cardiac dysfunction and the increased muscle mass leads to increased oxygen consumption and carbon dioxide production.
- Anabolic steroids can deplete clotting factors and induce fibrinolysis. A preoperative clotting screen is advisable prior to surgical procedures in these patients.

- Feelings of hostility and violence are not unusual in individuals withdrawing from anabolic steroids and these may cause management problems.
- Care must be exercised when using epinephrine (adrenaline)-containing local anaesthetics in those taking the sympathomimetic performance enhancers.

Key facts
Anabolic steroids

- This group of drugs can increase caries due to increased carbohydrate intake.
- They can affect general anaesthesia due to cardiovascular changes and increased muscle mass.
- Bleeding due to clotting-factor depletion is increased.

Conclusions

The misuse of drugs can produce orodental changes and affect management during dental treatment. Eliciting a full drug history is therefore important in diagnosis and treatment planning in dentistry.

Further reading

Brugger, J., Quenel, P., Leclerc, A., and Rodriguez, J. (1986). Differential effects of tobacco and alcohol in cancer of the larynx, pharynx and mouth. *Cancer*, 57, 391.

Dessler, F. A. and Roberts, W. C. (1989). Mode of death and type of cardiac disease in opiate addicts: analysis of 168 necroscopy cases. *American Journal of Cardiology*, 64, 909.

Duxbury, A. J. (1993). Ecstasy—dental implications. *British Dental Journal*, 175, 38.

26

Medical emergencies in dental practice

- Fainting
- Angina pectoris and myocardial infarction
- Cardiac arrest
- Asthma
- Acute allergic reactions
- Epilepsy
- Hypoglycaemia
- Adrenal crisis
- Further reading

Medical emergencies in dental practice

This chapter is concerned with the management of medical emergencies in dental practice. Surgical emergencies are not considered.

Before considering pharmacological methods of treating emergencies it must be stressed that it is essential that all members of the dental team are competent in basic life support, which is a drug-free means of maintaining the patient's vital functions. This is the least a patient can expect, and is required of a dentist as part of fitness to practise. It should be stressed that most of the medical emergencies considered in this chapter are likely to be very rare in the dental surgery. However, the practitioner must be familiar with methods of dealing with the immediate crisis. The treatment given by the dentist must be as simple as possible. An emergency kit of drugs must be available in every practice and should contain only a limited number of drugs *with which the practitioner is familiar*. It is pointless having an array of drugs whose actions are not known to the dentist and whose inappropriate use could worsen the patient's condition. The emergency kit suggested in Table 26.1 is satisfactory for most emergencies the practitioner is likely to encounter. All the drugs mentioned, with the exception of epinephrine (adrenaline), are unlikely to cause harm if used inappropriately. In addition to the drugs mentioned below *oxygen must be available in every dental surgery*. Another useful gas is nitrous oxide, either as a component of a relative analgesia machine or as Entonox (see Chapter 9).

Emergencies will be considered under the following headings:

(1) fainting;

(2) angina and myocardial infarction;

(3) cardiac arrest;

(4) asthma;

(5) acute allergic reactions;

(6) epilepsy;

(7) hypoglycaemia;

(8) adrenal crisis.

Local and general anaesthetic and sedation problems and those associated with bleeding have been dealt with in the appropriate Chapters.

Fainting

Fainting is likely to be the most common cause of loss of consciousness in the dental surgery. It is due to a transient lack of blood supply to the brain. Very often a fainting attack can be anticipated, and therefore prevented, by careful observation of the patient, particularly at the time of administration of a local anaesthetic. A patient who is pale, sweating, and feels sick and dizzy, is providing a warning. Such a patient may go quickly into unconsciousness. The pulse is weak at first, and slow, then it becomes fuller and bounding.

Fainting is less common today than in the past, because

Table 26.1 A simple emergency drug kit for dental practice*, together with recommended dosages for various emergencies

Drug	Dose	Route	Indication
Epinephrine (adrenaline) 1:1000	0.5–1.5 ml	IM	Anaphylactic shock/ life-threatening asthma
Hydrocortisone	100–500 mg	IV	Adrenal crisis/ anaphylactic shock/ acute asthma
Dextrose 50%	20–50 mL	IV	Hypoglycaemia
Glucagon	1 mg	IM	Hypoglycaemia
Chlorphenamine (chlorpheniramine)	10 mg	IV	Allergic reaction
Diazepam	5–20 mg	IV	Status epilepticus
Glyceryl trinitrate	0.4–0.8 mg	Sublingual	Angina
Salbutamol inhaler	1–2 puffs	Inhalation	Asthma
Morphine sulfate	10 mg	IV	Myocardial infarction

*When sedation and general anaesthesia are performed a more extensive list of drugs is required (see Chapter 9).
In addition, oxygen is essential and nitrous oxide is useful.

patients are now treated in the supine position. The sort of patient who is likely to faint is one who is unduly anxious, and the one who has decided not to eat before any dental treatment. A glucose drink should be provided for patients who have not eaten.

The treatment for fainting is to lie the patient flat with the head in a dependent position to allow the cerebral blood flow to be maintained.

Angina pectoris and myocardial infarction

Angina is a symptom of ischaemic disease; an attack is characterized by a sudden, very severe substernal pain that often radiates to the left shoulder and arm. Very occasionally the pain may radiate to the left mandible and teeth. The typical anginal attack is often brought on by exercise and by emotion, such as anxiety. Because of the anxiety association, an attack is a possibility in the dental surgery. The patient may have had anginal attacks for a long time and so will recognize the symptoms, and will be carrying his or her usual remedy, for example glyceryl trinitrate tablets or spray (see Chapter 16). It is probably sensible to keep glyceryl trinitrate in the surgery for emergencies, in case the patient does forget. It is better to have the spray formulation as the contents of a bottle of glyceryl trinitrate tablets must be discarded 8 weeks after opening. If an attack occurs they should have one to two puffs of the spray (0.4–0.8 mg) sublingually and then the mouth is closed or one tablet is placed under the tongue.

If a patient with recurrent angina pectoris develops an acute myocardial infarction, he or she may take several doses of glyceryl trinitrate in quick succession in an attempt to relieve the intractable pain. All this will do is produce a further reduction in myocardial blood flow, and this will clearly have a serious adverse effect. Patients should be advised that, in the event of very prolonged attacks of pain, taking excessive doses could be harmful.

If the patient has a myocardial infarct, the pain will be similar to that experienced during an attack of angina, but it will be more severe and persistent. The patient is often breathless and vomiting is common. The pulse will be weak and the blood pressure falls. They may become unconscious for a time, and may suffer cardiac arrest and die.

Once a myocardial infarct has been diagnosed the following steps should be taken:

1. An ambulance must be called for by an assistant.

2. Pain and anxiety must be relieved.

The nature of the pain experienced will provoke acute anxiety. This, in itself, will cause the outpouring of endogenous epinephrine (adrenaline) with the possible precipitation of cardiac ventricular fibrillation. Fibrillation is a cause of sudden death and should, as far as possible, be prevented by dealing effectively with the pain and anxiety. Morphine has been the drug of choice for a long time. Although it is a drug that can be held by dental surgeons, and can be administered by them, it is a controlled drug

(see Chapter 3) and is unlikely to be stored in the dental surgery by many practitioners.

The best treatment for myocardial infarction in this context is the use of Entonox, a premixture of gases—50/50 mixture of nitrous oxide and oxygen (see Chapter 9). This gaseous mixture provides more rapid pain relief than morphine. If Entonox is not available, nitrous oxide may be administered with oxygen, but the concentration of nitrous oxide must not exceed 70%, as anaesthesia and hypoxia may occur above this concentration. Nitrous oxide is a weak anaesthetic agent but possesses excellent analgesic properties. In addition, it has an euphoriant effect. The treatment should be explained to the patient as the anaesthetic mask may cause more anxiety.

The patient should be placed in the position that feels most comfortable. Pulmonary oedema is a possible consequence of infarction due to left ventricular failure and this causes dyspnoea. To lie the patient flat in these circumstances could cause the lungs to fill with fluid and make breathing virtually impossible. All tight clothing around the neck should be loosened.

Cardiac arrest

There are many causes of cardiac arrest, including myocardial infarction, anaesthetic agents, acute anaphylactic reactions, and adrenal crisis. Apart from the obvious fact that the patient will be unconscious, there are some signs to look for, namely:

- colour of the skin;

- absence of arterial pulse.

Pallor indicates underperfusion of the skin with blood. If the colour is white, then this may indicate a circulatory problem and could be the result of a mild cardiac infarct. If the colour is grey, this would indicate that the remaining oxygen tension in the peripheral vessels has been further reduced. A whitish-grey skin suggests circulatory collapse of some duration. Indications of such circulatory collapse would also include lack of pulse. Time is of the essence, and only the radial and carotid pulses should be felt.

There may also be lack of bleeding from a surgical wound, and the pupils will be dilated. However, eye signs should not be considered an essential feature of early diagnosis because they occur later on in the catastrophe. Do not waste time looking for eye signs!

Cardiopulmonary resuscitation

The brain is the organ most sensitive to oxygen deprivation. If its oxygen supply is cut off for 3 minutes, then brain death will occur, if the patient was in a reasonable condition beforehand. If he or she was in an agitated state, for example, where the oxygen demand would be raised, then the brain would suffer even more rapidly. Such a possibility may arise in the dental chair. So the emergency techniques must be well known and rehearsed, for no time can be spent reading them up in a book once the emergency has begun.

Procedures

1. *Aid the venous return.* Place the patient on the floor or on to a firm flat surface. Lift the feet up to help the flow of blood back to the heart.
2. *Open the airway.* The head is tilted, the chin lifted, and a finger sweep or mechanical suction is performed to clear any foreign bodies.
3. *Check breathing.* If no breathing then begin artificial ventilation.
4. *Artificial ventilation.* Two breaths are administered mouth to mouth, or via a mask, or two compressions given via an Ambu bag.
5. *Assess circulation.* If no pulse commence external cardiac massage.
6. *External cardiac massage.* The operator kneels by the side of the patient and depresses the sternum 1–1.5 inches (2.5–4.0 cm). One hand is placed over the other on the lower sternum and a forceful compression started. A rate of 60–70 should suffice for an adult. In very small children, the compression rate is about 100 and only the thumbs are used to press on the chest. When performing this procedure alone the ratio of compressions to artificial ventilation is 15:2. When two people are present 5:1 (compressions to ventilation) is suggested.

Medical help should be sought by an assistant, and the cardiopulmonary resuscitation maintained until there is a return to a good pulse or until the arrival of expert help. A patient who recovers will be admitted to hospital. It is no part of the dentist's job to try using drugs such as lidocaine (lignocaine) to deal with any dysrhythmias that may occur.

Asthma

An acute asthmatic attack can be induced by the stress of a visit to the dental surgery. If the patient has their bronchodilator inhaler (e.g. salbutamol) with them, then one or two puffs may suffice to counter the problem (see Chapter 17). As the patient may not have their inhaler, it is wise to have salbutamol in the surgery. If the patient cannot use the inhaler then, in the first instance, the dentist should spray salbutamol into a disposable cup used for mouth rinsing and place this over the patient's mouth and nose and ask them to breathe in. An alternative is to use nebulized salbutamol via an oxygen mask, but it is unlikely that many surgeries will have salbutamol in this form. If the asthma attack is severe and life-threatening then epinephrine (adrenaline) (intramuscularly) and hydrocortisone (intravenously) are administered in exactly the same fashion as described for the treatment of anaphylactic shock in Chapter 23.

Acute allergic reactions

See Chapter 23 and Table 26.1.

Epilepsy

Major epilepsy is a convulsive disorder with attacks that are characterized by an aura (a disorder of sensation), and a tonic and a clonic phase (see Chapter 15). In the tonic phase the patient is rigid and may stop breathing; in the clonic phase convulsions occur; in either phase patients may bite their tongue.

If the patient has an attack in the dental surgery, they must be prevented from injuring themselves during the seizure. All appliances should be removed from the mouth as quickly as possible. Recovery is fairly rapid—a matter of a few minutes. Whether or not dental treatment is continued can only be decided by the operator, taking into account the circumstances at the time. As some patients feel a little drowsy after recovery from a seizure, it is sensible to see they are accompanied home by a responsible adult.

It is important for epileptic patients to continue medication before attending for dental treatment.

If the patient does not recover in a few minutes, and seizures occur in rapid succession (status epilepticus), then an anticonvulsant drug must be given. The drug of choice is the benzodiazepine diazepam. Diazepam should be given IV as an emulsion (Diazemuls) as this minimizes the risk of thrombophlebitis. The dose is 5 mg min^{-1} up to 20 mg. If it is difficult to give the drug intravenously, it can be administered as a rectal solution. However, this route is not suitable for use by dentists because of their probable inexperience. Intramuscular injection provides too slow an absorption and is unsatisfactory. Urgent medical help is required, and the patient should be taken to hospital as soon as possible, as status epilepticus is a dangerous condition. The ultrashort-acting barbiturate thiopental (thiopentone) will also cut short an attack. However, it should be remembered that the ultrashort-acting barbiturate normally used in dental practice, methohexital (methohexitone), has convulsant properties *and should never be used.*

Hypoglycaemia

The patient most likely to develop hypoglycaemia is the Type 1 (insulin-dependent) diabetic. The diabetic patient's regimen can become unbalanced. Too much insulin will lead to hypoglycaemia, which happens if diabetics taking their medication have their diet disrupted; too little insulin can produce a state of diabetic ketosis. It is important to distinguish between hypoglycaemia and diabetic ketosis; both can cause the patient to become unconscious. However, it is extremely unlikely that diabetic ketosis would present with unconsciousness in the dental surgery as it takes several days to develop. The differential signs and symptoms are shown in Table 26.2.

One characteristic feature of hypoglycaemia is that the patient may become difficult to manage and even aggressive.

Patients experienced in the management of their condition may well be able to distinguish between the onset of a

Table 26.2 Differential signs and symptoms of ketosis and hypoglycaemia

Ketosis (lack of insulin)	Hypoglycaemia (excess of insulin)
Weakness	Weakness
Excessive thirst	Hunger
Dehydration (dry skin and mucous membrane)	Sweating
Decreased blood pressure	Blood pressure normal or elevated
Sweet breath–said to be acetone	Pulse—full and rapid
Deep laboured respirations	Patient anxious (epinephrine (adrenaline) release)
Later: coma (unlikely to be seen in dental surgery)	Later: coma

hypoglycaemic attack and ketosis. If there is any doubt about the diagnosis, a few lumps of sugar or sugar sweets will normally rectify the hypoglycaemia fairly rapidly. A hypoglycaemic attack requires urgent treatment and, if the patient is unable to swallow, glucose as an intravenous infusion (20–50 mL of a 50% dextrose solution) should be administered. Glucagon (1 mg intramuscularly) may be administered as an alternative if venous access cannot be achieved. Glucagon is a hormone secreted by the α-cells of the islets of Langerhans in the pancreas (the β-cells producing insulin). It raises plasma glucose concentration by mobilizing glycogen stored in the liver (see Chapter 20). Hypoglycaemia must be treated promptly: a prolonged hypoglycaemic coma is likely to lead to irreversible brain damage.

When there is doubt about whether the coma is hypoglycaemic or hyperglycaemic in origin, insulin *must not be administered* by the dental surgeon as it can be very dangerous in hypoglycaemic coma. The likelihood is that a coma occurring in the dental surgery in a diabetic patient will be caused by hypoglycaemia. Medical assistance must be obtained as quickly as possible.

Adrenal crisis

If the adrenal glands are unable to provide sufficient cortisol to meet the needs of 'stress', an adrenal crisis may occur. This is a state of profound shock, and a warning of such an occurrence would be weakness, vomiting, pallor, perspiration, tachycardia, weak pulse, and hypotension. Special precautions should be taken if surgery is to be carried out on a patient when there is this risk of an inadequate response to 'stress'. Adrenocortical function is likely to be depressed if the patient is taking corticosteroids as a prolonged course (1 month or longer), or has been taking corticosteroids regularly for a month or more during the last year. There is no general agreement on the time taken to restore normal adrenocortical function after prolonged steroid therapy has been discontinued. The approach to prophylactic steroid replacement was mentioned in Chapter 20

If, in spite of suitable prophylaxis, the patient shows signs of collapse, hydrocortisone (100 mg increments up to 500 mg) should be given intravenously and immediately. This is a very serious situation and the patient should be admitted to hospital as soon as possible, if not already an in-patient.

Patients who are considered to be vulnerable should have their blood pressure monitored; this may provide a reasonable guide to their general condition. For just how long this should be done, and at what intervals, has not been established with any certainty. It is recommended that the blood pressure should be measured in such patients at half-hourly intervals over a period of 2 hours. If, after this time, the blood pressure is still significantly low, the patient should be referred to hospital.

Further reading

General Dental Council (1996). *Professional conduct and fitness to practise.* General Dental Council, London.

Resuscitation Council (1997). *The 1997 resuscitation guidelines for use in the U.K.* The Resuscitation Council (UK), London.

27

Treatments for common dental conditions

- Dental hypersensitivity
- Acute pulpitis
- Periapical abscess
- Periodontal abscess
- Cellulitis
- Ludwig's angina
- Osteomyelitis
- Pericoronitis
- Acute necrotizing ulcerative gingivitis (ANUG)
- Acute herpetic gingivostomatitis
- Teething
- Herpes labialis
- Postoperative dental pain
- Postoperative swelling and trismus
- Dry socket (alveolar osteitis)
- Sinusitis
- Candidal infections
- Thrush
- Angular cheilitis
- Denture stomatitis
- Candidal leukoplakia
- Recurrent aphthous ulceration
- Other types of oral ulceration
- Xerostomia

Treatments for common dental conditions

This chapter discusses some of the common dental conditions that require treatment. The possible treatments are outlined as being either operative, that is a procedure done by the dental surgeon, or non-operative, that is the use of medication. In some conditions both are necessary. The list of non-operative measures is by no means exhaustive and only serves as a guideline. Many of the conditions have been discussed in the chapters on drug treatments. Since it is beyond the scope of this chapter to discuss the differential diagnoses of these conditions, the reader is referred to standard texts on oral surgery and medicine for details.

Dental hypersensitivity

Gingival recession, periodontal disease, or tooth-wear can result in the exposure of dentine to the oral environment. This can result in an increased sensitivity of the tooth to various chemical, thermal, or physical stimuli, which is commonly referred to as dentine hypersensitivity. This term should not be confused with hypersensitivity reactions which are described in Chapter 23.

Operative treatment

For cases that do not respond to desensitizing agents, the exposed dentine surface can be covered with an adhesive tooth-coloured restorative material such as glass ionomer cement or a dentine bonding agent. Root canal therapy may be indicated for persistent cases that do not respond to any form of conservative treatment. Laser therapy has been evaluated in the management of dentine hypersensitivity, however the results are somewhat inconclusive.

Many toothpastes contain active ingredients to treat dentine hypersensitivity, for instance strontium chloride and formaldehyde. Exposed dentine surfaces can be coated with Duraphat, a varnish preparation that contains 50 mg of sodium fluoride per millilitre of varnish. The latter may need to be applied several times before there is complete resolution of the dentine hypersensitivity.

Acute pulpitis

Inflammatory conditions of the pulp frequently arise as a result of caries. Acute pulpitis results in a severe throbbing pain exacerbated by temperature changes.

Operative treatment

Remove the pulp or extract the tooth.

Non-operative treatment

Ledermix contains 10 mg of triamcinolone acetonide and 30 mg of demeclocycline hydrochloride per gram of paste. It can be applied to the cavity floor if the pulpal inflammation causes inadequate anaesthesia. Analgesics are of little value for reducing the pain of acute pulpitis.

Periapical abscess

This is a localized infection confined to the apical tissues of a non-vital tooth.

Operative treatment

Establish drainage via the root canal or extract the tooth. If the tooth is already root-filled, an attempt can be made to refill it with or without an apicectomy and retrograde root seal.

Non-operative treatment

If the infection is not localized or treatment has been delayed, antibiotics and analgesics may be prescribed. However, only operative procedures provide a definitive cure. Most dental infections are treated empirically since bacterial cultures and antimicrobial sensitivity will not be available. The drugs of choice are amoxicillin (amoxycillin) or metronidazole. The traditional week-long course of antibiotics is not usually required, operative treatment can be performed when the acute infection is resolved and antimicrobial therapy stopped at that stage. Beginning treatment with a high loading dose of amoxicillin orally (such as 3 g) has been shown to be as effective as parenteral administration. Subsequent doses of amoxicillin are 250–500 mg three times daily. Metronidazole should be administered as a dose of 400 mg two to three times daily. The management of more severe infections arising from dental sources are discussed below.

Periodontal abscess

This is an acute localized infection in a periodontal pocket. These abscesses are often associated with posterior teeth, especially where there is furcation involvement.

Operative treatment

Establish drainage by curettage of the pocket and irrigate with 0.2% chlorhexidine.

Non-operative treatment

Hot, salt-water mouthbaths should be prescribed to encourage drainage. Severe cases should be treated with oral antibiotics: penicillin (250 mg four times daily for 5 days) or metronidazole (600–800 mg daily for 3–5 days) are both efficacious. Where possible, the patient should be instructed to irrigate the periodontal pocket with 0.2% chlorhexidine solution. Recurrent abscesses may respond to one of the local drug delivery systems such as metronidazole gel or the chlorhexidine gelatin chip. If these agents are to be used, then they must be applied 7–10 days after the initial debridement.

Cellulitis

This infection spreads along on the fascial planes, usually in the floor of the mouth, and is often the result of a streptococcal infection. It is not normally associated with a large collection of pus. If there is significant suppuration, this suggests a staphylococcal infection, often with anaerobes such as *Bacteroides* species.

Operative treatment

If suppuration is present then drainage should be established. If the cellulitis is due to a tooth, this should also be removed.

Non-operative treatment

Initial treatment is with intravenous amoxicillin (amoxycillin), 500–1000 mg every 8 hours, followed by oral amoxicillin 250–500 mg every 8 hours. Any pus obtained from the wound should be sent for culture and sensitivity, and the choice of antibiotic therapy depends on the findings. If a bacteroides infection is suspected, metronidazole (500 mg intravenously twice daily) is the drug of choice, whilst flucloxacillin is the treatment of choice for penicillinase-producing staphylococci.

Non-steroidal analgesics such as ibuprofen 200–400 mg three times daily are also needed.

Ludwig's angina

This is a serious and potentially life-threatening cellulitis simultaneously affecting the submandibular, submental, and sublingual spaces. It usually follows a submandibular infection caused by a periapical abscess or pericoronitis. The infection spreads into the sublingual space and around the deep part of the submandibular gland. From here, it passes into the opposite sublingual and the contralateral submandibular region.

Operative treatment

Establish surgical drainage and watch the airway. These patients may require a tracheostomy if the airway becomes compromised.

Non-operative treatment

Patients require immediate and intensive antimicrobial therapy. An intravenous infusion of metronidazole 500 mg and amoxicillin (amoxycillin) 500–1000 mg every 8 hours is a suitable regimen. If the patient is allergic to penicillin, they should be given clindamycin intravenously (150–300 mg every 6 hours), but only for a short period, and this should be stopped if diarrhoea occurs. Erythromycin may also be used but this must be administered as a slow intravenous infusion.

Appropriate analgesia is required, NSAIDs are usually suitable.

Osteomyelitis

This severe infection of bone is now rarely seen in the Western world. Patients susceptible to osteomyelitis include alcoholics, drug abusers, diabetic patients, the immunosuppressed, and those suffering from malnutrition. The most common cause of acute pyogenic osteomyelitis of the mandible is an odontogenic infection, usually of the staphylococcal type.

Operative treatment

If possible, remove the sequestra and any remaining portions of necrotic bone.

Non-operative treatment

Antimicrobial therapy should be instituted immediately, consisting of a broad-spectrum bactericidal drug combined with one resistant to staphylococcal penicillinase; for example amoxicillin (amoxycillin) 500 mg every 8 hours with flucloxacillin 250 mg every 6 hours. Both drugs are given orally. This regimen should be continued until the causative organism and its sensitivity is known. Patients who are allergic to penicillin should be treated with a combination of oral erythromycin 500 mg and sodium fusidate 500 mg every 8 hours.

Clindamycin 300 mg every 6 hours may be useful because of the drug's ability to diffuse into bone. However, treatment must be stopped if the patient develops diarrhoea (see Chapter 11).

Antimicrobial treatment should be maintained for a minimum of 2 weeks and may be continued for up to 8 weeks.

Pericoronitis

Pericoronitis is an infection in the soft tissues around an erupting tooth. Nearly all cases are associated with impacted lower third molars.

Operative treatment

Extract the opposing upper third molar, or reduce the cusps if they are traumatizing the swollen gingival tissue around the erupting lower third molar. Once the pericoronitis has resolved, the lower third molar should be removed.

Non-operative treatment

Hot, salt-water mouthbaths (one teaspoon of salt in a cup of hot water) may be of benefit in pericoronitis. They should be used every 2 hours until the inflammation resolves. Trichloroacetic acid can be placed under the gingival tissues and then immediately neutralized with glycerine. The efficacy of this treatment is not established and great care should be taken when the caustic is applied. A chlorhexidine mouth rinse or topical application of chlorhexidine gel is also useful.

Moderate cases of pericoronitis should be treated with oral antibiotics, either metronidazole 400 mg every 12 hours for 5 days, or amoxicillin (amoxycillin) 250 mg every 8 hours for 5 days. Severe cases with trismus, marked buccal swelling, pyrexia, and lymphadenopathy should be treated with 3 g oral amoxicillin followed by 250–500 mg orally every 8 hours. If the condition is embarrassing the airway the patient is admitted to hospital and treated in the same manner as described above for Ludwig's angina.

NSAIDs such as ibuprofen 200–400 mg three times daily will also be required.

Acute necrotizing ulcerative gingivitis (ANUG)

This is a specific infection of the gingival tissues, characterized by inflamed, ulcerated papillae, and a characteristic foul halitosis. ANUG occurs in patients with poor oral hygiene and ill-kept mouths. There is a higher incidence in smokers. The causative organisms are *Treponema* spp., *Selenomonas* spp., *Fusobacterium* spp., and *Prevotella intermedia*.

Operative treatment

This involves local debridement of the gingival tissues and the removal of supragingival calculus if possible.

Non-operative treatment

If the condition is mild then oxygen-releasing agents, such as hydrogen peroxide or sodium peroxyborate, may be of some benefit. For the moderate to severe cases, oral metronidazole is the treatment of choice (200–400 mg every 8 hours for 3–5 days depending on the severity). Antimicrobials should only be used if there are signs of systemic involvement and/or the infection is spreading.

Acute herpetic gingivostomatitis

Herpes simplex viral infection of the gingiva and oral mucosa is mainly seen in children, but it can also occur in adults, especially in immunocompromised patients.

Non-operative treatment

Reduce the pyrexia with either aspirin or paracetamol. (NB aspirin cannot be given to children under 12 years of age because of the risk of Reye's syndrome). The patient should be kept well hydrated. Severe infections should be treated with systemic oral acyclovir 200 mg five times daily for 5 days. If the patient is immunocompromised, the dose of acyclovir should be increased to 400 mg every 8 hours. A chlorhexidine 0.2% mouthwash should be used every 6 hours to reduce the incidence of secondary infection in the ulcerative area.

Teething

The eruption of the primary dentition is frequently associated with constitutional disturbances such as pyrexia, diarrhoea, and increased irritability as well as increased salivation and sleep disturbances.

Operative treatment

Massage the gums over the erupting tooth or allow the baby to chew on something hard.

Non-operative treatment

Choline salicylate (Bonjela) rubbed into the gums may be of some benefit. (The association between aspirin and Reye's syndrome does not apply to non-aspirin salicylates or to topical preparations found in teething gels.) Other proprietary agents used in the treatment of teething (Dentinox, Soothadent) contain a topical local anaesthetic agent such as lidocaine (lignocaine). They should be used sparingly because of the risk of anaesthesia of the oropharynx and the subsequent loss of protective reflexes. Paracetamol elixir (5–10 mL) can be prescribed to reduce the pyrexia that often accompanies teething.

Herpes labialis

This is a recurrent herpes simplex viral infection that affects the vermilion border of the lips.

Operative treatment

If patient is prone to herpes labialis, avoid trauma to the lips during dental procedures and keep the lips coated with Vaseline, also advise the patient to avoid excessive exposure to sunlight or the use of sunbeds.

Non-operative treatment

Acyclovir cream 5% shortens or aborts the recurrence of herpes labialis. For the drug to be effective, it must be applied in the early, prodromal phase.

Postoperative dental pain
Non-operative treatment

Pain after dental procedures is usually of short duration and responds to aspirin or any of the proprionic acid derivatives (e.g.

ibuprofen, ketoprofen, etc.). Medication should be taken every 4–6 hours. If the pain persists after 48 hours, then a secondary infection may have occurred and this should be treated with antibiotics. Analgesics recommended are aspirin 1 g, paracetamol 1 g, ibuprofen 400 mg, and for severe cases diclofenac 25 mg. IM may be useful.

Postoperative swelling and trismus

Non-operative treatment

Cold compresses applied buccally and hot, salt-water mouthbaths may be appropriate local measures to reduce swelling. Aspirin or one of the other NSAIDs will help to reduce postoperative swelling and trismus.

The preoperative administration of corticosteroids may be of some benefit in reducing the incidence and magnitude of swelling after dental surgical procedures (see Chapter 4). Steroids used for this purpose include intramuscular dexamethasone 20 mg, methylprednisolone 80 mg, and hydrocortisone 100 mg. They are administered 1–2 hours before surgery, and may be repeated 6 hours after surgery. Their value in reducing postoperative swelling and trismus remains equivocal.

Dry socket (alveolar osteitis)

This is a localized infection occurring in a tooth socket 2–3 days after extraction. Breakdown of the blood clot within the socket appears to be an important aetiological factor.

Operative treatment

The socket should be irrigated with warm saline to remove any remains of blood clot.

Non-operative treatment

A sedative dressing should be placed in the socket; examples include ribbon gauze soaked in Whitehead's varnish, bismuth iodoform paraffin paste (BIPP) or Alvogyl (Septodont; France). Alvogyl contains butyl-paraminobenzoate (a topical anaesthetic), iodoform (an antiseptic), and eugenol which provides further pain relief.

Alternatively, cotton wool impregnated with zinc oxide and eugenol may help to reduce the pain commonly associated with this condition. Dressings containing eugenol are not without problems and may cause bone necrosis.

Patients should be prescribed analgesics—aspirin or other NSAIDs—to help to reduce the pain.

Sinusitis

This infection, involving the mucosal linings of the sinuses, frequently follows an upper respiratory tract infection.

Operative treatment

Ensure that the antrum is free of foreign bodies, such as root fragments, and that there is no oroantral fistula present. Recurrent cases should be treated by antral washout.

Non-operative treatment

The patient should use inhalations with either menthol and benzoin 2%, or menthol and eucalyptus dissolved in hot water. Ephedrine nose drops 0.5% produce vasoconstriction of the nasal mucosa and facilitate drainage. However, ephedrine should only be used as a short-term measure (no more than 1 week). Acute cases should be treated with antibiotics—doxycycline 200 mg as an initial dose, followed by 100 mg daily, is particularly effective. Alternatively, any of the broad-spectrum penicillins can be used.

Candidal infections

Infections due to _Candida albicans_ are the most frequent oral fungal infections. Patients with persistent candidal infections must be investigated for any underlying cause. These include xerostomia, HIV infection, nutritional deficiency, diabetes mellitus, and immunosuppression.

Non-operative treatment

Most oral candidal infections respond to topical antifungal therapy. Systemic antifungals are reserved for severely ill patients with chronic mucocutaneous candidiasis, immunosuppressed patients, and those with candidal septicaemia.

Thrush

Non-operative treatment

Prescribe a 2-week course of nystatin pastilles (100 000 IU), one dissolved in the mouth four times a day; alternatively amphotericin lozenges (10 mg) or miconazole tablets (250 mg) should be allowed to dissolve in the mouth every 4–6 hours. For infants, treatment should be with sugar-free oral suspensions of either nystatin (100 000 IU), amphotericin (100 mg mL^{-1}) or miconazole oral gel (25 mg mL^{-1}). All preparations should be held in the mouth for as long as possible.

Angular cheilitis

Operative treatment

In edentulous patients, check that the vertical height of their dentures is correct. Investigate their blood for deficiencies of iron, folate, and vitamin B$_{12}$, since chronic fungal infections are frequently associated with haematological disorders.

Non-operative treatment

Sore areas should be treated with a topical antifungal agent. However, many of these infections are also infected with

Staphylococcus aureus or β-haemolytic streptococci. In these cases, topical miconazole gel (25 mg mL^{-1}) is efficacious because it has both antifungal and antibacterial activity. Alternatively, either nystatin ointment (100 000 IU g^{-1}) or amphotericin ointment 3% can be used in conjunction with sodium fusidate ointment 2%. All agents should be applied three or four times a day.

Denture stomatitis

Operative treatment

Advise patients to leave their dentures out as much as possible and keep them in a cleaning agent such as sodium hypochlorite. Dentures should be replaced when the condition resolves. Full haematological investigation should be carried out, as for angular cheilitis cases.

Non-operative treatment

The dentures should be left out, and the patient given nystatin pastilles or amphotericin B lozenges to dissolve in the mouth four times a day. However, patients will be reluctant to leave their dentures out for any length of time. When inserted the denture fitting surface should be coated with miconazole cream.

Candidal leukoplakia

Operative treatment

Biopsy or, if small, surgically excise and graft. Candidal leukoplakia is frequently associated with HIV infections.

Non-operative treatment

Fluconazole appears to be the antifungal of choice for this condition; treatment may have to be continued for 14 days.

Recurrent aphthous ulceration

The aetiology of this troublesome recurrent oral ulceration is uncertain. Factors implicated include deficiencies of iron, vitamin B$_{12}$, and folic acid. Some patients respond to a gluten-free diet, whilst others report allergy to certain food stuffs or constituents such as chocolate, benzoic acid, and cinnamaldehyde. Aphthous ulceration can also be related to menstruation.

Operative treatment

Remove any local causes of irritation, such as the sharp edges of teeth and restorations; check that the clasps of appliances or dentures are not traumatizing the oral mucosa. Investigate blood for deficiencies of iron, vitamin B$_{12}$, and folate.

Non-operative treatment

A chlorhexidine mouthwash 0.2% or a tetracycline mouthwash (made by dissolving the contents of a tetracycline capsule in 10 mL of water) may reduce the incidence of secondary infection associated with aphthous ulceration. Benzydamine mouthwash or oral spray 0.15% may help to reduce the pain of the ulceration. Carmellose gelatine paste, DPF, may provide mechanical protection of the oral mucosa. Hydrocortisone pellets (2.5 mg) are useful if the patient experiences a prodromal symptom, i.e. a tingling sensation in the oral mucosa prior to the ulcers occurring. The pellets should be applied to the area every 6 hours and allowed to dissolve. Once ulcers have occurred, triamcinolone acetonide 0.1% dental paste or betamethasone aerosol spray applied every 6 hours may help. Alternatively, betamethasone tablets (as sodium phosphate) 0.5 mg dissolved in 15 mL of water and used as a mouthwash four times a day may be an easier method of delivering steroids to the oral mucosa.

If there is an underlying haematological factor or vitamin deficiency, the following medications are of value: ferrous sulfate or gluconate tablets 200 mg twice daily; folic acid tablets 5 mg per day; vitamin B$_{12}$ injections 1000 μg weekly for 1 month; vitamin B$_1$ tablets 300 mg daily; vitamin B$_6$ tablets, 50 mg three times a day. Duration of therapy depends on the severity of the underlying problem and its response to medication.

Other types of oral ulceration

All forms of oral ulceration should be thoroughly investigated and if necessary biopsied. Many systemic diseases can cause oral ulceration, including white blood cell disorders, Crohn's disease, and HIV infection. Indeed, the oral manifestations may be the first signs of a systemic illness. Where there is no underlying factor, ulceration may be treated with topical corticosteroids as outlined above. However, it is more likely that severe oral ulcerations will require treatment with systemic corticosteroids. Prednisolone is the treatment of choice, and the dose regimen depends on the severity of the condition. Very severe cases may need treatment with azathioprine.

Xerostomia

Xerostomia, or dry mouth, may be due to a variety of factors. These include certain types of drug therapy, especially anticholinergics, antihistamines (H$_1$ receptor blockers), tricyclic antidepressants, and sympathomimetics. Other common causes of xerostomia are Sjogren's syndrome, type 1 diabetes mellitus, radiation to the salivary glands, mechanical obstruction, and infection.

Operative treatment

Investigate salivary glands for mechanical obstruction with calculi.

Non-operative treatment

If there is still some residual salivary function, diabetic sweets, sugar-free chewing gum, and citric and malic acids may promote some salivary flow. However, citric and malic acids may cause erosion. Pharmacological stimulation of the salivary glands can be achieved with cholinergic agonists such as bethanechol chloride, pilocarpine, and pyridostigmine. These drugs should only be used for a short time since they can have adverse effects on the gastrointestinal tract, cardiovascular system, and CNS.

Salivary substitutes are of value in patients where there is minimal or no salivary flow. Examples include Saliva Orthana (mucin based) and Glandosane (methylcellulose based), both of which are described in the *BNF*, and Luborant (carboxymethylcellulose based). Both Saliva Orthana and Luborant have a high pH. This property may help in the remineralization of carious lesions. In the edentulous patient, a glycerin and lemon mixture (50% glycerin and 50% water) may be of value since there is no risk of caries associated with the regular use of such a solution.

Patients with xerostomia are very susceptible to caries because they have lost the buffering capacity of their saliva. They should receive repeated applications of fluoride to prevent this problem. Xerostomia induced by irradiation therapy may be treated with pilocarpine hydrochloride 5 mg three times a day. However, this drug has many unwanted effects, and its use should be restricted to specialist centres.

Index